NURSING
RESEARCH
Theory and Practice

NURSING RESEARCH
Theory and Practice

NANCY FUGATE WOODS, R.N., Ph.D., F.A.A.N.

Professor and Chairperson,
Department of Parent-Child Nursing,
University of Washington,
Seattle, Washington

MARCI CATANZARO, R.N., Ph.D.

Assistant Professor,
Department of Physiological Nursing,
University of Washington,
Seattle, Washington

with **108** *illustrations*

THE C. V. MOSBY COMPANY

ST. LOUIS • WASHINGTON, D.C. • TORONTO   1988

A TRADITION OF PUBLISHING EXCELLENCE

Publisher Alison Miller
Editor Tom Lochhaas
Developmental Editor Terry Van Schaik
Assistant Editor Laurie Sparks
Project Manager Sylvia B. Kluth
Production Editors Florence Achenbach, John A. Rogers,
 Sheila Walker
Design Elizabeth Fett

The C. V. Mosby Company
11830 Westline Industrial Drive, St. Louis, Missouri 63146

Library of Congress Cataloging-in-Publication Data
Woods, Nancy Fugate.
 Nursing research.

 Includes bibliographies and index.
 1. Nursing—Research. I. Catanzaro, Marci. II. Title.
[DNLM: 1. Nursing. 2. Research. WY 20.5 W896n]
RT81.5.W65 1988   610.73′072   87-7336
ISBN 0-8016-5703-2

TSI/VH/VH 9 8 7 6 5 4 3 2 1 04B579

CONTRIBUTORS

JEANNE QUINT BENOLIEL, R.N., D.N.S., F.A.A.N.
Professor,
Community Health Care Systems,
University of Washington,
Seattle, Washington

CATHRYN L. BOOTH, Ph.D.
Research Assistant Professor,
University of Washington,
Seattle, Washington

OLGA MARANJIAN CHURCH, Ph.D., F.A.A.N.
Associate Professor,
Department of Psychiatric Nursing,
University of Illinois,
Chicago, Illinois

MARY DUFFY, R.N., Ph.D.
Assistant Professor,
Department of Mental Health, Community,
and Administrative Nursing,
University of California School of
Nursing, San Francisco, California

BARBARA HEDIN, R.N., Ph.D.
Assistant Professor,
Teachers College,
Columbia University,
New York, New York

MARGARET HEITKEMPER, R.N., Ph.D.
Associate Professor,
Department of Physiological Nursing,
University of Washington,
Seattle, Washington

NANCY EWALD JACKSON, Ph.D.
Research Associate Professor,
Department of Parent-Child Nursing,
University of Washington,
Seattle, Washington

MARCIA KILLIEN, R.N., Ph.D.
Associate Professor,
Department of Parent-Child Nursing,
University of Washington,
Seattle, Washington

PAMELA HOLSCLAW MITCHELL, R.N., M.S., F.A.A.N.
Professor,
Department of Physiological Nursing,
University of Washington,
Seattle, Washington

SANDRA K. MITCHELL, Ph.D.
Associate Professor,
Department of Parent-Child Nursing,
University of Washington,
Seattle, Washington

ELLEN OLSHANSKY, R.N., D.N.S.
Assistant Professor,
Department of Parent-Child Nursing,
University of Washington,
Seattle, Washington

JOAN FOWLER SHAVER, R.N., Ph.D.
Associate Professor,
Department of Physiological Nursing,
University of Washington,
Seattle, Washington

To Marjorie V. Batey
for her contributions to our
development as critical thinkers
and nurse investigators and for
her constructive review of
this manuscript

N.F.W.
M.C.

PREFACE

The special focus of the discipline of nursing is the health of individuals and their families, the influence of the environment on human health, and therapeutic measures to promote, maintain, and restore health. There is a great need for the generation and dissemination of knowledge that will help practitioners better understand human adaptation to health and illness and of clinical strategies to assist people to promote their own health or to cope with illness and its effects on their lives. Because nursing is a practice discipline, its need for a science of therapeutics is paramount.

The purpose of this text is to guide nurse investigators in their efforts to generate and disseminate nursing knowledge. The primary audience for the text is advanced undergraduate nursing students who are consumers of nursing research and who as graduates will become partners in research efforts; graduate students who are preparing to conduct research; and clinicians who are consumers of research, as well as investigators.

Contemporary nursing science emphasizes a holistic understanding of human beings in interaction with their environments. The complex nature of the questions relevant to contemporary nursing practice requires a pluralism of paradigms and methods. Current scientific work in nursing draws on the traditional positivist-empiricist perspective and on the naturalistic-inductive perspective. The contents of this text reflect the necessity for a pluralism of philosophical approaches and research methods to achieve an understanding of phenomena of central importance to nursing.

Nursing research has not had a dramatic effect on how nursing is practiced. Moreover, theory development efforts in nursing have not had a profound influence on nursing research. The mismatch between our scientific endeavors, theory-building efforts, and practice prompted us to emphasize in this text theory development tasks that will support nursing practice and their relationship to research methods and the dissemination of research findings to practitioners, consumers, and other investigators.

The text addresses five aspects of nursing research: conceptualizing nursing research, designing nursing studies, measuring phenomena of interest to the nursing profession, analyzing and interpreting research findings, and communicating about and critically evaluating proposed or completed nursing research. Unit One, Conceptualizing Nursing Research, focuses on the scope of nursing science; contemporary strategies for theory development in nursing and the paradigms that have guided nursing theory and nursing research; identifying nursing research problems; analyzing existing knowledge; and specifying conceptual frameworks for nursing studies. Unit Two, Designing Nursing Research, begins with consideration of human rights in research and quantitative and qualitative sampling strategies. Consideration of the selection of a research design in relation to a theoretical task precedes discussion of designs for studies to describe nursing phenomena, to explore associations and differences, to test hypotheses in small and large samples, and to test prescriptions for nursing care. Study designs reflecting positivist-empiricist and naturalistic-inductive orientations are included. Unit Three, Measurement and Data Production, includes guidelines for selecting and developing measures for nursing research. Qualitative and quantitative approaches to measurement provide a foundation for understanding concepts of validity and reliability. This section focuses on several methods for data production, including biological measures, observation, interviewing, and questionnaires. Guidelines for use of existing data sources including historical archives and existing databases complete this section. Unit Four, Analysis and Interpretation, addresses the logic of planning statistical analysis, preparation of data for computer and manual analysis, and use of descriptive, inferential, and advanced statistical techniques. In addition, this section addresses qualitative analytical techniques. Unit Four closes with a discussion of interpretation of research findings. Unit Five, Communicating Nursing Research, focuses on proposed and completed research. Preparation of research proposals, publication and presentation of completed research, and critical evaluation of research constitute the primary focus of this section. Guidelines for evaluating reports of completed and proposed research from positivist-empiricist and nat-

uralistic-inductive perspectives are included. Finally, new directions in nursing research are explored from a feminist perspective.

We acknowledge the special stimulus for this book: our students who have questioned the limits of current approaches to nursing science and theory development to guide practice. Colleagues whose works have provided examples illustrating nursing science at its best and those who have critically reviewed this book in its manuscript form deserve our special acknowledgment. Finally we extend our thanks and friendship to Terry Van Schaik, one of Mosby's finest editors.

Nancy Fugate Woods
Marci Catanzaro

FOREWORD

It is exciting while studying this volume to realize how much nursing research and the broader domain of nursing science have matured in a relatively few years. Only three decades have passed since in 1958 the American Nurses' Association House of Delegates designated research nursing's number one long-term goal. At that time a book such as this one could not have been envisioned, let alone written. Then, as now, nursing leaders were convinced that the professional practice of nursing is based on an evolving knowledge base and that research is one necessary means to that end. As expressed in the rationale for that 1958 research goal, nursing was searching for a clear conception of its province, one that represented more than only the performance of functional nursing tasks. Scientific principles were considered the basis for nursing practice, but what organizing image would bring some unity to those principles?

Without a conception of nursing to guide problem identification for research or nursing scientists who could engage in that research, the strategy in 1958 was to look to other disciplines in the search for scientific principles to prepare nurses in research. The relatively rapid evolution of nursing science and the discipline of nursing overall can be traced to that strategic turning point, as can also the controversies emerging from the markedly different perspectives as to what constitutes appropriate nursing research problems and methods for their investigation. Together, this progress and these controversies provide a foundation for this work by Professors Woods and Catanzaro and their associate authors.

If I were to single out one point to emphasize concerning the value of this text, it would be its integrated perspective of the relationship between the methods of inquiry for discovering, expanding, and verifying nursing knowledge and the goal of that knowledge: to contribute directly and indirectly to nursing practice. The authors consistently depict research methodologies for the scientific production of findings compatible with the criteria necessary for acceptance as scientific knowledge. They speak to methodologic issues within each stage of the research process—conceptualization through utilization—in the linkages of those stages. Throughout, research methods are depicted as scientific tools to investigate the research questions pertinent to nursing's knowledge base. In this context, the authors cut through a contemporary controversy concerning the merits or demerits of particular approaches to inquiry. They show that no one method has intrinsic merit that sets it apart from or above another, beyond the extent to which it addresses a particular research question and clarifies its relationship to existing knowledge.

Professors Woods and Catanzaro and their associate authors have assembled and analyzed an array of methodologies, including recent technologic advances, that are critical for the repertoire of scientific tools available to nurse researchers. They demonstrate the application of those tools by examining their use in recently reported studies, thus illustrating how the investigator's creativity plays a vital part in research development and implementation. They address issues of the uses of nursing science in professional nursing practice. Consequently, we become acutely aware that with an immense increase in nursing knowledge and improvement in scientific methods, we are in a prime position to move forward. Now we have a conception of nursing to guide our identification of problems. Now we have scientists who can pursue inquiry pertinent to that conception and engage in the dialogue necessary for its organization, expansion, or alteration. Yes, progress toward nursing's full research goal has been significant, but there is much we still need to explore. This text will contribute to the development of future nurse scientists, as well as provide a valued resource for more advanced scientists, as we search for knowledge and for means for utilization of that knowledge in nursing practice.

Marjorie V. Batey
Professor
School of Nursing
University of Washington
July 1987

TO THE READER

This textbook includes an extensive glossary of key terms used in nursing research. To expedite the learning process, terms defined in the glossary are italicized where they are first discussed in the text.

Two appendixes are included to provide up-to-date resource information for nurse researchers. The Software appendix is an annotated overview of computer programs useful for managing bibliographical citations, text and numerical data, and statistical analysis. We have selected programs that are widely used by nurse researchers, that are easily learned and used, and that have adequate documentation and technical support. The Research Instrument appendix offers an annotated listing of sourcebooks that provide comprehensive reviews and critiques of available paper-and-pencil and biomedical research instruments. Because tool development is complex and time consuming and thousands of instruments have already been developed, use of already available instruments can significantly improve research effectiveness. Researchers may begin the instrument selection process with this appendix and proceed to the more detailed compendia described here to locate a valid and reliable instrument that will measure the variables appropriate to their studies.

N.F.W.
M.C.

CONTENTS

1

GENERATING NURSING SCIENCE

NANCY FUGATE WOODS AND MARCI CATANZARO

Nursing's professional obligation is the provision of caring service to human beings. Providing effective nursing care in contemporary practice settings requires a broad knowledge base for understanding and promoting human health, which often must be complemented by knowledge of specialty areas of practice. The knowledge base for nursing practice is developed through research on the responses of individuals and groups to actual or potential health problems, the environments that influence health in humans, and the therapeutic interventions that affect the consequences of illness and promote health (American Nurses' Association [ANA], 1980). The scientific base for nursing practice is referred to as *nursing science*. Nursing science uses systematic inquiry to develop knowledge that will allow nurses to promote, maintain, and restore states of health in human beings (Benoliel, 1984). In this chapter we will consider some of the foundations on which nursing research is built and present an overview of the processes we use in research to discover, expand, and verify knowledge for nursing. We will explore the discipline of nursing, the scope of nursing science, sources of knowledge, and the process of inquiry. Finally, we will examine the historical

development of nursing research and consider where nursing research appears to be headed in the future.

THE DISCIPLINE OF NURSING
Definitions of nursing

Throughout history, nursing leaders have defined nursing in a variety of ways (see box, p. 4). Common to the definitions of contemporary nursing leaders is the notion of assisting individuals of all ages and social and cultural groups to accomplish the tasks of daily living. In 1980 the ANA published a Social Policy Statement that included the following definition: "Nursing is the diagnosis and treatment of human responses to actual or potential health problems" (p. 9). The statement defined the concern of nurses as observable phenomena within the target area of nursing practice that could be described or scientifically explained. Human responses are both health restoring and health supporting. Nurses direct these responses toward the reaction of individuals and groups to actual health problems and concern about potential health problems. The consequences of illness and the resulting need for self-care are

DEFINITIONS OF NURSING

Nightingale	1859/1946	Nursing proper is therefore to help the patient suffering from disease to live, just as health nursing is to keep or put the constitution of the healthy child or human being in such a state as to have no disease. (p. 133)
Henderson	1966	The unique function of nursing is to assist the individual, sick or well, in the performance of those activities contributing to health or its recovery (or to peaceful death) that he would perform unaided if he had the necessary strength, will or knowledge. (p. 15)
King	1971	A process of action, reaction, interaction, and transaction whereby nurses assist individuals of any age group to meet their basic human needs in coping with their health status at some particular point in their life cycle. (p. 27-31)
Rogers	1970	A discipline that aims to assist people in achieving their maximum health potential. Maintenance and promotion of health, prevention of disease, nursing diagnosis, intervention, and rehabilitation encompass the scope of nursing's goals. Nursing is concerned with people—all people—well and sick, rich and poor, young and old. (p. 86)
Orem	1985	Nursing is a response of human groups to one recurring type of incapacity for action to which human beings are subject, namely, the incapacity to care for oneself or one's dependents when action is limited because of health state or health care needs of the care recipient. (p. 39)
ANA	1980	Nursing is the diagnosis and treatment of human responses to actual or potential health problems. (p. 9)

examples of actual health problems. Concern about a potential health problem may focus on the risk of developing cardiovascular disease or the desire to promote well-being through exercise.

Components of nursing

Nursing is both a profession and a discipline (Fig. 1-1). A profession assists in efforts to improve the future quality of life by resolving the current problems that influence that quality. The profession of nursing is concerned with the activities of practitioners that are channeled toward improving the health and well-being of human beings. A discipline is a realm of learning, a distinct body of knowledge that evolves from a unique way of viewing phenomena. The discipline of nursing has emerged from a perspective that emphasized the health of whole human beings in relation to their environments (Donaldson & Crowley, 1979) and focuses on the entire spec-

trum of human responses to actual and potential health problems (ANA, 1980; ANA, 1985). The discipline of nursing includes both nursing science and professional foundations. As defined earlier, nursing science is the body of scientific knowledge that guides nursing practice. Professional foundations include knowledge about the value orientation of the profession, the nature of clinical practice, and the historical and philosophical underpinnings of the profession and professional practice. Knowledge and its application are explored through the process of scientific inquiry. Nursing not only generates knowledge for its own sake but also provides direction for the use of that knowledge in nursing practice.

THE SCOPE OF NURSING SCIENCE

Nursing science is knowledge gained through systematic study. Its purpose is to guide nursing practice through areas such as the following:

1. How individuals and families adapt to wellness and illness, including effective and ineffective means used to promote health, prevent disease and disability, and foster recovery from illness and rehabilitation to optimal functioning

2. How the physical, biological, psychological, and sociocultural environments affect development and maintenance of health or unhealthy states in humans

3. Physical and interpersonal interventions that assist patients and families in reducing the adverse consequences of illness, in coping with the physical, psychological, interpersonal, and social effects of ill-

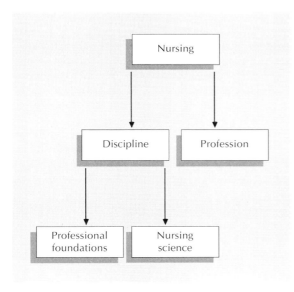

Fig. 1-1. Components of nursing.

ness, and in promoting health and health-related behaviors (Barnard, 1980)

The perspective of nursing scholars emphasizes the health of intact human beings, rather than isolated body systems or subsystems, and the constant interaction between humans and their environments (Donaldson & Crowley, 1979). Nursing literature reflects the perspective of nurse scholars, and much of it is concerned with principles or laws governing life processes and well-being, or optimal functioning, of people, whether they are well or ill. Nursing literature also emphasizes patterns of human behavior in interaction with the environment, especially in critical life situations. Finally, nurse scholars exhibit concern for the processes for effecting positive changes in health status (Donaldson & Crowley, 1979). The perspective of nursing is influenced by the value system evolving from its professional practice, which emphasizes the self-respect and self-determination of the individual and the fostering of self-caring behavior that leads to health and well-being. The work of some nurse scholars who are concerned primarily with philosophical, moral, and ethical questions links nursing to the humanities as well as the sciences (see box below) (Donaldson & Crowley, 1979).

CONTRIBUTIONS OF NURSING SCIENCE TO NURSING PRACTICE

Adaptation to wellness and illness

Research influences nursing practice by generating information that fosters our understanding of human health-related experiences. Burgess and Holmstrom's study of rape victims (1974) illustrates the contributions of nursing research to an understanding of people's health-related experiences. These investigators followed the progress of rape vic-

---

PERSPECTIVE OF NURSING SCHOLARS

Health of intact human beings
Patterns of health behavior in interaction with the environment
Laws and principles governing life processes
Well-being or optimal functioning of people
Processes for effecting positive changes in health status
Emphasis on self-respect and self-determination of individuals
Fostering self-caring behaviors

tims admitted to Boston City Hospital for a period of 2 years after they had been raped. Burgess and Holmstrom were the first to identify and describe rape trauma syndrome, a cluster of distressing and repetitive symptoms that women continue to experience long after the rape. These symptoms include mentally and physically reliving the rape, fear of seeing the assailant again, and fear of another attack.

Burgess and Holmstrom found two phases of the experiences of rape victims (1) immediate and acute responses, and (2) long-term processes. During these phases physical, emotional, and behavioral stress reactions occurred. The victims' physical responses included soreness, sleep disturbances, decreased appetites, and physical symptoms at the focuses of the attacks. Shock and disbelief characterized the immediate phase, and the victims either expressed or controlled their emotions. Expressed emotions were anger, fear, and anxiety. Women with controlled emotions were calm and subdued, seeming to mask their feelings. Emotional symptoms included fear, humiliation, degradation, guilt, shame, and embarrassment. These women felt self-blame, anger, and revenge, and thoughts of their assailants haunted them. They were preoccupied with how to undo what had happened.

Long-term responses among rape victims included changes in lifestyle, such as minimal functioning, seeking greater support from their families, moving to other homes, and changing their phone numbers. Many had dreams and nightmares of the rape or another situation from which they were unable to escape. Many became phobic of crowds or of being alone, or they developed other special fears. Some women were fearful of sexual experience and some experienced paranoia.

The importance of this study is reflected in the use of rape trauma syndrome as a diagnosis and the use of the Boston model in rape crisis centers around the country. Burgess and Holmstrom's work has had significant influence on psychiatric and emergency room nursing in the follow-up care of rape victims and, as such, is an important example of a study that expands our understanding of human health-related experiences.

Another study that illustrates how nursing research expands our understanding of people's health-related experiences addresses the problem of personal control among people with cancer. Concerned about the quality of life of late-stage cancer patients, Lewis (1982) assessed whether perceptions of personal control by these patients resulted in greater self-esteem, less anxiety, and a greater sense of purpose in life. As one means of supporting patients, nurses commonly have offered them greater control over treatment. Despite the intuitive appeal of the belief that more treatment control produced greater self-esteem, this relationship had never been tested. Lewis found that personal control over life in general was associated with greater self-esteem, less anxiety, and a greater sense of purpose in life. In contrast, perceived control over one's health was not related to anxiety or self-esteem and only weakly related to sense of purpose in life.

These results suggested that well-being for late-stage cancer patients is not a function of the perceived control they maintain over health but a more generalized sense of control over their lives. Perhaps late-stage cancer patients lose their concern about maintaining a sense of control over their health as their personal realities are resolved. This change may be a positive sign that the patients are dealing with the realities of their situation.

These two examples illustrate how nursing research is focused on the ways in which individuals and their families experience health-related situations and attempt to adapt them. Other studies have demonstrated how individuals and families adapt to such life events as pregnancy, birth, hospitalization, developmental changes, chronic and acute illness, trauma, and death.

Environmental influences

Nursing research also has expanded our awareness of the interrelationship between people and their environments in health-related situations. Nuckolls' classic study of pregnant women revealed that many were coping with extremely stressful life situations. She found that despite being highly stressed, women who had supportive people in their environments experienced significantly fewer pregnancy complications (Nuckolls, Cassel, & Kaplan, 1972). Similarly, Norbeck and Tilden (1983) found that a supportive network had protective effects on pregnant women. Other studies have demonstrated the role of social support in adaptation to hemodialysis (Dimond, 1979) and cancer (Dunkel-Schetter, 1984; Wortman & Dunkel-Schetter, 1979). Levy (1983) pointed out the relationship of social support to compliance with treatment regimens. As a result of these studies on the relationship between social support and health, nurses are becoming increasingly aware of the importance of assessing a person's support resources and of helping to identify new support networks when necessary.

Therapeutic intervention

Another way that nursing research influences practice is by contributing to our understanding of the therapeutic measures to promote health and minimize the negative consequences of illness. For example, extensive nursing research has been undertaken in the preparation of patients to cope with threatening events, ranging from a noninvasive procedure, such as cast removal, to major surgery. Early work by Lindeman and Van Aernam (1971) grew out of the clinician's concern for finding the best way to prepare patients for surgery. A growing body of nursing research has contributed to the development of a theory for helping people cope with threatening events. Jean Johnson's work has demonstrated that giving information to patients about the sensations they will experience in advance of gastroendoscopic examinations (Johnson & Leventhal, 1974; Johnson, Morrissey, & Leventhal, 1973) and cast removal (Johnson, Kirchoff, & Endress, 1975) reduced disruptive behavior during and after the procedure. Use of sensory information to prepare young women for breast and pelvic examinations resulted in significantly less distress during the examination (Fuller, Endress, & Johnson, 1978). When combined with instruction in relaxation, sensory information was even more effective.

In a later study, Johnson, Rice, Fuller, and Endress (1978a) contrasted the effects of instruction in coping behaviors (including postoperative deep breathing, coughing, turning, walking, and exercising) with the effects of giving three types of preparation. These three types of preparation were (1) information about the sensations people usually experience postoperatively, (2) the objective aspects of what people usually experience, and (3) no information. All patients received the instructions in coping behaviors the day before surgery. Among patients having cholecystectomy who were relatively fearful preoperatively, the combination of exercise instruction, procedural information, and sensory

information reduced negative mood states postoperatively. Furthermore, sensory information was related to shorter postoperative hospitalization and quicker return to routine activities at home (going out of the house). Exercise instruction alone did not affect rate of recovery, but when it was coupled with the sensory information, the shortest hospital stay occurred.

In a subsequent study, Johnson and her colleagues (Johnson, Fuller, Endress, & Rice, 1978b) found that a third component, temporal orientation (information about the duration and sequence of events) also had positive effects on patients' rates of recovery (length of hospital stay and venturing from home). These studies and others provide an important theoretical perspective for nurses who care for people coping with threatening events. The studies suggest that instructing people in activities such as turning, coughing, and deep breathing is insufficient, but that providing people with information about impending sensory experiences and the temporal sequence and duration of events can have an important impact on both their well-being and cost of care.

Similarly, research on the care of premature infants illustrates how therapeutic measures can promote their health development. Measal and Anderson (1979) observed that restless premature infants who develop intestinal distension can relax and be tube-fed more successfully if allowed to suck on a pacifier during and after each feeding. They tested this treatment by comparing infants using a pacifier with a group of infants receiving routine care that afforded few, if any, sucking opportunities. Infants using the pacifier showed readiness for bottle-feeding 3 days earlier than those without pacifiers, gained an average of 2.6 gm more per day, and were discharged 4 days sooner than the infants receiving routine care. This study demonstrated the value of capitalizing on the innate sucking responses of premature infants and provided nurses with scientific knowledge useful in the care of infants.

SOURCES OF KNOWLEDGE IN NURSING

Knowledge that makes up the science of nursing is only one component of the discipline of nursing. A broad scope of knowledge that emanates from humanitarian and scientific perspectives is required to understand the profession of nursing, the value orientation of the profession, and the nature and philosophical foundations of practice. Professional foundations in nursing are derived from modes of inquiry that include empirics, aesthetics, personal knowledge, and ethics (Carper, 1978). Although the major focus of this text is on empirical ways of knowing, it is important to appreciate the validity and significance of other patterns of knowing and to differentiate scientific inquiry from other forms of inquiry in nursing. Each pattern of acquiring knowledge represents a necessary but incomplete approach to the problems and questions facing nursing.

Empirics

In the context of the science of nursing, *empirics* refers to knowledge about the experienced (empirical) world. This knowledge is generally organized into laws and theories that help to describe, predict, and explain phenomena. Nurse scientists currently do not embrace a single scientific approach to guide their investigations. Instead, several traditions influence how nurses study nursing problems. In nursing, empirical work describes and classifies nursing phenomena that are open to observation and inspection. Examples of these phenomena include self-care limitations, strain related to life processes, such as birth, growth and development, and death, and impaired function in such processes as rest, sleep, ventilation, circulation, activity, nutrition, elimination, and sexuality (ANA, 1980).

Aesthetics

The *aesthetic* component of nursing knowledge is closely associated with the art of nursing. Aesthetic knowledge is acquired through instructional processes requiring exposure to and imitation of one who has mastered the art. Generating knowledge in this manner is common to learning such fine arts as music and painting. Knowledge gained through subjective experience cannot be organized according to logic or reason alone, because it involves perceptions of unique characteristics of an individual rather than of universal attributes that characterize a large group of individuals. Carper (1978) suggested that the development of empathy, the capacity for participating in or vicariously experiencing another's feelings, is an important mode in the aesthetic pattern of knowing.

Personal knowledge

Personal knowledge refers to knowing, encountering, and actualizing oneself. In therapeutic encounters, nurses develop authentic personal relationships with others, a process possible only from having learned about themselves. Personal knowledge can be characterized as a subjective, concrete, and existential pattern of knowing that is concerned with promoting wholeness and integrity in personal encounters and interacting with another person.

Ethics

Ethics refers to the moral component of nursing knowledge that influences difficult decisions that must be made in the context of increasingly complex health services. The ethical code of nursing emphasizes principles of obligation through concepts of service to people and respect for human life. Ethical knowledge includes not only an understanding of what ought to be done but also other normative judgments in relation to motives, intentions, or character traits. Our judgments concerning health reflect both values and understanding of health facts. The ethical pattern of knowing necessitates understanding various philosophical orientations about what is right, good, or desirable.

Each pattern of knowing contributes to the discipline of nursing by making possible an increased awareness of the complexity and diversity of nursing knowledge. The broad scope of nursing requires knowledge from all four domains: empirical, aesthetic, personal, and ethical. Empirical knowledge of human behavior in health and illness provides the scientific basis for nursing practice. The aesthetic perception of significant human experiences combined with a personal understanding of each person's unique individuality help to influence the artistic aspects of nursing practice. The knowledge that each individual possesses the ability to make moral choices in daily, practical situations influences routine patterns of behavior.

THE PROCESS OF SCIENTIFIC INQUIRY

Scientific inquiry and common sense

Science is concerned with the observation and classification of facts according to scientific principles. The goals of science are the discovery of new knowledge, the expansion of existing knowledge, and the reaffirming of previously held knowledge. Scientists seek to establish verifiable theories and general laws that are objective and unbiased. The scientific approach to inquiry is used to arrive at generalizations, not judgments about a single case. A single observation that a woman with multiple sclerosis is unable to find employment does not constitute a generalization; however, this observation may be representative of the generalization that people with chronic disease are the target of discrimination in the workplace. Further systematic observation is required before a generalization can be made.

A nurse may notice that a child in skeletal traction feels lonely. A generalization from this single case may be that immobility is associated with decreased sensory stimulation manifested by loneliness. More than one observation is necessary to establish the objective, unbiased truth that applies in many situations. Thus *generalizations* may be a summary of observed facts arrived at systematically (empirically) or derived from logical and abstract thinking (theoretically).

How does the scientific approach to knowledge differ from the commonsense approach we use in everyday life? Scientific inquiry differs from common sense in that the former is systematic and controlled, whereas common sense is based on loosely joined concepts. An example from research on acquired immunodeficiency syndrome (AIDS) can be used to illustrate some of the differences between common sense and scientific inquiry that are outlined in Table 1-1. AIDS is known to have a higher incidence among homosexual men than in the general popula-

tion; therefore, a commonsense approach might be to link this concept to the cause of AIDS and conclude that homosexuality causes the immune syndrome. A scientifically derived explanation, on the other hand, would systematically develop a framework of concepts and test this framework. A theory that a virus causes AIDS might be proposed and tested. The commonsense approach to testing the accuracy of the relationship between concepts often is done selectively rather than in a controlled, systematic manner. The commonsense testing of the theory that homosexuality causes AIDS may ignore the fact that other groups of people have AIDS. In other words, only evidence consistent with the hypothesis is proposed and tested. However, the scientist explores all other possible explanations for the proposed connections between the concepts and seeks out instances that are incongruous with previously held beliefs. The scientist is constantly seeking relationships between phenomena rather than being content to accept the first relationship that becomes apparent. A final difference between common sense and scientific inquiry is that observed phenomena rather than metaphysical explanations are the bases of science. For instance, it is not possible to observe that AIDS is God's punishment for homosexuality.

Research process

Scientific inquiry to discover, expand, and verify knowledge follows specific processes, involving movement that includes many changes and steps along the way. Process implies that a particular method of doing something exists. The process of scien-

---

TABLE 1-1. Scientific inquiry versus common sense

	COMMON SENSE	SCIENTIFIC INQUIRY
Concepts	Loosely joined	Systematically developed and tested
Testing	Selective	Systematic, controlled, empirical
Control	Accept findings congruent with belief	Control for extraneous influences
Relationships	Ignores relationships incongruent with belief	Seeks out exceptions
Explanation	Metaphysical	Observed phenomena

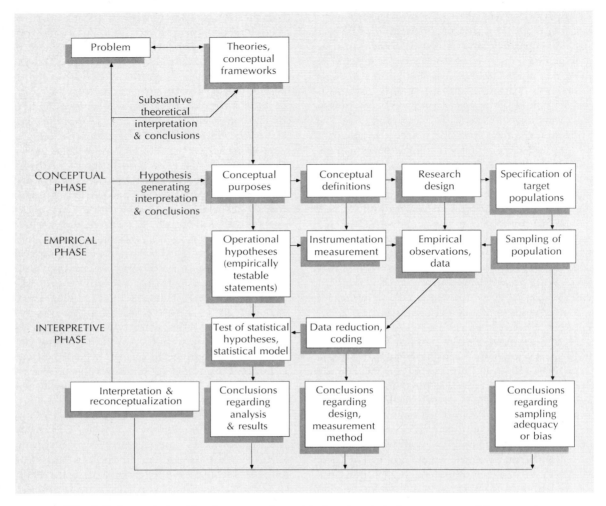

Fig. 1-2. Interrelationship of conceptual, empirical, and analytical components of the research process. (Modified from Batey, M.V., Conceptualizing the research project. ©, 1971, American Journal of Nursing Company. Reprinted with permission from *Nursing Research,* July-Aug., *20,* 296-301.)

tific inquiry is used to discover new knowledge and to verify old knowledge in nursing. Steps must be followed in the process of conducting nursing research. Sometimes these steps proceed in exact sequence; at other times many changes are made along the way. Throughout this book each step of the research process most commonly used in nursing (Fig. 1-2) will be explored in detail. Concern for detail, however, often obscures our perception of the whole. An overview of the research process will pro-

vide a conceptual map for the interrelationship of the conceptual, empirical, and interpretive components of the research process so that they can be examined in detail (Batey, 1971).

The research process described in this text involves three major phases: (1) the conceptual phase, (2) the empirical phase, and (3) the interpretive phase. The conceptual phase begins when the researcher formulates an idea for a research study. This idea may result from an observation or unanswered question in clinical practice, from reading nursing literature on a specific subject, or from the intuition of the researcher. Often the researcher will discover that the area of interest is too broad to address in a single research project. The topic will need to be limited so that it is feasible to study. A critical review of relevant literature provides the researcher with an understanding of the current state of knowledge or the level of theory already developed. Knowledge of previous work in the field will suggest to the researcher the type of question that is appropriate for study and the methods for approaching the question. A summary of the current state of knowledge is obtained by reading about the topic of interest. This is incorporated into the research process as a review of the literature, and it establishes the conceptual framework. The researcher then identifies one or more of the study's specific purposes. A purpose expresses the concepts to be studied and, if appropriate, proposes relationships between the concepts.

The empirical phase of the research includes the blueprint or design for the conduct of the study. Concepts that were expressed in the purpose are now treated as specific variables to be studied. Decisions are made and implemented about how these variables will be described or measured and what sample of people or situations will be studied. The design of the study is planned carefully to control for threats to *reliability* and *validity*. Once the investigator knows what will be studied and where, plans are made for the generation of data, for example, by observation, interview, or physiological instrumentation. When human or animal subjects will be involved in the research, plans must be drawn for protecting their rights. Regardless of the form in which data will be collected (words, numbers, electrical tracings), a format is needed to organize these data. The investigator will select and implement the specific qualitative or quantitative techniques for data analysis.

The final phase of the research process is the interpretive phase. During this phase the researcher interprets data and draws inferences about the findings of the study. The interpretive phase of the research process interacts with the conceptual and empirical phases. In other words, the findings of the study are examined for their credibility in the context of how the study was conceptualized, planned, and actually carried out. The results of the study may be presented in the form of a thesis or dissertation, a research article for publication, or a paper or poster for presentation at a professional or scientific meeting. Finally, the researcher and peers critically evaluate the entire study for potential use in subsequent research, and clinicians evaluate it for use in practice.

DEVELOPMENT OF NURSING RESEARCH
Practice sphere
Florence Nightingale's detailed observations, recorded during the Crimean War, may be considered the first effort at research in nursing. Through the use of detailed records of the effects of nursing actions on soldiers, Nightingale was able to effect changes in nursing care. However, little evidence exists in the historical literature that the research efforts begun by Nightingale were pursued by others. Nursing education occurred in hospitals that used an apprenticeship model of education. The demands of patient care and the lack of societal expectations for intellectual initiative in women contributed to the lack of nursing research.

Large-scale interest in biomedical research began in the 1940s. By the 1950s medical research was concentrated on the study of human responses to the environment. Nurse researchers lagged far behind in understanding knowledge about the prevention of illness and the health needs of society (Kalisch & Kalisch, 1978).

Early nursing research in the practice sphere focused on nurses rather than on nursing. Emphasis was placed on the roles and tasks that nurses performed in hospital settings, but little was done to explore the effect of nursing practice on patient care (Henderson, 1977).

Educational sphere
Although affiliation of schools of nursing with universities began in 1909 at the University of Minnesota, opposition to college-level education in nursing prevailed throughout the first quarter of this century. Physicians argued that intelligent and sound knowledge of theory would handicap the nurse. The first autonomous collegiate school of nursing that offered a Bachelor of Nursing degree opened in February 1924, at Yale University. Five years later, Yale University began offering a course of study leading to a Master of Nursing degree. However, master's degree programs grew slowly; by 1962 just over 1000

nurses were receiving master's degrees each year (Kalisch & Kalisch, 1978).

Doctoral degree preparation for nurses began in 1924 with a program designed for nurses in the School of Education at Teacher's College, Columbia University. A similar program was established in 1934 at New York University (Murphy, 1985). Because these early nurse researchers were prepared in education, it is not surprising that their research was conducted in nursing education, particularly in teaching methods for educating nurses.

In 1956 the federal government made available awards to assist institutions to develop nursing research competencies through a special predoctoral research fellowship program. The Faculty Research Development Grant (FaReDeG) program, in effect from 1959 to 1966, focused on the development of research competencies by faculty members in schools of nursing. The program was followed by the Research Development Program, which concentrated on developing the research undertaken by faculty. The second program was extended to 1976. The Nurse Scientist Program, initiated in 1962, provided funds to schools of nursing to support nurses seeking doctorates in such fields as anthropology, psychology, sociology, anatomy, physiology, and microbiology.

The evolution of doctoral programs in nursing was also slow. The University of Pittsburgh began offering a Doctor of Philosophy degree in maternal-child nursing in 1954, and in 1960 Boston University initiated a Doctorate in Nursing Science in psychiatric nursing. It was not until 1964 that the University of California at San Francisco offered a comprehensive Doctor of Nursing Science program in several nursing specialties (Kalisch & Kalisch, 1978). Since then, doctoral education, which has a strong concentration in nursing research, has continued to grow. By 1985, there were 34 doctoral programs in nursing in the United States and over 3500 nurses held doctorates. The trend today is for nurses to pursue postdoctoral education in research methodology or in substantive content areas with an emphasis on improving their research skills.

Publications

Nursing Research, the first major journal devoted exclusively to research reports, began publication in 1952. Thereafter, other journals concentrating on reports of nursing research began to appear in print (see box below). *The Annual Review of Nursing Research* initiated publication in 1983 for the purpose of providing an integrative review of published and unpublished research to help nurse scholars become familiar with the current state of knowledge in selected fields of study. The systematic, critical assessment of advances in the field provides nurse scholars with information about the availability and quality of research. This publication identifies gaps in knowledge and proposes suggestions for further study in the field (Werley & Fitzpatrick, 1983).

Reports of research in such areas as individual and family adaptation to health and illness, environments that support health and healthy living, and therapeutic nursing interventions are not confined to nursing research journals. Nursing specialty publications such as *Heart and Lung, Cancer Nursing, Public Health Nursing, Journal of Psychosocial Nursing and Mental Health Services, Journal of Nursing Education, Nursing Administration Quarterly,* and *Maternal-Child Nursing Journal* consistently include reports of nursing research. Proceedings from scientific meetings also present the results of nursing research.

Funding

In 1955 the ANA formed the American Nurses' Foundation, an organization devoted exclusively to the support and promotion of nursing research. The extramural grants program for nursing research of the United States Public Health Service began in 1956 and awarded nearly $500,000 to researchers for projects in nursing in the first year. In the same year federal support for research training for predoctoral fellows became available from the Division of

---

INCEPTION OF PUBLICATION OF NURSING RESEARCH JOURNALS

1952	*Nursing Research*
1964	*International Journal of Nursing Studies*
1978	*Research in Nursing and Health*
1979	*Western Journal of Nursing Research*
1979	*Advances in Nursing Science*
1983	*Annual Review of Nursing Research*

Nursing Resources of the United States Public Health Service.

The Division of Nursing within the United States Public Health Service and various institutes within the National Institutes of Health funded nursing research for many years. In 1986 the National Center for Nursing Research was established as a center within the National Institutes of Health. Other sources of research funding include the Veterans' Administration and private foundations such as the Robert Wood Johnson Foundation. Small grants for nursing research also are available through organizations such as International Sigma Theta Tau, the American Cancer Society, and the American Nurses' Foundation. (For further information about funding for nursing research see Chapter 32.)

PARTICIPATION OF NURSES IN RESEARCH

Educational preparation

Every nurse, regardless of educational preparation, can be involved in and benefit from nursing research. As the level of educational preparation increases, the sophistication of the nurse's participation is expected to increase (see box below). Guidelines to assist educators in preparing nurses to perform investigative activities appropriate to their academic program were set forth by the ANA (1976a; 1981b). These guidelines also encourage administrators to support nurses in their investigative pursuits.

The ANA recommended that nurses with an associate degree in nursing should understand the value of research in nursing. They could assist in identifying problem areas in practice and with collecting data within an established research protocol.

Nurses with baccalaureate preparation would be able to read, interpret, and evaluate research for its applicability to practice. Additionally, they would be able to assist in the identification of nursing problems in need of study and use the practice of nursing as a means of gathering data for refining and extending their effectiveness. Sharing research findings with colleagues and applying the findings of nursing and other health-related research to practice were outlined as other expectations of the baccalaureate graduate.

The ANA defined the role of nurses with master's preparation as one of analyzing and reformulating problems in nursing practice so that scientific meth-

---

LADDER OF INCREASING EDUCATION AND RESPONSIBILITY FOR RESEARCH

Doctoral degree
Extend scientific basis
Develop methods to measure nursing phenomena
Provide leadership

Master's degree
Conduct investigations
Facilitate access to clients
Collaborate with other investigators
Facilitate research
Provide consultation
Analyze and reformulate problems

Baccalaureate degree
Apply findings to practice
Share findings
Interpret and evaluate research for practice

Associate degree
Collect data
Identify problems
Appreciate the value of research

ods could be applied to their solutions. Nurses with master's degrees can enhance the quality and clinical relevance of nursing research by sharing their expertise in clinical problems and by providing consultation to investigators about the manner in which clinical services are delivered. A nurse with a master's degree can also facilitate investigation of clinical problems by contributing to a climate that is supportive of investigation, by collaborating with others in investigations, and by helping to provide contact with clients. At this level the nurse can conduct investigations to monitor the quality of practice and assist others in the application of scientific knowledge in nursing practice.

The nurse with a doctorate provides leadership for the integration of scientific knowledge with other sources of knowledge to advance the practice of nursing. Developing methods to monitor quality of nursing practice and to measure nursing phenomena is an extremely important contribution of the nurse with a doctorate. Finally, at this level of preparation, the investigator conducts studies to evaluate the contributions of nursing activities to the well-being of clients and broadens the scientific base supportive of nursing practice.

The nurse as investigator

Despite the fact that the primary concern of nurse researchers is intimately linked to the delivery of nursing care, the perspectives of clinicians and researchers are somewhat different (see box below). The focus of clinicians usually is on the individual. Indeed, nurses in clinical practice value individualizing patient care. Clinicians typically assess one patient or a group of patients at a time rather than thinking about an entire population. Clinicians ana-

lyze individuals, examining change within the person over time. They often deal with subjective data, focusing on feelings and the meanings of experience to people. The clinician examines patterns that reflect the whole of a person's reality, including individual–environmental interaction. Data often are collected and analyzed in collaboration with the client. The clinician usually generates some conclusions such as a nursing diagnosis.

Scientists, or nurse researchers, more often focus on collectives that allow them to arrive at some general law or rule. They frequently are concerned with objective measures and devote a great deal of effort developing valid and reliable measurement instruments. To study how one isolated factor relates to another without interference from the rest of the world, scientists try to isolate or stabilize the environment. This isolation of phenomena often does not provide a holistic view or preserve the connections between the phenomena and clinical reality. Many investigators measure the variables they study in a static way, often only once or just a few times. The analysis of data often is quantitatively oriented and may involve the use of statistical methods to assess outcomes. Increasingly, evidence indicates that nurse scientists are blending the clinical and scientific approaches in the study of human responses.

IMPORTANCE OF NURSING RESEARCH

In an earlier section of this chapter, we discussed the importance of nursing research in generating and testing knowledge to guide practice. The significance of the contribution of research to the profession is linked to the accumulation of new knowledge, the

---

PERSPECTIVES OF CLINICIANS AND RESEARCHERS

Clinician	*Researcher*
Focused on individual	Focused on population
Subjective data obtained in collaboration with client	Objective measurement developed and implemented by the investigator
Focus on individual–environmental interactions	Focus on two or more isolated factors
Data analyzed collaboratively with client	Analysis removed from setting of data generation

testing of old knowledge, and professional account-ability and autonomy. For a practice discipline to control the provision of its own services, research on those services and the knowledge research can yield are essential. Nursing, because of its broad range of services, requires a knowledge base paralleling the scope of its practice. Nursing practice requires knowledge of human beings from birth to death in health-related situations ranging from high-level wellness to critical illness. Moreover, nursing practice has a direct, significant impact on human health and human life. To make clinical decisions that preserve human life and promote health, nurses need access to valid information about caring for people. The development of knowledge through research is essential for accountability of the profession to clients and to society.

In addition to nursing practice, nursing education and administration are important domains of nursing knowledge. The special emphasis of nursing in the educative and administrative processes mandates the generation and testing of theory pertaining to these processes if nursing educators and administrators are to be truly accountable to their clients, students, patients, and staff.

Batey and Lewis (1982) defined autonomy as "freedom to make discretionary and binding decisions within one's scope of practice" (p. 13). Research efforts contribute to professional autonomy for nursing through the selection, generation, and testing of a unique body of knowledge. Knowledge provides a basis for professional autonomy and power. Research efforts that refine the knowledge for the discipline provide a source of focus for nursing, help to distinguish our body of knowledge from other sciences, and empower nurses. On an individual basis the use of research findings to justify or change practice empowers the nurse to challenge existing practice. For the profession, research findings justify nursing services by establishing their value to clients (Chinn & Jacobs, 1987).

Research that is directed at developing theory for nursing moves the discipline toward an explicit goal for the profession; it does not merely complement the practice of other health professions. Moreover, research that generates and tests nursing theory ultimately enables nurses in various roles within nursing (clinician, theorist, investigator, educator, administrator) to communicate their central concerns.

DIRECTIONS FOR NURSING RESEARCH

Priorities

The Cabinet on Nursing Research of the ANA periodically publishes a statement describing priorities for research in nursing (ANA, 1976b; 1981a). Through the years the Cabinet has consistently noted that nursing research develops knowledge about (1) health and health promotion over the full life span, (2) the care of persons with health problems and disabilities, and (3) nursing actions that enhance the ability of individuals to respond effectively to actual or potential health problems. The 1981 statement identified priorities that fell into two distinct areas: the practice of nursing and the profession of nursing. Guided by major social trends, these priorities will change over time.

In 1985 the Cabinet on Nursing Research of the ANA again stressed that nurse scientists emphasize the study of whole human beings in interaction with their environments rather than the study of isolated body systems or subsystems. It was noted that nurse scholars traditionally have exhibited concern for (1) laws and principles governing life processes and optimum functioning of human beings, (2) human behavior in critical life situations, and (3) ways in which positive changes occur in health status. It follows from these concerns that nurse researchers would become involved in generating knowledge about health and health promotion in individuals and families. The specific priorities for nursing research suggested by the Cabinet on Nursing Research and various nursing specialty organizations are presented in Chapter 3.

Societal trends

The influence of the social and physical environment on health and the interpersonal and physical therapeutic actions that enhance the individual's ability to respond to actual or potential health problems are key areas of interest to nurses. Further knowledge also is needed to determine the types of systems able to deliver health-care services to members of society in an increasingly technological world.

The changing character of our society further suggests direction for nursing research. As children and young adults survive trauma and diseases that previously resulted in death, a greater percentage of the population in the United States is shifting to an older age-group. It is anticipated that by the year 2000,

15% of our population will be over the age of 65 years and many will have one or more chronic illnesses. The increased prevalence of chronic health problems such as cancer, heart disease, arthritis, chronic pulmonary disease, and degenerative diseases of the nervous system will require considerable adjustment on the part of individuals and families and will command a major proportion of health resources.

John Naisbitt (1982), in his book *Megatrends,* identified several trends in the United States that have implications for nursing. The first of these is the shift from an industrial society to an information society. The importance of information in society continues to increase as shifts occur in the way in which people receive, process, and respond to information. How will this shift to an information society affect nursing practice? How can nurses use the available technology to exchange information with other health-care providers about those for whom they care? What influence will the shift to an information society have on patient teaching? On nursing education? What influence will the shift from a labor-intensive society have on the mental health of Americans?

As technology increases, human need increases for what Naisbitt called "high touch," the need for human-to-human physical contact. As more and more medical technology became available to monitor mother and infant during the perinatal period, the interest in home birth, birthing centers, and rooming-in increased (Naisbitt, 1982). The hospice movement has assumed great importance as advances in medicine and technology have made it possible to extend the life of terminally ill individuals. How can nurses best enact their caring role in such situations? What responsibilities do nurses have in high technology situations?

Another trend discussed by Naisbitt is the shift from institutional help to self-help. What role will nurses enact in meeting consumer demands for less hospital-based or other institution-based health care? What functions do self-help groups provide for chronically ill individuals? How can nurses take advantage of the interest of the American consumer in health and fitness to benefit their clients?

SUMMARY

Nursing research is the systematic inquiry into the phenomena of interest in nursing science, namely, the adaptation of individuals and groups to actual or potential health problems, the environments that influence health in humans, and the therapeutic interventions that affect the consequences of illness and promote health. Nursing research follows a more or less sequential process that includes the conceptual, empirical, and interpretive phases. Knowledge is derived from empirics, aesthetics, personal knowledge, and ethics. Empirics deals with the science of nursing and is the focus of this book.

Historically, developments in nursing practice and education have influenced the direction of nursing research. Because nurse researchers initially were prepared in education, their research centered on nursing education and the tasks and roles of nurses. Doctoral education in the basic sciences (e.g., physiology, microbiology, and sociology) underlying nursing practice and in nursing science (a discipline of its own) have resulted in more emphasis on research into adaptation to illness and into environments and therapeutic interventions that promote health. All levels of nursing education today include the preparation of nurses to participate in the research process.

References

American Nurses' Association. (1976a). *Preparation for nurses for participation in research.* Kansas City, MO: Author.

American Nurses' Association. (1976b). *Priorities for research in nursing.* Kansas City, MO: Author.

American Nurses' Association. (1980). *ANA social policy statement.* Kansas City, MO: Author.

American Nurses' Association Cabinet on Nursing Research. (1985). *Directions for nursing research: Toward the twenty-first century.* Kansas City, MO: Author.

American Nurses' Association Commission on Nursing Research. (1981a). *Priorities for research for the 1980's. Generating a scientific basis for nursing practice.* Kansas City, MO: Author.

American Nurses' Association Commission on Nursing Research. (1981b). *Guidelines for the investigative function of nurses.* Kansas City, MO: Author.

Barnard, K. E. (1980). Knowledge for practice: Directions for the future. *Nursing Research, 29,* 208-212.

Batey, M. V. (1971). Conceptualizing the research process. *Nursing Research, 20,* 296-301.

Batey, M. V., & Lewis, F. M. (1982). Clarifying autonomy and accountability in nursing service. *Journal of Nursing Administration, 12*(9), 13-18.

Benoliel, J. Q. (1984). Advancing nursing science: Qualitative approaches. *Communicating Nursing Research (Vol. 17).*

Burgess, A. W., & Holmstrom, L. L. (1974). *Rape: Victims of crisis.* Bowie, MD: Robert J. Brady.

Carper, B. (1978). Fundamental patterns of knowing in nursing. *Advances in Nursing Science, 1*(1), 13-24.

Chinn, P. L., & Jacobs, M. K. (1987). *Theory and nursing: A systematic approach* (2nd ed.). St. Louis: Mosby.

Dimond, M. (1979). Social support and adaptation to chronic illness: The case of maintenance hemodialysis. *Research in Nursing and Health, 2,* 101-108.

Donaldson, S., & Crowley, D. (1979). The discipline of nursing. *Nursing Outlook, 26,* 113-120.

Dunkel-Schetter, C. (1984). Social support and cancer: Findings based on patient interviews and their implications. *Journal of Social Issues, 40*(4), 77-98.

Fuller, S. S., Endress, M. P., & Johnson, J. E. (1978). The effects of cognitive and behavioral control on coping with an aversive health examination. *Journal of Human Stress, 4*(4), 18-25.

Henderson, V. A. (1966). *The nature of nursing.* New York: Macmillan.

Henderson, V. A. (1977). We've 'come a long way' but what of the direction? *Nursing Research, 26,* 163-164.

Johnson, J. E. & Leventhal, H. (1974). Effects of accurate expectations and behavioral instructions on reactions during a noxious medical examination. *Journal of Personality and Social Psychology, 2,* 55-64.

Johnson, J. E., Morissey, J. F., & Leventhal, H. (1973). Psychological preparation for an endoscopic examination. *Gastrointestinal Endoscopy, 19,* 180-182.

Johnson, J. E., Kirchoff, K. T., & Endress, M. P. (1975). Deterring children's distress behavior during orthopedic cast removal. *Nursing Research, 75,* 404-410.

Johnson, J. E., Rice, V. H., Fuller, S. S., & Endress, M. P. (1978a). Sensory information, instruction in coping strategy, and recovery from surgery. *Research in Nursing and Health, 1*(1), 4-17.

Johnson, J. E., Fuller, S. S., Endress, M. P., & Rice, V. H. (1978b). Altering patients' responses to surgery: An extension and replication. *Research in Nursing and Health, 1*(3), 111-121.

Kalisch, P. A., & Kalisch, B. J. (1978). *The advance of American nursing.* Boston: Little, Brown.

King, I. (1971). *Toward a theory for nursing: General concepts of human behavior.* New York: Wiley.

Levy, R. L. (1983). Social support and compliance: A selective review and critique of treatment integrity and outcome measurement. *Social Science and Medicine, 17,* 1329-1338.

Lewis, F. M. (1982). Experienced personal control and quality of life in late-stage cancer patients. *Nursing Research, 31,* 113-119.

Lindeman, C. A., & Van Aernam, B. (1971). Nursing intervention with the presurgical patient: The effects of structured and unstructured preoperative teaching. *Nursing Research, 20,* 319-332.

Measal, C. P., & Anderson, G. C. (1979). Nonnutritive sucking during tube feedings: Effect on clinical course in premature infants. *Journal of Obstetric, Gynecologic and Neonatal Nursing, 8,* 265-272.

Murphy, J. F. (1985). Doctoral education of nurses: Historical development, programs, and graduates. In H. H. Werley & J. J. Fitzpatrick, (Eds.). *Annual Review of Nursing Research (Vol. 3).* New York: Springer.

Naisbitt, J. (1982). *Megatrends.* New York: Warner Books.

Nightingale, F. (1860). *Notes on nursing: What it is and what it is not.* Philadelphia: Lippincott, 1946. (Facsimile of first edition. London: Harrison & Sons.)

Norbeck, J. S., & Tilden, V. (1983). Life stress, social support, and emotional disequilibrium in complications of pregnancy: A prospective, multivariate study. *Journal of Health and Social Behavior, 24,* 30-46.

Nuckolls, K. B., Cassel, J. C., & Kaplan, B. H. (1972). Psychosocial assets, life crises and the prognosis of pregnancy. *American Journal of Epidemiology, 95,* 431-441.

Orem, D. (1985). *Nursing: Concepts of practice* (3rd ed.). New York: McGraw-Hill.

Rogers, M. (1970). *An introduction to the theoretical basis of nursing.* Philadelphia: Davis.

Werley, H. H., & Fitzpatrick J. J. (1983). *Annual Review of Nursing Research* (Vol. 1). New York: Springer.

Wortman, C. B., & Dunkel-Schetter, C. (1979). Interpersonal relationships and cancer: A theoretical analysis. *Journal of Social Issues, 35*(1), 120-155.

2

DEVELOPING NURSING THEORY

MARCI CATANZARO AND NANCY FUGATE WOODS

Whereas Chapter 1 deals with the need for a scientific basis for nursing practice, nursing practice itself provides a basis for research that leads to the development of knowledge *for* practice, sometimes in the form of nursing theory. Thus nursing theory, in turn, provides the scientific basis for nursing practice. Since the beginning of organized health care, nurse clinicians have thought about the people they care for, the environment in which the care takes place, and the care they provide. Chapter 2 discusses the ongoing cyclical relationship among theory, research, and practice in the process of developing scientific knowledge relevant to nursing, beginning with a discussion of the need for theory and theory development in nursing. The chapter then considers definitions of nursing theory, the components of a theory, and the ways in which theory development proceeds. The nature of theory and its relationship to the development of the discipline of nursing are the central themes of this chapter.

INTRODUCTION TO THEORY

Theory is part of the vocabulary of nurses in all areas of practice. The word itself has many meanings and uses. We may say that we have a theory about why something happened when what we actually have is an idea or hunch about the connection between events. Nursing theory goes beyond this everyday meaning to include ideas that are formulated and tested carefully. A theory is a systematic vision of reality that serves a scientific purpose. The theory of gravity helps us to understand body mechanics and positioning. Developmental theories assist us in understanding the behavior of children. Psychiatric nurses are familiar with and often use concepts from psychoanalytical theory in client care. A theory consists of words or other symbols that are intended to represent something in the real world. The symbol is not the thing itself, only a label for the object, property, or event. The term "systematic" implies that the concepts are organized in an orderly pattern (Chinn & Jacobs, 1983).

Purposes of nursing theory

Nursing theory serves many purposes. Among these purposes are (1) to develop research propositions, (2) to serve as a reservoir for knowledge and research findings, (3) to explain observations and predict outcomes, and (4) to stimulate new directions in practice and in research. Theory provides frameworks that link research and practice and contribute to meaningful and generalizable scientific findings. Both practice and theory can be used to generate research questions. In addition, nursing theory can provide directions for the type of methods that are appropriate for seeking answers to research questions. Research is the way in which we prove, disprove, or modify a theory. The cycle is completed when a theory that has been supported through research is used to guide practice.

Jean Johnson's work serves as an example of the

various purposes of nursing theory. She used knowledge of theories pertaining to cognitive processes and distress reactions to threatening events to develop research propositions about how patients would respond to such threatening events as orthopedic cast removal or gastric intubation. Johnson and her colleagues designed a series of laboratory and clinical experiments to test the influence of information on coping with threatening events. Findings from each part of the research program were compared with the propositions set forth in the theory guiding the research. These findings consistently demonstrated that the content and the sequence of teaching influenced outcomes such as crying or early discharge from the hospital and provided a way of explaining and predicting outcomes in patients who were faced with threatening events. The relationship established between selected propositions in cognition theory and the real-life experiences of patients living through threatening events made a major contribution to how nurses teach patients (Leventhal & Johnson, 1983).

Nursing theory is a source of professional autonomy and power. Theory provides nurses with a sound basis to describe, explain, and predict factors that influence nursing care. The recurrent themes in nursing theory guide nursing education, research, and practice and differentiate nursing practice from other disciplines. As Chinn and Jacobs (1983) summarized it, theory provides a firm basis for planning and considering our actions and for challenging nursing practice and theory itself. Nursing theory enables nurses to predict the outcomes of what they are doing and to explain their selection of patient-care approaches.

Definitions of theory

Perhaps as many definitions of nursing theory exist as do nurse theorists. The personal and professional history of the theorist and that of the profession influence how an individual will view the world and the role of nursing in that world. These factors are just a few of the influences on theory development. Further confusion in defining theory arises from terminology when authors use words interchangeably, such as conceptual framework, conceptual model, paradigm, and theory.

Although many specific definitions of theory exist, social scientists generally agree that a theory is a set of concepts interrelated to form propositions that are useful for prediction and control. Chinn and Jacobs (1983) identified four focuses of theory definitions: structure, practice goals, tentativeness, and research. Definitions of nursing theory that focus on structure incorporate research as a significant step in theory development. McKay's definition (1969) of nursing theory is an example of a definition focusing on structure. She defined nursing theory as "logically interrelated sets of confirmed hypotheses" (p. 394). Research is required to confirm the hypotheses that constitute the theory and their relationship to each other. This approach to nursing theory emphasizes the fact that theory development is more than a mental process. According to Chinn and Jacobs (1983), none of the current nursing theories have been sufficiently tested to meet the structural definition of nursing theory; however, components of some nursing theories have been tested and validated in some situations.

Dickoff and James (1968) defined theory as "a conceptual system or framework invented for some purpose" (p. 198). This definition is focused on practice goals, outcomes, or consequences. Dickoff and James believed that all nursing theory should have as its purpose the prescription of actions for nursing. Definitions of nursing theory that emphasize tentativeness acknowledge that theories are always in the process of development and that invention of theory is as important as discovery of theory. Stevens (1979) provided a definition of nursing theory that focused on tentativeness when she stated that theory is "a statement that purports to account for the characterization of some phenomenon" (p. 1).

Another approach to the definition of nursing theory focuses on theory guiding research. Ellis (1968) defined theory as "a coherent set of hypothetical, conceptual, and pragmatic principles forming a general frame of reference for a field of inquiry" (p. 217). This definition of nursing theory emphasizes the cycle of practice guiding theory, theory guiding research, and research guiding practice.

Chinn and Jacobs (1983) defined nursing theory in a way that takes into account the multiple uses of theory. Their definition stated that theory is the following:

A set of concepts, definitions, and propositions that project a systematic view of phenomena by designating specific interrelationships among concepts for purposes of describing, explaining, predicting, and/or controlling phenomena (p. 70).

This definition makes clear that nursing theory is an integrated whole used for some specific purpose; it does not restrict theory to propositions verified by research.

Meleis (1985) noted that nursing theory must be articulated and communicated. The theory itself, according to her, can be invented or discovered. A theory is an articulation of how phenomena are conceptualized. A nursing theory also includes the relationships among the concepts as they pertain to nursing. Meleis believed that theory has as its purpose ". . . describing, explaining, predicting, or prescribing nursing care" (p. 29).

Components of a theory

Components of a nursing theory include concepts and a statement of propositions. *Concepts* are the building blocks of a theory. Concepts are abstract characteristics, categories, or labels of objects, persons, or events to be studied. A concept is a generalization about something particular and may have many degrees of abstraction, ranging from the very concrete to the very abstract. Height is an example of a concrete concept; it expresses numerous observations of things that are more or less short or tall. Other concrete concepts are stages of sleep, body temperature, and electrolyte balance. Caring, pain, and health are examples of abstract concepts.

Fawcett (1983) pointed out that any theory of nursing must contain the concept of nursing as an activity. Furthermore, inclusion of the concepts of person, health, and the environment helps to explain and predict how nursing actions interact with other concepts to produce a desired patient outcome. Various nurse theorists have viewed the person, society/environment, health, and nursing differently. A comparison of two theorists, Florence Nightingale (1860) and Sister Callista Roy (1976), is shown in Table 2-1.

A *construct* is a concept invented by the theorist or adopted from another source for a special scientific purpose. Locus of control, for instance, is a construct behavioral scientists have invented to describe the site of power within or outside an individual in relation to the control they believe they have over events.

Many authors use the words "concept" and "construct" interchangeably.

A statement of *proposition* holds concepts in a theory together by indicating a relationship between the concepts. Propositions may be stated in the form of an *axiom*, a summary of empirical evidence linking two concepts; or as a *postulate,* a statement of presumed relationship between concepts (Fawcett, 1984). A proposition may state that one concept is associated with another or is contingent upon another.

Scope of theory

Another way to view theory is in terms of its scope, ranging from broad to limited. Another term for *broad-range theory* is *grand theory.* A grand theory is one that takes into account all of nursing. Although not proposing a nursing theory as such, Florence Nightingale (1860) wrote of the inherent reparative powers that each individual possesses. As Table 2-1 shows, she pointed out that nursing was not a curative process but rather was intended to manipulate the environment, communicate with the patient and other care providers, and assist with the individual's reparative processes. She noted that all of society and the environment influenced life and well-being. She viewed health as a repair of disease. Grand theories such as Nightingale's are too broad and global to be tested. To test Nightingale's theory one would need to define the concepts of environment and health. Additionally, one would need to specify the propositions that relate the concepts to each other.

Middle-range theories are more likely to be testable than grand theories. Jean Johnson's work on cognitive preparation of patients for diagnostic and treatment procedures is an example of a middle-range theory (Leventhal & Johnson, 1983). Because the concepts were defined and their relationships were specified, Johnson could test the theory about the types of patient preparation in both the laboratory and the clinical setting. Phyllis Stern's work (1980) with stepfathers provides another example of middle-range theory. She used grounded-theory methodology to develop a theory about how a stepfather is integrated into a family consisting of a mother and child. The theory includes clearly defined concepts and propositions about strategies that stepfathers used. These propositions can be tested to determine which consistently lead to successful outcomes when

TABLE 2-1. Comparison of concepts as defined by two nursing theorists

	NIGHTINGALE (1860)	ROY (1976)
Person	Has vital natural powers for the reparative process	Biopsychosocial being Interacts with environment Adapts to environment through biopsychosocial mechanisms Adaptation determined by focal, contextual, and residual stimuli Modes of adaptation are physiological, self-concept, role function, and interdependence
Society/environment	Central concept All external conditions and influences affecting development and life Major areas: ventilation, warmth, effluvia (odors), noise, light	Central concept Provides matter, energy, and information Stimulates individual
Health	Disease is reparative process Cause of disease is environment Laws of health synonymous with laws and nature of nursing	State of function that allows adaptation to occur A continuum from peak wellness to death Poor health the result of maladaptation to environmental change
Nursing	Places individual in best possible conditions for nature to act Provides environment conducive to the reparative process Communicates with person in unhurried, uninterrupted manner Observes and collects data to prevent health problems Has goal of assisting reparative process	Interpersonal process initiated by individual's maladaption to changes in environment Takes action directed at reducing or removing stimuli Enhances adaptive level of individual

a stepfather enters an existing family of mother and child.

Narrow-range theory deals with one situation at one point in time. It has little usefulness for the development of nursing theory beyond providing ideas about further theory development.

In summary, grand theory is too broad and ill-defined for systematic testing. Middle-range theory is generalizable and yet specific enough to be testable. It is the most useful for the development of nursing science. Narrow-range theory, as its name implies, is too narrow to be useful in many nursing situations.

Paradigms for nursing science

A *paradigm* is a way of looking at the world, a general perspective. A paradigm presents a set of philosophical assumptions about the world that are interrelated in a way that helps break down the complexity of the real world (Kuhn, 1962, 1970). Paradigms are collections of assumptions about a domain of knowledge that guide and influence inquiry. Paradigms perform the following functions:

1. Structure the questions to be asked
2. Eliminate questions that are outside the conceptual boundaries of the paradigm
3. Imply a particular frame of reference common to many investigators
4. Provide a linkage to certain types of research methods
5. Suggest criteria by which to judge appropriate research tools
6. Provide criteria for evaluating the quality of the research effort

Two paradigms influence contemporary nursing research: positivist-empiricist and naturalistic-inductive.

Positivist-empiricist paradigm. The positivist-empiricist paradigm emerges from a tradition based on the physical sciences. Historical roots of this paradigm can be traced at least to Aristotle (384-322 BC), who believed that knowledge was acquired by passive observation. Polkinghorne (1983) pointed out that the craft guilds of the Middle Ages began a movement toward empirical investigation that Francis Bacon championed in *Novum Organum,* which was published in 1620. Knowledge was viewed as those things such as logical and mathematical truths, about which we could be absolutely certain. The

thrust of thinking that became known as realism and logical positivism guided scientific inquiry well into the eighteenth century.

The positivist-empiricist tradition, sometimes mistakenly referred to as the quantitative approach, assumes that a body of facts or principles exists to be discovered or understood and that these facts or principles exist independently of any historical or social context. Investigators who are influenced by this tradition seek universal, abstract, and general principles to understand phenomena. Generating understanding of causal relationships is an important purpose of research in this tradition, and the use of experimental methodology is common. The positivist-empiricist tradition is oriented to understanding and mastering the phenomena under study. Scientific detachment is desirable for conducting inquiry in this tradition (Tinkle & Beaton, 1983). Ideally, investigators are "removed" from the data, and their findings reflect the perspective of the scientist as an "outsider" rather than an individual with subjective knowledge about the topic.

Investigations in this tradition can be described as outcome-oriented. Measurement is oriented toward obtaining reliable and replicable data. The investigator, concerned about generalizing the study results, typically uses methods to ensure that the individuals studied are selected so that they represent the total population of interest. Usually the investigator seeks to study large numbers of people, objects, or events. The positivist-empiricist approach, in its most extreme case, assumes a stable reality and mechanistic relationships characterized as a law or principle. Investigations employed by scientists whose work is influenced by the positivist-empiricist tradition typically follow a series of steps, including stating a hypothesis, choosing measures of the concepts under study, collecting data, and analyzing the results (Fig. 2-1).

Pender (1984) used a positivist paradigm in her study of the effects of progressive muscle relaxation on the blood pressure of clients with hypertension. She drew a sample from participants in a hypertension-monitoring program who had a diagnosis of primary hypertension with no identified secondary changes. A comparison group of clients who met the criteria for inclusion in the study were matched with the experimental subjects on sex, age, number of medications, and systolic blood pressure.

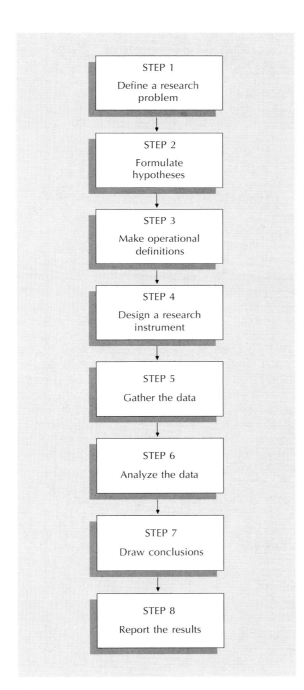

STEP 1

Define a research problem

↓

STEP 2

Formulate hypotheses

↓

STEP 3

Make operational definitions

↓

STEP 4

Design a research instrument

↓

STEP 5

Gather the data

↓

STEP 6

Analyze the data

↓

STEP 7

Draw conclusions

↓

STEP 8

Report the results

Fig. 2-1. Linear sequence in positive-empiricist research.

Pender obtained baseline measurements of blood pressure, heart rate, muscle tension, and temperature. She also collected data concerning medication regimen, medication and nutritional compliance, and level of physical activity. The experimental group members then participated in group training in relaxation.

Participants in the experimental and the comparison groups were seen throughout the study for monitoring and health counseling. Nurses who were uninformed about which clients were in the experimental and comparison groups did the monitoring. Follow-up data were collected at 2 and 4 months after the end of the relaxation training. Pender found that the experimental group had a lower mean systolic blood pressure than the comparison group at 4-month follow-up. The relaxation-trained group showed a significant decrease in diastolic pressure from baseline to follow-up, but the difference between the experimental and comparison groups was not significant. The investigator concluded that relaxation taught in groups with individual follow-up visits resulted in continued practice of relaxation and subsequent lowering of blood pressure in the participants with essential, uncomplicated hypertension.

Pender's study is an example of nursing research using a positivist-empiricist approach. She followed a linear sequence to design and test an intervention to lower blood pressure of hypertensive clients. She used objective measures of blood pressure, heart rate, muscle tension, and temperature. Control of the study design was introduced through a comparison group. Nurses who did not know the group assignment of the study participants collected the follow-up data.

Naturalistic-inductive paradigm. Rapid social change during the eighteenth and nineteenth centuries raised questions concerning the usefulness of positivism in understanding human beings. German idealists held that the mind was the source and creator of knowledge and that the social world was created by the individuals who lived in it (Filstead, 1979). The naturalistic-inductive paradigm is derived from a tradition that assumes that facts and principles are embedded in both historical and cultural contexts. Truth is seen as dynamic and derived from human interaction with real social and historical settings. This tradition emphasizes research conducted in naturalistic settings and the use of methods that will lead to a full understanding of the situation. Sociohistorical factors are considered an integral part of the phenomenon being studied, not a source of error to be controlled.

The naturalistic-inductive paradigm implies the use of qualitative methods. Investigators who use naturalistic-inductive paradigms are concerned with understanding human behavior from the person's own frame of reference, rather than imposing the scientist's frame of reference. Investigators influenced by this paradigm employ naturalistic and controlled observation; they value data from the perspective of those studied. Naturalistic-inductive research is discovery-oriented, explanatory, descriptive, and inductive in nature. It is process-oriented rather than outcome-oriented and has as its goal understanding rather than control. The investigator assumes a dynamic reality and a holistic rather than a reductionist understanding. Single case studies may be used to contribute to understanding of the phenomena under study. Generalizability of findings is less of

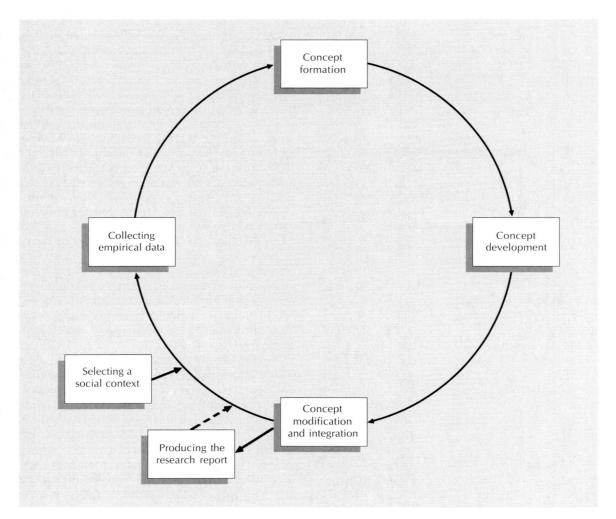

Fig. 2-2. Cyclical sequence in naturalistic-inductive research.

a concern to the investigator than is understanding of the particular case in point. The naturalistic-inductive approach to inquiry is concerned with the discovery of theory rather than with the verification of theory. This approach emphasizes a dynamic interchange among theory, concepts, and data, with feedback and modification of theory and concepts based on new data (Fig. 2-2). Emphasis is on understanding the social reality from an evolving, negotiated point of view (Tinkle & Beaton, 1983).

A naturalistic-inductive paradigm guided the investigation by Corbin and Strauss (1984) in the management by couples of chronic illness. The investigators' awareness of the prevalence of the difficulty couples experience in working together to manage chronic illness led to a detailed exploration of the problem. In-depth, unstructured interviews were conducted with 60 couples over a period of 2 years. Data were analyzed using an inductive technique known as *grounded-theory* methodology. These techniques involve the constant analysis of interview data as they are generated and the ongoing comparison of new and old data as the categories emerge (see Chapter 28).

"Biography," "trajectory," and "work" formed the conceptual framework of Corbin and Strauss's study. The concept of biography was defined as the progressive and at times overlapping phases of the life course, during which a series of expected and unexpected events and circumstances occurs. These events and circumstances require occupational, marital, domestic, and identity work. The concept of trajectory included the course of the chronic illness, the work that the couples did to manage the illness, and the impact that illness had on their lives. The management of each phase of a chronic illness described by Corbin and Strauss required work. Work associated with the biography and trajectory required a high degree of coordination between the husband and wife with regard to the type of work necessary to manage the illness, the tasks that needed to be accomplished in relation to the illness, and the individual's contribution to accomplishing the work. The investigators identified seven problems of coordinating the work required by the illness trajectory and biography that occur when the illness trajectory and the biography intersect. They explored how couples worked collaboratively to deal with these problems and identified three nursing interventions that

would help couples living with chronic illness to reduce disharmony: (1) assessing the source of the couple's conflict, (2) bringing the couple into open awareness of the problem, and (3) assisting the couple to resolve the problem by talking about it, talking it over, and talking it through.

Corbin and Strauss identified a problem of couples living with a chronic illness. They began to collect empirical data from couples and analyzed the interview data while continuing to collect data. They did not begin their study with concepts already defined nor did they attempt any intervention with their study participants. Rather, they explored the social context of living with a chronic illness from the perspective of their study participants and formulated, developed, modified, and integrated the concepts of biography, trajectory, and work as the study evolved.

Critical social theory is an example of a paradigm that is derived from the naturalistic-inductive paradigm. Critical social theory is derived from the belief that reality arises out of an analysis not distorted by power imbalances among the participants (Bernstein, 1978). Autonomous, responsible communication resulting in consensual reflection and analysis is the basis for critical theory. Critical theory uses history and theory to inform the researcher of the nature of the social contract we are living and to make us fully self-conscious of the contradictions implicit in our material condition. Research questions are derived from social problems that are critical to our lives. An example of critical theory is related to the feminist movement, which seeks to understand issues important to the lives of women. Women's ideas, needs, and experiences are accepted as valid. The purpose of the research is to understand the multiple truths that together explain the situation. Reflexive thinking is employed and includes the processing of social, political, biological, economic, and cultural factors as they interrelate with the phenomena of concern (MacPherson, 1983; Roberts, 1981). The investigator and the study participants are viewed as equal in status and power. Because the researcher assumes the validity of women's responses, no need exists to control or objectify them. Personal involvement of the researcher with the participants results in a sharing experience for both and increases the researcher's confidence in the data.

Early nursing leaders, including Nightingale, promoted nursing as an art and a science. The traditional blending of humanitarian and scientific values constitutes an important part of nursing tradition that is only beginning to be evident in contemporary nursing research. Historically, nurse scientists first employed a positivist paradigm in their research. The first generation of nurse scientists were prepared predominantly in education or educational administration. The second generation of nurse researchers were prepared for their role as scientists in such basic sciences as physiology, sociology, and microbiology; nurse researchers educated in these disciplines used positivist-empiricist paradigms. As preparation for advanced roles in nursing research has moved from related sciences to nursing science, nurse scientists have begun to integrate positivist-empiricist and naturalistic-inductive approaches to clarify unique phenomena of central interest to nursing. Methodological approaches to research are not irrevocably linked to a paradigm, nor are paradigms mutually exclusive (Goodwin & Goodwin, 1984). Contemporary nursing literature reflects an awareness of the nature of the nursing phenomenon. New paradigms are emerging, often a mixture of past ones, that better enable those phenomena to be studied more meaningfully.

OVERVIEW OF THEORY DEVELOPMENT

Process of theory development

The development of nursing theory requires a systematic process of inquiry. Components of that process include concept analysis, construction of theoretical relationships, testing of theoretical relationships, and practical validation of theory (Chinn & Jacobs, 1987). Concept analysis and construction of theoretical relationships are largely thought processes that may or may not involve the research process. One can sit in the quiet of the living room and analyze a concept and generate propositions that relate the concept to other concepts. However, as a practice discipline nursing requires that the theoretical relationships be tested and that the theory be validated in the real world.

Concept clarification

A theory is a collection of concepts and propositions that relate those concepts. One of the first steps in theory development is clarification of the concepts. Concept clarification is also an essential part of developing a research project; it is the process of examining the characteristics of a concept. Methods for clarifying concepts in nursing vary among theorists. Qualitative or inductive methods such as phenomenology, ethnoscience, and grounded theory are among the methods used. These methods use interview data, participant observation, and written communications to understand a phenomenon within a contextual situation. A discussion of these methods may be found in Chapter 9.

A theoretical perspective such as a general systems theory can be used to clarify concepts. A system is a set of components that interact with each other. Systems theory takes into account the inputs, throughputs, and outputs of the system and the broader environment (suprasystem) in which all this occurs (e.g., eating and drinking behaviors can be studied by using general systems theory [Norris, 1982]).

Evans (1979) used systems theory to describe the concept of depleted health potential by reviewing the literature that described various health states and conducting personal interviews with clients. She characterized a state of depleted health by overall increased stress and increased requirements for energy expenditure. People were viewed as open, living systems that can take from and give to the environment in which they live. The criteria to describe depleted health potential include impositions on the processes of adaptation and integration. These criteria are listed in the box (top right). Evans concluded that "the concept of depleted health potential directs inquiry into the vulnerabilities and weaknesses that attend one's health status" (p. 73). Minimizing the effects of depleted health potential requires that intervention be directed toward capitalizing on personal strengths and mobilizing the system's internal and external supportive processes.

In a different study, Rawnsley (1980) clarified dimensions of privacy and reviewed its historical and cultural origins. She viewed privacy as a legal right, a social privilege, and a psychological function. She concluded that these dimensions were more than additive and that further exploration of the phenomenon of privacy could be achieved through clarification of related spatial concepts of territory, interpersonal distance, and visual exposure and from the perspective of personal autonomy, emotional release, self-evaluation, and limited and protected communication. Thus the clarification of one concept can require examination of how it is different from, similar to, and related to other concepts.

DESCRIPTIVE CRITERIA FOR DEPLETED HEALTH POTENTIAL

1. The person experiences an overall decreased, or limited, ability to negotiate with the environment to obtain and retain necessary "goods" and/or to keep external and dispose of various "goods" that threaten proficient adaptation.
2. A state in which resources are not available or are significantly decreased may exist.
3. Social contacts may be characterized by increased tension.
4. Disengagement, the mutual withdrawal resulting in decreased interaction between a person and others in the social system, may occur.
5. Decreased physical and/or social mobility may limit opportunities for interaction and negotiation with the environment.
6. Depletion of health may precipitate a confrontation of "self with self."
7. The ability to exercise personal will and control over one's life decreases.
8. Problem-solving ability decreases.
9. Depletion of health interferes with the process of growth and change.

Modified from Evans, S.K. (1979.) *Advances in Nursing Science, 1*(4), 67-74. © Reprinted with permission of Aspen Publishers, Inc.

Forsyth (1980) examined the concept of empathy, using the techniques of concept analysis outlined by Wilson (1963). These techniques include:

1. Description and analysis of model cases or analysis of empirical events that most observers can say represent an instance or occurrence of the abstract concept
2. Description and analysis of alternative cases that represent the occurrence of contrary, related, and borderline concepts
3. Review of existing literature to extract explicit or implicit meanings
4. Extraction of provisional criteria that may be used in naming the occurrence of the phenomenon
5. Examination of such factors as social context, underlying anxieties, and application of varying means in different social situations

To analyze empathy as a concept, Forsyth used the following case study* of a 4-year-old child hospitalized with a tentative diagnosis of blood dyscrasia.

The child was accompanied by both parents. The mother remained with the child. Visiting hours are from 2 PM until 4 PM. At 4 the announcement is made over the public address system that visiting hours are over. The mother rushes to the nurses' desk and, bursting into tears, she implores, "I can't leave. He has never been away from me."

N. "You are concerned about how he will react to your leaving?"

M. "Yes, and I'm afraid to leave. I don't know what will happen if I do."

At this time the nurse comes from behind the desk and, putting her arm around the woman, leads her toward a lounge area.

N. "You are afraid that something will happen?"

M. "I may never see him again. The doctor is afraid he has a terrible sickness. He told us two weeks ago we could not delay in bringing him in. Oh, if anything happens. . . ."

N. "You believe you delayed and that you may be responsible for a serious outcome?"

M. (Sobs uncontrollably.) (Forsyth, 1980, pp. 34-35)

Analysis of the concept of empathy using this case as a model reveals six conditions or provisional criteria that may be essential components of empathy: consciousness, temporality, relationship, validation, accuracy, and intensity. Consciousness was present when the mother approached the nurse's desk and invited her attention. The nurse interrupted her work and became aware of the mother and her distraught condition. Temporality involves the "here and now" response that is necessary before the situation changes. What would have happened if the

Advances in Nursing Science, 2(2), 33-42. © 1980. Reprinted with permission of Aspen Publishers, Inc.

nurse had ignored the mother? The criteria of relationship require mutual exchange. In the example the nurse attended to the mother's words and initiated a response. The nurse became involved in a relationship by removing the physical barrier of the desk and by placing an arm around the mother. The nurse sensed the mother's distress and her plea for attention and provided validation by listening and providing comfort to the mother. The mother in turn accepted the action of the nurse. Accuracy of the interpretation of the mother's feelings is evident; the nurse interpreted that the mother believed her delay in bringing the child to the hospital may have had serious consequences. The mother's response of sobbing confirmed the nurse's understanding.

Forsyth's description and analysis of this case illustrate the first of Wilson's steps in concept clarification. In addition to the abstract analysis of the case, Forsyth used a scale from the literature for measuring empathic understanding to determine the intensity of the interaction between the mother and the nurse.

The second step in concept clarification presented by Wilson is to describe contrary, related, and borderline concepts. Forsyth implemented this step by questioning how empathy differed from sympathy, pity, and compassion. The criteria of objectivity and freedom from value judgment were added during the process of differentiating empathy from the other concepts. Forsyth then tested the consistency of her conceptualization of empathy by comparing her work with the literature from a broad range of fields of inquiry. Provisional criteria for empathy were identified and the related concepts of empathy, sympathy, pity, and compassion were compared on these criteria (Table 2-2). Finally, Forsyth examined the social contexts and anxieties underlying empathy. She concluded that in everyday usage the concept of empathy cannot be differentiated from sympathy.

In summary, concept clarification can be accomplished by various means. Analysis of a concept from a general systems theory perspective was illustrated in Evans' work (1979). Rawnsley (1980) used a different approach, the review of the historical and cultural origins of the concept of privacy. Forsyth (1980) used the techniques for concept clarification suggested by Wilson (1963) to clarify the concept of empathy.

Constructing and testing theoretical relationships

Constructing theoretical relationships involves suggesting propositions that link the concepts. The process of linking concepts through statements about how the concepts fit together gives form and structure to the theory. Many ways of developing propositions exist (Dubin, 1978; Jacox, 1974; Newman, 1979). What is already known about the phenomenon of interest, the purpose of the theory, and the theorist's philosophy of nursing will guide the approach used to develop propositions. If little is known about the phenomenon, a descriptive system of central and related categories of concepts may be used. One way of organizing such a description is through use of a relational taxonomy. If extensive knowledge already exists about the phenomenon, an explanatory or predictive theory is appropriate.

TABLE 2-2. Comparison of observed criteria of related concepts with the essential criteria of empathy

PROVISIONAL CRITERIA	EMPATHY	SYMPATHY	PITY	COMPASSION
Consciousness	X	X	X	X
Temporality	X	X	X	X
Relationship "I-thou" objective	X	X	X	X
Validation	X			
Accuracy	X			
Intensity	X	X	X	X
Objectivity	X			
Subjectivity		X	X	X
Freedom from value judgment	X			

From Forsyth, G. L. (1980). *Advances in Nursing Science*, 2(2), 33-42. Reprinted with permission of Aspen Publishers, Inc.

Propositions may link two concepts or, if complex, link many concepts (Chinn & Jacobs, 1983).

Nursing theory must be useful for the practice of nursing. Because a theory is an abstraction of reality, the theory must be tested to ensure that it represents the real world. The research process validates the theory. This process of theory testing involves defining the concepts so they can be measured, that is, developing operational definitions of the concepts; formulating specific statements about how the concepts are linked, that is, developing propositions; and then validating the statements through systematic methods (Chinn & Jacobs, 1983).

Analyzing and evaluating a theory

Analysis of a theory is intended to clarify statements in the theory and to indicate the relationships and relative hierarchy of concepts. Analysis involves an objective breakdown of statements into component elements. Such a breakdown allows us to recognize the unstated assumptions that may be contained in the theory and to detect any logical fallacies in the theory. Analysis focuses on achieving an objective presentation of what the author of the theory has expressed, rather than evaluating or making judgments about the author's work (Fawcett, 1984).

Fawcett (1984) has proposed questions for the

ANALYZING CONCEPTUAL MODELS IN NURSING

Questions for analysis

What is the historical evolution of the conceptual model?
What approach to development of nursing knowledge does the model exemplify?
How are nursing's four metaparadigm concepts explicated in the model?
   How is person defined and described?
   How is environment defined and described?
   How is health defined? How are wellness and illness differentiated?
   How is nursing defined? What is the goal of nursing? How is the nursing process described?
What statements are made about the relationships among the four metaparadigm concepts?
What areas of concern are identified by the conceptual model?
What is the source of these concerns?

Questions for evaluation

Are the assumptions underlying the conceptual model made explicit?
Does the conceptual model provide complete descriptions of all four concepts of nursing's metaparadigm?
Do the propositions of the conceptual model completely link the four metaparadigm concepts?
Is the internal structure of the conceptual model logically congruent?
   Does the model reflect more than one contrasting world view?
   Does the model reflect characteristics of more than one category of models?
   Do the components of the model reflect logical translation of diverse perspectives?
Is the conceptual model socially congruent?
   Does the conceptual model lead to nursing activities that meet social expectations, or do the expectations created by the conceptual model require societal changes?
Is the conceptual model socially significant?
   Does the conceptual model lead to nursing actions that make important differences in the client's health status?
Is the conceptual model socially useful?
   Is the conceptual model comprehensive enough to provide guidelines for practice, education, administration, and research?
   Does the conceptual model generate empirically testable theories?
Do tests of derived theories yield evidence in support of the model?
What is the overall contribution of the conceptual model to nursing knowledge?

From Fawcett, J. (1984). *Analysis and evaluation of conceptual models of nursing.* Philadelphia: Davis.

analysis of conceptual models in nursing that are relevant to the analysis of theories (see box below).

The theorist's work is placed in the context of earlier work, as well as the general climate of science. Of interest in analysis is the historical evolution of the theory. Questions are asked that will assist in identifying the elements of the theory and their relationships. Because middle-range theory cannot address the entire scope of nursing, analysis is concerned with identifying the nurse-patient situations or problems in the person-environment interaction the theory addresses. The reader interested in the analysis of conceptual models for nursing is referred to Chinn and Jacobs, 1983; Fawcett, 1984; Fitzpatrick and Whall, 1983; and Meleis, 1985.

Evaluating a theory involves making judgments about the theory in relation to set criteria. Chinn and Jacobs (1983) presented a guide for evaluating a theory that is shown in the box below. This guide includes questions one can ask to determine if the theory meets the criteria for clarity, simplicity, generality, empirical precision, and derivable conse-

quences. *Clarity* refers to how well the boundaries of the theory are communicated and to the sense of orderliness and consistency throughout the theory. Semantic and structural clarity and consistency are of concern.

Theoretical simplicity, also referred to as parsimony, refers to the number of concepts and their interrelationships. Untested theories often have complex structures because the truly unnecessary has not yet been recognized, tested, and eliminated. Ideally, a theory has a minimum number of descriptive components.

Generality is achieved when no limit exists to the application of the empirical facts and situations to which the theory applies. Chinn and Jacobs (1983) noted that generality is assessed by considering the scope of concepts and goals within the theory. In the initial stages of theory development, generality is limited. Because nursing is concerned with the broad concepts of individuals, society, health, and environment, nursing theory is expected to have generality.

GUIDE FOR THE EVALUATION OF THEORY

Clarity
Are all major concepts defined?
Are significant concepts not defined?
Are definitions confusing? Competing? Inconsistent?
Are words coined? Are coined words defined?
Are words borrowed from other disciplines and used differently in this context?
Are there unnecessary explanations?
Are examples or diagrams needed and not present?
Are examples and diagrams used meaningful?
Are basic assumptions consistent with one another? With goals?
Is the view of humanity and environment compatible?
Are the same terms defined differently?
Are different terms defined similarly?
Are the same terms defined incompatibly?
Are concepts used in a manner inconsistent with their definition?
Are diagrams and examples consistent with the text?
Are competing and irreconcilable structures suggested for different parts of the theory?
Can the theory be followed? Can an overall structure be diagramed?
Where, if any, are gaps in the flow? Do all concepts fit?
Are there any unclarities due to sequence of presentation?
Are there faulty premises or conclusions?
Does the theorist accomplish what she or he sets out to do?

From Chinn, P.L., & Jacobs, M. (1987). *Theory and nursing: A systematic approach* (2nd ed.). St. Louis: Mosby.

Guide for the Evaluation of Theory—cont'd

Simplicity

How many relationships are contained within the theory?

How are the relationships organized?

How many concepts are contained in the theory?

Are some concepts differentiated into subconcepts and others not?

Can concepts be coalesced without loss of theoretical meaning?

Is the theory complex in some areas, not in others?

Does the theory tend to describe, explain, or predict?

Is there an imbalance of description in relation to explanation or prediction?

Generality

How specific are the goals of this theory? That is, does it apply to all or some nurses, and at which time?

Could only a nurse utilize this theory? If not, who else could use it, and what allows for that usage?

Is the goal justifiably a nursing goal?

If subgoals exist, are they nursing actions?

How broad are the concepts within the theory?

Empirical applicability

Are concepts broad or narrow?

How specific or associative are definitions within the theory?

Are the concepts' empirical indicators identifiable in reality? Are they within the realm of nursing?

Do the definitions provided for the concepts adequately reflect the concepts' meanings?

Is a very narrow definition offered for a broad concept? A broad meaning for a narrow concept?

If words are coined, are they defined?

Consequences

Given the goal of the theory and its orientation, has anything of significance for nursing or health care been omitted?

Is the stated or implied goal one that is important to nursing?

Will use of the theory help or hinder nursing in any way? If so, how?

Will application of this theory resolve any issues in nursing? Will it resolve any problems?

Will research based on the theory answer important questions?

Are the concepts within the domain of nursing?

Empirical precision requires that the concepts contained in the theory be linked with observable reality, particularly if the theory is intended to be used for predicting and controlling some aspect of practice. Empirical precision is linked to the ability to test the theory and the utility of the theory.

Derivable consequences refers to the extent to which the theory results in or produces valued nursing outcomes. Nursing theory, according to Chinn and Jacobs (1983), should generate ideas and serve as a guide for research and practice. Additionally, nursing theory ought to differentiate the focus of nursing from other service professions.

Evaluation of theory requires comprehensive and precise thought. The evaluation criteria are hierarchical in that generality and simplicity are directly dependent upon the extent to which the theory possesses clarity. The purpose of evaluating theory is to determine whether the theory can guide research or practice and to determine what type of research is required to increase the extent to which the theory meets the evaluation criteria.

Relationship of nursing theory to nursing research

Nursing research is intricately related to theory development. Dickoff and James (1968) identified four levels of theory based on the level of existing knowledge about a phenomenon. These levels can be used to direct an investigator toward the appropriate level of research question for a given study and provide guidance for the design, method, and analysis appropriate to answer the research question (Diers, 1979). These levels of theory are (1) factor-isolating, (2) factor-relating, (3) situation-relating, and (4) situation-producing (Table 2-3).

Factor-isolating theory

A factor-isolating, descriptive, or concept-naming theory focuses on identification and classification of concepts. The ability to name and to describe the concepts of interest is prerequisite for all subsequent levels of theory. When little or no knowledge exists about a phenomenon, the purpose of the research will be to answer the question, "What is this?" Before the researcher can propose a theory of helping patients cope with threatening events, it is essential to understand coping, patient teaching, and the outcome variables such as crying or early hospital discharge. Nurses in intensive care units noted that patients consistently developed aberrant behavior,

TABLE 2-3. Relationship between levels of theory and research questions

LEVELS OF THEORY	RESEARCH QUESTION
Factor-isolating	What is this?
Factor-relating	What is happening here?
Situation-relating	What will happen if?
Situation-producing	How can I make "X" happen?

but what this phenomenon represented was unknown. The first step in understanding the phenomenon was to describe or characterize the situation as fully as possible so a clear picture of the events and situations existing in the intensive care unit would be presented. Factor isolation requires the precise examination of the parts and operations of a given phenomenon. Concept clarification is another term sometimes used to refer to factor-isolating theory. Examples of concept clarification from the nursing literature are discussed earlier in this chapter. An exploratory or descriptive design, also called factor-searching design, is appropriate to answer the question, "What is this?" It would use a broad approach to data collection, such as unstructured observations or open-ended questionnaires. Data will be analyzed and reported descriptively so that the concepts are fully identified and described.

Factor-relating theory

Factor-relating theories take the isolated concepts one step further and identify how they are related. The researcher is interested in finding out "What is happening here?" At this level, theory has some explanatory function because it provides information about how the concepts are associated with each other. Description is still the purpose of the study, but on this level the description is about the relationships between or among the concepts. Such a theory is called relationship-searching.

After the aberrant behavior of patients in the intensive care unit was fully described, the next step was to determine what variables seemed to be important in understanding what was going on. Do age, gender, diagnosis, medication, or the presence of visitors make a difference? Relating factors is a process of exploring possible relationships to see if, in fact, a relationship exists.

The design of a factor-relating study would be

more controlled than a factor-isolating study, observations more structured, and questions more precise. Inferential statistics would be used to explain the relationship and differences among and between the concepts.

Situation-relating theory

If a theory is going to have any practical value for nursing, the proposed theoretical relationships must be tested. Situation-relating studies are appropriate when the factors have already been named and good reasons exist to believe that the factors are related. The researcher asks the question, "What will happen if?" Hypotheses that predict the relationship among or between the variables are stated and tested. In the situation of aberrant patient behavior in the intensive care unit, the suspected relationship was between the continuous presence of noise and light and the observed patient behavior. The nurse researcher may ask, "What will happen to aberrant patient behavior if the environment of the intensive care unit is altered to provide a light-dark cycle?"

The nurse researcher attempting to answer the question, "What will happen if?" designs a study that imposes maximum control over the concepts and uses statistical tests to test the hypothesis. Johnson related the provision of information about the sensations that patients would experience during a threatening event with increased ability to cope with the event. This relationship was tested both in the laboratory and in clinical settings.

Situation-producing theory

Situation-producing theories involve the practical validation of a theory. Because action is directed toward a specific end, situation-producing theories are referred to as prescriptive theories. A prescriptive nursing theory includes what the nurse must do to bring about certain desired goals. Situation-producing theories require specification of the goal for a given activity and a prescription for activity to achieve the goal. The question of concern is, "How can I make 'X' happen?" Situation-producing theory is qualitatively different from situation-relating theory in that it is goal-oriented. Rather than asking if a light-dark cycle influences patient behavior, a situation-producing theory would state that providing a light-dark cycle in the intensive care unit will decrease aberrant patient behavior.

Nursing, a practice discipline, focuses on knowledge that impinges directly on practice. Nursing theory, then, must have the goal of improving clinical judgment. We cannot just understand phenomena; we must know how to change a situation to bring about the desired outcome. The extent of nursing knowledge varies considerably. In some cases we know what to do to make something happen. In other situations we do not even know what the phenomenon is with which we are dealing. Theory development can begin with any one of the components: concept analysis, construction of theoretical relationships, testing of theoretical relationships, or practical validation of the theory. Ultimately, all four components are essential for theory in a practice discipline.

SUMMARY

The relationship among nursing practice, research, and theory is ongoing and cyclical. The development of nursing theory arises from questions about the practice of nursing, is tested through research, and is used to inform the practice of nursing. A theory is a set of interrelated concepts that are useful for prediction and control. Concepts are the building blocks of theory and are linked together by propositions. Concepts are abstract characteristics, categories, or labels of objects, persons, or events. Propositions state the relationship among the concepts. Theory ranges in scope from broad to narrow. Broad-range or grand theory takes into account all of nursing. Grand theory is too broad and global to be tested. Middle-range theories are most likely to be of use to nursing because the concepts are sufficiently defined and the propositions specified so that they can be tested. Narrow-range theories may provide a basis for developing middle-range theories but are too restricted to be generalizable to many nursing situations.

The approach used to develop a theory will depend on the theorist's paradigm or way of looking at the world. The positivist-empiricist paradigm assumes that a body of facts or principles exists independently of any historical or social context. The naturalistic-inductive paradigm derives from a tradition that assumes that facts and principles are necessarily historical and contextual. Contemporary nursing research uses the positivist-empiricist and naturalistic-inductive paradigms to clarify phenomena of interest to nursing.

The development of nursing theory requires a systematic process of inquiry, including concept analysis, construction of theoretical relationships, testing of theoretical relationships, and practical validation of theory. The level of knowledge about the phenomenon of interest directs the level of theory development and the type of question asked of our research. Factor-isolating theory asks the question, "What is this?" and is used when little is known about the phenomenon. Factor-relating theory concerns the relationship among the concepts and is developed after the concepts have been named and described. Factor-relating research asks, "What is happening here?" Situation-relating theory is appropriate when good reason exists to believe that the concepts are related in the proposed way. Research questions focus on "What will happen if?" and test the proposed relationships. Situation-producing theory is prescriptive. It answers the question, "How can I make 'X' happen?" and is used to prescribe nursing activity.

In subsequent chapters, we will explore research designs that are used by nurse researchers to develop nursing theory. The positive-empiricist and the naturalistic-inductive approaches to theory development will be integrated.

REFERENCES

Bernstein, J. (1978). *Experiencing science: Profiles in discovery.* New York: Dutton.

Chinn, P.L., & Jacobs, M. (1983). *Theory and nursing: A systematic approach.* St. Louis: Mosby.

Corbin, J.M., & Strauss, A.L. (1984). Collaboration: Couples working together to manage chronic illness. *Image: The Journal of Nursing Scholarship, 16,* 109-115.

Dickoff, J., & James, P. (1968). A theory of theories: A position paper. *Nursing Research, 17,* 197-203.

Diers, D. (1979). *Research in nursing practice.* Philadelphia: Lippincott.

Dubin, R. (1978). *Theory building* (rev. ed.). New York: Free Press.

Ellis, R. (1968). Characteristics of significant theories. *Nursing Research, 17,* 217-222.

Evans, S.K. (1979). Descriptive criteria for the concept of depleted health potential. *Advances in Nursing Science, 1*(4), 67-74.

Fawcett, J. (1983). Hallmarks of success in nursing theory development. In P.L. Chinn (Ed.), *Advances in nursing theory development* (pp. 3-17). Rockville, MD: Aspen.

Fawcett, J. (1984). *Analysis and evaluation of conceptual models of nursing.* Philadelphia: Davis.

Filstead, W.J. (1979). Qualitative methods: A needed perspective in evaluation research. In T.D. Cook & C.S. Reichardt (Eds.), *Qualitative and quantitative methods in evaluation research* (pp. 33-48). Beverly Hills: Sage.

Fitzpatrick, J., & Whall, A. (1983). *Conceptual models of nursing.* Bowier, MD: Brady.

Forsyth, G.L. (1980). Analysis of the concept of empathy: Illustration of one approach. *Advances in Nursing Science, 2*(2), 33-42.

Goodwin, L.D., & Goodwin, W.L. (1984). Qualitative vs. quantitative research or qualitative and quantitative research? *Nursing Research, 33,* 378-380.

Jacox, A. (1974). Theory construction in nursing: An overview. *Nursing Research, 23,* 4-13.

Kuhn, T. (1962). *The structure of scientific revolutions.* Chicago: Phoenix.

Kuhn, T. (1970). *The structure of scientific revolutions* (2nd ed.). Chicago: University of Chicago Press.

Leventhal, H., & Johnson, J.E. (1983). Laboratory and field experimentation: Development of a theory of self-regulation. In P.J. Wooldridge, M.H. Schmitt, J.K. Skipper, & R.C. Leonard (Eds.), *Behavioral science and nursing theory* (pp. 189-262). St. Louis: Mosby.

MacPherson, K.I. (1983). Feminist methods: A new paradigm for nursing research. *Advances in Nursing Science, 5*(2), 17-25.

McKay, R. (1969). Theories, models and systems for nursing. *Nursing Research, 18,* 393-399.

Meleis, A.I. (1985). *Theoretical nursing: Development and progress.* Philadelphia: Lippincott.

Newman, M. (1979). *Theory development in nursing.* New York: Davis.

Nightingale, F. (1860). *Notes on nursing: What it is and what it is not.* Philadelphia: Lippincott, 1946. (Facsimile of first edition. London: Harrison & Sons.)

Norris, C.M. (1982). *Concept clarification in nursing.* Rockville, MD: Aspen.

Pender, N.J. (1985). Effects of progressive muscle relaxation training on anxiety and health locus of control among hypertensive adults. *Research in Nursing and Health, 33,* 378-380.

Polkinghorne, D. (1983). *Methodology for the human sciences: Systems of inquiry.* Albany: SUNY Press.

Rawnsley, M.M. (1980). The concept of privacy. *Advances in Nursing Science, 2*(2), 25-31.

Roberts, H. (1981). *Doing feminist research.* Boston: Routledge & Kegan Paul.

Roy, S.C. (1976). *Introduction to nursing: An adaptation model.* Englewood Cliffs, NJ: Prentice-Hall.

Stern, P.N. (1980). Grounded theory methodology: Its uses and processes. *Image, 12,* 20-23.

Stevens, B. (1979). *Nursing theory: Analysis, application, evaluation.* Boston: Little, Brown & Co.

Tinkle, M.B., & Beaton, J.L. (1983). Toward a new view of science: Implications for nursing research. *Advances in Nursing Science, 5*(2), 27-36.

Wilson, J. (1963). *Thinking with concepts.* New York: Cambridge University.

3

IDENTIFYING PROBLEMS FOR NURSING RESEARCH

MARCI CATANZARO

As a part of the history of scientific inquiry, nursing research is a very young discipline. As a result, to build a scientific basis for nursing practice, many questions need investigation. In fact, so many topics need investigation that nurse researchers are confronted with a situation not unlike children in a candy store wondering where to begin. Selecting a problem for research may be difficult because too much exists from which to choose. Because nursing is a practice discipline, problems for nursing research are related to understanding the human responses to health and illness and the nursing, therapeutic, and environmental factors that contribute to wellness. Identifying a problem for study is the important first step in the research process and provides direction for all subsequent research steps. In this chapter we will discuss sources of research problems and priorities for nursing research. Processes of identifying and refining a problem for study will be presented, and the chapter will conclude with a discussion of criteria for evaluating a research problem statement and the process of writing a research problem statement.

SOURCES OF RESEARCH PROBLEMS

The research problem for study involves an implicit or explicit question that reminds the researcher what answers are sought. The words "question" and "quest" are derived from the Latin word "quaerere," which means "to seek." We continually pose questions in our personal lives and our work. What

should I wear to work? Should I apply for that new job? How can I make this patient more comfortable? These questions prompt us to start our problem-solving process, but they seldom require a high degree of precision and control of research to answer them. Identifying problems for nursing research is a fundamental first step in the research process, and often it is difficult and challenging (Valiga & Mermel, 1985). Taking the time to think creatively about particular interests and discussing research ideas with another researcher help to clarify interests and generate ideas about the researchability of the problem. Problems that require research to answer are derived from many sources, including previous research, cultural stereotypes and popular conceptions, empirical interests, practical needs and interests of others, political concerns, and topical priorities of those who fund research.

Previous research

The organized body of nursing knowledge contains information about previous research. The investigator may have read something that did not make sense or work as predicted. A nurse may have read a variety of studies that report inconsistent findings on a specific topic. These discrepancies between published reports, as well as in everyday experience, provide a source of problems for study. For example, patient education programs have been shown to foster understanding and reduce anxiety in patients undergoing surgery. Patient teaching programs have included such teaching strategies as group instruction, audiotapes or videotapes, printed material, and individual instruction, but the literature offers no consensus concerning the best mode of presenting information (Barborowicz, Nelson, DeBusk, & Haskell, 1980; Christopherson & Pfeiffer, 1980; Devine & Cook, 1983). Such a discrepancy can serve as the basis for further study. Reports of research often suggest questions for further study. As research reports are read, the nurse researcher may think of an alternative explanation for the research findings and wish to test this idea. Previous research may have been done with a small sample or a sample that was homogeneous in terms of certain participant characteristics. The investigator may wonder if the findings will hold up with larger, more heterogenous groups.

Popular conceptions

Other sources of research problems are cultural stereotypes and popular conceptions. For example, health-care providers frequently believe that bathing the patient in bed consumes fewer physiological resources on the part of the patient than those required for either a tub bath or a shower. Consequently, patients who have had a myocardial infarction are routinely given a bed bath based on this assumption. Is this belief about bathing accurate? Winslow, Lane, and Gaffney (1985) used oxygen uptake and cardiovascular responses to investigate the physiological costs of tub bath, basin bath, and shower with a group of healthy volunteers and a group of patients recovering from myocardial infarction. They concluded that the physiological costs of the three types of baths were similar and that differences in responses to bathing seemed more a function of the participant's characteristics. These researchers challenged a popular belief and found evidence that contradicted the belief. Numerous beliefs guide nursing practice, and they need to be examined through research.

Empirical interests

The sudden insight, which may arise from seeing things in a different way, is another source of research problems. Fig. 3-1 illustrates how we can see things differently. Some persons see a rabbit heading east; others see a duck facing west.

Early in this century a mold that interfered with the growth of bacterial colonies in petri dishes was a common nuisance in the laboratory. The British bacteriologist, Sir Alexander Fleming, saw this phenomenon not as a nuisance but as something to be explored further. He won the Nobel prize for medicine for the discovery of penicillin.

Sudden awareness of something that had not been noticed before is another source for nursing research. A nurse who was interviewing people with neurological disease realized that although a woman could describe in biomedical terms the cause of her neurological disease, she attributed a symptom of her disease to her son's inappropriate conduct. How do people with chronic disease explain their symptoms? Does this explanation differ from their explanation for the underlying disease process? Guided by this type of research problem, investigators demonstrated that a significant portion of people studied did not associate their urinary bladder dysfunction with their multiple sclerosis (Catanzaro & Halter, 1985).

Curiosity about everyday clinical practice is a rich source for nursing research. For example, why is a procedure done in a certain way? Nurses working in a critical care area frequently determine cardiac output by use of the thermodilution technique. Why is iced injectate used in some settings and room temperature injectate used in others? Vennix, Nelson, and Pierpont (1984) compared cardiac outputs obtained with iced versus room temperature injectate and found that cardiac output results were equivalent with either method. Other studies have replicated this finding but raised other questions about the comparison between prefilled syringes and a closed injectate delivery system (Barcelona, Patague, Bunoy, Gloriani, Justice, & Robinson, 1985).

A review of nursing care plans and nursing care protocols, team conferences, and discussion with other nurses and members of the health-care team can be a source of research problems. Questions may

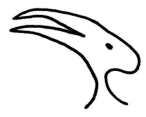

Fig. 3-1. Gestalt figure.

arise about why things are done in a particular way. We may question whether a better way exists to perform a procedure, plan care for a group of clients, or administer a nursing unit.

Practical needs

Nurses have noted that diarrhea commonly develops among patients receiving lactose-based tube feedings. Hansen and her colleagues undertook a series of studies concerning patient responses to tube feedings. One of those studies was to determine whether nurses could alter the development of diarrhea by manipulating the flow rate and temperature of the feedings (Kagawa-Busby, Heitkemper, Hansen, Hanson, & Vandenburg, 1980; Heitkemper, Hanson, & Hansen, 1977; Heitkemper, Martin, Hansen, Hanson, & Vandenburg, 1980.) Another practical concern of nurses is that of drawing blood samples for analysis from indwelling catheters. How much blood must be discarded before accurate laboratory values can be obtained? Underhill and colleagues have explored this question using different types of peripheral and central catheters (Burns, Gregerson, & Underhill, 1985; Carlson, Snyder, Wallace, Underhill, Ashwood, & Detter, 1986; Snyder et al., 1986; Wallace, Carlson, Snyder, Underhill, Ashwood, & Detter, 1986). Answers to these kinds of questions are necessary to deal with real-world problems of nursing care.

Political concerns

The political climate, which places emphasis on constraining health-care costs, has provided many avenues for nursing research. Do the diagnostic related groups (DRGs) relate to the amount of nursing care required by patients? What services can registered nurses versus lower-paid technicians best provide? Issues of women and of minority groups are other areas of political concern that may provide ideas about research questions. What is the effect of providing child care on maintaining women in the work force? Does available child care decrease stress-related illness in women? Does the removal of disincentives to employment, such as loss of medical care benefits, increase employment of disabled persons?

Priorities

Various groups within nursing have identified priorities for nursing research that, if followed, could result in the creation of knowledge that nurses need to care for future generations. These lists of priorities can serve as a source of research problems for the nurse investigator.

The American Nurses' Association Cabinet on Nursing Research (1985) identified priorities for nursing research (see box, p. 38). These priorities take into consideration that the population in the United States is socially and culturally diverse and that the demographic shift is toward an older group of citizens. Also considered is the trend toward high technology and the need for delivery of health care that balances high quality and cost-effectiveness.

Another source of priorities for research emanates from the agencies that provide funding for nursing research. Based on its policy decisions regarding how its monies will be spent, an agency may generate a formal list of priorities for a given time period, a special emphasis for funding by the agency or organization, or a special call for proposals that respond to a particular research need. For example, the Division of Nursing in the Bureau of Health Professions, Health Resources Services Administration, cooperated with the National Institute on Aging, National Institutes of Health, to carry out a special initiative on behavioral therapies for urinary incontinence in the elderly. A nurse who has an interest in a specific topic may get ideas for refining the scope of a research project from the guidelines for funding provided by an agency from which research funds will be sought.

Priorities for nursing research also have been set for some nursing specialty practices. In 1978 Oberst published a list of priorities for cancer nursing research. Gerber and Mellard (1985) suggested research priorities for rehabilitation of the learning-disabled adult, and Thomas (1984) published priorities for prepared childbirth research. Brower and Crist (1985) conducted a *Delphi survey* (questioning experts in the field) to determine the priorities in gerontological nursing for long-term care. A review of the literature will reveal many current priority lists of topics that groups of nurses have decided should be studied.

Lewandowski and Kositsky (1983) reported the results of a nationwide Delphi survey that identified 74 priorities for critical-care nursing research. These priorities are focused on specific questions about the influence of nursing interventions on patients in critical-care settings. Also of interest are ways to effectively and efficiently utilize nurses in critical-care

AMERICAN NURSES' ASSOCIATION PRIORITIES FOR NURSING RESEARCH

Promote health, well-being, and ability to care for oneself among all age, social, and cultural groups.

Minimize or prevent behaviorally and environmentally induced health problems that compromise the quality of life and reduce productivity.

Minimize the negative effects of new health technologies on the adaptive abilities of individuals and families experiencing acute or chronic health problems.

Ensure that the care needs of particularly vulnerable groups, such as the elderly, children with congenital health problems, individuals from diverse cultures, the mentally ill, and the poor, are met in effective and acceptable ways.

Classify nursing practice phenomena.

Ensure that principles of ethics guide nursing research.

Develop instruments to measure nursing outcomes. Develop integrative methodologies for the holistic study of human beings as they relate to their families and life-styles.

Design and evaluate alternative models for delivering health care and for administering health-care systems so that nurses will be able to balance high quality and cost-effectiveness in meeting the nursing needs of identified populations.

Evaluate the effectiveness of alternative approaches to nursing education for the kind of practice that requires broad knowledge and a wide repertoire of skills, and for the kind of practice that requires specialized knowledge and a focused set of skills.

Identify and analyze historical and contemporary factors that influence the shaping of nursing professionals' involvement in national health policy development.

From American Nurses' Association. (1985). Cabinet on Nursing Research: *Directions for nursing research.*

areas. The priorities listed are in the form of specific questions that can be answered by nursing research. The 10 highest-ranked questions follow:

1. What are the most effective ways of promoting optimum sleep-rest patterns in the critically ill patient and preventing sleep deprivation?
2. In light of the nursing shortage, especially in critical-care nursing, what measures can be taken to prevent or lessen burnout among critical-care nurses?
3. What type of orientation program for critical-care nurses is most effective in terms of cost, safety, and long-term retention?
4. What effects do verbal and environmental stimuli have on increased intracranial pressure in the patient with a head injury?
5. What are the most effective, least anxiety-producing techniques for weaning various types of patients from ventilators?
6. What types of patient classification systems are the most valid, reliable, and sensitive in determining staffing ratios in critical-care units?

7. What types of incentives (e.g., wage scales, recognition programs, "clinical ladders") will retain nurses in critical-care areas?
8. What are effective ways of reducing staff stress in critical-care areas?
9. What are effective nursing interventions with patients who have impaired communication (e.g., intubated patients, aphasic patients) to minimize anxiety, helplessness, and pain?
10. What are the effects of patient positioning on cardiovascular and pulmonary function of various types of critically ill patients?

The Nurses' Association of the American College of Obstetricians and Gynecologists (NAACOG) established a list of research priorities in the areas of obstetrical nursing, women's health nursing, and neonatal nursing. Rather than address specific research questions, the priorities identified by NAACOG are stated as broad topic areas. Examples are shown in the box p. 39.

For beginning researchers, priority lists such as those described here can stimulate ideas for their own research problems. Priority lists also can be useful to an investigator in evaluating the significance of

EXAMPLES OF PRIORITIES ESTABLISHED BY NAACOG

Concepts basic to obstetric nursing practice in family-centered care; life-cycle changes/demands, decision-making skills for clients/professionals; ethics of technology use and abuse; educational strategies; and individual and family interactions

Effect of changes in documentation (i.e., use of nursing diagnosis) of delivery of nursing services on outcomes, interdisciplinary prestige, and the public's image of nursing

Women's adaptations to life transitions such as parenthood, retirement, widowhood, alternative life-styles

Nursing practice models for populations vulnerable because of age, economic status, cultural heritage, alternative life-styles, and incarceration

Impact of evolving societal changes (e.g., technology, cost controls, and philosophies of care on neonatal outcomes desired from nursing practice)

Factors related to the profession of nursing (e.g., burnout, job availability, job satisfaction, credentialing, marketing the products of neonatal nurses, cost of staff development, and delineation of the responsibility for cost of achieving and maintaining competent neonatal nurses)

From Raff, B.S., & Paul, N.W. (Eds.). (1985). *NAACOG invitational research conference. Birth defects: Original article series* (Vol. 21, No. 3).

the problem of personal interest or practical need. Remember that priority lists represent only the point of time when they were generated. The lists should not be used to deter an investigator from an area of inquiry. After all, major breakthroughs in knowledge have occurred in the past through investigations that transcended the consensus.

SELECTING A PROBLEM FOR RESEARCH

The myriad sources from which research problems can be generated have potential to suggest far more problems than can be investigated in a lifetime.

How, then, does a researcher select the problem for study that is of greatest interest and importance? One approach to identifying a problem that will maintain the investigator's interest sufficiently to complete the research is to think curiously about everyday experiences. The person standing in line at the grocery store who is annoyed at being prevented from doing "more important things" might wonder if people are annoyed when they need to wait to see a doctor, to have laboratory tests performed, or to receive attention from a nurse. Some people do not mind using an automated teller at the bank but hate to leave a message on a telephone answering machine. Why do people like some forms of automation and not others? How much automation will hospitalized patients accept?

A strategy that can be used when the investigator finds it difficult to identify a problem for research is to think curiously throughout the day and to try to generate questions about everyday experiences that might relate to nursing care, recording each question that comes to mind on a separate index card. At the end of the day, the researcher in search of a problem for study can take a few minutes to think about what precipitated emotional reactions such as anger or joy (Gordon, 1978). The nurse may have been angry that the mother of a young child with leukemia was not administering prednisone as prescribed. Reassuring words to a patient experiencing pain may have brought an expression of gratitude from the patient and given the nurse a sense of joy that caring was communicated. Again, write these incidents on index cards. Try to complete five cards a day. When about 50 index cards containing curiosities and emotional reactions have been accumulated, sort the cards according to topic. The 50 cards probably will fit into about three categories reflecting the researcher's perspective, special interests, and concerns. These categories can be used as a basis for focusing on a problem that is sufficiently interesting and important to be pursued to completion.

EVALUATING A PROBLEM FOR RESEARCH

Researchability

The problem must be researchable; that is, it must be capable of being empirically investigated as described in Chapter 1. A philosophical question or an issue of a moral or ethical nature is not amenable to scientific investigation. For example, it is not possible to empirically test the question, "Is it God's will that people with Parkinson's disease become disabled?" It is not practical to investigate the effects of antigravity on patient adherence to an exercise regimen. The investigator cannot send a group of Parkinson's clients beyond the forces of gravity to study exercise adherence.

The variables of interest must be defined. For example, the concept of quality of life is not defined well enough to allow it to be studied. An investigator interested in quality of life will need to define a problem for study in terms that can be defined, such as the ability to carry out activities of daily living. The ability to measure variables also determines whether a problem can be researched. One can measure how well clients with Parkinson's disease dress, cook, walk, and perform other activities of daily living.

Feasibility

Exploring the feasibility of a study before it is begun is good insurance that one will identify many preventable problems early in the research process, therefore taking steps to eliminate them. We will discuss the critical analysis of problem statements in Chapter 4. Of concern now is evaluating a potential problem for its feasibility. Questions of concern include: Is the problem significant? In other words, will it help fill in the fabric of nursing knowledge or contribute to clinical practice? Will the findings have a broad application in nursing or be linked to theoretical knowledge? Who is interested in the findings of the study? Will it be of interest to other health-care professionals?

A nurse researcher who is interested in studying the effects of an exercise group on the daily activities of persons with Parkinson's disease must first determine the significance of the problem. Those with Parkinson's disease typically develop movement disorders (tremor, rigidity, bradykinesia, postural fixation) that clinical experience and research have indicated are very incapacitating. Attempts to decrease movement disorders have been approached pharmacologically and surgically, and various therapeutic and adverse outcomes have occurred. Regular exercise is recommended for persons with Parkinson's disease. A specific problem for study could be the following: Does a nurse-facilitated exercise group decrease the effects of movement disorders on daily

living in individuals with Parkinson's disease?

Further evidence of the significance of the problem comes from the American Parkinson Disease Association, which estimates that over 1 million Americans have Parkinson's disease (Lieberman, Gopinatham, Neophytides, & Goldstein, n.d.). The disease is progressive and ultimately results in difficulty moving about and accomplishing required activities of daily living. Thus nursing intervention that improved mobility and overall functional ability of persons with Parkinson's disease would be a significant benefit to persons with Parkinson's disease. Other progressive neurological diseases, such as multiple sclerosis, result in disorders of movement; persons with these diseases may likewise benefit from regular exercise. A study that demonstrated the effectiveness of exercise in improving functional ability in persons with movement disorders could stimulate further study into the mechanisms responsible for the improvement in functional ability.

The feasibility of solving a problem through nursing research depends on the availability of resources in terms of study participants, technology, and investigators necessary to implement the study. A problem that lacks these resources is not feasible. The feasibility of a problem for study is influenced by the availability of many resources, including: (1) time and timing, (2) money, (3) cooperation from others, (4) availability of participants, (5) facilities and equipment, (6) the experience of the researcher, and (7) ethical constraints (Cormack, 1984).

Time and timing. The time and timing of the study are important considerations for determining the feasibility of a study. Things always take longer than anticipated, so the investigator will need to consider realistically how long it will take to recruit participants, administer the exercise intervention over a set period of time, and administer the follow-up tests of ability to perform activities of daily living (ADL). How long should the intervention last? Should the ADL evaluation be done immediately after the intervention, at some specified interval after the end of the intervention, or a combination of these? When is the best time to do this study? The local weather during the winter may prevent people with impaired mobility from traveling to a group exercise class. How many potential subjects are likely to be away on vacation during the summer months? In some instances responses to these questions can result in rejecting a study idea as not feasible. In other instances feasibility might be increased by reducing the scope of the research problem.

Money. What will the study cost? In the previous example, there will be expenses for printing and postage to recruit participants and printing the evaluation instruments. The investigator or a research assistant will need to travel to the intervention site and conduct the exercise group. The researcher may need to rent space in which to hold the exercise classes and complete activity of daily living assessments. Will participants be paid for their participation? If laboratory tests will be done, how much will these cost and how can they be paid for?

Cooperation of others. The cooperation of others is another important consideration in determining feasibility of a study. Will others cooperate with this project? Will the American Parkinson Disease Association be willing to assist in recruiting participants? Will the local support group leaders encourage participation? Historically, are people with Parkinson's disease willing to participate in research? Sometimes the investigator may need the cooperation of a hospital laboratory to obtain information such as blood chemistry or other serum values. Studies that are planned for a clinical nursing unit will need the cooperation of the staff nurses and administrators. For instance, the study of wet versus dry environments in the treatment of decubitus ulcers required that staff nurses follow the research protocol.

Availability of participants. The researcher must ask if persons will give their time and energy to participate in this study. If hundreds of persons with Parkinson's disease live in the researcher's geographic area and if the local Parkinson's support groups are willing to assist in recruiting participants for the study, the researcher can conclude that this large pool will provide enough available participants for the study and that those who may be interested will be contacted. Other kinds of research will raise other questions. If an animal experiment is planned, will the particular breed of animal be available for study? If records are to be used, are these records complete and are they accessible to the researcher?

Facilities and equipment. The feasibility of a study also depends on the availability of facilities and equipment. Will special space be necessary, such as an observation room with a one-way mirror? Is there a quiet room on a busy hospital unit in which to conduct interviews? Is special equipment needed, such as an electrocardiogram monitor or a video recorder? In the study of persons with Parkinson's disease, the investigator must determine the need for and availability of such things as exercise mats and technical equipment required to assess functional ability. The study of treatment protocols for decubitus ulcers may require two types of dressing trays and a heat lamp.

Experience of the researcher. The experience of the researcher also will determine the feasibility of a planned research project. Does the investigator know something about the substantive area of study? For example, a knowledge of the physiology of wound healing is required for studying treatment of decubitus ulcers. An understanding of the pathophysiology of Parkinson's disease is essential to recognize whether regular exercise might contribute to improved performance of activities of daily living. Nurses with no experience in a critical-care unit may be at a decided disadvantage when trying to study the reliability of advanced monitoring equipment in a critical-care unit unless they are well trained in equipment calibration. The nurse's expertise in research is another consideration in the feasibility of the study. Can other, more experienced, persons, such as a statistical consultant, help?

Ethical considerations. A final consideration in determining the feasibility of a study is the ethics of the proposed study. Are there any risks to the participants? Is it likely that the proposed exercises for the patients with Parkinson's disease will stress the cardiovascular system? In studying treatments for decubitus ulcers, withholding all treatment from one group of patients would not be ethical. Kurzuk-Howard, Simpson, and Palmieri (1985) solved this ethical dilemma by studying the differences between two types of treatment. Other ethical considerations in deciding the researchability of a problem are discussed in Chapter 6.

WRITING A RESEARCH PROBLEM STATEMENT

When the problem is identified and the researchability and feasibility of studying the problem have been established, a statement must be written that communicates to others the phenomenon to be studied. The problem statement is a focused description of the area under investigation. The problem is not synonymous with the broad topical area or general research topic, nor is it the same as the specific purpose of the particular study. A research problem is a situation or circumstance for which the solution is to be described, explained, or predicted. The *problem statement* presents the situation that needs solution, improvement, or alteration. The problem is associated with the purpose of the study, but it is not identical. The *purpose* of the study is the specific aim or goal of the study—the task to be accomplished—not the problem to be solved. For example, a nurse working in a long-term care setting may be disturbed by the high incidence of decubitus ulcers. Decubitis ulcers is the general topical area of concern. He or she may wonder about the problem: "What is the optimum frequency of turning comatose patients to reduce the incidence of decubitus ulcers?" If this nurse were to design a study, its purpose might be to determine: "What is the difference between a 2-hour and a 4-hour turning schedule in preventing decubitus ulcers in comatose patients?" Another nurse may be interested in the general topic of cardiovascular nursing. A problem area is the hemodynamic changes that occur during position changes in the course of normal nursing care. The specific question or purpose of the research project may be: "What is the effect on PaO_2 of a turn to the lateral position?" (Table 3-1). Note that each of these specific research purposes, if answered through a study, would contribute to understanding something about the phenomenon represented in the research problem. Thus a research problem could be the basis for multiple research purposes.

Writing a research problem statement is not as simple as it may seem. The researcher must know what answers are needed before an adequate problem statement can be constructed. Unsure of where she wanted to go, Alice in Wonderland asked the Cheshire Cat which way she ought to go. The wise cat replied that if she did not care where she wanted to go, it really did not matter which way she went.

A nurse may be in the same situation as Alice when posed with the question, "Who is the patient who was just admitted?" The answer may provide the patient's proper name, a description of the admitting diagnosis, or a thumbnail description of previous medical history and admissions to the unit. The question itself did not provide a clue to the answer the questioning nurse really wanted. Any one of these responses may answer the question adequately for the nurse or may provide a point for further inquiry. In any case, to receive the correct answer, one must first ask the correct question. Not every sensible reply is an answer to a question. The nurse may ask, "What is a good way to prevent decubitus ulcers?" The answer to this question may be, "There isn't any" or "That's a good question." Neither of those responses really answers the nurse's question. A better way to phrase the question may be, "Can positioning prevent decubitus ulcer formation?"

No single correct way exists to approach the writing of a research problem statement. Some useful steps include: (1) identify a general topic area that is of genuine interest to you; (2) write some ideas about the problems or unanswered questions in this area; (3) review the literature to determine the state of the knowledge about the topic and to get ideas about how the question might be answered; (4) talk with colleagues to clarify thinking; (5) evaluate the feasibility of researching the problem; and (6) write the problem statement.

The investigator who is interested in developing a nursing intervention that will decrease or prevent the incidence of decubitus ulcers has started on the road to writing a research problem statement by identifying this general topic area. The next step is to write some ideas about the problem. The nurse working on an orthopedic unit knows from experience that elderly patients develop decubitus ulcers more often

TABLE 3-1. **Relationship between topic, problem, and purpose**

TOPIC	PROBLEM	PURPOSE
Decubitus ulcers	Prolonged pressure and decubitus ulcers	2-hr vs. 4-hr turning schedule on incidence of ulcers
Cardiovascular nursing	Hemodynamic change and position change	Effect on PaO_2 of turning to lateral position

than young adults. It has also been noted that people who are immobile for extended periods of time have a high incidence of skin breakdown. A brief review of the literature may indicate that much of the research is on preventing the development of decubitus ulcers, yet prevention of decubitus ulcers has not been effective. When prevention fails, methods of caring for decubitus ulcers are necessary. Many techniques have been suggested, including the application of insulin, collagenase, sugar, and Elase. Frequently, these recommendations are not supported by controlled studies. While talking with colleagues, the nurse may learn of other nursing interventions used in the management of decubitus ulcers. Uncertainty also exists about whether a wet or dry environment promotes healing. These steps will help the investigator understand the current state of knowledge about the general topical areas of wound healing and care of decubitus ulcers and come to some conclusions about where further study is needed.

Kurzuk-Howard, Simpson, and Palmieri (1985) focused their study on the problem of determining whether a wet or dry environment in the treatment of decubitus ulcers would reduce healing time and nursing care time. The problem statement for their study follows.

Decubitus ulcers continue to be a major problem in hospitalized patients who are confined to bed. The patient's rehabilitation is often delayed, increasing the time away from both job and daily activities, and nursing care hours are increased, thereby contributing significantly to the escalation of overall health care costs.

The rising incidence of decubitus ulcers is largely attributed to our aging population, which is most susceptible to them (Barton, 1977). Providing the most intensive care in decubitus ulcer prevention for the elderly does not mean in all cases that the ulcer will be prevented. New medical and surgical techniques frequently used in the older population can result in decubitus ulcers. It is estimated that 30% of elderly patients experience decubitus ulcers following a total hip replacement or repairs to the upper shaft of the femur (Barton, 1977). When prevention of decubitus ulcers in the elderly fails, one must look to a safe and effective treatment.*

*Kurzuk-Howard, G., Simpson, L., & Palmieri, A., "Decubitus ulcer care: a comparative study," *Western Journal of Nursing Research*, *7*, 1 (Feb. 1985), p. 58. Copyright (C) 1985. Reprinted by permission of Sage Publications, Inc.

The authors identify the clinical problem of decubitus ulcers in hospitalized patients in the first sentence. The writers then explain why this is an economic problem: decubitus ulcers delay rehabilitation, increase time away from usual activities, increase nursing care requirements, and escalate health-care costs. The percentage of elderly patients who have been reported to develop decubitus ulcers after orthopedic surgery is noted. Finally, the need is identified to develop a safe and effective treatment for decubitus ulcers in the elderly. This problem statement presents the unanswered question that started the investigator thinking and identifies the area where answers are needed (Batey, 1971).

A problem may be stated in a declarative form, as the researcher in the previous example did, or in an interrogative form. Stating the problem in the interrogative form is often advantageous because questions invite answers. Stating a problem in interrogative form may assist the investigator to think about the kind of answer required to solve the problem. In the previous example the investigators could have ended the problem statement with the question, "What is a safe and effective treatment of decubitus ulcers in the elderly?" Examples of research problems stated in interrogative and declarative forms are shown in Table 3-2.

The written problem statement includes: (1) the information about the issue or concern that provoked the study or about which further knowledge is

TABLE 3-2 Interrogative and declarative problem statements

INTERROGATIVE	DECLARATIVE
What are the effects of chronic illness during midlife?	The effect of chronic illness during midlife are unknown.
What volume of blood must be withdrawn from arterial catheters to ensure accurate plasma chemistry?	It is unknown what volume of blood must be withdrawn from arterial catheters to ensure accurate plasma chemistry.
What types of staffing patterns will decrease burnout in critical-care nurses?	Research has not demonstrated that the type of staffing patterns prevent burnout in critical-care nurses.

needed, (2) the scope of the problem area, for example, how many people are affected by it or how pervasive it is—the nature and scope of the problem to be studied, (3) why it is important to study the problem, (4) how nursing science or practice would be influenced by the study, and (5) the overall goal of the proposed research or question to be answered. The specific way in which the question will be answered is part of the purpose statement.

SUMMARY

Sources of research problems include previous research, popular conceptions, empirical concerns, practical needs, political concerns, and priorities for nursing research. Selecting a problem for study from a long list of potential problems requires that the researcher focus on personal perspective and recurrent themes of interest and wonderment that arise from curious thinking about the world of nursing.

The process of writing a research problem can be facilitated by identifying a general topical area of interest, writing ideas about the problem or unanswered questions, understanding the current state of knowledge about the topic, and clarifying thinking with colleagues. The written problem statement must clearly and explicitly define the problem and provide some guidelines for the type of answer that is expected. Finally, the problem statement will convey to the reader the importance of the problem for study.

The researcher will consider the significance, researchability, and feasibility of a problem. Feasibility includes the resources to solve the problem, the experience of the investigator, and the ethics of conducting the study. Attending to each of these issues in the initial phases of identifying a problem for study will increase the likelihood of undertaking a study that can be completed.

References

American Nurses' Association Cabinet on Nursing Research. (1985). *Directions for nursing research: Toward the twenty-first century.* Kansas City, MO: Author.

Barborowicz, P., Nelson, M., DeBusk, R. F., & Haskell, W. L. (1980). A comparison of in-hospital education approaches for coronary bypass patients. *Heart and Lung, 9,* 127-133.

Barcelona, M., Patague, L., Bunoy, M., Gloriani, M., Justice, B., & Robinson, L. (1985). Cardiac output determination by the thermodilution method: Comparison of ice-temperature injectate versus room-temperature injectate contained in prefilled syringes or a closed injectate delivery system. *Heart and Lung, 14,* 232-235.

Batey, M. V. (1971). Conceptualizing the research process. *Nursing Research, 20,* 296-301.

Brower, H. T., & Crist, M. A. (1985). Research priorities in gerontologic nursing for long-term care. *Image: The Journal of Nursing Scholarship, 17,* 22-27.

Burns, P. K., Gregerson, R. A., & Underhill, S. L. (1985). Adequate discard volume determinations to obtain accurate coagulation studies from heparinized arterial lines, *Circulation, 72* (Part 2), p. III-24.

Carlson, K. K., Snyder, M. L., Wallace, H. H., Underhill, S. L., Ashwood, E. R., & Detter, J. C. (1986). Obtaining reliable plasma sodium and glucose determinations from pulmonary artery catheters. *Heart and Lung, 15,* 307-308.

Catanzaro, M., & Halter, C. (1985). Perceived cause of symptoms in chronic illness. Influencing the future of nursing research through power and politics. *Communicating Nursing Research, 18,* 87.

Christopherson, B. C., & Pfeiffer, C. (1980). Varying the timing of information to alter preoperative anxiety and postoperative recovery in surgery patients. *Heart and Lung, 9,* 854-861.

Cormack, D. F. S. (Ed.). (1984). *The research process in nursing.* Boston: Blackwell Scientific Publications.

Devine, E. C., & Cook T. D. (1983). A meta-analytic analysis of effects of psychoeducational interventions on length of postsurgical hospital stay. *Nursing Research, 32,* 267-274.

Gerber, P. J., & Mellard, D. (1985). Rehabilitation of learning disabled adults: Recommended research priorities. *Journal of Rehabilitation, 51*(1), 62-64.

Gordon, M. J. (1978). Research workbook: A guide for initial planning of clinical, social, and behavioral research projects. *The Journal of Family Practice, 7,* 145-160.

Heitkemper, M., Hanson, R., & Hansen, B. C. (1977). Effects of rate and volume of tube feeding in normal human subjects. *Communicating Nursing Research, 10,* 71-89.

Heitkemper, M., Martin, D. L., Hansen, B. C., Hanson, R., & Vandenburg, V. (1980). Rate and volume of intermittent enteral feeding. *Journal of Parenteral and Enteral Nutrition, 5,* 125-129.

Kagawa-Busby, K. S., Heitkemper, M. M., Hansen, B. C., Hanson, R. L., & Vandenburg, B. (1980). Effects of diet temperature on tolerance of enteral feedings. *Nursing Research, 29,* 276-280.

Kurzuk-Howard, G., Simpson, L., & Palmieri, A. (1985). Decubitus ulcer care: A comparative study. *Western Journal of Nursing Research, 7*(1), 58-79.

Lewandowski, L. A., & Kositsky, A. M. (1983). Research priorities for critical care nursing: A study by the American Association of Critical Care Nurses. *Heart and Lung, 12,* 35-44.

Lieberman, A. N., Gopinatham, G., Neophytides, A., & Goldstein, M. (n.d.). *Parkinson's disease handbook.* New York: American Parkinson Disease Association.

Oberst, M. (1978). Priorities in cancer nursing. *Cancer, 1,* 281-290.

Raff, B. S., & Paul, N. W. (Eds.). (1985). *NAACOG invitational research conference. Birth defects: Original article series* (Vol. 21, No. 3).

Snyder, M. L., Gregersen, R., Underhill, S., Carlson, K., Wallace, H., Chandler, W., & Detter, J. (1986). Partial thromboplastin and thrombin time blood specimen collection through pulmonary artery catheters. *Heart and Lung, 15,* 315.

Thomas, B. S. (1984). Identifying priorities for prepared childbirth research. *Journal of Obstetrics and Gynecological Nursing, 13,* 400-408.

Valiga, T. M., & Mermel, V. M. (1985). Formulating the researchable question. *Topics in Clinical Nursing, 7*(2), 1-14.

Vennix, C. V., Nelson, D. H., & Pierpont, G. L. (1984). Thermodilution cardiac output in critically ill patients: Comparison of room temperature and iced injectate. *Heart and Lung, 13,* 574-578.

Wallace, H. H., Carlson, K. K., Snyder, M. L., Underhill, S. L., Ashwood, E. R., & Detter. J. C. (1986). Obtaining reliable plasma glucose and potassium values from intra-arterial catheters. *Heart and Lung, 15,* 317.

Winslow, E. H., Lane, L. D., & Gaffney, F. A. (1985). Oxygen uptake and cardiovascular responses in control adults and acute myocardial infarction patients during bathing. *Nursing Research, 34,* 164-169.

4

ANALYZING EXISTING KNOWLEDGE

NANCY FUGATE WOODS

A researcher analyzes existing knowledge before delving into a new area of study, while conducting a study, when interpreting the results of the study, and when making judgments about application of new knowledge in nursing practice. In short, investigators, clinicians, educators, and administrators must read the professional literature and avail themselves of other sources of knowledge. This chapter considers the processes involved in a critical analysis of scientific literature and the methods available for communicating a review. First we will examine the purpose of a literature review, sources of relevant literature, and information retrieval systems available for nursing research. Next, we will discuss approaches to reading and analyzing individual research reports, as well as the body of literature related to a specific topic. We will conclude with a description of approaches to communicating results of the review, including organizational, stylistic, and content options.

CRITICALLY ANALYZING EXISTING LITERATURE

Purposes of review

The typical purposes for analyzing existing literature are to generate research questions, to identify what is known and not known about a topic, to identify conceptual or theoretical traditions within bodies of literature, and to describe methods of inquiry used in earlier work, including their successes and shortcomings. Sometimes investigators discover exciting

unanswered questions by reading a body of literature. For example, while reading in the area of postpartum adaptation, Killien and Lentz (1984) discovered that investigators had devoted little attention to women's sleep patterns before and after they gave birth. This discovery, combined with a knowledge that women experience postpartum fatigue, led them to study the sleep and sleep disruption patterns during the immediate postpartum period in the hospital. Similarly, reading literature in two or more topic areas may help the investigator identify concerns that have been ignored in earlier work but that emerge when one simultaneously considers more than one topic. For example, Lee (1985) explored literature related to women's postpartum adaptation, particularly that related to postpartum depression. She noted important connections between postpartum hormonal changes and both depression and sleep disturbances.

A second purpose for reviewing the literature in a specific area is to identify what is known and not known about the topic. For example, Ritchie, Caty, and Ellerton (1984) found information related to behavioral adjustment of chronically ill school-aged children and adolescents, but they found little information related to the experiences of chronically ill preschool children. Consequently, these investigators designed a study of the concerns of healthy, acutely ill, and chronically ill preschool children in both short- and long-stay hospitalizations.

Another important purpose for conducting a critical analysis of the existing knowledge about a topic is to identify the theoretical traditions or conceptual frameworks used to study the problem. This analysis involves appraisal of the perspectives that have guided past studies rather than the research methods used or the actual research findings. As background for her study of personal control in late stage cancer patients, Lewis (1982) identified two dominant conceptual frameworks that organized the concepts of control. In the literature, she found an existential framework and a reinforcement framework. The existential framework emphasized the individual's concerns as they emerged from his or her experiences with cancer; the reinforcement framework emphasized the relationship between an individual's action and the results of that action. Individuals learn through experience that they can have some effect on their situation, that their experience results from their own behavior, or that the situation is beyond their control.

A fourth purpose for reviewing the literature is to explore the methods other investigators have used to study the topic. Often one benefits from knowing which methods have been effective and which have been ineffective. For example, McGuire's selection of an instrument to measure pain in clinical research (1984) illustrates the value of reviewing earlier work. She contrasted six approaches to pain measurement, illustrating that each differed in the dimension of pain it measured, its reliability and validity, the type of pain it was best suited to measure, its ease of understanding, the time required for explanation and administration, and the time required for scoring (Table 4-1). An investigator contemplating a study of pain would find this information helpful in selecting a method of assessing pain experience.

The purposes of analyzing existing knowledge also vary throughout the course of a research project or program. In the early phases of planning a research project, investigators analyze existing knowledge in the topic area so they can answer such questions as these: Have others already studied the question? If so, did they address it adequately? Is there another perspective on the problem? Should another study be conducted to explore the problem or some special aspect of the problem? Should another study be conducted using alternative methods? Should a previously reported study be replicated?

During the course of conducting a study, investi-

gators frequently turn to the scientific literature to ensure that they consider new findings in the current study. At this stage investigators may look for answers to these questions: Do any new findings indicate the study should focus on an additional variable? Is there justification for a design change? Does new evidence indicate that the study being conducted may have harmful effects to the participants? Should the instrumentation be changed or adjusted during the course of the study?

During the interpretation phase of a study investigators again review relevant literature to ensure that they are using the most recent knowledge to make sense of the results. At this stage investigators may ask these questions: Does new evidence support or fail to support the findings of the study? Does evidence suggest that a variable not considered in the original design may be important? Does a new theory account for the findings or account for the findings better than that on which the present study was based? Does new theoretical or empirical evidence suggest an alternative interpretation?*

In sum, investigators review the literature constantly, often repeatedly, and for different reasons throughout the conduct of a single study. In the following pages we will explore some of the sources of knowledge available to investigators and ways to gain access to them.

Sources of professional literature

Many sources of knowledge are available to investigators, including professional journals, abstracts of research reports, books, and published reports of presentations at professional meetings (often referred to as "proceedings"). These sources are accessible through indexes, bibliographies, and computerized search systems in many libraries. Personal communication with other investigators is another important source of information, particularly about unpublished work or work in progress. This communication can be cited in a formal literature review and

---

*Clinicians and administrators concerned with research findings also need to review literature continuously as a basis for modifying practice. The issues considered in reviewing research for its use in practice differ somewhat from those issues relevant to planning a study. A detailed discussion of critical appraisal of research findings for use in practice appears in Chapter 31.

TABLE 4-1. Comparison of instruments to measure pain

INSTRUMENT	DIMENSION(S) MEASURED	RELIABILITY / VALIDITY	TYPE OF PAIN BEST SUITED FOR	EASE OF UNDERSTANDING	TIME REQUIRED FOR EXPLANATION & ADMINISTRATION	TIME REQUIRED FOR SCORING
Verbal Descriptor Scale	Intensity	Good / Probable	Clinical acute chronic progressive	Very easy	<5 minutes	0
Visual Analogue Scale	Intensity	Good / Probable	Clinical acute chronic progressive	Easy to difficult, depending on sample	<5 minutes	<2 minutes
Chambers-Price Pain Rating Scale	Intensity Anxiety Attention paid to pain Physiological parameters	Probable / Questionable	Clinical acute	Moderately easy	5-15 minutes	<5 minutes
Johnson's Two-Component Scales	Physical intensity Emotional distress	Unclear / Unclear	Experimental and probably clinical	Moderately easy	<5 minutes	<2 minutes
McGill Pain Questionnaire	Location Sensation Affective aspects Evaluation Intensity Pattern	Good / Good	Clinical acute chronic progressive	Moderately easy to very difficult	15-30 minutes	5-10 minutes
Card sort method	Sensation Affective aspects Evaluation Intensity	Probable / Probable	Clinical acute	Moderately easy to difficult	10-20 minutes	5-10 minutes

From McGuire, D. (1984). Reprinted with permission from *Nursing Research, 33*, 152-156. © 1984, American Journal of Nursing Company.

indicates the investigator's interest in pursuing new ideas before their widespread publication. In addition to professional literature, the lay literature can provide valuable perspectives on human responses to health problems. Personal accounts such as *Last Wish* (Rollin, 1985) and *Anatomy of an Illness as Perceived by the Patient* (Cousins, 1979) include vivid descriptions of individual experiences with health problems and the health-care system. Contemporary and historical lay literature can contribute an understanding of a problem as seen by people who are not strongly influenced by the health sciences. Moreover, these sources, which can enhance awareness of contemporary theories about health, health problems, and health care, offer a broad view of the phenomena we study.

Journals

Professional literature related to human responses to health problems crosses the boundaries of several disciplines. Therefore the investigator must search professional literature from several disciplines and review many types of articles. The general nursing research literature is published in journals such as *Nursing Research, Advances in Nursing Science, Research in Nursing and Health, Western Journal of Nursing Research*, and *International Journal of Nursing Research*. These journals publish research reports, papers dealing with research methods, and conceptual or theoretical papers of interest to nurse researchers. Specialty nursing journals such as *Cancer Nursing, Heart and Lung, Public Health Nursing, Journal of Psychiatric Nursing and Mental Health, Journal of Obstetric, Gynecologic and Neonatal Nursing, Journal of Maternal Child Nursing, Journal of Neuroscience Nursing, Journal of Nursing Education, Journal of Nursing Administration*, and *Nursing Administration Quarterly* contain nursing research reports and other types of papers, such as review articles on topics of clinical relevance to the specialty. Theoretical and research literature from related disciplines such as physiology, psychology, sociology, and anthropology provides useful information, including research findings, methods for studying particular phenomena, and discussions of theoretical perspectives from that particular discipline.

Indexes and abstracts

Because so many professional journals are available to nurse investigators, selecting the appropriate journal and locating relevant articles may seem overwhelming. However, many resources are available to help investigators identify pertinent literature, including published indexes and abstracts and computerized information retrieval systems (Table 4-2). Indexes contain literature citations cross-classified by keywords and authors' names. They provide investigators with a quick enumeration of citations classified under the keyword or keywords the investigator wishes to search. For example, "pain" and "measurement" are two keywords that could have been used to identify the articles in which the instruments discussed in Table 4-1 were found. Many indexes, such as *Cumulated Index Medicus* and the *Cumulative Index to Nursing and Allied Health Literature*, publish an extensive listing of keywords that can be used to structure the literature search.

Indexes are usually updated several times each year. A typical literature search involves finding the citations in the most recent volume of the index and working backward to identify earlier citations. The *Cumulative Index to Nursing and Allied Health Liter-*ature, the *International Nursing Index to Periodical Literature, Nursing Studies Index*, and *Cumulated Index Medicus* are commonly used indexes for identifying nursing citations. *The Cumulative Index to Nursing and Allied Health Literature* includes citations from nursing and related health fields; formerly the *Cumulative Index to Nursing Literature*, it covers the period from 1956 to the present. *The Nursing Studies Index*, prepared by Virginia Henderson and colleagues, is the only index of nursing studies published between 1900 and 1959. *The International Nursing Index to Periodical Literature* contains citations for nursing articles from several thousand nursing and non-nursing journals, beginning with those published in 1966. *Cumulated Index Medicus* contains citations from several thousand biomedical journals, as well as from several nursing journals.

Computerized literature searches. Some of the more commonly used computerized searches for nursing studies include Medline/Medlars, HEIRS, PAIS, ERIC, and DATRIX. Medline/Medlars allows a search of several thousand biomedical and nursing journals. *Health Education Information Retrieval System* (HEIRS) searches journals across several disciplines for articles related to health education. *Psychological Abstracts Information Services* (PAIS) provides a computerized search of psychology literature, and *Educational Resources Information Center* (ERIC) searches education literature. *Direct Access to Reference Information* (DATRIX) allows the search of dissertation abstracts.

Many sources of abstracts of nursing research and research from related fields also are available. Abstracts were included in issues of *Nursing Research* from 1960 to 1978 and currently appear in *Advances in Nursing Science*. In addition, abstracts from nursing and related fields can be found in such diverse publications as *Index Medicus, Dissertation Abstracts, Psychological Abstracts, Sociological Abstracts, Abstracts for Social Workers, Child Development Abstracts and Bibliographies, Excerpta Medica, Hospital Abstracts, Hospital Literature Index*, and *Research Grants Index* from the U.S. Government Printing Office. These references are available in most university libraries.

Computerized literature searches can be applied to many of the databases discussed. For example, Medline, developed and maintained by the National Library of Medicine, in Bethesda, Maryland, is the major bibliographical database for biomedical journals in the United States. It contains citations perti-

TABLE 4-2. Selected indexes, abstracts, and bibliographies: nursing sources

TITLE	CONTENTS	FREQUENCY
Cumulative Index to Nursing and Allied Health Literature (CINAHL) 1956-	Indexes approximately 300 English language journals including nursing and allied health; selectively indexes from over 2600 biomedical journals indexed in *Index Medicus;* and also selectively indexes from popular journals. Separate subject and author sections List of journals indexed List of subject headings and cross references (in annual) List of audio-visual materials (in annual) List of book reviews (in annual) List of pamphlets (in annual) Online 1983-	Bimonthly Annual cumulation
International Nursing Index (INI) 1966-	Indexes over 200 English and foreign language nursing journals. Selectively indexes from over 2600 biomedical journals indexed in *Index Medicus* Separate subject and author sections List of publications indexed List of subject headings (MeSH) List of publications of nursing organizations and agencies List of nursing books received by INI List of doctoral dissertations by nurses (in annual) Online as part of the Medline Database 1966-	Quarterly Annual cumulation
Nursing Research Abstracts 1979-	Abstracts of United Kingdom published research or ongoing research by or about nurses and nursing Separate subject and author indexes	Quarterly
Nursing Studies Index 1900-1959	Indexes and annotates English language materials pertaining to nursing Separate subject and author indexes List of journals indexed List of firms, agencies, and institutions for book entries	vol. 1, 1900-1929 vol. 2, 1930-1949 vol. 3, 1950-1956 vol. 4, 1957-1959
Bibliography of Nursing Literature 1859-1970	Indexes English language materials pertaining to nursing, covering its history, biography, the profession, knowledge specialities and practice, and hospitals Author index in vol. 2	vol. 1, 1859-60 vol. 2, 1961-1970
Index Medicus 1894-	Indexes over 2600 U.S. and foreign biomedical journals including 20 nursing journals List of journals indexed MesH (medical subject headings) Bibliography of medical reviews Separate subject and author sections Online database, Medline 1966-	Monthly Annual cumulation

Modified from materials provided by University of Washington Health Sciences Library.

nent to human medicine and health, basic sciences, biomedical research, veterinary medicine, dentistry, nursing, and communication disorders. Medline indexes 3200 journals in all languages from 1966 to the present. Medline contains the same citations as those found in the printed versions of *Index Medicus, Index to the Dental Literature,* and *International Nursing Index.*

To use the computerized literature indexes, the librarian or the investigator searches databases, using appropriate terms to describe the subject of interest. Medline contains citations classified by thousands of keywords, which the investigator can specify to aid in the search for relevant citations. The search produces citations —in some instances an abstract or even a full text record—of the article.

Sometimes obtaining the desired article is possible only through a search—particularly when local library resources are limited. The results of a search can be printed on paper or saved on a computer disk. Researchers can even use special computer programs that allow them to conduct a literature search using their own personal computer.

When evaluating the usefulness of a computer search, one should consider such factors as experience with the database, time, cost, and ability to obtain the article. Online searching requires knowledge of the database and use of the associated computer programs and the ability to think quickly and creatively about the search. Searches cost from a few dollars to a few hundred dollars per hour of computer time. Experience increases the effectiveness and efficiency of the search.

Reference librarians of most health sciences libraries can provide invaluable assistance in using these resources. Indeed, early in the review process the researcher should consult a librarian who is aware of the scope of resources available. The librarian also can help decide when to use a manual search or computerized search, what databases or abstracts are likely to be most useful, which ones overlap, and what search strategies are most likely to be effective.

A reference librarian can be especially helpful in conducting searches when the researcher (1) cannot find much information about the topic, (2) wants a complete listing of all references on the topic, (3) cannot find a specific desired reference, (4) does not know where to start with a search, and (5) needs information not contained in the databases described here.

ANALYZING INDIVIDUAL RESEARCH REPORTS

Once the investigator has identified the appropriate research reports, the next task is a critical review of their content. Often the first attempt to read a research report is confusing because the reader is unfamiliar with the scientific language and the format. The following is a discussion of the format used for most research reports, the information typically included in each section, and some of the terms frequently encountered in research reports.

Components of research reports

Most published research reports are divided into several labeled sections. The typical format used by *Nursing Research* and *Research in Nursing and Health* (and many other journals) is the format described in the Publication Manual of the American Psychological Association (1985) and includes the following:

1. Title
2. Abstract
3. Introduction (usually not labeled)
4. Methods
5. Results
6. Discussion
7. References

Title

The title should clearly indicate the contents of the research report. Often a title conveys much more than the topic of the study and frequently the reader can determine the type of study from the title. Usually a study whose title begins with "Description of . . ." will describe some phenomenon. A study whose title contains the words "Relationship of . . ." often explores the relationships among phenomena. Studies with titles beginning "Effects of . . ." often report on experimental studies or studies testing hypothesized effects of one phenomenon on another. The title usually names the phenomenon of primary interest. Sometimes the reader can identify the population studied from the title, for example, "Cancer Patients' Experiences of. . . ."

Abstract

Most research articles begin with an abstract that

briefly summarizes the report. Abstracts contain a statement of the study's purpose, a brief description of the participants, the ways data were collected and analyzed, and the most important findings. Because the abstract conveys a synopsis of the study, it can be useful for screening articles rapidly to determine which the researcher should read in detail and which are less pertinent to the topic. In the box below, Ritchie, Caty, and Ellerton's abstract (1984) gives the reader an overview of the study's aims, methods, and findings.

Introduction

The body of a research report usually begins with an introduction to the topic, which may or may not be labeled "Introduction," "Problem Statement," or "Review of the Literature." This section conveys four kinds of information: a problem statement, a review of the literature, a conceptual framework, and a purpose.

Problem statement. The problem statement describes what the investigator will study; it tells the focus of and the justification for the study. Usually, the problem statement describes the scope of the problem, such as the groups of people the problem affects, how widespread it is, and how long it has remained unsolved. A problem statement often highlights the theoretical and practical significance of studying the topic and its importance to nursing science and practice. Usually, this portion of the research report does not employ extensive technological terminology. In the box below, Ritchie, Caty, and Ellerton (1984) tell the reader how they identi-

---

CONCERNS OF ACUTELY ILL, CHRONICALLY ILL, AND HEALTHY PRESCHOOL CHILDREN

Abstract

Judith A. Ritchie, Suzanne Caty, and Mary Lou Ellerton

The study was designed to determine if the concerns of 2 to 5 year old children hospitalized for chronic illness differ from the concerns of other children. Interviews were conducted with 32 short-stay chronically ill, 10 long-stay chronically ill, 20 acutely ill, and 20 healthy children. Narrative recordings were analyzed using a categorical system of 10 developmental and hospital-related concerns. Differences between groups in mean proportion of concerns expressed were examined for each interview using analysis of variance techniques. The major concerns expressed by each group on all interviews were Autonomy and Exploration and, in the chronically ill children, Intrusion. Increased age was associated with increased expression of Intrusion in all groups except the long-stay chronic illness group.

PROBLEM STATEMENT

Chronically ill young children who are frequently hospitalized must cope with the developmental stress normal to their age in addition to the stress of illness and the environmental stress of hospitalization. While caring for young children with chronic renal disease, observations confirmed reports of nurses that these children develop negative behaviors, such as apathy or belligerence, negativism, and tantrums. These behaviors may be manifestations of struggles and frustrations in striving to meet normal developmental drives while in an abnormal environment. It seemed that the children were attempting to grapple with more than the usual concerns of hospitalized preschool children so frequently cited in the literature. As the first stage in a project to develop methods of assessing hospitalized children's coping behavior, this study was undertaken to determine whether 2- to 5-year-old, chronically ill, hospitalized children differ in their concerns from healthy or acutely ill children.

Surveys in Great Britain and the United States indicated that 5% to 10% of children have a chronic physical illness (Pless & Pinkerton, 1975; Rutter, Tizard, & Whitman, 1970).

fied the problem, its dimensions, and its importance to nursing.

Literature review. The literature review contains a summary of earlier work on the same or related topics. This section contains a critical analysis of earlier work that identifies what is known and not known about a topic. Although usually not exhaustive, it includes the most important work in the area.

Conceptual framework. The introduction will explain the *conceptual framework* used in the study. The conceptual framework is like a pair of glasses that helps the reader see the problem in a special perspective. This section often explains the meaning of the concepts used in the study, thus conveying the investigator's particular perspective. For example, the concept "health" may be viewed from several perspectives. One investigator may emphasize a clinical perspective of health, defining it as the absence of disease or levels of biological indicators that are within normal limits. Another may emphasize a functional perspective of health, defined as the ability to perform certain roles. Still another might emphasize an adaptive perspective of health, defined as the ability of the person to cope with the stressors in the environment.

In addition, the conceptual framework often contains *propositions*, statements about how the concepts may be related. This section of a report is theoretical in nature. Sometimes an author will trace the historical development of the concept or perspective; in other cases an author may compare and contrast different schools of thought about the concept. This section of the report is not a summary of previously developed ideas of other investigators, rather it contains an expression of the investigator's particular orientation to the study. Sometimes this section is merged with the conceptual framework, and sometimes it stands alone.

The conceptual framework and literature review can be combined in a single section in which the investigator's conceptual orientation to the problem is grounded in the literature. The decision to present the conceptual framework and the literature review as a single section depends on personal orientation to the problem, the complexity of the literature being reviewed, and the investigator's reasoning style. Personal orientation to the problem may involve applying a new frame of reference to the study of an older problem. In this case, one may prefer to present a

summary of earlier literature first and an exposition of the conceptual framework after the literature review. In some instances the literature about a topic is very complex and may contain several conceptual frameworks. To simplify matters for the reader, the investigator may separate the literature review according to the dominant frameworks that characterize it. The personal preference or reasoning style may be to separate the presentation of the literature review and the conceptual framework.

Ritchie, Caty, and Ellerton (1984) combine the review of the literature and the conceptual framework. The categories of concerns that one might expect to hear from children are drawn from earlier research and clinical papers (see the box below).

Statement of purpose. The final section contained in the introduction to a research report is a *statement of the purpose*. The purpose statement describes exactly what the investigator intended to accomplish in the current study. Authors usually try to show the logical connection between the earlier

LITERATURE REVIEW AND CONCEPTUAL FRAMEWORK

Geist (1979) reported that during the onset of their chronic illness, 50 children of unspecified age exhibited specific and similar responses including: (a) mourning the loss of healthy body parts, of present or future abilities, and of self or body image; (b) rage resulting in aggression and guilt or depression; (c) developmental precocity, or acting out of unmanageable anger; and (d) concern about loss of masculine and feminine self images.

Several authors theorized that hospitalized chronically ill children show the same pattern of concern as acutely ill children (Freud, 1952: Korsch, 1978). The predominant concerns of young, hospitalized, acutely ill children have been reported repeatedly as: separation from parents, loss of familiar environment and experience, intrusion, body integrity, and punishment (Brown, 1979; Douglas, 1975; Erickson, 1972; Prugh, 1967).

work in an area, the conceptual framework for the study, and the purpose of the study they are reporting. The purpose statement often follows a summary of earlier thinking and research findings about the topic. Notice the links between the state of knowledge revealed in the literature review and the purpose statements in Ritchie, Caty, and Ellerton's example in the Purpose box below.

Method

The next major division of a research report is usually labeled "Method." This section is often subdivided into sections such as "Design," "Sample" (or participants), "Instruments," and "Procedure."

Design. The section labeled "Design" tells the reader the organizational plan for the study. In this section the author describes whether the study was organized as a description of things as they naturally occur or whether it was planned as an experiment in which some new procedure was tested. In their study, Ritchie, Caty, and Ellerton (1984) tell us that they observed the children during play interviews at varying frequencies (see Design box below).

Sample. The section labeled "Sample" refers to the cases (e.g., persons, groups, organizations) that are the focus of the study. In it the author describes the cases identified for inclusion in the study, the

---

PURPOSE

Although there is an increasing number of reports on the behavioral adjustment of the chronically ill school-aged child and adolescent, there is scant information on the concerns or coping behaviors of hospitalized, chronically ill preschool children in comparison to those who are healthy or who are hospitalized for acute illnesses. There is equally scant documentation regarding the relation of the chronically ill child's concerns, coping pattern, and eventual adjustment. Therefore, this study was designed to answer the following questions:

1. What are the dominant concerns expressed by preschool healthy children, acutely ill children, or chronically ill children in short-stay hospitalizations (less than 21 days) and by chronically ill children in long-stay hospitalizations (more than 21 days)?
2. Do the concerns expressed vary with age, previous hospital experience, previous experience with needles or surgery, or with parental visiting pattern?
3. Does the pattern of expression of concerns vary over time?

From Ritchie, J., Caty, S., & Ellerton, M. (1984). *Research in Nursing and Health, 7,* 267-268. Copyright © 1984. Reprinted by permission of John Wiley & Sons, Inc.

DESIGN

The play interviews were repeated every 5 to 7 days up to a maximum of six interviews for the long-stay chronically ill and the healthy children. Two hundred and one play interviews were done. With the short-stay acutely ill children, an average of 1 to 2 interviews were conducted. With the short-stay chronically ill children, 2 play interviews were the average. Long-stay chronically ill children had 4 to 6 interviews. Variation in the number of interviews with hospitalized children was the result of a child being discharged or too ill to play; only one hospitalized child refused to play on any occasion. Variation in the number of interviews with healthy children occasionally was the result of the child's absence from the center but frequently of the child's refusal to play.

From Ritchie, J., Caty, S., & Ellerton, M. (1984). *Research in Nursing and Health, 7,* 266-267. Copyright © 1984. Reprinted by permission of John Wiley & Sons, Inc.

SAMPLE

The subjects, 20 healthy children and 62 hospitalized children, ranged in age from 2 years to 5 years 11 months. Males and females were fairly evenly divided across all groups except in the acutely ill group where there were 14 boys and 6 girls. The healthy children were randomly chosen from one class list, having been judged by the head teacher to have normal cognitive development and no history of severe emotional disturbance.

The hospitalized children were chosen by convenience sampling if, according to the charge nurse, they had: (a) normal cognitive development, (b) no history of severe emotional disturbance, (c) an anticipated hospital stay of 8 to 10 days, (d) a physical condition permitting an initial play interview within 5 days of admission, (e) a physical condition expected to permit a second play interview within 5 to 7 days of the first interview, and (f) no requirement for sterilization of toys before and after the interview. The children were hospitalized for various medical and surgical conditions, and composed three groups: short-stay, acutely ill, hospitalized for less than 21 days ($n = 20$); short-stay, chronically ill, hospitalized for less than 21 days ($n = 32$); and long-stay, chronically ill, hospitalized for at least 21 days ($n = 10$).

MEASURES

Data were collected using the play interview method described by Erickson (1958). This technique involved providing the child with a suitcase containing clinical equipment, hospital figures, familiar toys, and family figures, and inviting the child to play.

The child's verbal and nonverbal activities were recorded in detailed running narrative by the researchers who knew whether the child was acutely ill, chronically ill, or healthy. To assure interobserver reliability, the researchers were trained in observing and recording behaviors using videotaped play interviews. Following the training period, the interobserver agreement was assessed on a new videotape. Interobserver agreement across the three researchers was 86% as calculated by the formula:

$$\frac{\textbf{Number agreed upon behaviors}}{\textbf{Total number of behaviors}} \times \textbf{100}$$

The narrative recordings of the children's play were divided into units of behavior for content analysis. Units of behavior were actions of the child in the form of vocalizations, verbal, and nonverbal behaviors. The units of behavior were categorized according to the type of concern expressed in the play. All behaviors were considered meaningful and reflective of a concern.

A concern was defined as a matter in which a child invests interest or energy in the course of development or in particular situations. The categories of concern were developed from published reports of concerns of this age group in relation to hospitalization and normal development. To ensure exhaustive groupings the categories and their definitions were derived from a preliminary analysis of the narrative recordings. Every observed behavior was coded within the category system and yielded frequency counts of behaviors in each category. The categories of concern were labeled Autonomy, Body Integrity, Caretaking, Exploration, Interpersonal Communication, Intrusion, Mobility, Punishment, Separation, and Violence.

To ensure uniformity in coding and categorizing units of behavior, the researchers underwent extensive training in the content analysis procedure before the actual coding of data. The three-way interjudge percentage of achieved agreement was: units of behavior 82% and categories of concern 78.2%.

reasons for excluding some cases from the study, and the way in which he or she selected participants for the study. This section also describes the study's actual participants. Ritchie and her associates (1984) described their sample and explained how the participants were entered into the study. (See Sample box p. 55).

As we will discuss in Chapter 7, the sample does not necessarily consist of persons only. Often a researcher may obtain a sampling of observations, such as observations of sleep or temperature.

Measures. The section labeled "Measures" contains a description of the measurement devices used to obtain the information from the participants. These devices may be interview guides, questionnaires, observation guides, or biomedical instruments such as electrocardiographs. The author usually discusses how the instruments were selected or constructed and describes their characteristics, such as their likelihood of producing valid and reliable data. Ritchie and her associates described the measures they used in their study of preschool children (see Measures box p. 55).

Procedure. The section labeled "Procedure" tells how the study was actually done. The information in this section usually conveys the sequence of events followed in the study and is designed to be sufficiently specific to allow another investigator to follow the same procedure (see box below left).

As part of a published report, the researcher outlines the means used to protect the welfare of human participants or animal subjects. Typically, authors include information on the assurance of confidentiality or anonymity of participants and the methods used for obtaining their consent to participate. Investigators studying animals outline procedures used to ensure the comfort and humane treatment of research animals. See Chapters 6 and 16 for further discussion of these issues.

Results

The "Results" section of a research report describes what the investigator found. This section usually

---

PROCEDURE

Interviews with the hospitalized children were conducted in the child's room with the curtain drawn or in a small private room on the same hospital floor. Interviews with the healthy children were conducted in a small room near the child's classroom. The research plan was approved by appropriate committees within the research settings, and informed consent obtained from the parents of the children.

The initial interview with the child began with the researcher picking up and naming each object in the suitcase. The child was then told that he/she could play with the toys while the researcher would do some writing. If the child had questions, they were answered with minimal direction. For example, to "What's this?" the researcher responded. "It can be whatever you want it to be." Requests to participate in the play were declined. When the child persisted and indicated a need to perform certain actions on a live person, rather than a doll, the researcher became a passive participant and took directions from the child. The researcher neither interfered with nor directed the child's play unless the play became dangerous. At times, parents of hospitalized children were present during the play interview. The play interviews lasted up to 45 minutes and the child was free to refuse to play or to stop playing at any time.

From Ritchie, J., Caty, S., & Ellerton, M. (1984). *Research in Nursing and Health 7,* 269. Copyright © 1984. Reprinted by permission of John Wiley & Sons, Inc.

RESULTS

Behaviors classified as Autonomy or Exploration consistently occur in high proportions in all four groups and, when all interviews are combined, rank first or second in the short-stay acute illness group, the short-stay chronic illness group, and the healthy group. The children in the long-stay chronic illness group expressed more concerns relating to Intrusion which ranks second for each interview. The average ranking of expressed concerns as determined by mean percentage for all interviews within each group is shown in Table 4-3.

From Ritchie, J., Caty, S., & Ellerton, M. (1984). *Research in Nursing and Health 7,* 269-270. Copyright © 1984. Reprinted by permission of John Wiley & Sons, Inc.

TABLE 4-3. **Average ranking of concerns expressed by ill and healthy children**

RANK	SHORT-STAY ACUTE ILLNESS (%) $n = 20$		SHORT-STAY CHRONIC ILLNESS (%) $n = 32$		LONG-STAY CHRONIC ILLNESS (%) $n = 10$		HEALTHY (%) $n = 20$	
1	Exploration	(38)	Exploration	(42)	Exploration	(31)	Autonomy	(37)
2	Autonomy	(29)	Autonomy	(18)	Intrusion	(23)	Exploration	(36)
3	Caretaking	(8)	Intrusion	(13)	Autonomy	(22)	Body integrity	(7)
4	Intrusion	(7)	Caretaking	(8)	Body integrity	(7)	Caretaking	(6)
5	Violence	(7)	Violence	(7)	Caretaking	(6)	Intrusion	(5.2)
6	Separation	(5)	Body integrity	(5)	Violence	(5)	Violence	(4.5)
7	Body integrity	(4)	Interpersonal	(2.2)	Mobility	(3.2)	Interpersonal	(1.4)
8	Mobility	(1.2)	Mobility	(2.0)	Interpersonal	(1.5)	Mobility	(1.3)
9	Interpersonal	(0.6)	Separation	(1.5)	Separation	(1.5)	Separation	(1)
10	Punishment	(0.2)	Punishment	(0.09)	Punishment	(0.3)	Punishment	(0.6)

From Ritchie, J., Caty, S., & Ellerton, M. (1984). *Research in Nursing and Health, 7,* 270. Copyright © 1984. Reprinted by permission of John Wiley & Sons, Inc.

DISCUSSION

The marked decrease in expressions of Autonomy in both groups of chronically ill children confirms clinical observations and merits attention. It was expected that an increased proportion of behavior related to any one concern would be reflected in a proportionate decrease in expression distributed across other concerns. However, this pattern did not occur and Autonomy consistently occurred in smaller frequencies in the chronically ill children. Depletion of energy by the illness does not account for this pattern because only two children were too ill to play, and the play activity of the long-stay group of chronically ill children in particular was vigorous and intense. It may have been that the children's illnesses had interfered with their normal developmental achievements in relation to Autonomy. However, because some illnesses were of relatively recent onset, it is more likely that the combination of chronic illness and hospitalization contributed to the decreased expression of Autonomy. Several factors may lead to a relative absence of opportunities for autonomous or independent activity in these children, for example, the illness itself and the tendency by staff and parents to limit the children's participation in self-care and decision-making. It seems such lack of opportunity may inhibit or discourage the expression of Autonomy. Such inhibition is alarming because of the importance of Autonomy in developing a sense of self, self-esteem, and ability to learn and manage the social and technical world in which these children, if they survive, will have to live. The findings suggest that, although expression of Autonomy is decreased in the group, it remains a concern, and that we must strive to develop programs of care that will foster the development and expression of autonomy in chronically ill children.

From Ritchie, J., Caty, S., & Ellerton, M. (1984). *Research in Nursing and Health, 7,* 272-273. Copyright © 1984. Reprinted by permission of John Wiley & Sons, Inc.

contains a logical presentation of the findings in words and often in tables or graphic illustrations. Frequently, the author discusses what the study revealed, as well as what it did not reveal. In this section the author states the study's factual outcome. The boxed excerpt (see Results box p. 56) from Ritchie, Caty, and Ellerton (1984) describes the types of concerns most frequently expressed by each of the four groups of children studied.

Discussion

In the final section, "Discussion," the author discusses the results in light of previous work, the study's conceptual framework, and the methods of research used in the study. Findings relative to the sample, measures, and procedures are discussed in relation to their adequacy and appropriateness and to the purpose of the study. In the discussion of the study, the author identifies the study's limitations and links these limitations to a proposal for the next study or series of studies. Many authors discuss the limitations of the study in relation to the findings of the study, for example, how the results might have been affected by the nature of the sample, measures, and procedures. The author may recommend that the research findings be implemented in nursing practice or indicate that the topic needs more research before nurses can use the findings in practice. Ritchie and associates (1984) discussed the infrequent expression of autonomy in both groups of chronically ill children and the implications of these findings for the children's development (see Discussion box p. 57).

References

A section labeled "References" follows the body of the research report. This section contains a listing of journal articles, books, and other resources that provided the background material for the study. The reference citations are useful in guiding reading in the topic area. The citations excerpted from the Ritchie, Caty, and Ellerton paper (1984) illustrate the special format for references recommended by the American Psychological Association (see the box on upper right).

Reading research reports critically

Of the many modes for reading research reports, each is appropriate for a different purpose. The first mode is reading the words to literally understand what the author has said. Usually this mode is useful when getting acquainted with a new area of litera-

References

Erickson, F. E. (1958). Play interviews for four-year-old hospitalized children. *Monographs of the Society for Research in Child Development, 23*(3), 77.

Erickson, F. E. (1972). Stress in the pediatric ward. *Maternal-Child Nursing Journal, 1,* 113-116.

Erikson, E. H. (1963). *Childhood and society* (2nd ed.). New York: Norton.

Freud, A. (1952). The role of bodily illness in the mental life of children. *Psychoanalytic Study of the Child, 7,* 69-82.

Geist, R. A. (1979). Onset of chronic illness in children and adolescents: Psychotherapeutic and consultative intervention. *American Journal of Orthopsychiatry, 49,* 4-23.

Hymovich, D. (1979). Assessment of the chronically ill child and family. In D. Hymovich & M. U. Barnard (Eds.), *Family health care* (Vol. 1). New York: McGraw-Hill.

From Ritchie, J., Caty, S., & Ellerton, M. (1984). Research in Nursing and Health, *7,* 274.

ture. Reading in a critical fashion to analyze what the author meant is a second mode. Critical analysis of the report is important when considering the adequacy of the study and requires reading between the lines. Critical analysis of a research report requires that the reader apply a set of standards or criteria to judge the adequacy of the report, such as the following questions. These criteria are based on guidelines published by Downs (1979), Fleming (1974), Leininger (1968), Norbeck (1979), and Ward and Fetler (1979).

Problem statement

1. What is the problem that was studied? Is it explicitly identified?
2. Is the problem stated precisely and clearly?
3. Is the problem delimited in scope?
4. Is the problem justified in light of theoretical and empirical work relevant to the topic?
5. Is the theoretical and practical significance of the problem discussed?
6. Of what importance is the problem to nursing science and practice?

Conceptual framework
1. What are the major concepts guiding the study and how are they defined?
2. Are the concepts linked to one another? How?
3. What theoretical perspective has been used to better understand the problem? Is a theoretical or conceptual perspective clearly identified?
4. Does the conceptual framework accurately reflect the state of nursing science?

Purpose
1. What is the purpose of the study? What concepts or variables are specified in the purpose?
2. Is the purpose logically linked to the conceptual framework?
3. Is the purpose linked to earlier empirical work?
4. Does the purpose precisely indicate how the study will contribute to new knowledge? For example, will the study contribute description of a phenomenon, explanation of a relationship between two or more concepts, or predict an outcome?

Design
1. What is the study design?
2. Is the design consistent with the stated purpose of the study?
3. Is the design appropriate given the state of knowledge about the topic or the current understanding of research design?
4. Is the design too complex or inadequate for the purpose?
5. Are threats to the validity of the study identified? Are they corrected where possible?

Sample
1. What is the sample? Is it described clearly?
2. How was the sample selected? Was the method of selection appropriate given the purpose of the study?
3. Is the sample representative of the groups to which the study findings should be applied? If not, how does it differ? What are the consequences of the difference?
4. Was the sample size large enough to support the use of the statistical tests employed in the study?

Instruments
1. What instruments were used to measure the concepts? Were they adequate reflections of the concepts being studied?
2. Are the validity and reliability of the instruments adequate for their application?
3. Were the instruments appropriate for the population being studied?
4. If the instruments were developed for the study, what were the procedures used to assess their adequacy?

Procedure
1. What procedure was used for data production? Is it clearly described? Were the procedures appropriate?
2. Could another investigator repeat the same study, given the description of the procedures?

Analysis
1. What procedures were used to analyze the data?
2. Are the analyses described appropriate for the purposes of the study?
3. Are the analyses appropriate for the type of data?
4. Are negative and positive findings presented where appropriate?
5. Are factors that might have influenced the results taken into account in the analyses?

Discussion
1. How are the findings related to previously cited research?
2. How are the findings related to the conceptual framework?
3. Are the generalizations appropriate?
4. Are the conclusions valid? Are they justified by the results presented?
5. What are the limitations of the study?
6. What recommendations for further study are appropriate?
7. What recommendations for implementing the research are appropriate? Is more work needed before the findings can be appropriately applied in nursing practice?

In addition to the critical review of each section of the research report, the reader evaluates the report as a whole. In holistic analysis, the reader evaluates research reports to determine if logical consistency exists between the components of the study. This type of analysis involves sophisticated processes and becomes much easier to do as one becomes knowledgeable in a special area of literature.

Table 4-4 is a modification of the approach initially suggested by Hinshaw (1979) for assessing the logical consistency of a report's theoretical, design, and analysis components. When little is known about a problem, the research is usually concerned with identifying and describing relevant concepts. The theoretical structure of such a report most appropriately would be concerned with that concept or concepts. The research purpose usually is posed as a question or statement rather than a hypothesis. In addition, the design would be descriptive in nature; often qualitative methods, including interviews and observation, would be appropriate. The data analysis methods for concept identification studies (as described in Chapter 9) usually include the development of taxonomies or classification systems related to the concept or frequencies and percentages reflecting how often instances of the concept(s) were observed or what the average value for the phenomenon was.

If the concept being studied was defined and its properties were described through prior research, then an exploratory study is appropriate. This type of study is described in Chapter 10 as a study designed to explore associations and differences. Usually the theoretical structure for an exploratory study links two or more concepts as they relate to or differ from one another under given circumstances, but the structure does not state a cause-effect relationship. The relationship of one concept to another concept is explored but unknown. Usually a research question or statement guides this type of study. The design is exploratory, and often investigators can use instruments that have been assessed for their reliability and validity. Usually researchers use statistics that describe average values, their variability, and their associations.

When an area of knowledge is well developed, a theoretical framework can guide the study. In this

TABLE 4-4. Guidelines for assessing consistency among three structures for different types of investigation

STRUCTURES	TYPE OF INVESTIGATION		
	DESCRIPTIVE	EXPLORATORY	HYPOTHESIS-TESTING
Theoretical structure	Concepts undefined or vague	Concepts defined, relationships between concepts not defined, or direction of relationship not defined	Concepts defined specifically, relationships between concepts defined specifically
Theoretical task	Define, describe concept	Explore relationship between concepts	Test hypothesized relationship
Research problem or purpose	Research question or statement	Research question or statement	Hypothesis
Design structure	Descriptive (Chapter 9)	Exploratory (Chapter 10)	Hypothesis-testing (Chapters 11 and 12)
Data collection	Unstructured techniques, open-ended questions	Structured instruments tested for reliability and validity	Precise measurement of variables
Analysis structure	Content analysis, descriptive statistics	Descriptive statistics	Inferential statistics to test hypotheses

Modified from Hinshaw, A. (1979). Planning for logical consistency among three research structures, *Western Journal of Nursing Research, 1* (Summer 1979), 250-253. Copyright © 1979. Reprinted by permission of Sage Publications, Inc.

instance the relationships between concepts can be suggested, including their direction (positive or negative) and magnitude. The statement of purpose generally is expressed in the form of one or more hypotheses that link the concepts. Hypothesis-testing designs—including experimental, as well as non-experimental, designs—are employed to test theory in this type of study. The investigator usually uses instruments developed in previous work. The analysis focuses on testing the hypotheses by using inferential statistics.

The final mode for reading research reports requires projection of the consequences of the research. Evaluation of the research report for its application to practice or for its application in one's own research requires projection of the consequences of these applications. The considerations for application of research findings are discussed in Chapter 31.

Techniques for recording review of individual reports.

Once investigators have reviewed an individual research report, most record the complete citation, some information about the study's problem, conceptualization, methods, impressions about the work, and its relationship to the topic of interest. A good practice is to record this information about the study even when it initially seems only remotely related to one's topic. Retrieving the information from the library is more difficult than retrieving it from personal records. Many investigators use note cards to record their citations and notes. In addition, several microcomputer programs allow the investigator to create a computer file for cross-referencing (see Appendix). A notation for the Ritchie, Caty, and Ellerton (1984) study is given in the box on the right.

Analyzing a body of literature

In addition to analyzing single studies, for many reasons the investigator must frequently analyze a large body of literature related to a specific topic. First, an investigator may search for patterns of findings, such as a consistent influence of one concept on another. Over the years several studies have documented the importance of social support in reducing the negative effects of exposure to stress. An investigator reviewing these studies could readily discern the pattern of protective effects of social support. Second, the investigator may be able to identify common

conceptual or theoretical perspectives in studying a specific topic. For example, several theoretical perspectives have been offered to explain the experience of depression, among them the theory that depression results from learned helplessness and the theory that depression is the product of biochemical processes. An investigator may search for inconsistencies among several studies that point to a key factor to consider in future work. When the investigator uncovers inconsistencies among findings of different studies, an analysis may explain why these occurred. They may be due to variability in the concepts used to frame the study or in some aspect of the method, such as a difference in the sample, design, instruments, or procedure used in earlier studies.

Sometimes using a chart to compare the methods and results of studies helps to discern consistencies or inconsistencies across the studies. Consider the prev-

NOTE CARD

Citation. Ritchie, J., Caty, S., and Ellerton, M. (1984). Concerns of acutely ill, chronically ill, and healthy preschool children. *Research in Nursing and Health, 7,* 265-274.

Problem. Concerns of preschool children not known, especially chronically ill, hospitalized children.

Framework/literature. Concerns: manner in which child invests energy/interest; includes autonomy, body integrity, caretaking, exploration, interpersonal, communication, intrusion, mobility, punishment, separation, and violence. Adjustment/coping linked to concerns.

Purpose. Identify concerns.

Sample. Healthy ($n = 20$), hospital—short-stay chronically ill ($n = 32$), long-stay chronically ill ($n = 10$), acutely ill ($n = 20$).

Measures. Play interview (Erickson); recorded in running narrative; content analysis coded.

Procedure. Child-directed; interview, researcher passive.

Results. Major concerns, autonomy and exploration. Intrusion, major for chronically ill. Autonomy lowest for children with chronic illness.

Comment. Low autonomy with chronically ill children suggests need for follow-up. Does it occur after hospitalization? What programs would foster autonomy?

TABLE 4-5. **Percentage estimates of the prevalence of perimenstrual distress by different investigators**

	TIMONEN AND PROCOPE (1971)				BERGSJØ, JENSSEN, AND VELLAR (1975)	SHELDRAKE AND CORMACK (1976)		TAYLOR (1979)	
Sample	748 female university students, including 136 physical education (PE) students from Helsinki				234 Norwegian industrial electrical/technical textile workers	3323 women university students, Edinburgh University		65 Australian women, mainly hospital staff, median age 19 years	
Method	Questionnaire including 60 yes/no items sent to two groups of students				Questionnaire asking about specific menstrual symptoms shortly before or during menstruation	Questionnaire, 9 symptoms listed		Daily symptom rating scale from items used in previous studies and Moos MDQ (retrospective)	
Symptom	PE students		Others						
	P	M	P	M		P	M	P	M
Mood swings	—	—	—	—	—	—	—	45	29
Depression	30.2	—	43.2	—	21[†]	31	15.4	40	21
Irritability	57.5	—	70	—	—	32.5	21.6	40	22
Weight gain	32	—	30	—	16[†]	—	—	40	21
Tension	—	—	—	—	—	11.8	10.4	33	—
Swelling	57	—	49	—	—	—	—	28	—
Fatigue	30	—	43	—	—	—	—	22	29
Cramps	—	92	66[§]	75	61[††]	20.8*	25.4*	—	47
Backache	33	—	45	54	—	12.1	26.2	—	22
Headache	11.4	—	26.8	21.6	15[†]	24.0	12.4	—	21
Nausea	6	—	11	18	—	4.6	12.3	—	—
Painful or swollen breasts	43	—	47	—	—	—	—	—	—

From Woods, N., Most, A., & Dery, G. (1982). *Research in Nursing and Health, 5,* 123-136.
P, premenstruum, M, menstruum.
*Reported as "stomach ache."
[†]Cycle phase not differentiated.
[‡]Reported as "dysmenorrhea."
[§]Reported as "pelvic pain."

alence of perimenstrual symptoms indicated in the four studies in Table 4-5. Two of the studies involved university students, and the other two involved working women. Three used questionnaires, and one used a daily symptom rating scale. Notice the different percentage of women reporting irritability and cramps. One wonders whether these inconsistencies are due to differences in certain biological characteristics of the samples, differences in methods, or cultural variation across the samples.

Another method for summarizing the results of several studies addressing the same topic is *meta-analysis*. Meta-analysis is a formalized method for statistical analysis of a large collection of results from individual studies. Its purpose is to integrate the findings of several studies. Of the two meta-analysis approaches, the first involves using the original raw data, which are combined from several studies, that meet certain criteria for comparison (Light and Smith, 1971). The second approach relies on use of the outcomes of several studies rather than the raw

data; this approach is quicker and less expensive. A statistic is calculated to summarize the magnitude of effect of one variable on another (Glass, 1976). These techniques are not part of a typical literature review, but they are useful when the object of the research is to address a large body of research findings rather than to conduct a single study. Examples of research that employ meta-analysis are appearing more commonly in the nursing literature. (See box below).

The researcher who is interested in exploring more about meta-analysis can consult Brown (1984), Cooper (1984), Hunter (1982), and Strub and Hartmann (1983). Many studies of nursing therapeutics have been done with small numbers of patients. Meta-analysis provides a statistical method of integrating the findings of these studies in a way that allows for greater generalization.

COMMUNICATING A REVIEW OF THE LITERATURE

The review of literature does not merely summarize findings; it also identifies empirical and theoretical patterns and inconsistencies, interprets earlier literature, and relates earlier literature to one's own work. Communicating a review of the literature involves consideration of the review's content, organization of the content, and style. The content of the review includes the investigator's recounting and interpretation of the literature that forms the foundation for the current study. Including both theoretical and empirical literature in the review is appropriate. The scope of the review may vary considerably with the type of problem and the space limitations for the review. Nevertheless, the investigator needs to discuss the most important studies and theoretical papers that form the background for the study. Studies that are particularly relevant to the current work can be discussed in detail, with specific information about the conceptual, methodological, and analytical approaches included in that discussion. Usually, the information is paraphrased from the original sources, but in some instances verbatim quotations are included. Most important is inclusion of the investigator's interpretation of the earlier work and its relationship to the current study.

Initially, organizing the review into an outline is

META-ANALYSIS

Devine and Cook (1983) reviewed 102 published and unpublished studies on the effects of psychoeducational interventions on length of postsurgical hospital stay. Each of the studies reviewed had an experimental group who received some form of preoperative teaching and a control group who received no structured teaching. The meta-analytical review, in which the investigators calculated an effect size for the reported outcome of each study, demonstrated that patients who received some form of preoperative teaching were discharged ½ day sooner than those patients who did not receive teaching. The method of delivering the instruction (e. g., verbal, written, slides), did not influence the outcome of shorter hospital stay. This study demonstrated that preoperative teaching has a positive effect on patient length of stay across many types of patients, in different hospitals, and under different conditions.

helpful. Creating an outline of major concept areas or major relationships that have special relevance to the current study allows the investigator to insert material on each study or theoretical paper at an appropriate point in the review. In some instances historical organization, proceeding from earliest to most contemporary work, is quite effective in illustrating the progression of scientific thought. In other instances organization according to specific conceptual or theoretical positions is more appropriate.

The style for presenting the results of a literature review and analysis will vary according to the style requirements for courses, journals, theses and dissertations, and grant proposals. However, each of these styles requires documentation of the citations that support the statement the investigator makes. For example, references pertinent to the statement follow the statement, as illustrated throughout this text. Inclusion of tables, figures, and lists can be very helpful to the reader, particularly when the investigator reviews several studies in a similar area. Usually reviews do not include many illustrations, but in certain situations pictorial representation of a complex set of relationships is extremely helpful. Finally, a summary of the review that points out areas of consistency and inconsistency and leads the reader to understand the importance of the study being proposed or reported is recommended.

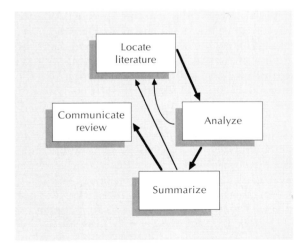

Fig. 4-1. Cycle of literature review.

SUMMARY

Investigators review literature for several purposes: to generate research questions, to identify what is known about a problem, to identify theoretical traditions for studying a problem, and to describe methods used in earlier work. Both professional and lay literature contribute to an understanding of the problems nurses study.

Exploration of scientific literature proceeds in a cyclical fashion (Fig. 4-1). Investigators begin by locating relevant literature, often searching literature through indexes such as the *Cumulative Index to Nursing and Allied Health Literature* and the *Cumulated Index Medicus.* They proceed by analyzing and summarizing the individual research reports, considering their components and the report as a whole. Next, investigators analyze and summarize a body of literature. Finally, they complete the cycle by communicating the results of their own work.

REFERENCES

American Psychological Association. (1974). *Publication Manual of the American Psychological Association* (2nd ed.). Washington, D.C.: Author.

Athens, L. (1984). Scientific criteria for evaluating qualitative studies. *Studies in Symbolic Interaction, 5,* 259-268.

Brown, J., Tanner, C., & Padrick, K. (1984). Nursing's search for scientific knowledge. *Nursing Research, 33,* 26-32.

Cooper, H. (1984). *The integrative research review: A systematic approach.* Beverly Hills, CA: Sage.

Cousins, N. (1979). *Anatomy of an illness as perceived by the patient.* New York: Norton.

Devine, E., & Cook, T. (1983). A meta-analytic analysis of effects of psychoeducational interventions on length of postsurgical hospital stay. *Nursing Research, 32,* 267-274.

Downs, F. (1979). Elements of a Research Critique. In F. Downs & J. Fleming (Eds.), *Issues in nursing research.* New York: Appleton-Century-Crofts.

Fleming, J., & Hayter, J. (1979). Reading research reports critically. *Nursing Outlook, 22,* 172-175.

Fox, F. (1982). *Fundamentals of research in nursing* (4th ed.). New York: Appleton-Century-Crofts.

Glass, G. (1976). Primary, secondary, and meta-analysis of research. *Educational Researcher, 5*(11), 3-8.

Hinshaw, A. (1979). Planning for logical consistency among three research structures. *Western Journal of Nursing Research, 1,* 250-253.

Hunter, J., Schmidt, F., & Jackson, G. (1982). Meta-analysis: Cumulating research findings across studies. Beverly Hills, CA: Sage.

Killien, M., & Lentz, M. (1985). Sleep patterns and environmental interference with sleep among postpartum mothers. Unpublished manuscript.

Knafl, K., & Howard, J. (1984). Interpreting and reporting qualitative research. *Research in Nursing and Health, 7*, 17-24.

Lee, K. (1984). Adaptation to the maternal role: A predictive theory of maternal health. Unpublished manuscript.

Leininger, M. (1968). The research critique: Nature, function, and art. *Nursing Research, 17*, 444-449.

Lewis, F. (1982). Experienced personal control and quality of life in late-stage cancer patients. *Nursing Research, 31*, 113-119.

Light, R. (1979). Capitalizing on variation: How conflicting research findings can be helpful for policy. *Educational Researcher, 8*(9), 7-14.

Light, R., & Smith, P. (1971). Accumulating evidence: Procedures for resolving contradictions among different research studies. *Harvard Educational Review, 41*,(4), 429-471.

McGuire, D. (1984). The measurement of clinical pain. *Nursing Research, 33*, 152-156.

Norbeck, J. (1979). The research critique: A theoretical approach to skill development and consolidation. *Western Journal of Research in Nursing, 1*, 296-306.

Polit, D., & Hungler, B. (1983). *Nursing research: Principles and methods* (2nd. ed.). Philadelphia: Lippincott.

Ritchie, J., Caty, S., & Ellerton, M. (1984). Concerns of acutely ill, chronically ill, and healthy preschool children. *Research in Nursing and Health, 7*, 265-274.

Rollin, B. (1985). *Last wish*. New York: Linden Press.

Selltiz, C., Wrightsman, L., & Cook, S. (1976). *Research methods in social relations*. New York: Holt, Rinehart, & Winston.

Strauch, K., & Brundage, D. (1980). *Guide to library resources for nursing*. New York: Appleton-Century-Crofts.

Strub, M., & Hartmann, D. (1983). Meta-analysis: Techniques, applications, and functions. *Journal of Consulting and Clinical Psychology, 51*(1), 14-27.

Turabian, K. (1973). *A manual for writers of term papers, theses, and dissertations* (4th ed.). Chicago: University of Chicago Press.

Ward, M., & Fetler, M. (1979). Evaluating research reports. *Nursing Research, 28*, 120-125.

Wilson, H. (1985). *Research in nursing*. New York: Addison Wesley.

Woods, N., Most, A., & Dery, G. (1982). Toward a construct of premenstrual distress. *Research in Nursing and Health, 5*, 123-136.

5

SPECIFYING A CONCEPTUAL FRAMEWORK

MARCI CATANZARO

Conceptualizing a study begins with the first idea about a research topic. That idea becomes crystallized as the researcher writes a problem statement about the topic of interest and searches the literature to learn what is already known about the topic. The framework for a study is a product of the investigator's creative integration of the existing body of knowledge about the topic. The framework sets the stage for the specific purpose of the study and provides direction for the study design. This part of a study is called the *conceptual framework*. Conceptual framework has different meanings, depending on the context in which it is used. In some cases a conceptual framework refers to the beginning of a grand theory for nursing practice. The works of nurse theorists such as Rogers, Orem, and Roy are variously referred to as nursing theories, conceptual models for nursing practice, or conceptual frameworks. In research, conceptual framework refers to the part of the study that integrates otherwise scattered and unrelated information in a way that clarifies our assumptions, suggests variables and relationships to be considered in the study design, and clarifies the meaning of the research goal. A conceptual framework provides a network of concepts and relationships within which questions are asked and data are integrated (Newman, 1979). In this chapter we will discuss the components, functions, and formulation of a conceptual framework; the role of conceptual models for nursing practice as sources of frameworks for nursing research; and finally, the last step of conceptualizing a study, specifying the purpose.

COMPONENTS OF A CONCEPTUAL FRAMEWORK

Concepts are the building blocks of a conceptual framework. A *concept* is an abstract way of describing the real world; it is acquired by generalizing from particulars. For example, we might define a book as organized pages contained within covers for the purpose of communicating information. To further define a book in terms of its content, size, color of cover, and so forth alters the concept in terms of observable characteristics. A *construct* is formed when the meaning of the concept is modified by limiting the concept to certain observable, measurable characteristics (Newman, 1979). For example, a book is a concept; a 350-page nursing research textbook is a construct. A construct may be tested, whereas a concept may refer to a category or to a class of objects not amenable to testing, such as a ball, cardiac output, or social support. We cannot, for example, observe cardiac output directly, but we can compute the integral of temperature change versus time curve after the injection of an indicator solution through a special pulmonary artery catheter and calculate cardiac output by using a standard formula. The bonding of mother and infant is a generalization that cannot be measured; however, we can measure the construct of the mother-infant interaction patterns.

Concepts are linked together to form a framework by statements of interrelationships or propositions. An interrelationship is a general statement that specifies what the relationship is, whereas a proposition specifies values and states the predicted values of the units (Dubin, 1978). For example, an interrelationship may state, "Social support is positively related to maternal well-being." A proposition based on that relationship might be, "As the level of social support increases, there will be an increase in maternal well-being."

In summary, a conceptual framework is made up of concepts (generalizations) that are linked by statements of interrelationships or propositions. This matrix of concepts defines the focus of inquiry and provides an organized image of the phenomenon to be studied. A construct includes the meaning of the concept but is limited to the measurable characteristics.

FUNCTIONS OF A CONCEPTUAL FRAMEWORK

A conceptual framework serves three important functions in nursing research. (1) It clarifies the concepts on which the study is built. (2) It identifies and states the assumptions underlying the study. (3) It specifies relationships among the concepts.

Clarifying concepts

We use concepts every day to organize the world around us. Our own implicit conceptual frameworks about how the world is ordered guide our interpretation of and interaction with the world. Because each researcher has a biased view of the world, the conceptual framework of the study should be explicit. Specifying a conceptual framework for study helps the investigator explicate the concepts, assumptions, and linkages that will guide the investigation. Additionally, specifying the conceptual framework allows the investigator to communicate the focus of the inquiry to others who may have different assumptions and hypotheses about the phenomenon.

Through the use of concept analysis, the formation and expression of a conceptual framework helps to clarify concepts and to make otherwise elusive and abstract ideas more concrete. Mager (1972) recounted a fable from the land of Fuzz that is reproduced in the box at right. This story has important implications for nurse researchers. Concepts are abstractions (i.e., fuzzy). Broad statements of intent can be achieved only to the degree that their meaning is understood. The researcher who cannot describe

FABLE FROM THE LAND OF FUZZ

Once upon a time in the land of Fuzz, King Aling called in his cousin Ding and commanded, "Go ye out into all of Fuzzland and find me the goodest of men, whom I shall reward for his goodness."

"But how will I know one when I see one?" asked the Fuzzy.

"Why, he will be *sincere,*" scoffed the king, and whacked off a leg for his impertinence.

So, the Fuzzy limped out to find a good man. But soon he returned, confused and empty-handed.

"But how will I know one when I see one?" he pleaded.

"Why, he will be *dedicated,*" grumbled the king, and whacked off another leg for his impertinence.

So the Fuzzy hobbled away once more to look for the goodest of men. But again he returned, confused and empty-handed.

"But how will I know one when I see one?" he pleaded.

"Why, he will have *internalized his growing awareness,*" fumed the king, and whacked off another leg for his impertinence.

So the Fuzzy, now on his last leg, hopped out to continue his search. In time, he returned with the wisest, most sincere and dedicated Fuzzy in all of Fuzzland, and stood him before the king.

"Why, this man won't do at all," roared the King. "He is much too thin to suit me." Whereupon, he whacked off the last leg of the Fuzzy, who fell to the floor with a squishy thump.

The moral of this fable is that . . . *if you can't tell one when you see one, you may wind up without a leg to stand on.*

From Mager, R. F. (1972). *Goal analysis.* Belmont, CA: Fearon Publishers. © 1984 by David S. Lake Publishers.

the concept to be studied will not "know it when (he or she) sees it." If the phenomenon to be studied is described in fuzzy terms, the researcher, like Ding, may end up without a leg to stand on. That is what conceptual frameworks are all about. They help investigators and consumers of research to understand the meaning of the research goal, whether the goal deals with attitudes, appreciations, understandings, or physiological measurements. The process of concept development, as it relates to theory development, is discussed in Chapter 2. Many of the strategies presented there are useful to the investigator who wishes to clarify concepts for research.

Specifying assumptions

Another function of a conceptual framework is to specify the assumptions underlying the study. An assumption is a statement or principle that is accepted as true on the basis of logic or reason. Some assumptions we hold are within our awareness, while others are not. Assumptions that are so much a part of our belief system that they operate on a subconscious level make specifying a conceptual framework difficult. For example, each of us has a set of assumptions about women. One person may believe that women are passive, that they allow themselves to be pursued in relationships with men, and that they are passive participants in sexual encounters. Another may believe that women's lives are dominated by a willingness to suffer and sacrifice for the benefit of others. Still another may believe that women are equal to men in all respects. Our assumptions about women may be so much a part of our socialization that we do not consciously think about them in our daily life. Yet these assumptions must be made explicit in the framework for a study about women. In a study of rape victims, for example, any assumptions about women must be made clear, or confusion will arise about the context of the study and the interpretation of the findings.

Some black persons in the United States may be disadvantaged in terms of education, income, and social status in ways that make their performance on some standardized tests invalid. The researcher who plans to use a standardized intelligence test with black children must make explicit, through the framework for the study, the conceptual reasoning that allows standardized intelligence tests to be used. Research can be clearly understood only when the researcher specifies assumptions and hypotheses about the concepts to be studied.

Williams (1980, p. 48) identified some assumptions about human behavior that underlie nursing research (see box). Assumptions such as these may come from previous research, from society, or from accepted nursing practice. We may not agree with each of these statements; however, they must be specified so that the consumer of the nursing research can understand what the researcher has assumed to be true for the purposes of the study.

Specifying relationships

A third function of a conceptual framework is to specify relationships among the concepts. For example, building a house must begin with the foundation, not the roof; the basement, windows, and interior walls cannot be done all at once. A blueprint is needed that shows the builder how to put everything together in a way that achieves the desired outcome.

ASSUMPTIONS ABOUT HUMAN BEHAVIOR

1. People want to assume control of their own health problems.
2. Stress should be avoided.
3. People are aware of the experiences that most affect their life choices.
4. Health is a priority for most people.
5. People in underserved areas feel underserved.
6. Most measurable attitudes are held strongly enough to direct behavior.
7. Health professionals view health care in a different manner than do lay persons.
8. Human biological and chemical factors show less variation than do cultural and social factors.
9. The nursing process is the best way of conceptualizing nursing practice.
10. Statistically significant differences relate to the variable or variables under consideration.
11. People operate on the basis of cognitive information.
12. Increased knowledge about an event lowers anxiety about the event.
13. Receipt of health care at home is preferable to receipt of care in an institution.

After the concepts for study are identified and defined, the investigator draws on creative appraisal to construct a blueprint for how the concepts fit together. The plan for the study is built within the context of existing knowledge obtained through a review of the literature. The investigator uses facts that have been classified, organized, and analyzed, and rounds out the blueprint with first-hand knowledge (Batey, 1977).

FORMULATING A CONCEPTUAL FRAMEWORK

Formulating a conceptual framework is also like building a house. The architect considers the building materials to be used, how parts of the house will be assembled, and a vision of the finished house. The researcher will identify the concepts to be studied, the relationship among the concepts, and the desired outcome or purpose of the study. Formulating a conceptual framework is an interactive process that involves specifying the building blocks (concepts) and drawing a blueprint (suggesting ways that the concepts are related).

Identifying concepts

The first step in formulating a conceptual framework is to identify the concepts (the building blocks). Remember that a concept is a generalization about a category or class of objects. We may define concepts differently, depending on our feelings, values, attitudes, and perceptions. The word "cup" may bring to mind a tea cup, a measuring cup, a hip socket, a cup hook, or a brassiere size. "Cup" may also remind us of the last great cup of tea we enjoyed or conjure images of tea with a good friend or high tea in London. Social status may be conceptualized to include income, occupation, neighborhood of residence, gender, or marital status. Exactly which of these meanings is relevant to the research? The researcher must go beyond identification of the concept and further clarify it.

Concepts emerge from the problem to be studied and serve as a springboard for deriving specific variables for investigation (Fawcett, 1984). For example, in a study of network structure, social support, and psychological outcome of pregnancy, the outcome (dependent variable) is the psychological responses to parenthood (Cronenwett, 1985). The

conceptual framework for this study discusses the relationships between health and social support, as well as the relationships among network structure, social support, and parenting (Fig. 5-1). Cronenwett considered all the things that might influence the outcome of psychological response to parenthood. She then selected constructs that would be measured in her study and postulated which were related. The double arrows indicate that the constructs influenced each other.

In an experimental study the *independent variable* is the intervention, treatment, or condition that the investigator manipulates; it has an effect on the *dependent* or *outcome variable*. In a study by Pender on the effects of progressive muscle relaxation training on various physiological and psychological variables in persons with hypertension, the independent variable was the intervention of progressive muscle relaxation (PMR). Pender was interested in how biofeedback might be used to decrease anxiety. Since anxiety is a concept that cannot directly be measured, physiological and psychological variables that served as an indicator of anxiety were used (Fig. 5-2). These indicators could be measured as outcome variables.

Nonexperimental studies may also have independent variables. When Cronenwett (1985) studied pregnancy outcomes, she did not provide a treatment for her study participants. Instead, she used a naturally occurring event, parenthood, to study the relationships among properties of the individual, properties of the social network, perceived social support, and psychological responses to parenthood.

The first factor that influences the investigator's choice of concepts to be included in the framework for a study is the research problem. Additional factors influence how the investigator might look at that research problem. These might include (1) professional socialization, (2) experience as a practitioner, (3) relevant literature, (4) personal or professional philosophy, (5) assumptions about humanity, and (6) personal insights. For example, a nurse who is concerned about obtaining accurate laboratory values from indwelling vascular catheters has many options. The initial interest may have stemmed from a concern for patients who have repeated venipunctures, because it is unknown if accurate coagulation studies can be obtained from indwelling catheters. Clinical experience has indicated that coagulation

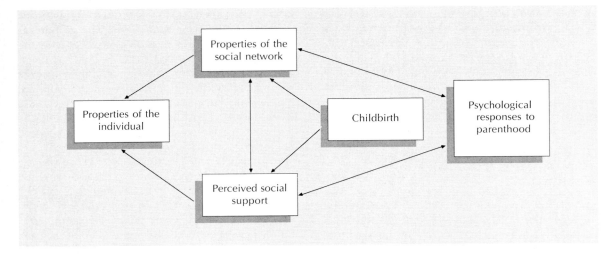

Fig. 5-1. Relationships among network structures, social support, and psychological responses to parenthood (From Cronenwett, L. R. [1985]. Reprinted with permission from *Nursing Research, 34,* 93-99. ©, 1985, American Journal of Nursing Company.)

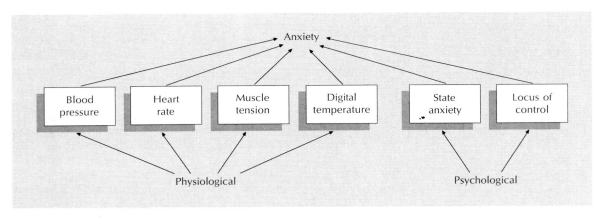

Fig. 5-2. Relationships among physiological and psychological indicators of anxiety.

tests on serum are performed several times daily and are often repeated, because practitioners lack confidence in the reported laboratory values. The nurse researcher suspects that many catheter variables may affect the accuracy of coagulation studies drawn from intravascular catheters: the material, the coating, the number of lumens, and the location of ports. Additionally, infusates, both through the indwelling catheter and in the circulatory system proximal and distal to the indwelling catheter, may alter laboratory values. Indwelling vascular catheters can be located in a vein or artery and can be in the peripheral or the central circulation. A review of the literature will point out those variables that have already been studied and point to where further research is needed. The process of thinking about all these things will lead the investigator to specify the concepts and variables specific to this study.

The review of the literature is an essential part of bringing meaning to the concepts (Batey, 1977). Previous studies will give the investigator ideas about how others have specified and studied the phenomenon of interest. What is already known about the concepts? Under what conditions have the concepts been studied? Lewis (1982) noted that a reinforcement paradigm and an existential understanding of the concept of control were two dominant frameworks that had been used to organize the concept of control. After reviewing the previous work in the area of control, she chose to use the reinforcement paradigm for her study on experienced personal control in cancer patients.

Beyond the research literature, many other resources in the library contribute to the development of a conceptual framework. Newspapers, magazines, popular nonfiction, diaries, letters, and ethnographies can provide many ideas about important concepts that previously may not have been considered. Beyond learning how others have conceptualized the problem for study, the researcher can use certain strategies for identifying concepts of importance to the proposed study. Wicker (1985) suggested four strategies that are useful for expanding conceptual frameworks: (1) playing with metaphors, (2) attending to process, (3) considering the context, and (4) probing assumptions.

Wicker (1985) cited as an example of playing with metaphor McGuire's application of the theory of inoculation, in which the body's defenses are increased by inoculation with a weakened form of virus. McGuire translated this principle to the possibility of strengthening a person's resistance to persuasion by first presenting weak arguments. Another example is creating a metaphor based on applying characteristics of magnetic fields to the exploration of interpersonal relationships.

An additional strategy for identifying concepts is to focus on process. For example, the noun "social support" has a static connotation. What would happen to our ideas about social support if we thought of it as an active verb? How does one go about supporting another? Would social support be measured in the same way if it were perceived as a verb rather than a noun?

Considering the context includes placing the problem in a larger domain, making comparisons outside the problem domain, and considering the implications of the research. Is the proposed study a part of a larger picture? Does a study of noise in the intensive care unit have implications for other environmental factors in the unit or for noise in other settings? What is known about the effect of industrial noise on worker performance? What is the source of the noise? Is all noise equally noxious? What factors might compound the effects of noise (poor lighting, increased stress)? Does noise affect men and women equally? How will nursing care be influenced by the findings of this study? Will the implications extend beyond the study setting?

Probing assumptions is another way of stimulating thinking. We noted earlier that some assumptions are implicit; they are imbedded in our language or tied into our sensory and nervous system (Wicker, 1985). One way to uncover hidden assumptions is to consider alternative or competing perspectives. An investigator studying adaptation to chronic illness may assume that persons with a physical impairment will strive to overcome disability and to normalize daily living. An alternative view is that the physically impaired give up the continual struggle to compete with able-bodied individuals. Both responses may occur in some circumstances. The chronically ill person may attempt to normalize relationships at work but not in other social situations. Assumptions also can be probed by recasting. Recasting involves taking the opposite stance. For example, things that are assumed to be disorganized are assumed to be organized, assumed cause is considered to be an effect, or unrelated things are assumed to be related and vice versa (Davis, 1971).

In summary, concepts are generalizations that emerge from the problem to be studied. Professional socialization, experience, literature, philosophy, insights, and assumptions about humanity influence how concepts are defined. Strategies for expanding our conceptual thinking include playing with metaphors, attending to process in things that appear to be static, considering the context, and probing assumptions by recasting and considering alternative assumptions.

Specifying relationships

The way in which concepts are linked is limited only by the investigator's imagination. One way of making the connections between concepts concrete is to draw a picture of how the concepts are believed to fit

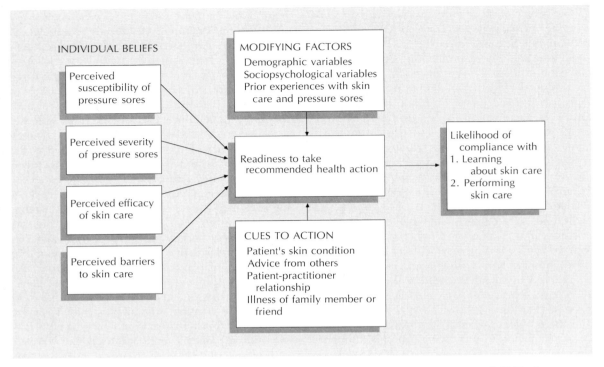

Fig. 5-3. Health belief model for compliance to skin care in paraplegics. (From Dai, Y-T., & Catanzaro, M. [1987]. *Rehabilitation Nursing, 12,* 14.)

together. Pender's study (1984, 1985) of anxiety linked the concept of anxiety to physiological and psychological variables as shown in Fig. 5-2. Anxiety cannot be measured directly. Previous research had demonstrated that people who reported subjective feelings of anxiety experienced physiological changes such as increased blood pressure and heart rate and had increased muscle tension and cold extremities (digital temperature). Pender used these physiological variables as dependent or outcome variables to determine the effect of a nursing intervention. The psychological variables of state-anxiety and locus of control also were believed to be associated with anxiety and were considered by Pender to be covariables in determining anxiety.

Dai and Catanzaro (1987) modified the Health Belief Model (Rosenstock, 1974) for use with paraplegic men and compliance to skin care and diagramed the model depicted in Fig. 5-3. These investigators believed that many factors influenced the readiness of men to take recommended health

actions to prevent the development of decubitus ulcers. These factors included individual beliefs about pressure sores and skin care, modifying factors including demographic and socio-psychological variables, and prior experience with skin care and pressure sores. Cues to take action also contributed to readiness to take action. The likelihood of the paraplegic's compliance with learning about and performing skin care resulted from readiness to take action.

Fig. 5-1 shows the model used by Cronenwett (1985) in her study of parenthood. She conceptualized her study in terms of parenthood and believed that many interrelationships existed among the variables in the study, as indicated by the arrows pointing in both directions. These properties of the individual contributed to the properties of the social network and to perceived social support. All the concepts in the model influenced social network and perceived social support.

Many ways exist to illustrate the relationship

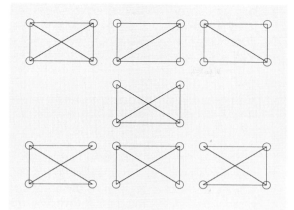

Fig. 5-4. Examples of patterns of relationships involving four concepts. (From Crawford, G. [1982]. *Advances in Nursing Science*, 5[1], 1-6. Reprinted with permission of Aspen Publishers, Inc.)

among concepts. Crawford (1982, pp. 4-5) illustrated 11 ways of connecting four elements. Seven of those ways are illustrated in Fig. 5-4. One way to develop relationships among concepts in a study is to think of all possible connections. Do these connections make sense? Does the existing knowledge support these connections? Are there connections that have not yet been explored? Questions such as these will help the investigator think creatively about structuring a conceptual framework for research. A combination of circles, triangles, and rectangles, and straight, curved, solid, and broken lines provides limitless possibilities for drawing a picture of how the investigator believes the concepts for a study to be related.

Another way to see relationships among concepts is to change the scale, in other words, to see things as bigger or smaller than they actually are (Wicker, 1985). What might it be like to work in an intensive care unit with 200 beds? What if we had no electronic equipment to monitor patients? What would life be like if everyone lived to be 150 years of age? How would child raising be different if, from the time of birth, children remembered everything they heard and saw? What if nurses had unlimited time for patient teaching? What if the nursing unit budget for the new fiscal year was onl~ ~~% of the current bud-

get? What would happen if it were assumed that the opposite assumption was true? What if things assumed to be unrelated are related or things we thought were positively related are, in fact, negatively related? What if the presumed cause was actually the effect?

In summary, specifying relationships among concepts requires that the investigator make connections between the generalizations that underlie the study. Drawing a picture of how the investigator perceives the concepts to be linked often is a useful strategy. Strategies to expand thinking about relationships include consideration of other ways to link concepts and to change the scale of thinking about the relationship among concepts.

CONCEPTUAL MODELS FOR NURSING PRACTICE

Many nurse theorists have developed conceptual models for nursing practice. These models are useful during the conceptual phase of a study because they provide an understanding of basic conceptual issues and suggest instrumental rules and methodological approaches (Fawcett, 1984). Chinn and Jacobs (1983) noted that research problems can be derived from conceptual models or studies can be undertaken to develop theoretical propositions. Theory-linked research, according to Chinn and Jacobs (1983), is conceived and conducted within the framework of an abstract model and is designed to develop or to test that model. There are many evolving conceptual models for nursing practice. Among the best known are Johnson's Behavioral Systems Model (1980), King's Open System Model (1981), Levin's Conservation Model (1973), Newman's System Model (1982), Orem's Self-Care Model (1980), Rogers' Life Process Model (1970), and Roy's Adaptation Model (1976). Portions of these global models can be tested through research. Additionally, these models may provide the investigator with ideas about concepts that are useful for the planned investigation.

Rothlis (1984) used Orem's Self-Care Model as a conceptual umbrella for her study of the effects of a self-help group on feelings of hopelessness and helplessness. Orem's framework suggested that the goal of the nurse is to assist the individual to learn to provide for personal universal and health-deviation needs. Rothlis conceptualized reactive depression as a health-deviation self-care deficit and established a self-help group that assisted the person with reactive depression to provide for self-care. The self-help group was seen as the nursing intervention technique in a supportive-educative-developmental system that helped the depressed person arrive at self-care.

Newport (1984) used Levine's Conservation Model as a framework for her study on conserving thermal energy and social integrity in the newborn. She compared different methods of thermal energy conservation: (1) drying infants after delivery, (2) avoiding placing the infants on solid surfaces that were cooler than the uterus, (3) covering the infants with a blanket, (4) placing the infant on a heated surface in the neonatal unit, and (5) placing the infant on the mother's chest. This latter intervention was believed to conserve social integrity (mother-infant bonding). Newport found that conservation of energy could be maintained efficiently by placing the infant on the mother's unclothed chest and covering both with a warmed blanket.

WRITING A CONCEPTUAL FRAMEWORK FOR RESEARCH

Batey (1977) pointed out that the conceptual phase of a study guides the consumer—whether the reviewer of the research proposal or the reader of a published report of the study—about the dimensions of knowledge related to the phenomenon of study and the researcher's image of how that phenomenon appears in the real world. The conceptual phase of the study includes the problem or phenomenon to be addressed, the current state of knowledge about the phenomenon, the framework of concepts and their relationships, and the specific part of the conceptual relationships that will be examined in the study (Batey, 1977). The process of identifying the problem for study is discussed in Chapter 3. Identifying the current state of knowledge through a review of the literature about the phenomenon is presented in Chapter 4. In this chapter we are concerned with specifying a conceptual framework. This framework is variously termed the conceptual framework, the theoretical framework, or the rationale for the study.

A written account of the study framework will make explicit the investigator's meanings and reasoning (Batey, 1977). It will include the concepts and their relationships and will use references to published materials to bring the concepts into focus and to identify any areas of ambiguity or incompleteness in the current level of knowledge. Findings of previous studies are used to illustrate what is known about the phenomenon and the conditions under which the concepts and their relationships have been studied (Batey, 1977).

The logical development of the framework for study must be evident, and the concepts must be clear. Assumptions upon which relationships are constructed must be made explicit. If the researcher has determined that insufficient knowledge exists about the phenomenon to suggest relationships, the conceptual framework must make explicit the logical basis for that decision. The investigator may choose to diagram the hypothesized relationships among the concepts and include this diagram in the written report. Writing a conceptual framework requires that the investigator exercise creativity in identifying concepts and specifying relationships.

PURPOSE OF THE STUDY

When the investigator has reviewed the literature and constructed a framework for the proposed study, the specific purpose of the study can be identified. The problem that started the investigator thinking and planning the study, the review of previous work in the field, and the intensive thought processes that integrate what is known about the problem lead the investigator to identify the level of knowledge that exists about the topic and the next step for research. If little is known about the phenomenon, a factor-describing study is indicated. The researcher will write a purpose for the proposed study that essentially asks, "What is this?" If little is known about the experience of people with progressive neurological disease, the investigator may state, "The purpose of this study is to describe how middle-aged women with multiple sclerosis who live in the community manage the illness in their daily lives." The investigator would describe how a sample of women between the ages of 30 and 59 years talk about managing the demands of their illness and the demands of daily living.

If the daily experience of balancing the demands

of illness with other demands such as working, living with a partner, and raising children have already been described, a factor-relating study that asks, "What is happening here?" will be done. In our example, the purpose would state. "The purpose of this study is to relate how middle-aged women with multiple sclerosis describe themselves to themselves before and after a change from being independently ambulatory to using a wheelchair."

Situation-relating studies are undertaken when factors have been isolated and related. The question "What will happen if . . ." is appropriate at this level of knowledge development. The purpose of situation-relating studies may be to study something as it naturally occurs, such as, "Greater changes in personal identity will occur among middle-aged females with a sudden onset and rapid progression of multiple sclerosis than among middle-aged females with slow, steadily progressive multiple sclerosis." Situation-relating studies can also be done in settings where a variable is manipulated or a treatment is introduced. For example, we might have as the purpose of a study to test the hypothesis that "Middle-aged males with multiple sclerosis who participate in a social support group of peers will be significantly more likely to maintain employment than those who do not participate in a social support group."

Prediction is the aim of situation-producing research. The purpose of a study built on previous work that has isolated and described the concepts of interest and determined how things are related would be to see if the desired outcome consistently can be produced. The researcher might test the hypothesis: "Participation in a peer-facilitated self-help group for 10 weeks will significantly increase the length of time persons with multiple sclerosis remain employed." For both situation-relating and situation-producing studies, the purpose of the study is expressed in the form of a hypothesis.

The complete statement of the purpose of the study should contain information about the type of study, the setting in which the study will be conducted, and the sample to be used for the study. Kelly and Cross (1985) studied stress and coping behaviors in intensive care and medical surgical ward registered nurses. Their stated purpose could be to compare intensive care unit nurses and ". . . medical surgical ward nurses at two large urban acute care teach-ing hospitals examining stress levels, the frequencies of stress factors, coping behaviors to deal with stress, and recommendations for coping effectively with stress" (p. 322).

SUMMARY

The conceptual framework for a research study presents the reasoning on which the purposes of the proposed study are based. The framework provides the perspective from which the investigator views the problem and is not merely a restatement of previous research but an integration of the existing theoretical traditions and knowledge about the topic. A conceptual framework consists of concepts and the propositions about how those concepts are related. The concepts that form the basis of the study are clarified so that others will be able to understand the study from the same frame of reference as the investigator. The conceptual framework sets forth the state of the science in the problem area and identifies whether the phenomena still need description, whether connections between concepts need to be made, or whether knowledge is needed about how to produce desired outcomes. The purpose of the study is dictated by the conceptual framework, which has indicated the current level of knowledge about the phenomenon of interest.

REFERENCES

Batey, M. V. (1977). Conceptualization: Knowledge and logic guiding empirical research. *Nursing Research, 26,* 324-329.

Chinn, P. L., & Jacobs, M. K. (1983). *Theory and nursing: A systematic approach.* St. Louis: Mosby.

Crawford, G. (1982). The concept of pattern in nursing: Conceptual development and measurement. *Advances in Nursing Science, 5*(1), 1-6.

Cronenwett, L. R. (1985). Network structure, social support, and psychological outcomes of pregnancy. *Nursing Research, 34,* 93-99.

Dai, Y.-T., & Catanzaro, M. (1987). Health beliefs and compliance to skin care. *Rehabilitation Nursing, 12,* 13-16.

Davis, M. S. (1971). That's interesting: Toward a phenomenology of sociology and a sociology of phenomenology. *Philosophy of the Social Sciences, 1,* 309-314.

Dubin, R. (1978). *Theory Building.* New York: Free Press.

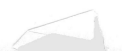

Fawcett, J. (1984). *Analysis and evaluation of conceptual models of nursing.* Philadelphia: Davis.

Johnson, D. E. (1980). The behavioral system model for nursing. In J. P. Riehl & C. Roy (Eds.), *Conceptual models for nursing practice* (2nd ed.) (pp. 207-216). New York: Appleton-Century-Crofts.

Kelly, J. G., & Cross, D. G. (1985). Stress, coping behaviors, and recommendations for intensive care and medical surgical ward registered nurses. *Research in Nursing and Health, 8,* 321-328.

King, I. M. (1981). *A theory for nursing: Systems, concepts, process.* New York: Wiley.

Levine, M. E. (1973). *Introduction to clinical nursing* (2nd ed.). New York: Wiley.

Lewis, F. M. (1982). Experienced personal control and quality of life in late-stage cancer patients. *Nursing Research, 21,* 113-119.

Mager, R. F. (1972). *Goal analysis.* Belmont, CA: Fearon Publishers.

Newman, M. (1979). *Theory development in nursing.* Philadelphia: Davis.

Newport, M. A. (1984). Conserving thermal energy and social integrity in the newborn. *Western Journal of Nursing Research, 6,* 176-190.

Orem, D. E. (1980). *Concepts of practice* (2nd ed.). New York: McGraw-Hill.

Pender, N. J. (1984). Physiologic responses of clients with essential hypertension to progressive muscle relaxation training. *Research in Nursing and Health, 7,* 197-203.

Pender, N. J. (1985). Effects of progressive muscle relaxation training on anxiety and health locus of control among hypertensive adults. *Research in Nursing and Health, 8,* 67-72.

Rogers, M. E. (1980). Nursing: A science of unitary man. In J. P. Riehl & C. Roy (Eds.), *Conceptual models for nursing practice* (2nd ed.) (pp. 329-337). New York: Appleton-Century-Crofts.

Rosenstock, I. M. (1974). Historical origin of the health belief model. *Health Education Monograph, 2,* 329-335.

Rothlis, J. (1984). The effect of a self-help group on feelings of hopelessness and helplessness. *Western Journal of Nursing Research, 6,* 157-169.

Roy, C. (1976). *Introduction to nursing: An adaptation model.* Englewood Cliffs, NJ: Prentice-Hall.

Wicker, A. W. (1985). Getting out of our conceptual ruts. *American Psychologist, 40,* 1094-1103.

Williams, M. A. (1980). Assumptions in research. *Research in Nursing and Health, 3,* 47-48.

6

CONSIDERING HUMAN RIGHTS IN RESEARCH

JEANNE QUINT BENOLIEL

A basic value in modern Western society is that the advancement of scientific knowledge is inherently good and desirable because of the benefits it brings to human existence. Yet the free exploration of intriguing ideas through scientific inquiry and methods has been tempered by the importance of other values in society. In the twentieth century, societal controls have appeared in response to research that has resulted in (1) harm to people, such as occurred in the Tuskegee study in which black men with syphilis went untreated in order to understand "the natural history of the disease" (Barber, 1976; Rothman, 1982), and (2) damage to the environment, such as when DDT was found to destroy certain wildlife by interfering with the natural food chain (Edsall, 1975).

Concern about the welfare of human beings and their environment has not been the rule according to history, and often captive populations and other vulnerable groups were used freely for human experimentation (Beecher, 1959). Today, according to Davis (1979a), research with human subjects poses special problems for the investigator in balancing three competing social interests: (1) protection of individual human subjects, (2) needs of society for the benefits of research, and (3) the need to encourage and foster research as a means for garnering systematic knowledge. Nurses who participate in research involving human subjects need to be aware that human considerations are matters of serious importance in the planning, implementing, and reporting of such research. Although protection of research subjects is a primary concern, human considerations also require attention to study design, special populations of interest to nurses, measurement issues, and rights and responsibilities of investigators and staff in collaborative research.

PROTECTION OF HUMAN SUBJECTS

The ethical principles underlying the use of human beings as research subjects were identified by the National Commission for the Protection of Human Subjects of Biomedical and Behavioral Research (NCPHSBBR) (1978) as threefold: (1) respect for persons as autonomous agents, (2) beneficence, referring to a maximizing of benefits and a minimizing of harms for the research participants and society, and (3) justice, referring to equitable sharing of the benefits and burdens of research by the population in general. These principles have been translated into federal policies and procedures for the protection of human subjects in general and for special populations in need of extra safeguards because of their extreme vulnerability to exploitation by others (Department of Health and Human Services [DHHS], 1981; Levine, 1981, p. 248). These principles, policies, and guidelines provide direction to the nurse investigator in planning research that will involve human subjects.

Human participation in research

The basis for human participation in research rests on the notion that autonomous agents have the right of self-determination about whether to permit an invasion of personal privacy for research purposes. Consent to participate, however, is not unconditional; the investigator is expected to ensure certain protections and safeguards: (1) consent is informed and voluntary, (2) the subject can withdraw without penalty, (3) benefits of the research outweigh the risks, and (4) the investigator is qualified to perform the research (Davis, 1979b).

Informed consent

The concept of informed consent places special responsibility on the investigator to make appropriate information available to potential participants, to ensure that these persons are competent according to accepted legal standards, and to develop ways to ensure that the subjects understand what is expected of them and what will be done with the information obtained. A key assumption underlying informed consent is that it requires a noncoercive environment in which the individual is given all information essential for making an informed decision about whether or not to participate.

The information deemed essential for informed consent includes the purpose of the study, procedures to be used, nature and amount of risk or discomfort, anticipated benefits, assurance of confidentiality, opportunity to ask questions, and alternative procedures when therapy is involved (DHHS, 1981). In the majority of studies a written consent

---

UNIVERSITY OF WASHINGTON
Consent Form for Men
Coping with Infertility

Mary Ann Draye, R.N., F.N.P., Assistant Professor
Community Health Care Systems

Nancy Woods, R.N., Ph.D., Professor
Physiological Nursing

Purpose

Despite the fact that nearly 20% of American couples are infertile, health professionals know little about the kinds of problems these women and men experience in everyday living and the ways in which they cope with these problems. The purpose of this study is to describe the difficulties experienced by infertile couples in their personal lives, relationships with a female partner/spouse, family and friends, in their work and with the health care system during the year after their first infertility clinic appointment. In addition, the study will explore how couples cope with these problems and what resources help them cope.

Benefits

Although participating in this study will not be of immediate benefit to you, the information you contribute may benefit other infertility patients in the future.

Procedures, Risks

If you choose to participate in the study, you will be asked to complete the same questionnaire on 3 occasions, once right away and then in six months and in one year. The questionnaire will take about 30 minutes to complete each time. The questions will relate to the influence of infertility on your relationships with a female partner/spouse, family and friends, your work, the health care system, and your personal life. You will also be asked about how you cope with these experiences and about the support you receive from others. Some of the questions may make you feel anxious and some may seem of a personal nature, for example, "Since our infertility problem, I feel sex is more for reproductive purposes than for pleasure." You are free to skip questions that you do not wish to answer.

Continued.

form is used to convey information to the potential subject and to obtain a signature of agreement (see box). Yet the use of written forms in no way ensures that the subject comprehends the information. Factors found to affect the comprehension of information include (1) the amount and complexity of the information, (2) the method of presentation of information, (3) demographic factors such as sex and education, and (4) personal factors such as status of health, patterns of recall, and attitudes toward the informed consent process (Silva & Sorrell, 1984).

Other factors influencing the subject's willingness to participate include the setting in which investigator and potential subject meet and the nature of their preestablished relationship. Individuals who are captive subjects in the sense of "feeling an obligation to the investigator" may not be free to consent voluntarily. The patient who has known the investigator as a nurse involved in health care may feel an obligation to participate in the study because of this feeling (Benoliel, 1975). This sense of wanting to reciprocate, in itself, may not be wrong, but it places special burdens on the investigator to use practices and procedures that foster freedom of choice and allow opportunities for questions and discussion.

Sensitivity to factors that interfere with informed consent is especially important when the potential subjects are representatives of deprived socioeconomic groups or of certain ethnic minorities who tend to comply unquestioningly with requests of persons in authority or who fear that nonparticipation will block their access to health care (Hayter,

---

Voluntary Participation, Confidentiality

Your participation in this project is completely voluntary and you may withdraw from the study at any time without penalty or loss of benefits to which you are otherwise entitled. Your questionnaire will be marked with a number, not your name, and the questionnaires will be kept in a locked file cabinet. Only the investigators and their research assistant will have access to the questionnaires, and the information will be destroyed when reports of the study are completed.

Costs, Reimbursement

You will not be paid for your involvement. There are no financial costs associated with your participation.

_____   _____
Signature of Investigator   Date

Participant's Statement

The study described above has been explained to me, and I voluntarily consent to participate in this activity. I have had an opportunity to ask questions and understand that future questions I may have about the research or about subjects' rights will be answered by one of the investigators listed above.

_____   _____
Signature of Subject   Date

I agree to have the investigators send me a second questionnaire 6 months and one year from now.

_____   _____
Signature of Subject   Date

_____
Copies to: subject
           investigators' file   Mailing Address

1979). Sensitivity of this nature is also imperative when potential subjects are patients whose illness has contributed to a serious mental or emotional disorder that could interfere with understanding the investigator's request (Drane, 1984).

Responsibilities of the investigator

The investigator's responsibilities in relation to informed consent include activities to foster comprehension of information by the persons considering participation in a project. Silva and Sorrell (1984) noted the merits of the following: (1) a written statement of essential information that is brief, clear, and direct, (2) allowance of sufficient time to absorb the information, (3) provision of special help when education and vocabulary limitations may interfere with understanding, (4) recognition that persons in disruptive life circumstances may need extra help with interpreting information, (5) recognition that forgetting comes easily when information is threatening, and (6) awareness that comprehension and memory need to be assessed independently.

When full disclosure of information about a study would compromise the validity of its findings, the investigator has responsibility to indicate to potential subjects that some information is being withheld at the time of consent but will be made known when the study is completed (NCPHSBBR, 1978). In this situation, the decision to withhold information must be essential for the goals of the research, and any undisclosed risks are expected to be minimal. Decisions of this sort are components of the study design and must incorporate a careful analysis of the risks and benefits associated with the projected research.

The investigator has responsibility for determining the criteria for judging the competency of potential subjects. These criteria are very important when the persons to be studied are vulnerable to difficulties in understanding information because of severity of illness (Benoliel, 1980), institutionalization (Mitchell, 1980), cultural interpretations (Meleis, 1980), and the effects of aging (Wolanin, 1980). Development of such criteria are important in general, but they are essential when the investigator relies on project staff to obtain consent.

Since privacy and confidentiality are also components of respect for the individual, the investigator has responsibility to establish procedures that demonstrate respect for the privacy of persons during the

data production process. In addition, the investigator needs to provide adequate storage for any records and documents that contain identifying information about the participating subjects. Precautions for the storage of research data are especially important when the subject under investigation is a sensitive one and the information obtained could be deleterious to the well-being of those who gave it. Nurse investigators need to be aware that research data are not immune from the subpoena process, and this possibility needs to be considered in designing research that deals with complex social problems, for example, illegal drug use, child abuse, or criminal behaviors (Reynolds, 1979, pp. 304-316).

Responsibilities of the institution

To counteract abuse of human rights in research, the United States Public Health Service in 1966 established a policy requiring prior approval by a peer review committee of all research proposals involving human subjects and requesting federal monies (Hayter, 1979, p. 135; Reynolds, 1979, pp. 262-274). As a result of this policy, most institutions have established institutional review boards (IRBs) that have responsibility to review proposed research and the progress of ongoing studies, usually on an annual basis. These reviews are guided by policies and guidelines from the various federal agencies from which research monies are requested, and particular attention is directed toward the measures used to protect the rights of participating human subjects. The effectiveness of IRBs in reviewing and monitoring research is directly related to the institutional standards set for the conduct of research, the consistent application of these standards to all proposals, and the adequacy of membership from all representative groups, including the general public (Levine, 1981, pp. 226-238). An example of a human subjects review committee application is shown in boxed material on pp. 83-88.

Because of the importance of human subject considerations, similar research review boards or committees composed of representative scientists are appointed in an advisory capacity to various funding agencies and foundations. These committees provide peer review of all research applications, critiques of the proposals, and priority scores based on scientific merit and subject importance. Many health service agencies have established institutional committees to review proposals for research involving their clien-

Form UW 13-11 (Revised 1/78)

UNIVERSITY OF WASHINGTON
Human Subjects Review Committee Application

Date _____8/10/82_____

CONFIDENTIAL

Please type; use supplemental sheets as needed. Submit 9 copies, including the signature copy, and all relevant materials, e.g., consent form(s), questionnaires, other, to the Human Subjects Office AD-22. Students should submit one copy of thesis proposal, as well. For information call.

| | Name and position | Department/Division | Mail Stop | Telephone |

I. [Application will be filed under name of first person listed.]

Investigator: Mary Ann Draye, FNP, M.S.
Assistant Professor   Community Health Care
Systems

Associates: Nancy Woods, Ph.D., R.N.
Associate Professor   Physiological Nursing

II. Names of other persons responsible for performing or supervising procedures.

Research Assistant, Masters prepared, to be named.

III. Title of proposed activity.

Coping With Infertility

IV. Beginning date of proposed activity.

October, 1982

V. Grant and contract information. List all relevant grants and contracts.
ATTACH ONE COPY (without budget) unless "other training grant."

A. Activity related to: research grant __X__, contract _____, fellowship _____, other training grant _____, other (specify) _____, none (if "none," proceed to Section VI.) _____.

B. Has proposal been submitted through Grant and Contract Services? Yes __X__, No _____.

C. Has award been made? Yes __X__, No _____.

D. Name of Principal Investigator shown (or to be shown) on proposal:

Rheba de Tornyay, Ed.D.

E. Name of agency to which proposal was (or will be) submitted:

Division of Research Resources, NIH

F. If continuation (or already awarded), what is the agency's grant or contract number?
_____RR05758-09_____

Continued.

G. Title of proposal shown (or to be shown) on GC-1 form:

Biomedical Research Support Grant

H. Inclusive dates of grant or contract:

From _____4/1/82_____, through _____3/31/83_____.

I. Will activity be performed if funding is not received? Yes _____, No _____. N/A

VI. Recommendations and action: Date   Approve   Disapprove

A. Department _____ _____ _____ _____
    Chairman   Typed name, plus signature

B. Faculty Sponsor _____ _____ _____ _____
    (for student)   Typed name, plus signature

C. Human Subjects _____ _____ _____ _____
    Review Committee   Chairman's signature

Subject to the following conditions: _____

_____

Period of approval from _____, through _____

Valid only as long as approved procedures are followed.

VII. Outline of activity (circle OPTION you will use in responding):

FIRST OPTION: Provide answers in spaces below (add sheets, when needed).

SECOND OPTION: Provide answers on separate sheet(s) and reference page and paragraph below.

A. Background or rationale for this activity.

Infertility affects 20% of the U.S. couples of childbearing age. It may constitute a major life crisis with resultant decreased self-esteem, anger, isolation, and marital strain. Little has been done to study the problems of infertile couples and how they cope. The estimated outcome of this research is the generation of knowledge which will allow nurses and others who care for infertile couples to provide anticipatory counselling and facilitate these patients' coping efforts.

B. Objectives.

1. To describe the problems which infertile couples experience in the areas of their personal and marital lives, relationships with family and friends, in the work environment, and the health care system when workup is initiated, while their workup is in progress, and one year after they have begun treatment.
2. To compare and contrast how women and men cope with the problems enumerated in #1.
3. To explore the factors (in particular the personal and social resources) influencing how women and men cope with these problems.

Continued.

C. Procedures involved. Provide a short description of the sequence and methods to be used. (Which of these will be performed primarily for the purpose of this activity, e.g., volume of blood, size of biopsy, questionnaire, name of psychological test?)

We will employ a longitudinal design to describe the experiences of infertile couples over a one year period. Couples will be asked to complete a questionnaire at entry into treatment, and six months and one year later. Each woman beginning a workup at the UW Infertility Clinic will be given a brief written description of the study as she registers for her clinic appointment (see attachment 1). If she is interested in participating in the study, one of the investigators (M. Draye or N. Woods) or the research assistant will review the study in greater detail with her and obtain her written consent (see attachment #2). If the woman agrees to participate in the study she will be given a written questionnaire to complete and mail back to the investigators (see attachment #3). She will also be given a questionnaire for men to take to partner/spouse. He will be asked to fill in the questionnaire and mail it back to the investigators. We will ask both the woman and her partner/spouse for permission to contact them 6 months and 12 months later to complete a questionnaire containing parts 2 through 9, and parts 11 and 12 of the questionnaire appended.

D. Identify alternative procedures, if any, that are not included in the study but might be advantageous to the subject.

    N/A

E. If any deception (withholding of complete information) is required for the validity of this activity, explain why this is necessary and attach debriefing statement.

    N/A

F. Subjects.

1. Approximate number and ages:

	How many	Age Range
normal		
patient	50	21-40 women + 50 male partners
either		

2. Criteria for selection and exclusion.

All new female patients 21-40 beginning infertility workup and their male partners/spouse will be asked to participate. Patients seeking tubal ligation reversal will be excluded.

3. Source of subjects (including patients).

University of Washington Infertility Clinic

4. How subjects will be approached and by whom.

Women will be given a brief written description by clinic staff when they register. If they indicate an interest in the study one of the investigators or the RA will obtain informed consent and administer the questionnaire.

Continued.

5. Steps taken to avoid causing potential subjects to be or feel coerced?

Use of intermediary to inquire re: study, stressing that participation is voluntary and won't affect their care.

6. Will subjects receive an inducement, e.g., payment, services without charge, extra course credit? If so, what amount or how? What is the reason for the inducement?

No

7. Location where procedures will be carried out.

Women may complete the questionnaire in the UW Infertility Clinic or at home as they choose.

G. Risk.
1. Nature and amount of risk (include side effects), substantial stress, discomfort, or invasion of privacy involved.

Respondents may feel some anxiety as they respond to the questions and may find some items to be of a personal nature.

2. Describe the expected benefits of the activity (for individual and/or society) and explain how they outweigh the risks.

There is little knowledge about the problems infertile couples experience and how they cope with them over time. This study should yield information that will help professionals give anticipatory guidance and support to such couples.

3. Follow-up planned as part of the procedures.

Follow-up questionnaires will be sent to subjects at 6 and 12 months after initial questionnaire. At each follow-up, informed consent will be obtained for each questionnaire from each respondent.

4. Plan for handling possible adverse effects.

None anticipated

5. Arrangements for financial responsibility for adverse effects.

N/A

H. Confidentiality and anonymity.
1. Will participation be anonymous (that is, investigator will have no way to identify subjects by appearance, name, or date)? Yes _____, No __X__. If yes, how assured?

The investigators will be aware of subjects' names & addresses, but no names will be attached to data

2. Where participation is not anonymous, steps to insure confidentiality.

Only an ID number will be placed on questionnaires.

Continued.

3. Provision for controls over access to documents and data.

Data will be kept in a locked file cabinet & only seen by the investigators & RA.

VIII. Checklist to be completed by investigator:

	Yes	No
A. Will any group, agency, or organization be involved? If yes, please specify.	X	

UW Infertility Clinic; staff have given permission for the study to be conducted in the clinic.

B. Will materials with potential radiation risk be used, e.g., X-rays, radioisotopes? If yes,   X
   1. Status of annual review by Radiation Safety Committee (RSC). (If approved, ATTACH ONE COPY of approval.)

   2. Title of application submitted to RSC.

C. Will an investigational new drug (IND) be used?   X
   If yes, name, source, proposed dosage, how administered, status with Food and Drug Administration, and IND number. ENCLOSE ONE COPY of: 1. available toxicity data; 2. reports of animal studies; 3. description of human studies done in Europe or other countries; 4. a concise review of the literature prepared by the investigator; and 5. the drug protocol.

D. Will other drugs be used: N/A
   If yes, names, sources, dosages, how administered, and side effects.

E. Will medical or academic records be used: X

F. Will audio-visual or tape recordings, or photographs be made?   X

G. Should this activity be covered by the adverse effects insurance?   X

H. Will written consent form(s) be used? Written consent is required in most   X
   cases (in addition to an oral explanation).
   1. If no, explain why a written consent form will not be used.

   2. If no, is a statement attached describing what particpants will be told? Participants should be informed of elements of I., below.

I. Does (Do) the consent form(s) include "University of Washington" heading?   X

Name, position, department, and telephone number of investigator(s)?   X

Copy for subject?   X

Signature and date lines to be completed by investigator, subject, parent   X
or legal guardian, and subject advocate, as applicable?

The following information in simple language appropriate to the reader:

   1. Purpose—what the objectives are and why the study is being conducted?   X

   2. Benefits to be expected or knowledge hoped to be gained?   X

   3. Procedures to be followed, time involved for each, and total time   X

   4. Nature and amount of risk, substantial stress, discomfort, or invasion of privacy involved?   X

Continued.

5. Appropriate alternative procedures that might be advantageous or available to subject?	X	_____
6. Costs the subject may immediately or ultimately be forced to bear?	X	_____
7. Reimbursement of costs or other inducement the subject will receive?	X	_____
8. Voluntary nature of participation and freedom to withdraw at any point without penalty or jeopardizing medical care?	X	_____
9. Opportunity to ask questions before consenting?	X	_____
10. Assurance that subject's identity will remain confidential or is anonymous?	X	_____
11. Who will have access to subject's responses?	X	_____
12. How the information will be used?	X	_____
13. How long the data will be retained by investigator?	X	_____

tele, and sometimes investigators must have their proposals reviewed by several different institutional groups before approval to conduct the study is complete. Within many large hospitals, departments of nursing research have been organized to monitor the excessive use of patients and personnel in various projects and to approve research activities affecting the nursing department. Nursing departments in general have responsibility to establish policies and guidelines that assist all nurses in knowing their obligations and rights regarding participation in clinical studies in medicine or nursing and protection of patients whose rights appear to be threatened.

Institutional review boards also play an important role in determining whether a secondary analysis of data collected originally for another purpose is covered by the initial approval or requires a new consent procedure. Institutional review committees in health service agencies have a special responsibility to determine that access to patient records for research purposes has been based on appropriate consent procedures. Physicians and nurses who have access to patient records in their roles as providers of care do not have access to these data sources for research purposes unless prior approval by the appropriate reviewing body has been granted. Because care providers have easy access to patient records, they sometimes need reminding that the patient's record is a privileged document. Nurses in practice also need written guidelines on the appropriate action to take when an unauthorized person requests access to a patient record.

Despite the development of these various social mechanisms for protection of human subjects in research, evidence indicates that some studies involving human beings are not reviewed by IRBs, monitoring of human protection protocols after the initial review is cursory at best, and some investigators are lax in their use of appropriate consent procedures (Barber, 1976; Hayter, 1979). Ultimately, respect for the rights of research subjects depends on the personal integrity of the investigator and the project staff who implement the established protocols and procedures for a given research study.

Responsibilities of the profession

The expansion of health-related and behavioral research involving human beings led to the development of written policies and codes of ethics by many professional organizations. The Code for Nurses was adopted by the American Nurses' Association (ANA) in 1950 and is updated from time to time to incorporate new ideas and information (ANA, 1985a). The *Code for Nurses with Interpretive Statements* provides nurses and the public with specific statements relative to nurses' responsibilities in relation to patients and their well-being, competence in practice, improvement of standards of practice, and participation in the development of new knowledge.

To guide nurses in matters specifically related to research activity, the ANA published *Human Rights Guidelines for Nurses in Clinical and Other Research* in 1975. The current version of that document focuses attention on human rights considerations for nurses and potential subjects, the functions of review boards and sponsors in the conduct of research, and various mechanisms to safeguard the protection of human subjects in research (ANA, 1985b). These written policies by the ANA have been very influential in promoting the appointment of nurses to institutional review boards and the active involvement of nurses in research activity.

Publication of sensitive subject matter

A general principle governing the use of humans in research is that the data be considered confidential and be reported anonymously. Implementation of this principle means that data will not be shared with people other than appropriate members of the project staff, and special procedures will be used to safeguard information that is highly sensitive. In *longitudinal studies* involving multiple contacts with the respondents, special care is needed to separate the data to be used from identifying information about the subjects. Transfer of the data into coded form for computer storage is one approach to ensure anonymity, and specific guidelines governing data management activities are essential when the research team is large and responsibilities are diverse.

The commitment to ensure anonymity in public reports of research involves more than concealment of the names of participating subjects. Authors of research articles are obligated to present information in such a way that participants could not be identified by someone reading the report. Much of the time protection of confidentiality and anonymity poses no major problem in reports based on survey data from large samples. Even here, however, investigators need to present sensitive findings in a manner that reflects a respectful attitude toward those who provided the data.

Protection of anonymity in public reports can be problematic in research involving small samples, organizations, small communities, or groups whose values differ from the majority. Often fictitious names are used in published reports, but this step may not be adequate protection if basic descriptive information about the group, community, or organization makes concealment nearly impossible. Some of the ethical problems associated with publication of community studies include (1) individuals upset at the way they are portrayed in the report, (2) unwanted publicity by individuals or groups, (3) hazards of published information about identifiable groups being used for exploitation, (4) depiction of individuals in ways embarrassing to the larger group to which they belong, and (5) harm done to individual investigators, science, and future scientific opportunities (Johnson, 1982, p. 71).

All authors of research reports need to be aware that how they present their research results can have both positive and untoward effects on sponsors, funding agencies, publishers, other investigators, society, subjects, and themselves. Careful thought must be given to whether a publication will be unnecessarily harmful to the subjects or to the scientific community. Sometimes a delay in publication for months or even years may be necessary. If the investigator believes that anonymity cannot be guaranteed or that ownership of the data is controlled by others (e.g., the funding agency), communication of these possibilities to the research participants is imperative. When the research centers on a special group or community, it is wise to seek validation of the findings from members of that group before pursuing publication.

Research based on fieldwork or participant observation is particularly vulnerable to violations of confidentiality: the subjects themselves may decide to reveal their participation in research. Similar problems in control of data can take place when investigators disagree on what is an ethically acceptable use of a particular set of data (Johnson, 1982). Communication and agreement on standards and procedures appear to be essential for responding to ethical problems in collaborative research. These agreements may be especially important when the results of research are likely to be used by others, deal with sensitive or embarrassing subjects, and to be incorporated into public statements in the mass media (Johnson, 1982; Reynolds, 1979, pp. 396-400).

Growing public concern about human rights has affected the media through which research is generally reported. Increasingly, editorial boards of health-care and nursing journals insist on adherence to established ethical standards as a requirement for publication of a manuscript. Johnson, 1982, pp. 87-88) proposed a set of "ethical proofreading" guidelines for evaluating fieldwork manuscripts in terms of concealment of identity, judgmental comments, unflattering observations about participants, and investigator biases affecting objectivity of reporting. These guidelines might be useful for evaluating any research report about sensitive issues in people's lives.

CONSIDERATIONS IN STUDY DESIGN

Ethical as well as technical issues are important considerations in planning and implementing research about human beings and their behaviors. These issues affect choices and decisions about research design, access to subjects, informed consent concerns, and use of the role of the nurse in research.

Research design

The ethical principles of beneficence and justice are centrally important in guiding decisions about research design and the overall study plan. The NCPHSBBR (1978, p. 6) defined beneficence as an obligation to secure the benefits of research by doing no harm to participants in the process and maximizing possible benefits while minimizing potential harms. The principle of justice requires that fair procedures be used in the identification and selection of research participants within the framework of the proposed research such that no one group is used disproportionately as subjects.

A basic first step in any research is a judgment that the phenomenon of interest is sufficiently important to justify systematic study. Once the investigator has selected a design appropriate to the problem to be studied, a determination of the possible benefits and risks associated with the proposed research must be done. The risks associated with a given study may be to the participating subjects, their families, or the society at large. The types of risk can be one or several and may include physical, psychological, social, and economic insults and injuries (Levine, 1981, pp. 28-37). The benefits associated with the study can pertain to the anticipated knowledge to be gained and to the personal gains experienced by the participating subjects. Reynolds (1979, p. 43) proposed several questions to ponder relative to the central problem of finding a balance between benefits and risks:

1. What are the positive and negative effects associated with the conduct of a specific research project?
2. What are the positive and negative effects of an individual's participation in a research project?
3. Are the major positive and negative effects of research distributed evenly among different social groupings? If so, is the distribution unjust?
4. What features of the research procedure provide confidence that the rights and welfare of the participants will be respected?

Federal guidelines require that investigators carefully evaluate the potential risks in relation to benefits in a proposed investigation and provide evidence that the benefits outweigh the identified risks. Careful risk-benefit analysis appears to be critically important, for at least two reasons, in research proposals using experimental design. First, the research generally requires a control group of people who do not receive the experimental treatment but whose human rights must be considered. Second, the risks associated with a projected experimental treatment may not always be completely anticipated or their possible negative effects may be more than minimal. Evaluation of the risks and benefits of using patients for randomized clinical trials of lifesaving treatments is especially problematic; these treatments have been judged by Marquis (1983) to be unethical as presently conducted.

In any research proposal, plans for responding to anticipated and unanticipated adverse effects on research participants must be explicated. For example, subjects in double-blind studies of new drugs may need to carry a wallet card or wear an identification bracelet containing information on persons to contact in case of emergency, and the attending providers may need to know the medications being taken (Levine, 1981, p. 42). If information must be withheld from participating subjects to ensure validity of the results, the research design must incorporate plans for debriefing those subjects at some time during the study—most commonly at its completion. Further, care must be taken that the randomization procedures for assigning subjects to treatment or control groups are used in an appropriate manner, such that the results will present a valid picture of the treatment effects and potential participants will not be assigned in a biased fashion (Boruch & Cecil, 1982, pp. 219-232).

Access to subjects

Successful research depends on the investigator's access to a pool of potential subjects whose characteristics make a good fit with the problem being studied. Because nurses are often interested in using patients as research subjects, they are likely to encounter "gatekeepers" who serve as obstacles to contacting potential subjects. Often physician approval will be required by IRB protocols when patients are used as subjects in nursing research. Nurses need to recognize the importance of sponsorship in the process of obtaining an adequate sample or gaining access to the proposed research site (ANA, 1985b; Benoliel, 1975). Negotiation for access to the desired sample may require effective communication at several different levels within an organization (Mitchell, 1980) or complex family group (Benoliel, 1983, p. 165).

Access to potential subjects can be especially problematic when the topic under study—such as cancer—causes strong and ambivalent feelings in patients, family members, and health-care providers. For example, during the enrollment period of a longitudinal study of patients' adaptations to living with lung cancer, 73 potential subjects were lost to the research before written consent was obtained. In over 40% of these cases, a decision that the patient should not participate was made by the physician, someone designated by the physician, or a family member. The major reasons given for refusal were the patient's health status, the intrusiveness of the interview on the patient's time and situation, and concerns for the appropriateness of home–nursing care (the treatment being tested) (McCorkle, Packard, & Landenburger, 1984). It appeared that caregivers who denied patients the opportunity to participate did not fully understand the purposes and benefits of the study. The experience illustrates the importance of budgeting adequate time and personnel for communication with key individuals who can influence the possibilities of obtaining an adequate sample.

Informed consent issues

In the conduct of research, it is important to recognize that informed consent is more a process than a contractual agreement made at one point in time. This reality is clear in ethnographic and field research in which the investigator often makes observations of people from whom formal consent has not been requested or exchanges information with a variety of people as part of the process of data production. Wax (1982) argued that the rigid consent protocol that evolved in biomedical research is inappropriate for fieldwork studies in which investigators must enter into ongoing negotiations with the networks of reciprocity of the home community. He noted further that members of the populations being studied focused their attention on the sponsorship of the investigator, the character and disposition of the investigator, and the benefits and utility of project activities on their lives, rather than on the goals and design of the research.

Given this human tendency to pay attention to information that is personally relevant, it is not surprising that many subjects have difficulty recalling full details of a consent agreement (Silva & Sorrell, 1984). Because of this the investigator in any study must allow the subject opportunities for clarification of information and be sensitive to behavioral indicators that the person may wish to withdraw from participation. The complexities of communication and respect for human rights are especially problematic in cross-cultural studies, because the researcher and the participant may differ greatly in language, value systems, and beliefs about agreements. Such research requires careful attention to the values of the host society, protection of confidential data, and care to avoid exploitation of innocent people (Davis, 1980; Meleis, 1980).

The meaning of deception in research raises interesting questions. The investigator does not always share complete information with subjects about the research design, procedures for data production, and methods of data manipulation and analysis. On the matter of informed consent, federal guidelines do emphasize the importance of voluntary participation, specific information about the nature of the study and its benefits and risks, and avoidance of coercive circumstances (NCPHSBBR, 1978). According to these ethical standards, research that makes use of people without their knowledge and consent would be deceptive and clearly unacceptable. Also of questionable value would be the deliberate manipulation of research subjects without concern for their well-being and health or the disclosure of secrets that the subjects do not wish to have shared.

From a pragmatic point of view, however, deception can be a factor in day-to-day decisions about the conduct of research. For example, the investigator's decision to dress in a manner that conveys an acceptable image to potential subjects is a common strategy to gain access to a suitable sample. Is such behavior politeness or hypocrisy? In research as in daily life, people engage in transactions in which the rules of communication include the acceptance of certain "social lies" as essential to the maintenance of social order. Cassell (1982) proposed two possible criteria for situations in which deceptive behavior by the investigator might be acceptable: (1) when the behavior is in keeping with local rules of propriety and (2) when the behavior protects those being studied from social, psychological, or legal harms.

Nurse role conflicts of interest

A conflict of interest exists between the physician-as-therapist and the physician-as-researcher, and available evidence suggests that patients are unlikely to consider fully the risks of participation in research when the physician occupies both roles concurrently (Gray, 1975). In other words, the patient-subject in this context is prone to view the physician in the provider role and to overlook or discount the conflicting demands of the researcher role. In a sense, the patient-physician relationship can be viewed as setting up a coercive set of circumstances such that the patient cannot freely consent to participate in that physician's research. Davis (1980) argued that a similar conflict of interest exists when the nurse is known to a patient-subject as both practitioner and investigator. In contrast, May (1980) suggested that most laypersons have no concept of a nurse-researcher and are likely to consent to participate in research because they relate to the nurse (caregiver) role.

In planning nursing research, the investigator needs to be aware that use of the nurse role influences both the subjects who participate and the staff who function as nurse-observers (data collectors). In a study of women who had experienced mastectomy, for example, it was necessary to set limits on how much active nursing care was to be provided by the nurse-observers and to provide counseling when they were tempted to move into caregiver roles (Benoliel, 1975). In research of this nature, the investigator needs to formulate explicit protocols and plans for using the nurse role in a responsible manner and for guiding the nurse-observers in situations in which the obligations of the nurse and those of the observer are in conflict (Benoliel, 1980).

It is important to recognize that nurses are not the only investigators who experience conflicting demands in the performance of research. Minority investigators in minority communities may be asked to intervene in a local problem or to withhold information from curious bystanders (Zinn, 1979). Use of the nurse role as entree for studying certain types of clinical nursing problems may be an important research strategy, but the complexity of its use needs to be recognized, appreciated, and built into the research design.

STUDY OF SPECIAL POPULATIONS

Because of the past exploitation of certain populations, federal guidelines and policies have been formulated to guide the research use of such vulnerable groups as children, fetuses, and the mentally retarded (Pothier, 1980) and persons defined as legally or mentally incompetent or members of captive populations (Hayter, 1979). Investigators with interest in studying any high-risk population need to familiarize themselves with the current policies and guidelines governing consent practices, risk requirements, and acceptable procedures for research involving that population. In general, federal policy has justified the use of high-risk groups when there is no alternative population of subjects and when the research is likely to bring benefits in knowledge about the treatment of serious diseases. Further, even when the subjects are defined as legally or mentally incompetent and others (such as parents or guardians) are responsible for the formal consent agreement, obtaining assent from the index person is generally recommended as essential support of the self-determination of that individual (NCPHSBBR, 1978).

Because nurses wish to expand knowledge about the health, health needs, and well-being of many individuals and groups who are considered high-risk populations, nurse-investigators need to find creative ways of designing research that can provide understanding of these special people and their circumstances of living. Two concerns of critical importance in research on vulnerable individuals are judgments of the person's ability to give informed consent and determinations of the competency of the person to consent and provide data according to the research plan.

Judgments about informed consent

From a legal perspective decisions by individuals defined by law as old enough to give consent for research or treatment are based on voluntary agreement, competency to make an informed choice, and understanding of the essential information (Watson, 1982, p. 45). When the proposed research centers on people who are considered a captive population, special care must be taken to develop a consent protocol that facilitates free choice between consent and refusal. When the potential subject is considered legally or mentally incompetent, it is important to obtain consent from both the subject and a relative or legal guardian.

In nontherapeutic research that does not directly benefit the subject, a need may exist for careful monitoring of proxy consent procedures to determine that the parent, spouse, or guardian has the best interests of the subject in mind (Pothier, 1980). "Best interests of the other" is not a simple concept, however, and the special circumstances of the person need to be considered with care in these evaluations. There is no reason to think that caregivers are able to make better judgments about the "best interests" of vulnerable people than are family members. Systematic review of these proposals in terms of benefits and harms to potential subjects is an important responsibility of review committees and may require the appointment of someone to serve as an advocate for the potential subjects.

Determinations of competency

For some populations of interest to nurses, the competency of the person to enter into a research contract may be an important consideration. In the case of mental illness, the courts increasingly have made a distinction between the status of being institutionalized and mental competence in the legal sense (Reynolds, 1979, p. 328). This trend permits mentally ill persons to participate in research if they can give informed consent and are judged to be competent. In general, the more the research poses risks for the participating subjects, the more stringent are the requirements for judging the competency of the persons being asked to participate.

Applebaum and Roth (1982) conceptualized four groups of standards to be used for assessing the competency of a mentally ill subject. These groups are identified as providing a hierarchically ordered set of standards, each more stringent than its predecessor, to guide the desirable level of competency in relation to the potential risks of a study. In order of complexity these groups center on (1) evidence of a choice, (2) factual understanding of the issues, (3) rational use of information for decision making, and (4) appreciation of the nature of the situation. The first two groups appear to require only a concrete level of cognitive functioning whereas the latter two imply the ability to draw distinctions and make judgments.

In a carefully designed study Davidhizar and Wehlage (1984) found that institutionalized persons with chronic schizophrenia were able to meet some of the criteria for each of these four categories of standards. Equally important, the study offers a model of well-planned research with protocols and procedures tailored to respect the self-determination of the patients and to minimize the influence of the interviewer on the ongoing process of treatment.

MEASUREMENT ISSUES

The difference between observation in research and observation in everyday life is that the former makes use of systematic rules, procedures, and technological devices to ensure that the outcomes of observation are narrowly defined, delimited, and precise in meaning. Kaplan (1964, pp. 171-176) pointed out that the functions of measurement in science are to promote standardization such that equivalences exist among objects of diverse origins and to make possible increasingly precise discriminations and descriptions of objects of interest. To that end, a variety of techniques have been developed to increase the validity, reliability, and sensitivity of observations by scientists and to take into account their human errors and biases.

The technical problems of measurement are especially problematic when the objects of study are other human beings, because the technical merits of data are affected by the idiosyncratic, situational, and cultural biases of both participants and investigators in the research enterprise. For any investigator, it is important to recognize that the meaning of data collected through human interactions, whether by questionnaire or interview, is based on the investigator's use of commonsense knowledge, everyday language, and selective judgment that certain events or words are important (Cicourel, 1964; Garfinkel, 1967). Nursing research that provides sensitive and valid information about human beings requires the ability to make technical, procedural choices that take into account human, as well as technical considerations.

These choices could involve selection of instruments appropriate to the population being studied, instructions that take language and cultural differences into account, and sensitivity to personal biases in perceptions of words, people, and events. Scales with words that are not understood by the respondents are unlikely to result in valid information. Invitations that fail to take into account local customs of politeness can interfere with obtaining an adequate sample. Insensitivity to personal bias in perception can contribute to a one-sided view of a situation by the investigator rather than an openness to different explanations. For example, a nurse who views patient behavior only in terms of compliance to medical regimen may have difficulty in interpreting the behavior from a different frame of reference.

When patients are the focus of nursing research, the investigator needs to give attention to procedures that minimize the possibility of harm while maximizing the validity of the results. In a practical sense, these concerns may require the use of brief instruments, the allowance of extra time for the data collection process, and opportunity for rest in case of fatigue. Regardless of the populations studied, however, the nurse investigator needs to plan for measurement that incorporates respect for the respondents as persons and provides for variations in ability to respond to diversified instruments and procedures.

RIGHTS AND RESPONSIBILITIES IN COLLABORATIVE RESEARCH

Respect for the individual is also a factor affecting working relationships among investigators. In this regard, the principal investigator carries responsibility to provide a research plan that is both morally and scientifically honest. The project staff should not be expected to perform acts that are illegal or immoral, and any requirements to withhold information from subjects should have a sound rationale and be explained carefully to the staff members. The research process usually functions best when the division of labor among participants is clear and problems in communication are dealt with expeditiously.

Ownership of ideas and publication rights often can be a problem in team research if guidelines for these matters are not spelled out in written form. Even with guidelines, difficulties can arise when there are differences of opinion as to the appropriate use of the ideas or when someone leaves the project before it is completed. Various disciplines have identified different ways of establishing credit for authorship of publications, and individuals joining a research team would do well to ascertain the guidelines that govern the particular piece of research (Krueger, 1980). It probably is important also for the principal investigator to learn whether or not cooperating agencies wish to be identified in any research reports. Some may wish to be acknowledged; others may not.

A serious ethical problem occurs when data are falsified or misused in research reports. In team research, the investigator who carries principal responsibility for the conduct of the study must accept the blame for any data fabrication (Davis, 1984). To guard against these possibilities, the research should be done with an abundance of discussion among the research staff and established procedures for regular review of the data records.

Theft of scientific ideas is a serious matter in the research community, and every effort must be made by investigators to maintain personal integrity and to support it in others. Acknowledgment of the work of others is a valued practice in research activity and is expected to appear in research reports. Most of all, freedom of communication among investigators is essential for the critical validation or invalidation of the findings and the conduct of scientific research. The development of sound, systematic knowledge through research appears to require an atmosphere of goodwill and respect that facilitates accountability among all involved (Edsall, 1975).

SUMMARY

Research on human beings requires policies, plans, and procedures that protect individual rights of self-determination, privacy, and confidentiality. Promotion of informed consent in research imposes special responsibilities on investigators, institutions, and concerned professions. The principle of beneficence demands research design that maximizes the benefits of any study to the participating subjects and society and minimizes the harms to both. Careful risk-benefit analysis is essential in preparing the proposal. Human considerations are also necessary for the effective accrual of research subjects, the maintenance of informed consent throughout the research process, and decisions to use the nurse role in scientific studies. Research involving high-risk populations requires special attention to judgments that informed consent procedures protect the rights of vulnerable people and that subjects are competent to participate in research. Decisions about measurement devices and techniques need to take variations in the characteristics of different human populations into account and provide for the special risks of subjects who happen to be patients. Human considerations are also important in working relationships among members of a research team, and they include attention to the ownership of ideas and publication rights.

REFERENCES

American Nurses' Association (1985a). *Code for nurses with interpretive statements.* Kansas City, MO: Author.

American Nurses' Association (1985b). *Human rights guidelines for nurses in clinical and other research.* Kansas City, MO: Author.

Applebaum P., & Roth, L. (1982). Competency to consent to research, a psychiatric overview. *Archives of General Psychiatry, 39,* 951-958.

Barber, B. (1976). The ethics of experimentation with human subjects. *Scientific American, 234*(2), 25-31.

Beecher, H. (1959). Experimentation in man. *Journal of American Medical Association, 169,* 461.

Benoliel, J. Q. (1975). Research related to death and the dying patient. In P. J. Verhonick (Ed.), *Nursing Research* (pp. 189-227). Boston: Little, Brown.

Benoliel, J. Q. (1980). Research with dying patients. In A. J. Davis & J. C. Krueger (Eds.), *Patients, nurses, ethics* (pp. 119-128). New York: American Journal of Nursing Company.

Benoliel, J. Q. (1983). Grounded theory and qualitative data: The socializing influences of life-threatening disease on identity development. In P. J. Wooldridge, M. H. Schmitt, J. K. Skipper, & R. C. Leonard (Eds.), *Behavioral science and nursing theory* (pp. 141-187). St. Louis: Mosby.

Boruch, R. F., & Cecil, J. S. (1982). Statistical strategies for preserving privacy in direct inquiry. In J. E. Sieber (Ed.), *The ethics of social research: Surveys and experiments* (pp. 207-232). New York: Springer-Verlag.

Cassell, J. (1982). Harms, benefits, wrongs, and rights in fieldwork. In J. E. Sieber (Ed.), *The ethics of social research: Fieldwork, regulation, and publication* (pp. 7-31). New York: Springer-Verlag.

Cicourel, A. V. (1964). *Method and measurement in sociology.* New York: Free Press.

Davidhizar, R., & Wehlage, D. (1984). Can the client with chronic schizophrenia consent to nursing research? *Journal of Advanced Nursing, 9,* 381-390.

Davis, A. J. (1979a). Ethical issues in nursing research. *Western Journal of Nursing Research, 1,* 70-73.

Davis, A. J. (1979b). Ethical issues in nursing research. *Western Journal of Nursing Research, 1,* 145-147.

Davis, A. J. (1980). Ethical issues in nursing research. *Western Journal of Nursing Research, 2,* 760-762.

Davis, A. J. (1982). Ethical issues in nursing research. *Western Journal of Nursing Research, 4,* 111-112.

Davis, A. J. (1984). Ethical issues in nursing research. *Western Journal of Nursing Research, 6,* 452-454.

Department of Health and Human Services. (1981). Basic HHS policy for the protection of human research subjects. *Federal Register, 46,* 8366-8392.

Drane, J. F. (1984). Competency to give informed consent. *Journal of American Medical Association, 252,* 925-927.

Edsall, J. T. (1975). *Scientific freedom and responsibility* (Report of the Committee on Scientific Freedom and Responsibility). Washington, D. C.: American Association for the Advancement of Science.

Garfinkel, H. (1967). *Studies in ethnomethodology.* Englewood Cliffs, NJ: Prentice-Hall.

Gray, B. H. (1975). *Human subjects in medical experimentation.* New York: Wiley.

Hayter, J. (1979). Issues related to human subjects. In F. S. Downs & J. W. Fleming (Eds.), *Issues in nursing research* (pp. 107-147). New York: Appleton-Century-Crofts.

Johnson, C. G. (1982). Risks in the publication of fieldwork. In J. E. Sieber (Ed.), *The ethics of social research: Fieldwork, regulation, and publication* (pp. 71-91). New York: Springer-Verlag.

Kaplan, A. (1964). *The conduct of inquiry.* San Francisco: Chandler.

Krueger, J. C. (1980). Intra- and interprofessional cooperation. In A. J. Davis & J. C. Krueger (Eds.), *Patients, nurses, ethics* (pp. 177-191). New York: American Journal of Nursing Company.

Levine, R. J. (1981). *Ethics and regulation of clinical research.* Baltimore: Urban & Schwarzenberg.

Marquis, D. (1983). Leaving therapy to chance. *Hastings Center Report, 13*(4), 40-47.

May, K. A. (1980). Informed consent and role conflict. In A. J. Davis & J. C. Krueger (Eds.), *Patients, nurses, ethics* (pp. 109-115). American Journal of Nursing Company.

McCorkle, R., Packard, N., & Landenburger, K. (1984). Subject accrual and attrition: Problems and solutions. *Journal of Psychosocial Oncology, 2,* 137-146.

Meleis, A. I. (1980). Cross-cultural research. In A. J. Davis & J. C. Krueger (Eds.), *Patients, nurses, ethics* (pp. 137-147). New York: American Journal of Nursing Company.

Mitchell, A. E. (1980). Research with women prisoners. In A. J. Davis & J. C. Krueger (Eds.), *Patients, nurses, ethics* (pp. 129-135). New York: American Journal of Nursing Company.

National Commission for the Protection of Human Subjects of Biomedical and Behavioral Research. (1978). *The Belmont report: Ethical principles and guidelines for the protection of human subjects in research* (DHEW Publication No. (05) 78-0012). Washington, DC: U.S. Government Printing Office.

Pothier, P. C. (1980). Research involving children, fetuses, and the mentally retarded. In A. J. Davis & J. C. Krueger (Eds.), *Patients, nurses, ethics* (pp. 149-162). New York: American Journal of Nursing Company.

Reynolds, P. D. (1979). *Ethical dilemmas and social science research*. San Francisco: Jossey-Bass.

Rothman, D. (1982). Were Tuskegee and Willowbrook "studies in nature?" *Hastings Center Report, 12*(2), 5-7.

Silva, M. C., & Sorrell, J. M. (1984). Factors influencing comprehension of information for informed consent: Ethical implications for nursing research. *International Journal of Nursing Studies, 21,* 233-240.

Watson, A. B. (1982). Informed consent of special subjects. *Nursing Research, 31,* 43-47.

Wax, M. L. (1982). Research reciprocity rather than informed consent in fieldwork. In J. E. Sieber (Ed.), *The ethics of social research: Fieldwork, regulation, and publication* (pp. 33-48). New York: Springer-Verlag.

Wolanin, M. O. (1980). Research and the aged. In A. J. Davis & J. C. Krueger (Eds.), *Patients, nurses, ethics* (pp. 163-174). New York: American Journal of Nursing Company.

Zinn, M. B. (1979). Field research in minority communities: Ethical, methodological and political observations by an insider. *Social Problems, 27,* 209-219.

7

SAMPLING

NANCY FUGATE WOODS

In the earliest phases of planning a study, an investigator precisely defines the problem to be studied and the frame of reference that will guide the investigation. In the process of specifying the problem and purpose of the study, an investigator considers not only the phenomenon to be studied but also the sources of data regarding the phenomenon. This chapter will focus on a series of decisions that investigators make about the source of data and decisions related to the process of sampling—selecting the people or things that will be included in the study as sources of data. We will begin by considering some basic concepts related to the topic of sampling. Then we will consider several sampling strategies useful in nursing research. We will conclude with a discussion of methods in estimating sample size and implementing a sampling plan.

BASIC CONCEPTS

Sampling is the process of selecting a subset of a population in order to obtain information regarding a phenomenon in a way that represents the entire population. The concepts, population, sample, sampling unit, and element are essential to understanding sampling.

A *population* is an aggregate of elements sharing some common set of criteria, for example, all adult women, all children attending a preschool, or all epochs of sleep during the course of a night. Investigators distinguish between the target population and the accessible population in planning a sampling strategy. The *target population* refers to the popula-

tion that the researcher wishes to study, the population about which the researcher wishes to make a generalization. The *accessible population* is that aggregate that meets the criteria for inclusion in the study and that is available to the investigator. Because investigators rarely have access to the entire target population, the population that is actually studied usually differs from the target population on one or more characteristics. Although the target population for a study might be the United States population of women giving birth in birthing rooms, the accessible population is likely to be restricted to a more limited geographic area such as a single city or region. Implications of the differences between the target population and the accessible population will be discussed later in this chapter.

A *sample* is a subset of the population of interest, for example, every tenth woman, every third preschooler, or every other sleep epoch. A *sampling unit* is the entity used for selecting the sample, for example, the United States population of women, a specific group of preschoolers, or a night's collection of sleep epochs. The nature of the study sampling unit may alter the generalizability of the results. If the investigator studies only those women treated for breast cancer at a teaching hospital, the sample probably will be quite different in many ways from a sample of women treated at small community hospitals lacking university affiliations. Women treated at the teaching hospital are likely to be sicker: they may have been referred for specialty treatment from practices that treat less seriously ill patients. As a result, the research findings from this sample may not

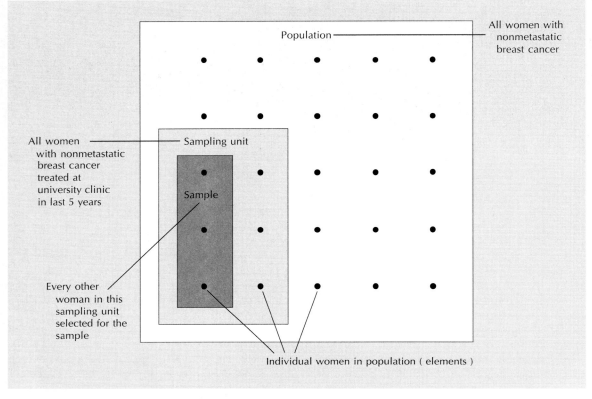

Fig. 7-1. Relationships between the population, sampling unit, and elements in the sample.

TABLE 7-1. Relationship between population, sample, sampling unit, and element

POPULATION	SAMPLING UNIT	ELEMENT
All adult women	U.S. population of all adult women	1 woman
All preschoolers	Selected preschools	1 preschooler
All epochs of sleep	Night's collection of epochs	1 epoch

resemble those from a population of women who are treated in community hospitals. It is often desirable and not unusual to select several sampling units (e.g., several clinics or several neighborhoods). By using several sampling units the investigator decreases the homogeneity of the sample, that is, makes the sample more heterogeneous, and usually increases the generalizability of the results to a broader population.

An *element* is the most basic unit of the population about which information can be collected, for example, one woman, one preschooler, or a single epoch of sleep. Although the sampling element is frequently a person, it may also be an animal, a group, a family, an organization, or an observation. An investigator interested in studying sleep may study a sample of sleep epochs occurring during the course of the night. In this example the sample consists of observations rather than individuals or animals. An investigator studying community health nursing might sample communities from populations of communities rather than sampling individuals within a community.

The relationships between population, sample, sampling unit, and element can be seen in Table 7-1. To illustrate further the relationships between these concepts, consider the following example. The investigator has selected a target population of women with nonmetastic breast cancer. The sampling unit for the study is a clinical practice at a teaching hospital. The element is each woman. The sample consists of every second woman in the practice who has been treated for breast cancer during the last 5 years (Fig. 7-1).

SPECIFYING THE POPULATION

One of the earliest challenges facing the investigator in sampling is specification of the population to be studied. Several considerations guide the decision: (1) the problem and the purpose of the study, (2) the study design, and (3) the accessibility of the potential participants of interest.

The *problem statement* and purpose of the study usually imply the people or things to whom the results of the study are expected to be applicable. The investigator plans carefully to include those individuals in whom the phenomenon of interest can be studied. For example, if the study addresses the impact of a community health nursing intervention program on the rates of adolescent pregnancy, the population to be studied must be composed of adolescents who are at risk of pregnancy.

The study design is another important consideration in selecting a population. An investigator studying patients' responses to preparation for threatening events such as surgery will need to specify a population of individuals who are anticipating surgery and who will have the opportunity to participate in the preparation being studied. Investigators use sampling criteria to exclude characteristics that may confound study results or to facilitate control for these confounding variables in the analysis. If age were a variable likely to alter the relationship between preparation for childbirth and adaptation to parenthood, the investigator might choose only women in their early twenties to participate in the study in order to control for the influence of age on the relationship being studied. On the other hand, the investigator might wish purposely to include women who range in age from 20 to 40 so that the influence of preparation for childbirth and adaptation to parenthood could be studied across several age groups.

Another consideration is the investigator's access to the potential participants for the study. In nursing, investigators frequently concern themselves with special populations, for example, those undergoing open-heart surgery or those chronically ill with arthritis. In some instances the best access to individuals is through health-care agency records such as those of hospitals or community health clinics. Selecting individuals with special health problems or concerns from the community at large may be impractical because it may require screening thousands of individuals to find one person who meets the study criteria. The sample selected from a health-care setting, however, may reflect those people treated for a health-care problem in some special way. It is important to realize that these individuals have access to care and thus may not resemble the individuals with arthritis who are not being treated or they may resemble a very special subset of people receiving care for arthritis at a university teaching hospital (Fig. 7-2). Nevertheless, these approaches to accessing a sample may be quite defensible given the nonfeasible alternatives.

Once the investigator has identified the potential population for the study, he or she will need to stipulate carefully the inclusion and exclusion criteria. These criteria are important guidelines for considering each possible sampling element. Typically the inclusion criteria specify those characteristics required for each element of the sample, for example, a certain age range. Likewise, excluding some potential participants is often desirable to control or eliminate characteristics that would interfere with interpreting the results of the study. For example, an investigator interested in adaptation following a myocardial infarction may wish to concentrate only on those individuals who have experienced their first myocardial infarction and exclude those who have had previous attacks.

In a study of mothers' health beliefs and use of well-baby services among a high-risk population, investigators explored experiences of poor and minority women (Kviz, Dawkins, & Ervin, 1985).

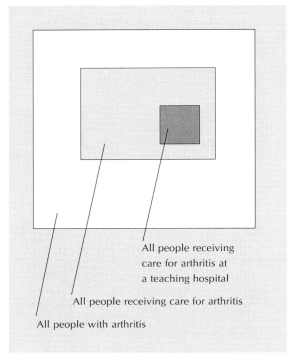

All people receiving
care for arthritis at
a teaching hospital

All people receiving care for arthritis

All people with arthritis

Fig. 7-2. Relationships between the population of all people with arthritis, all people receiving care for arthritis, and the sample obtained from a teaching hospital.

They studied 61 clients attending a maternal child health clinic located in a predominantly black, low-income, inner-city community. A large proportion of the clients were unmarried adolescents. The investigators clearly specified the inclusion and exclusion criteria.

Mothers were identified for eligibility as subjects by a clinic record audit according to the following criteria: (a) first-time (primiparous) mother, (b) absence of chronic disease, (c) no history of congenital health problems, and (d) normal progress during pregnancy. Once selected for the study, mother-child dyads were eliminated from continued participation if: (a) the mother had a complicated delivery, (b) the mother had multiple births, (c) the mother or child became serious-ly ill or injured during the study period, (d) the pair changed residence to outside the clinic's service area, (e) the mother and child became separated, or (f) the moth-er or child died during the study period. These eligibil-

ity criteria were imposed to avoid potential confound-ing influences of relatively atypical concomitant circum-stances that might be related to mothers' health beliefs and/or health behaviors. Also, subjects were limited to first-time mothers to eliminate potential effects of pre-vious parenting experiences. (Kviz, Dawkins, & Ervin, 1985)

The following excerpt describes the extent to which the accessible population, as reflected in the actual sample that was studied, resembled the target population.

All the mothers were black and ranged in age from 14 to 25, with a median age of 18; most (78.6%) were less than 20 years old. None of the mothers reported their marital status as married and living with a spouse. Almost all (98.2%) had never been married, while the others reported themselves as separated. Almost all (96.6%) were unemployed and most (58.9%) mothers were attending school. The median annual household income reported by the mothers was $5000. (Kviz, Dawkins, & Ervin, 1985)

In summary, specifying the population involves consideration of the problem statement, study design, and access to participants. The inclusion and exclusion criteria detail the characteristics required for each element of the sample.

PURPOSES OF SAMPLING

In most situations the investigator's primary concern in selecting a sample from a population is whether the individuals (or elements) who make up the sample will possess the characteristics to be studied and will be representative of the population of interest. To achieve representativeness, investigators select sampling strategies that enhance the generalizability of the research results. The primary motivation in selecting a sample for some studies is to obtain find-ings that can be applied to the population that inter-ests the investigator. Sampling strategies permit an investigator to measure or control some characteris-tics from a subset of all possible observations in ways that ensure a close approximation of measurements that would have been obtained had all possible observations been studied.

An investigator rarely has access to all possible observations. Even if total access were possible, studying every possible observation probably would be impractical because of time and expense. Sampling strategies ideally allow the investigator to maximize the representativeness of the observations while minimizing the cost of the sampling process.

In some cases, however, the investigator is not concerned with the generalizability of the results. Instead, the investigator's goal may be to describe the sample, not to generalize the results beyond the sample. Sometimes the investigator must choose between gathering detailed information from a nonrepresentative sample or gathering less detailed information from a representative sample. For example, an investigator studying the influence of high-technology care in the home on the family's functioning and coping might choose to study a few families in which one member in the home is ventilator dependent. The investigator could study these families intensively, gathering a great deal of information from each family member as opposed to gathering superficial information from a representative sample of families.

In some instances, an investigator is interested in studying specific individuals or groups that, for some reason, are very unusual. For example, the investigator might select individuals because they have had a particularly favorable response to treatment or because they are atypical, such as extremely healthy individuals who have been exposed to extremely unhealthy conditions. These unusual individuals are not representative of the total population, and for just that reason they may be particularly informative. Next we will explore the array of options available to investigators.

SAMPLING STRATEGIES

Several sampling strategies are available for application in nursing research. Generally, these sampling strategies can be classified as either probability or nonprobability sampling strategies.

Probability sampling

A characteristic of *probability samples* is that every element in the population has a known, nonzero probability of being included in the sample. The researcher using probability sampling can estimate the probability of each element of the population being included in the sample, hence the name. The goal of probability sampling is to ensure that the sample represents the population of interest. Probability sampling procedures involve some form of random selection in choosing the sampling elements. This approach maximizes the representativeness of the sample, minimizes the risk of gross distortion of estimates for the target population, allows the investigator to estimate sampling error, and permits the appropriate use of inferential statistics. In probability sampling each element has an equal chance of selection. Because the elements are selected at random, the risk of overrepresentation or underrepresentation of certain subsets of the population generally will be minimized. As a result, estimates based on data from the sample should accurately reflect the value for the population.

Probability sampling procedures allow an investigator to estimate a characteristic of the population from the sample, for example, the mean or median temperature and pulse in newborns. The investigator cannot measure the values of blood pressure and pulse for every newborn; instead, estimates of the parameter (population value) are made from the statistics for the sample. The investigator ultimately wishes to infer the parameter of pulse or blood pressure for the population from the statistics for the sample. The parameters for the population are the theoretically "true" values that are inferred from statistics obtained from the sample.

The process of *inferential statistics* allows the investigator to infer the value for the whole population, based on the information for the sample. Thus the mean for a sample *(M)* is an estimate of the population mean (μ); the sample variance *(s)* is an estimate of the population variance (σ) (Fig. 7-3).

Sample statistics best approximate the population parameters when the sample is representative of the population. Thus, the more different the sample from the target population, the less accurate will be the estimates of the true population parameter. Bias refers to the difference between the true but unknown value for the population and its estimate based on data from the sample:

Bias = True, unknown value − Sample estimate

Bias is indirectly proportional to the validity of the estimate. The smaller the bias, the greater the validity of the estimate.

Probability sampling also permits the investigator to estimate the *sampling error*, that is, the tendency

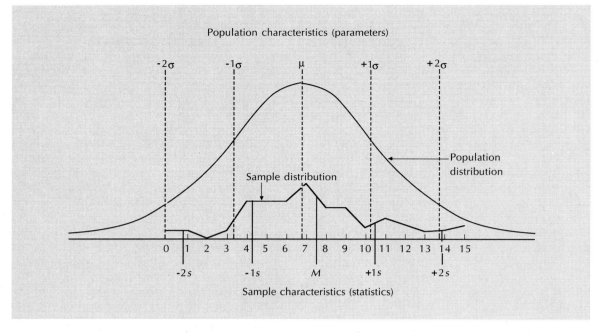

Fig. 7-3. The sample statistics are estimates of the population parameters. *M* is the sample mean, which approximates the population mean μ. The variance of the sample (standard deviations labeled *s*) approximates the population variance (standard deviations labeled σ).

for statistical estimates to fluctuate from one sample to the next. The reproducibility of the estimate on subsequent sampling of the population reflects the *reliability* of the estimate (Fig. 7-4). The standard error of the estimate can be computed as an indicator of the reliability of the estimate. The smaller the standard error of the estimate, the more reliable will be the estimate. The *standard error of the mean* reflects the magnitude of the standard or average sampling error. The standard error of the mean is computed by

$$S_{\bar{x}} = \frac{\text{SD}}{\sqrt{n}}$$

where *SD* is the standard deviation of the sample, *n* is the sample size, and $S_{\bar{x}}$ is the standard error of the mean. For a sample of 200 with a standard deviation of 20, the standard error of the mean would be 1.43. For a sample of 20 with a standard deviation of 20, the standard error of the mean would be 4.5. The smaller the standard error, the less variable is the

sample mean, and the more accurate is the mean as an estimate of the population value.

Although probability sampling is desirable to achieve generalizability of results, it is important to recognize that bias is still possible and typical because of deviations from probability sampling procedures. Bias does occur even when probability sampling procedures are used, for example, when elements with certain characteristics, such as people too ill to participate in clinical studies or those who believe they are too busy to participate in a telephone survey, are excluded systematically.

Keeping in mind the features of probability sampling, we will now focus on sampling strategies used to obtain a probability sample. These include simple random sampling, systematic sampling, stratified sampling, and cluster sampling.

Simple random sampling

The *simple random sample* is the most basic type of probability sample. Selecting the simple random sample is a strategy that ensures that each element in

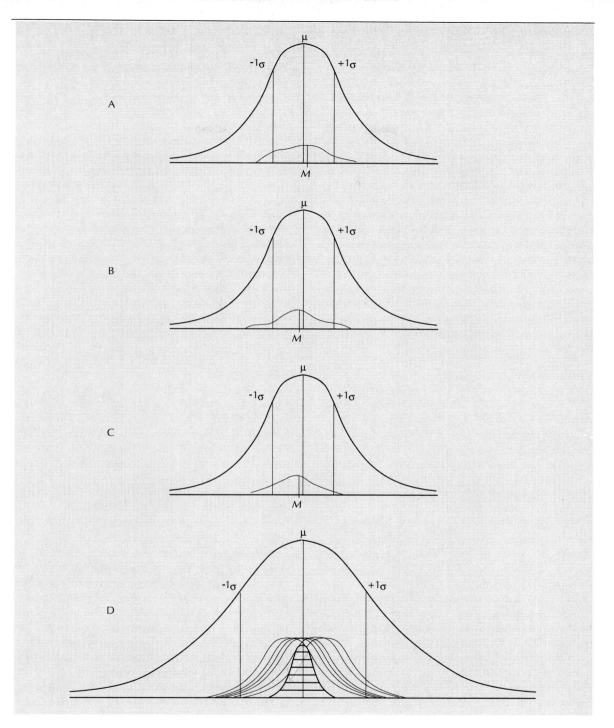

Fig. 7-4. Multiple samples vary in reliability for estimating the population parameters. In **A**, the sample mean *(M)* is higher than the population mean *(μ)*, whereas in samples **B** and **C** the sample mean is lower. **D** shows how when many samples are averaged together, the sampling mean approaches the population mean, thereby reducing sampling error. From *Reasoning with statistics,* 2nd ed., by Frederick Williams. ©, 1979, 1968, by Holt, Reinhart, & Winston. Reprinted with permission from Holt, Reinhart, & Winston, Inc.

the population has the same likelihood of being selected as any other.

After the investigator specifies the target population and inclusion and exclusion criteria, the next step is to develop the sampling frame for the study. The *sampling frame* is an enumeration list of each element of the population from which the sample will be selected. Developing the sampling frame involves identifying each possible element, for example, every household resident in a neighborhood, every patient discharged from a state-sponsored psychiatric facility during a specified time period, or every person enrolled in a health maintenance organization. The investigator prepares the sampling frame by listing each individual and assigning each a consecutive identification number (see box on facing page). Using a table of random numbers found in most statistics and sampling textbooks (see box on facing page), the investigator randomly selects a starting place in the table of random numbers. The starting place can be identified by simply closing your eyes and placing your pencil on the page. The number under the pencil will be the starting point.

Suppose you wished to select 20 of the 50 individuals whose names are given in the box. Using the two-digit combinations of numbers from the table, the investigator would begin at the starting point and read the table in any direction. As a number between 1 and 50 is encountered, the individual assigned to that number on the enumeration list is selected for inclusion in the sample.

Reading across row 1, the first number in the table of random numbers is 46, corresponding to Turner, M; the second number is 29, corresponding to Nelson, H; the third, 50, corresponding to Zborowski, F. The investigator continues in this manner until twenty individuals have been selected from the enumeration list. In this way a subset of elements is identified for inclusion in the sample. Using the enumeration list of clinic patients and the table of random numbers as illustrated, the investigator's sample would be comprised of those individuals whose numbers are circled.

Systematic sampling

A *systematic random sample* is achieved by selecting every *k*th case from an enumeration of all elements. Instead of selecting elements strictly in random order, the investigator begins sampling at one point, selected at random, and proceeds to select every sec-

ond, fifth, or *k*th element. The size of the interval, *k*, is a function of

$$k = \frac{N}{n}$$

where *k* is the interval, *N* is the size of the population available for study, and *n* is the desired sample size. When the population is large relative to the desired sample size, *k* will be large. When the population is small relative to the desired sample size, *k* will be small. Thus a population size of 2000 from which 50 elements will be selected will yield an interval (*k*) of 40. By contrast, for a population of 60 with a desired sample of 20, the interval for selection is 3.

The systematic sampling technique is appropriate when the elements are arranged in an order that would not introduce some bias in the selection process. For example bias could occur in a list of married couples in which the husband's name always preceded the wife's name. The investigator who selected every second element could select a list comprised entirely of either men or women.

The systematic sample also can be considered a *nonprobability sample* (a sample for which it is not possible to estimate the probability of each element being included) when every element does not have the same chance of being selected. For example, studying every third college student who comes into the student health service would not give the investigator a random sample of all students who attend a university, but it could yield a random sample of students who use the health services if a random start were used.

Sometimes it is not possible to enumerate in advance each element in the sampling frame, for example, all the people being admitted to an emergency room as a result of motor vehicle accidents. An investigator could choose every third patient admitted as a result of such accidents, but a systematic random sampling could not be applied without an enumeration of the total population. Nevertheless, this can be a useful strategy for sampling, and it can produce results similar to random sampling approaches provided a random start also is used.

Stratified sampling

Stratified random sampling is a type of sampling in which the investigator first divides the population into subgroups called "strata" and then obtains a random sample from within each stratum. The aim of

TABLE OF RANDOM NUMBERS APPLIED TO AN ENUMERATION LIST

Underlined numbers are those between 1 and 50 chosen to select the sample of 20 from the 50 elements in the sampling unit. Circled numbers on the enumeration list are those chosen by using the table of random numbers.

Excerpt from a table of random numbers

82	<u>46</u>	73	<u>29</u>	<u>50</u>	54	53	67	90	99	74	<u>21</u>	<u>25</u>	<u>17</u>	<u>19</u>
88	73	89	66	55	<u>38</u>	72	<u>47</u>	90	<u>27</u>	<u>24</u>	<u>36</u>	96	74	<u>25</u>
<u>25</u>	96	<u>43</u>	<u>33</u>	57	96	<u>25</u>	95	73	<u>46</u>	58	<u>25</u>	57	68	52
<u>33</u>	<u>23</u>	56	94	72	56	<u>39</u>	<u>50</u>	63	92	<u>07</u>	<u>08</u>	<u>36</u>	56	<u>23</u>
82	<u>09</u>	<u>16</u>	06	23	74	77	09	03	52	44	25	36	74	98

Enumeration list

1. Abbot, P	26. Madsen, D
2. Ackerman, W	(27.) Milbank, S
3. Ainsley, H	28. Neary, D
4. Beardsley, G	(29.) Nelson, H
5. Buckley, R	30. Olson, O
6. Cassill, D	31. Owens, A
(7.) Clark, A	32. Park, M
(8.) Darrow, M	(33.) Porter, S
(9.) Donaldson, G	34. Powell, P
10. Emery, E	35. Quinn, P
11. Evenson, W	(36.) Reagan, P
12. Ford, B	37. Rowell, R
13. Funk, F	(38.) Rice, D
14. Goodfellow, J	(39.) Sampson, S
15. Gregory, J	40. Smith, B
(16.) Haggert, S	41. Spaulding, T
(17.) Hartung, H	42. Sullivan, I
18. Ingle, T	(43.) Swanson, I
(19.) Ives, C	44. Taylor, C
20. Jennings, J	45. Thomas, P
(21.) Jones, J	(46.) Turner, M
22. Keith, K	(47.) Ulrich, S
(23.) Kellogg, C	48. Wagner, P
(24.) Lamont, C	49. Young, J
(25.) Luth, S	(50.) Zborowski, F

stratified random sampling is to ensure that sub-groups of the population are represented. For example, an investigator may desire a sample that includes both men and women. To achieve this, the investigator first divides, or stratifies, the population into strata of men and women. Next, the investigator selects elements at random from each stratum.

Stratification may be based on one or more characteristics, such as age, gender, and race. A major challenge is identifying which characteristics of the individuals in the sample to use as a basis for stratification. Often enumeration lists do not include information necessary for assigning an individual to a stratum. For example, patient rosters may only include hospital numbers and names, not the gender or race of the patient. Telephone directory listings often do not include enough information to allow the investigator to determine the gender or ethnicity of the residents.

The characteristics used to stratify the population are expected to produce homogeneity. This is simple in the case of gender, but it is considerably more challenging to stratify on the basis of a characteristic such as ethnicity because some individuals identify themselves with more than one ethnic group.

The procedure for drawing the stratified random sample involves grouping the elements into homogeneous strata and randomly selecting the desired number of elements from each stratum. The investigator may employ a table of random numbers to select the elements within the strata. Alternatively, the investigator may select the elements within each stratum by using a systematic random sampling procedure in which every *k*th element is selected.

An investigator may select a proportionately stratified or a disproportionately stratified sample. A *proportional stratified sample* could be drawn from two strata (one of men and one of women, both of whom had recent myocardial infarctions) by choosing a number of elements from the male and the female strata in proportion to their numbers in the population. For example, if 90% of the people with myocardial infarctions were male, the investigator would choose 90% of the sample from the male stratum and 10% from the female stratum.

The investigator may choose to use a *disproportional sampling strategy* in which the number of elements selected from the two strata does not reflect the proportion of males and females in the population. Because the number of elements in each stra-

tum is disproportionate to the underlying population, the investigator will find it necessary to weight the values for the strata by using a mathematical formula to estimate a parameter for the entire population. (See Fleiss, 1981, for further information about weighted estimates.) For example, the incidence of cholecystectomy is greater among women than among men. To ensure an accurate estimate of the amount of nursing-care time for the entire population of individuals recovering from cholecystectomy, the investigator would need to weight the estimate for women more heavily because they constitute a larger proportion of the population than do men.

To ensure adequate representation of individuals from differing strata in a study, an investigator may find it advantageous to use a disproportional stratified sampling strategy. For example, because the proportion of men and women having myocardial infarctions differs, the investigator who wishes to ensure adequate representation of women in a study of recovery from myocardial infarction might find it advantageous to select 10% of the men but 50% of the women who had myocardial infarctions during the last year.

The size of the sample within each stratum is guided partially by plans for analysis of the data. A particular concern is whether the number of elements in each stratum will be adequate to support the planned analysis. For example, when only a small proportion of the total sample is composed of ethnic minorities, it is difficult to cross-tabulate two variables such as stressful life events and depression because often too few individuals may be available to support the analysis. For this reason investigators anticipate the analyses to be performed within a stratum and use these to determine the minimum number of elements in each stratum.

Investigators may select a stratified sample on the basis of multiple variables such as age, gender, and ethnicity. However, the procedure for selection demands a complex database for the enumeration list, including data regarding each characteristic. In addition, finding an adequate number of elements for each stratum is difficult unless the sampling frame is very large.

Cluster sampling

Cluster sampling involves the successive random sampling of units. The first units to be sampled are the largest, followed by smaller and smaller units. Because the investigator samples successive units in several stages, this strategy is also termed "multistage sampling." Rather than studying a random sample of children from all schools, an investigator wishing to study children in school could draw a sample of schools within a region, within them randomly select classrooms, and within classrooms randomly select children. Another application of cluster sampling is selecting a random sample of the population at large. An investigator interested in studying health behaviors of a representative sample of families within a community could begin by randomly selecting census tracts within the city, then blocks of households from within the census tracts, and finally families within the household blocks. The investigator can select the clusters using stratified methods as well as random sampling procedures.

Cluster sampling is particularly useful when obtaining a complete enumeration of the elements in a population is not possible. Enumerating the entire United States population of preschool children would be impractical, but using a cluster sampling approach to identify children within census tracts, within cities, and within selected regions would help assure the representativeness of the sample of the nation's children.

Cluster sampling requires specific statistical techniques for data analysis. Moreover, because estimates based on this type of procedure have a higher sampling error than those based on simple random selection, the sample size required for cluster sampling is somewhat larger than that required for a simple random sample. (Levy & Lemeshow, 1980)

Random digit dialing is a special variation of cluster sampling. In this approach an enumeration of all possible telephone numbers is generated. First existing telephone exchanges within a geographic area of interest are enumerated. Then a computer program is used to generate all possible combinations of 4-digit numbers by which a random sample of phone numbers within randomly selected telephone exchanges is identified. This approach is used frequently for market research, and its use is becoming increasingly prevalent among health researchers. Uhl (1985) employed random digit dialing to identify elderly residents for a survey of support and health among the elderly. More detailed information about the use of random digit dialing is available (Waksberg, 1978). Examples of the application of probability sampling to health-related studies from current nursing literature are given in Table 7-2.

Nonprobability sampling

Nonprobability sampling procedures do not assure that each element in the population has the same chance for inclusion in the sample. Nevertheless, a variety of nonprobability sampling techniques are used in nursing research with sound justification for their application. First, completely enumerating all elements in a population is not always possible. Second, when it is possible, the enumeration is expensive and inconvenient. For example, an investigator needing to identify everyone living in a specific census tract cannot simply refer to a city directory, inasmuch as parts of this document may be obsolete by the time of publication. Instead, the investigator would need to identify every individual living in each household.

Another justification for using nonprobability sampling techniques is the rarity or unpredictability of the phenomenon being studied. To illustrate, so few individuals experience coma each year that the likelihood of being able to select them randomly for study is low. Moreover, anticipating the occurrence of some of the phenomena nurses study is difficult. Studying trauma in persons as they are admitted to an emergency room precludes the creation of an enumeration list before selection of the sample.

Convenience sampling

The *convenience sample* is obtained by accessing individuals who are easy to identify and contact. An investigator might recruit volunteers from a day-care center, clinic, or university by handing out questionnaires to individuals who use these facilities during a specified period of time. Sometimes a special technique called "snowballing" is useful: the investigator asks the first participant to refer friends to the study, and these new participants are asked to recruit their friends, and so on. Convenience sampling is commonly used despite the fact that the available subjects might be atypical of the population with respect to the phenomena being studied. For example, patients who are accessible to an investigator for a study of preoperative teaching may differ from all preoperative patients in certain characteristics that also may influence their responses to preoperative teaching. Convenience sampling is particularly useful for studies of phenomena seemingly homogeneous with respect to the characteristic being studied. Usually the phenomena nurses study are quite heterogeneous, making the choice of this strategy less desirable. Nevertheless, there are situations in which no

TABLE 7-2. Application of probability sampling strategies

SAMPLE TYPE	ARTICLE USING SAMPLE TYPE	DESCRIPTION OF SAMPLING PROCEDURE
Simple Random Sample	Walsh, V. (1985). Health beliefs and practices of runners vs. nonrunners. *Nursing Research, 34,* 353-356.	A sample of 150 runners was drawn at random from the membership of a running club. A comparative sample of 150 students enrolled in a university was chosen at random.
Systematic Random Sample	Woods, N. (1985). Self-care practices among young adult married women. *Research in Nursing and health, 8,* 227-233.	A systematic random sample of married women between 20 and 40 years of age was selected from a population of women clients at a family health clinic.
Stratified Sample	Chapman, D., & Holzemer, W. (1985). College choice among prospective health professions majors: Implications for nursing education. *Research in Nursing and Health, 8,* 339-346.	Questionnaires were administered to graduating seniors in a stratified random sample of all high schools in New York. Stratification was by geographical region, urban/suburban/rural location, and district expenditure per pupil.
Cluster Sample	Ryder, S. M. (1985). Environmental support for autonomy among the institutionalized elderly. *Research in Nursing and Health, 8,* 363-371.	Four nursing homes were chosen randomly from proprietary facilities in the Minneapolis area. The target was a random sample of 120 residents, 15 of these on intermediate care and 15 on skilled care in each facility.

reasonable alternative exists. Aside from saving time, money, and effort, little else can be said for convenience sampling because it neither contributes to generalizability of the findings nor ensures a full array of responses.

Quota sampling

Quota sampling is useful to ensure adequate representation of underlying groups within the population, such as age and ethnic groups. Quota sampling requires knowledge of the structure of the population being studied. The investigator uses knowledge about the composition of the population to specify a certain desired number of participants (quota) from each of several segments of the population.

The variable used to define the strata in quota sampling is the one that, according to the investigator, would influence the variable being estimated, or the dependent variable. An investigator studying several cardiac rehabilitation programs could enhance the representativeness of the sample by studying a quota of individuals from programs selected because they vary in some way thought to influence cardiac function in response to exercise. For example, some may encourage more vigorous exercise than others.

The major difference between the quota sample and the stratified random sample is that elements are not randomly selected in the strata of a quota sample. Although quota sampling introduces the same biases as convenience sampling and the selection process is similar, this approach increases the representativeness of the sample of the underlying population.

Purposive sampling

The *purposive sample,* also known as a *judgmental sample,* is one in which the investigator handpicks the cases based on a judgment of the extent to which the potential participants meet the selection criteria. In some instances the investigator may wish to interview individuals who reflect different ends of the range of a particular characteristic, as for example, very young and very old individuals who receive nursing care from the same home health-care agency. In other instances, the investigator may judge that certain individuals have special information about the experience of certain segments of the community or about certain health-related experiences. For example, the investigator may wish to obtain information about a new nursing-care clinic from potential clients and from potential professionals in the referral network. In another case, the investigator may wish to select individuals who have extremely good responses to a health-promotion regimen and contrast them with individuals who have extremely poor responses to the same regimen.

The *Delphi method* is used when an investigator wishes to sample experts who have special knowledge about the phenomenon being studied. Purposive sampling is often used with the Delphi method. In this method several rounds of questionnaires are sent to experts to elicit their opinions. The investigator analyzes data from the questionnaires after each round and provides feedback about the preceding round to the participants. The Delphi method provides a means of achieving experts' consensus about an issue.

The five types of cases selected for purposive sampling are (1) extreme or deviant cases, (2) typical cases, (3) those with maximum variation, (4) critical cases, and (5) politically important or sensitive cases (Patton, 1980). Extreme or deviant cases are sought when information is desired about particularly troublesome or enlightening instances of the phenomenon. For example, to describe the impact of diagnostic related groups (DRGs) on nursing care, the researcher may want to select a sample from a nursing unit that has experienced problems as a result of the prospective payment system and a sample from a unit that has found the new system advantageous. Typical cases are important to include so that the findings of the study are not dismissed as representing only the extreme, unusual, or deviant perspective. In the example of DRGs, it is important to sample those hospitals that represent the typical experience of nursing units using DRGs. Selecting a sample for maximum variation of factors believed to influence the subject of study will increase confidence in common patterns that cut across categories. The investigator studying DRGs may sample along a continuum of age of staff, educational background of administrators, the types of patient diagnosis, and the institution's previous experience with change. Sampling critical cases permits the maximum application of information to other cases by pointing out that something that is true in this particular case is likely to be true in other cases. If DRGs have positive outcomes on a nursing unit known to provide leadership for the remainder of the hospital, sampling from that unit may give the investigator a good idea of what is likely to follow from other nursing units in that hospital. Sampling important or sensitive cases is a way of attracting attention to the study. If, for example, media attention has been given recently to early and apparently inappropriate discharge of elderly patients, inclusion of nursing units with a high percentage of elderly clients may provide data to support or refute media claims about the adverse effects of DRGs on the elderly.

A limitation of the purposive sampling approach is that it is impossible to assess the representativeness of the individuals who participate. Nevertheless, this approach is defensible when the investigator is not concerned with the typical experience of the population but is more concerned with understanding the experiences of special segments of the population. Examples of nonprobability sampling techniques as applied in contemporary nursing research are included in Table 7-3.

A comparison of probability and nonprobability sampling

When probability sampling techniques are used correctly, the probability sample is most representative of the underlying population, because bias in population estimates is minimized, and the sampling error can be estimated. Probability sampling makes it possible for the investigator to use inferential statistics correctly. On the other hand, nonprobability sampling procedures tend to be less expensive and require less time than probability sampling techniques. For example, the creation of complete enumeration lists of a population is very time consuming, inconvenient, and sometimes impossible. Finally, probability sampling can only ensure representativeness in the sample selection process; it has little

TABLE 7-3. Examples of nonprobability sampling

SAMPLE TYPE	ARTICLE USING SAMPLE TYPE	DESCRIPTION OF SAMPLING PROCEDURE
Convenience Sample	Magilvy, J. (1985). Experiencing hearing loss in later life: A comparison of deaf and hearing impaired older women. *Research in Nursing and Health, 8,* 3245-353.	Populations from a center on deafness, two speech and hearing centers, two audiology practices, and several senior residences were the sources for the convenience sample of 66 women.
Quota Sample	Hilbert, G. (1985). Spouse support and myocardial infarction. *Nursing Research, 34,* 217-220.	The sample of 60 convalescing male patients with myocardial infarction and their wives was drawn from those who had attended or were attending one of three cardiac rehabilitation programs, a private exercise program and two programs associated with large metropolitan hospitals. Twenty patients from each program, including 10 who were active and 10 who stopped attending, were studied.

effect on participation. The most carefully drawn probability sample provides no guarantee against bias caused by selective participation of individuals from the population.

CHOOSING THE SAMPLING PLAN

Investigators consider several criteria in selecting a sampling plan for a study, including accuracy, cost, and feasibility. *Accuracy* refers to the reliability and validity of the estimates obtained from the sample. The *reliability* of an estimate of a population parameter refers to how reproducible it is likely to be over repetitions of the sampling process. Reliability is reflected in the standard error of an estimate, with the smaller standard error indicating higher reliability. The validity of the estimate refers to the extent to which it differs from the true value of the population. Bias reflects the difference between the true value and the value obtained from the sample. The smaller the bias, the greater the validity of the estimate. Ideally, investigators choose a sampling plan that maximizes the reliability and validity of estimates of the phenomena under study.

Cost and feasibility are both important considerations. Ideally the investigator chooses the sampling plan that maximizes accuracy and allows completion within the limits of the budget for the project. Ele-

gant sampling plans that maximize accuracy may not be feasible. Balancing accuracy with cost and feasibility is the central challenge in choosing a sampling approach.

IMPLEMENTING THE SAMPLING PLAN

Implementing the sampling plan in studies with human participants requires several processes: (1) enumerating the elements of the sampling unit, (2) identifying the elements of the sample, (3) contacting the individuals in the sample, and (4) assessing the sampling approach.

Enumerating the elements

Most probability sampling approaches require the identification or enumeration of elements in the population being studied. The investigator must generate or obtain an enumeration list, often referred to as a sampling frame, for each sampling unit in the study. Enumerating the elements creates a special challenge for investigators studying clinical populations. Although investigators easily can obtain names of individuals from clinical rosters, medical record reviews, or lists of people admitted to health-care facilities, frequently they encounter difficulties associated with these enumeration sources, such as incomplete databases and missing medical records.

Further, the investigator must obtain permission from the clinical agency for access to health records and must sign an assurance that any information gleaned from these records will remain confidential.

In studies of individuals in community settings, investigators might use city directories or telephone books, but these sources usually are incomplete because of problems such as unlisted telephone numbers and transience of residents in neighborhoods. Nearly complete identification and enumeration of all elements in the population is possible only with techniques, such as those used by the United States Census Bureau, in which detailed protocols are established for contacting households at varying times of the day and on varying days of the week.

Random digit dialing is one technique that affords a random sample of all possible households with telephones and yields complete enumeration of all the possible telephone numbers within a given telephone exchange. One problem associated with random digit dialing is that an exchange may cover a geographic area larger than that from which the investigator may wish to draw the sample. In addition, some telephone exchanges contain business numbers rather than household numbers almost exclusively. Complete enumeration of all the elements in the population is not an easy task regardless of the method the investigator uses or the population of interest.

Regardless of the source, the investigator must consider several questions in evaluating the enumeration list. The first consideration is the completeness of the list. What systematic omissions, such as individuals without telephones, will influence the study findings and generalizability? Will individuals who are very ill or socially disadvantaged be overlooked and what are the implications of their exclusion? Second, the investigator considers what proportion of the population will be missed by this enumeration method. Will only a small fraction be omitted or will a sizable proportion be omitted? If an investigator obtains a sample through telephoning households, what percentage of households lack telephones? Third, the investigator considers the possibility of any systematic ordering of the enumeration list. For example, the list may be ordered by age or gender in such a way that individuals with special characteristics are more likely to be selected than others. This concern is especially important when using a system-atic sampling strategy in which alternate names may be associated with one gender or age group. Fourth, the investigator considers whether any unusual circumstances may influence the enumeration list. Is the list likely to be affected by events that are linked to certain seasons or days of the week? Events such as emergency room admissions for trauma are linked closely to social activities related to day of the week, and infectious diseases can be associated with seasons of the year. Both of these factors may affect an enumeration list obtained for special days of the week or seasons of the year. Finally, the investigator considers the extent to which the potential participants on the enumeration list resemble the population of interest to the study. Will the use of the enumeration list generated by random digit dialing really yield a population of individuals with low incomes? Will the listing obtained from a university teaching hospital really provide information about the average woman's labor and delivery experiences? All these considerations are significant if the investigator is to be assured of having a fairly representative sample of the population desired.

Identifying the elements for the sample

After the investigator has identified the population of interest, specified inclusion and exclusion criteria, and enumerated the elements of the sampling unit, the next challenge is choosing the elements or potential participants. Random selection of individuals from an enumeration list can be obtained most readily by numbering each element and using a table of random numbers to select the elements to be included in the sample. Alternatively, the investigator can use a systematic random sampling strategy. In this case, the investigator simply chooses a name at random from the entire listing and then selects every kth name from the enumeration list for inclusion in the study.

Contacting the sample

The investigator may contact potential participants in one of several ways, most commonly through personal contact, the telephone, or the mail. Each of these approaches has relative advantages and disadvantages. Usually participants respond most readily to personal contact, such as in a home interview, while the telephone approach and the mailed questionnaire yield respectively lower response rates. Clearly the cost of contacting the potential participants varies with the approach. Usually the personal contact is most expensive, followed by the telephone contact and the mailed questionnaire. These issues are discussed in more detail in later chapters addressing questionnaires and interviews (see Chapters 18 and 19).

When the investigator is studying individuals whose names have been released through a health-care agency, using an intermediary to make initial contact is customary. The intermediary is an individual who normally has access to the names of the individuals in the sample and can ask the prospective participants for their permission to be contacted by the investigator. The investigator then has access only to individuals who agree to have their names released to the study personnel. The investigator subsequently is responsible for interpreting the study to the potential participants and for obtaining their consent to participate.

Assessing the sampling approach

After the participants are entered in the study, the investigator assesses the extent to which the sampling approach produced a representative sample. The investigator can compare the characteristics of the sample with other known values for the population of interest. For example, are the participants better educated, more economically advantaged, or healthier than the population of interest? One alternative for the investigator is to compare the sample with the population characteristics described by other investigators or experts in the field. For example, do the elderly nursing-home residents in one study resemble those in another study with respect to the value they place on personal control over activities of daily living? Another alternative is to collect data from those individuals who chose not to respond to the study. An investigator using a clinical enumeration list might be able to obtain permission to review records of individuals who chose not to participate in an interview. Alternatively, the investigator could ask those individuals who chose not to participate to complete an abbreviated interview or questionnaire describing demographic characteristics or other information of particular interest to the investigator. The approaches outlined here do not repair bias that is created in selecting participants or in the selective participation of individuals, but they do afford the investigator some data that allows inferences about the biases.

ESTIMATING SAMPLE SIZE

Estimating sample size is an important consideration in any investigation. Investigators ultimately must weigh the reliability of the population estimates associated with the sampling approach with the cost of studying the sample.

General guidelines

In general, the larger the sample size, the more likely it is that estimates of the population parameters will be reliable. Larger samples permit randomness to work in offsetting any error that may occur in representing the population with smaller samples. Size alone, however, does not guarantee representativeness. A very large sample can underrepresent segments of the population, such as certain economic groups or individuals who are not well enough to participate in a study. Simply gathering data from more people will not eradicate the bias of ignoring the poor or ill.

In addition to the general guideline of maximizing sample size to maximize reliability, there are other important considerations. When estimating sample size, the investigator considers the purpose of the study, homogeneity of the phenomenon being studied, and the proposed study design. The investigator assesses the precision required by the purpose of the study. Is it necessary to generate a precise estimate of the phenomenon, or can a large degree of error be tolerated? Little error can be tolerated when very precise estimates are necessary, for example, an estimate of the amount of blood that must be withdrawn from a premature infant to obtain accurate electrolyte levels without compromising the blood volume of the infant. In this instance the investigator would be concerned with maximizing the sample size to minimize the error in the estimate.

In addition, the investigator considers the homogeneity or heterogeneity of the phenomenon being studied. If the parameter being studied is relatively homogeneous, such as the potassium level in a rat bred for homogeneity and housed under controlled conditions, studying a large number of rats is not necessary. Moreover, when the parameter is believed to be quite homogeneous, such as in the specially bred strain of rats, sampling procedures such as those described in this chapter are unnecessary for selecting the rats to be studied. Similarly, if the parameter in humans is likely to be quite homogeneous, such as diurnal temperature patterns in healthy newborns during their first day of life, the sample size required for the study would be very small and probability sampling procedures would be unnecessary. However, humans are notoriously heterogeneous, and the nature of many of the parameters that nurses investigate is highly variable. Consequently, investigators must consider how variable the phenomena are. Health values, blood pressure, mental status, speed of recovery from trauma, and pain are parameters that are likely to be quite heterogeneous in humans. In general, studies of homogeneous phenomena require smaller samples than studies of heterogeneous phenomena.

Investigators also consider the study design when determining sample size estimates. For example, the number of elements necessary for a longitudinal investigation involving intensive data collection on individuals over many years is greater than that required for a cross-sectional survey of a population studied at only one time. In this case, the longitudinal investigation requires a substantially larger sample than the cross-sectional survey. A larger sample size for the longitudinal study is essential to compensate for the anticipated number of participants who will drop out of the study over the course of many years. Unless some adjustment is made for loss of participants, the final sample size may be inadequate for the planned analyses. Certain designs, such as experimental or factorial ones, require a minimum number of elements per group. Guidelines for the number of participants per group range from 10 to 30.

On the other hand, the number of informants or participants in a descriptive study designed to identify concepts, such as in a grounded theory approach, is difficult to determine in advance. Data are generated until the researcher experiences repetition of statements describing the phenomenon under study. Stern (1985) proposed that the best the investigator can do at the beginning of the study is to determine its scope and suggest a number that seems reasonable—enough but not too many.

Calculating sample size

Calculation of sample size requires consideration of (1) the amount of variance in the parameter being studied, (2) the statistical test selected and its significance criterion and power, and (3) the anticipated outcome of the study, sometimes referred to as an effect size. Let us consider each of these in turn.

Variance in the phenomenon

When a large amount of variance exists in the parameter being estimated, the sample size must be large in order to achieve a precise estimate. An estimate of the variance in the parameter can be obtained from results of applications of the measure previously reported in the literature or from preliminary studies conducted by the investigator. In some instances, however, no such estimates are available, and the investigator is faced with the necessity of making an estimate independently, based optimally on a trial of the measure with a sample from a population similar to that being studied. The variance in the parameter is a function of both true variance in the population value and measurement error. The presence of measurement error, whether the result of unreliable electronic equipment, observer fatigue, or poor psychometric properties of scales, reduces the precision of sample estimates because it increases the variability of the observations beyond their true variability (Cohen, 1969).

Some formulas for calculating sample size require the investigator to estimate the anticipated variance of the phenomenon within the sampling unit and the amount of sampling error that can be tolerated. These formulas are derived from the relationship

$$\text{Sampling error} = \frac{\text{Variability of the parameter}}{\sqrt{\text{Size of the sample}}}$$

Sampling error is represented in these formulas by the standard error, and the variability of the parameter is represented by the estimated standard deviation for the phenomenon. The investigator specifies the sampling error based on the precision of the estimate required for the study. The greater the sampling error that can be tolerated, the smaller the sample size that is needed. Other formulas for calculating sample size are based on consideration of the statistical test, the desired significance level and power associated with the test, and the anticipated effect size.

Statistical test

Cohen (1977) has generated a collection of tables for estimating sample size for a variety of statistical tests. The sample size estimates in the tables are based on consideration of the significance level and the power associated with the test and the anticipated effect size.

Significance level. The *significance level* (sometimes referred to as a significance criterion or *p* value) represents the probability that the investigator mistakenly will reject the null hypothesis (an assertion that no difference exists between variables); in other words, the investigator will infer a statistically significant difference or association exists when, in fact, it does not. The smaller the *p* value selected by the investigator, the stronger the evidence needed to reject the null hypothesis in favor of the alternative. If the investigator selects a *p* value of .01, the risk of false rejection of the null hypothesis is lower than if a *p* value of .05 is used. (See also Chapter 26.)

Power. The *power of a statistical test of a null hypothesis* is the probability that the test will lead to the rejection of the null hypothesis. The power of a statistical test refers to its ability to detect small but important findings, such as differences or associations. Statistical power refers to the value $1 - B$ where B is the probability of *type II error*, the probability of failing to reject the null hypothesis when the effect really exists.

One cannot maximize the chance of rejecting the null hypothesis when it is false and at the same time maximize the likelihood of detecting small but important effects for a given sample size. In other words, the more difficult it is to reject the null hypothesis, the easier it is to overlook a small, important finding. The power of the statistical test is inversely related to the *p* value (also referred to as the alpha level). Increasing the sample size makes it easier to detect small, important effects and to reject the null hypothesis when it is false. (The concepts of significance and power are discussed in greater detail in Chapter 26.)

Effect size

A final consideration in estimating sample size is the effect size. *Effect size* refers to the magnitude of the findings, such as the degree to which the phenomenon is present in the population being studied, or the degree of departure from the null hypothesis. When the effect size is large, for example, when the degree of influence of prelabor preparation on pain during childbirth is large, the sample size necessary to detect the effect is smaller than when the effect size is small. Simply stated, when the investigator anticipates a large effect size, a smaller sample size is necessary; conversely, a suspected small effect will require a larger sample for detecting the effect.

In summary, as the sample size estimate becomes larger, both the power of the test and the ability to detect small effect sizes increase. Moreover, as the

sample size becomes larger, the ability to obtain statistically significant findings (low *p* values) becomes easier. Several formulas for estimating sample size exist, and the selection of the appropriate formula depends on the choice of statistical test and study design.

Investigators can use a variety of approaches to estimate sample size, basing their estimates on data related to the desired precision of the sample estimates and the estimated variance of the parameter or, as an alternative, basing their estimates on the estimated effect size, the choice of statistical test, and the associated significance level and power. Regardless of the approach, the investigator reviews the choice of measures, the study design, and the statistical estimate or statistical test for the study, specifies either the degree of precision required for the estimate or the significance criterion and power associated with the test, and then either calculates the sample size or refers to tables of sample size such as those in Cochran (1977), Cohen (1977), Fleiss (1981), and Levy and Lemeshow (1980).

Once the investigator has identified the desired sample size, further adjustments are necessary. The investigator needs to consider the probable participation rate of the individuals being sampled. When the sample consists of individuals who may choose to be involved in a study, the investigator needs to predict a likely response rate. For example, if the investigator anticipates that 50% of the individuals invited to participate in the study actually will do so, the size of sample drawn would need to be twice as large as the sample size estimates. Even when the sample consists of measurements on inanimate objects or animals, some adjustments must be made for missed observations or the inevitable, unanticipated glitch in data collection.

SUMMARY

In this chapter we have examined the concept of sampling, the process of selecting a subset of the population in order to obtain information regarding some phenomenon in a way that represents the entire population. Major considerations in choosing a sampling method include maximizing representativeness of the population, so that findings can be applied to the population of interest, and minimizing cost. In some cases, the purpose is to gather intensive information from a sample that may not be representative of the underlying population. Two general sampling strategies are probability and nonprobability sampling (see Table 7-4). Probability sampling strategies are those in which every element in the population has a known, nonzero probability of being included in the sample, with the goal of ensuring that the sample represents the population of interest. Procedures of selection involve some form of random selection of the sampling elements. Probability sampling methods include simple random sampling, systematic sampling, stratified sampling, and cluster sampling. Nonprobability sampling strategies such as convenience sampling, quota sampling, and purposive sampling do not require each element to have a known, nonzero probability of selection. Probability sampling strategies maximize representativeness of the sample to the underlying population but typically are more expensive and less convenient than nonprobability sampling strategies. Implementing a sampling plan involves several processes: (1) enumerating elements of the sampling unit, (2) identifying the elements for the sample, (3) contacting the prospective participants, and (4) assessing bias in the study sample. Estimating sample size requires consideration of the purpose of the study, the homogeneity of the phenomenon being studied, and the proposed study design. Larger sample sizes are necessary when the variance in the parameter being estimated is large, when the desired significance level associated with a statistical test (p value) is small, and when the effect size is small. Although larger samples increase the reliability of the data, even the largest possible sample will not eradicate bias in participation.

TABLE 7-4. Type of sample and sampling approach for probability and nonprobability samples

TYPE OF SAMPLE	SAMPLING APPROACH
PROBABILITY	Each sampling element has equal probability of selection
Simple random sample	Investigator uses random numbers or random draw to guide selection of elements
Systematic random sample	Investigator selects each kth unit from an enumeration list of the units in the population
Stratified random sample	Investigator selects elements at random within each of many mutually exclusive strata
Cluster sample	Sampling units are successively randomly sampled from larger to smaller units
NONPROBABILITY	No assurance that each element has equal probability of selection
Convenience sample	Investigator selects elements that are readily accessible
Quota sample	Investigator specifies desired number of elements from several strata of the population
Purposive sample	Investigator selects elements from carefully defined units that represent a spectrum of qualities

REFERENCES

Chapman, D., & Holzemer, W. (1985). College choice among prospective health professions majors: Implications for nursing education. *Research in Nursing and Health, 8,* 339-346.

Cochran, W. (1977). *Sampling techniques.* New York: Wiley.

Cohen, J. (1977). *Statistical power analysis for the behavioral sciences.* New York: Academic Press.

Fleiss, J. (1981). *Statistical methods for rates and proportions.* New York: Wiley.

Hilbert, G. (1985). Spouse support and myocardial infarction. *Nursing Research, 34,* 217-220.

Kish, L. (1967). *Survey sampling.* New York: Wiley.

Kviz, F., Dawkins, C., & Ervin, N. (1985). Mothers' health beliefs and use of well-baby services among a high-risk population. *Research in Nursing & Health, 8,* 381-387.

Levy, P., & Lemeshow, S. (1980). *Sampling for health professionals.* Belmont, CA.: Lifetime Learning.

Magilvy, J. (1985). Experiencing hearing loss in later life: A comparison of deaf and hearing impaired older women. *Research in Nursing and Health, 8,* 324-353.

Patton, M. Q. (1980). *Qualitative evaluation methods*. Beverly Hills, CA: Sage.

Ryder, S. M. (1985). Environmental support for autonomy among the institutionalized elderly. *Research in Nursing and Health, 8,* 363-371.

Slonim, M. (1966). *Sampling: A quick, reliable guide to practical statistics*. New York: Simon and Schuster.

Stern, P. N. (1985). Using grounded theory method in nursing research. In M. M. Leininger (Ed.), *Qualitative research methods in nursing*. Orlando: Grune & Stratton.

Uhl, J. E. (1985). *Health-related outcomes of marital status and social support among the elderly*. Unpublished doctoral dissertation, University of Utah, Salt Lake City.

Waksberg, J. (1978). Sampling methods for random digit dialing. *Journal of the American Statistical Association, 73,* 40-46.

Walsh, V. (1985). Health beliefs and practices of runners vs. nonrunners. *Nursing Research, 34,* 353-356.

Woods, N. (1985). Self-care practices among young adult married women. *Research in Nursing and Health, 8,* 227-233.

8

SELECTING A
RESEARCH DESIGN

NANCY FUGATE WOODS

The early conceptual work of a study consists of specifying a research problem, linking it to a conceptual framework constructed from earlier relevant theoretical and empirical work, and stating the purpose of the study. Whereas these activities occur in the investigator's mind, designing the study is a pivotal activity that marks the transition from the conceptual to the empirical (real world) phase of research.

In this chapter we will introduce the concept of research design and explore its functions. After examining the elements of research design, we will consider designs appropriate for different research purposes: identification of concepts and description, exploration of differences or associations, explanation and prediction, and prescription or control. Finally, we will consider several factors investigators need to weigh when choosing a research design.

DEFINITIONS AND PURPOSE

Designing a nursing study is the creative process of planning the empirical aspects of an investigation. Research designs link the investigator's abstract thinking about a topic with the realities of studying a topic. Designs guide investigation. A research design is analogous to the musical score for a symphony. Just as the score indicates to the conductor and musicians what notes various sections of the orchestra should be playing and the sequence and manner in which the music should be played, research designs indicate what activities the investigator and partici-

pants should be performing and the order in which they should occur. Without a research design, the investigator's activities may not suit the purpose of the study.

The many types of research design

Because different research purposes exist, different research designs are necessary. Consider the following questions:

1. What is the experience of families with a member who is recovering from open-heart surgery?

2. What is the relationship between maternal anxiety, length of labor, and epinephrine levels?

3. What is the course of development of premature infants from birth to entry into grade school?

4. What is the effect of a home-care program on the incidence of rehospitalization of elderly people who are being treated for cancer?

Each of these questions implies a different research purpose and thus a different design. The first question implies a description of what families experience as one of their members recovers from open-heart surgery; for example, the investigator may study their problems, concerns, and adaptations in family life. The second question implies an examination of relationships among a pregnant woman's anxiety, the length of her labor, and the epinephrine levels. Do women with high levels of anxiety have longer or shorter labors? Is the epinephrine level related to anxiety level? Are high epinephrine levels associated with longer or shorter labors? The third question implies the study of premature infant development from birth until they enter school. The investigator will ask what these infants experience as they grow and develop to school-age children. The fourth question implies the testing of a home-care program to determine if the program can reduce the incidence of readmission of elderly patients with cancer. Is the home-care program more effective than usual care?

Many designs are available for studying each of these questions. We will discuss the relationship between theory development, or the kind of knowledge being generated, and the nature of research designs.

THEORY DEVELOPMENT AND RESEARCH DESIGN

The relationship between theory development and research can be depicted as a spiral with research refining theory and theory refining research (Fig. 8-1). As theory development and research influence one another, they broaden the boundaries of knowl-

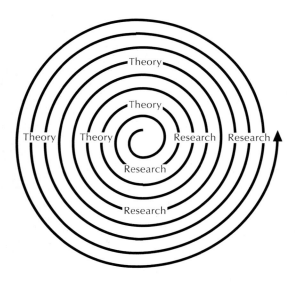

Fig. 8-1. Theory-research spiral of knowledge. (From Chinn P., and Jacobs, M. [1987]. *Theory and nursing: A systematic approach* [2nd ed.]. St. Louis: Mosby.)

edge (Chinn & Jacobs, 1983). Research contributes to theory development in two ways: by generating theory and by testing theory.

Theory-generating research

Theory-generating research is designed to discover and describe phenomena and their observed relationships. It often employs *inductive reasoning*, that is, the inference of a general conclusion from a set of particular observations. For example, the investigator may observe that a number of women who experience pregnancy—a developmental crisis—also experience instances of personal growth. One woman may learn to give in new ways, another to transcend the physical changes of her body, and still another to feel power in generating a new life. From observing these particulars, the investigator can generalize that personal growth is associated with the developmental crisis of pregnancy.

Because an investigator's task is theory generation during the early stages of investigation, researchers often are concerned with identification or careful description of a phenomenon. Identification of relevant concepts, description of prevalence or frequency, estimation of the value, or description of stability or change over time can be achieved through various descriptive designs.

Once the phenomenon has been clearly described, investigators begin to explore its relationships to other phenomena or to compare how the phenomenon differs in varying conditions. This can be achieved by correlation or comparison, by studying certain cases in depth, or by studying large groups. The results of these studies may suggest hypotheses that relate the phenomenon of central interest to other phenomena, leading to theory-testing research.

Theory-testing research

Theory-testing research attempts to determine how accurately a theory accounts for observed facts. This research translates theoretical relationship statements, also known as theoretical propositions, into hypotheses. *Hypotheses* are statements of theoretical relationships that can be tested empirically. The researcher identifies empirical indicators that correspond to abstract concepts in theoretical relationships or propositions. As shown in Fig. 8-2, a hypothesis may contain one or more empirical indicators for each abstract concept. The translation of

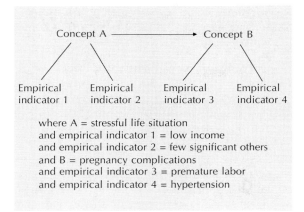

where A = stressful life situation
and empirical indicator 1 = low income
and empirical indicator 2 = few significant others
and B = pregnancy complications
and empirical indicator 3 = premature labor
and empirical indicator 4 = hypertension

Fig. 8-2. Relationship between concepts and empirical indicators. The hypothesis is that stressful life situations such as having low income and having few significant others may be related to such pregnancy complications as premature labor or hypertension.

abstract concepts to empirical indicators is discussed in detail in Chapter 14.

Theory-testing studies usually address only some of the relationships included in a theory; that is, they may test a few hypotheses, not the entire theory. Over time, some relationships that derive from the theory are tested and refuted. Others may be tested and not refuted. As the results of many studies accumulate, the theory can be revised or discarded.

Theory-testing research usually employs *deductive reasoning,* that is, the inference of a particular conclusion from a set of general observations. The research begins with a statement of general relationship that is translated into an empirically testable statement about a particular situation. The process of reasoning begins with a general observation and a set of initial conditions that in turn explain the conclusions. For example:

General observation: Persons confronting developmental crises have opportunities for personal growth.
Initial condition: Pregnancy is a developmental crisis.
Explanation: People confronting pregnancy have opportunities for personal growth.

A hypothesis derived from this reasoning might be that during pregnancy, women experience increased personal power and readiness to learn.

We may explain why a phenomenon occurs or predict its occurrence through studies that are designed to test hypotheses. Some of these studies involve experimental manipulation under highly controlled conditions, whereas others involve naturalistic observation.

Testing prescriptive theory, producing or controlling phenomena such as health and well-being, can be achieved through trials of the nursing therapeutics that are described in the theory. These studies involve constructing empirical conditions that represent the theory and then validating the theory through research in a clinical setting.

Although this schema is a useful way of relating theory development and empirical testing of theory, a one-to-one correspondence does not always exist between theory and research design. Some designs meet many types of research purposes. Each design has inherent merit, none is more important or valuable than the others, and each serves special purposes. Theory development does not proceed from a single study but from the convergence of knowledge derived through the application of many research designs.

ELEMENTS OF RESEARCH DESIGN

Research designs include several elements: (1) a description of participants (who), (2) observations of variables (what), (3) measures of time (when), (4) selection of setting (where) and (5) role of the investigator.

Participants

Participants are the individuals who take part in the study. Designs specify who the participants will be and what the *unit of analysis* (elements of the sample) will be. Participants in nursing research studies may be individual human beings, couples, families, groups, communities, or animals. Sometimes, instead of the individual, these larger aggregates or groups are considered the unit of analysis. Moreover, more than one group of participants may enter the study. Participants may be included from groups who differ according to health status or some other variable of interest. For example, a group of participants may represent persons who have a particular response to a health problem (pain) and another group may represent persons without the response (no pain).

Groups may enter a study at different times. These groups may be a *cohort* of individuals, a group of persons who share a common experience within a defined time period. A birth cohort is a group of individuals all born within a specific time span, for example, between 1940 and 1945. Persons who were diagnosed with specific health problems within a certain time span might also constitute a cohort.

Variables

Variables are the focus of the study and reflect the empirical aspects of the concepts being studied; the investigator measures variables. Research designs are univariate or multivariate. Univariate designs address only one variable. Nursing investigators more commonly study two or more variables (multivariate), which is not suprising in view of the complexity of human health.

Time

The time element of design is the frequency (how often) and the order (when) in which observations are made. In some designs variables are observed at only one point in time. In studies in which time functions are of primary concern, for example, the study of changing health values with age, time becomes a crucial dimension. Considering the rate of change is also important when planning studies of change over time. In some studies the timing of measurements must allow the investigator to capture rapidly changing processes, such as electroencephalographic measurements in sleep. In others, measurements may be made at longer intervals, such as over several menstrual cycles, to reflect more slowly changing processes. When the investigator is interested in the pattern of occurrence, such as oscillation of a variable or simultaneous variation of two or more variables, the time dimension must allow for both rapid and slow processes. For example, an investigator who is studying temperature rhythms in women would need to consider the circadian temperature rhythm as it changes over 24 hours, as well as the monthly temperature changes attributable to the menstrual cycle. Studies of trends must include several measures over time. Time also is used to describe certain types of study designs. In prospective studies, measures are made from the present to some point in the future.

Retrospective studies involve looking backward in history with measures reflecting events that occurred in the past.

Convergence of participants, variables, and time

The three-dimensional figure (Fig. 8-3) illustrates how participants, variables, and time converge to describe research design. The variables being studied are represented on the vertical dimension from $V1$ to Vn; persons participating in the study are represented on the horizontal dimension from $P1$ through Pn; and the timing of measurements is represented on the third dimension from $T1$ to Tn. The total number of observations in the study is the product of the number of variables multiplied by the number of times measurements are made multiplied by the number of participants.

Setting

The setting is often a neglected element in the description of research designs, yet it may vary con-

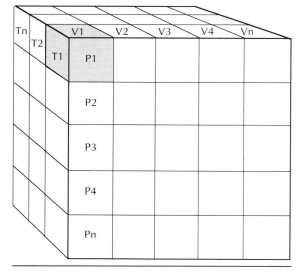

T = Time
P = Participant
V = Variables

Fig. 8-3. Three-dimensional matrix for research designs. Shaded area represents possible observation of one variable for one participant at one time.

siderably. Some research occurs in natural settings with the investigator attempting not to alter any aspect of the setting. The natural setting is a particularly important element in studies that describe naturally occurring events. Some research, directed at observing how only a single variable affects another, is conducted under highly controlled conditions in an artificial setting such as a laboratory. Whatever the setting, the researcher provides a careful description of the setting that enables other investigators to replicate the study. This description is particularly important for investigators who are conducting studies in natural settings, such as care settings, because it enables clinicians to assess the likelihood that use of the research findings will be effective in their own environments.

Investigator's role

Another element of research design is the role of the investigator. In some studies the investigator remains unobtrusive, attempting not to influence the variables being studied. In other studies the investigator imposes control on many variables, actively manipulates some of the variables being studied, and allocates the participants to different conditions.

DESCRIPTION OF RESEARCH DESIGNS

Describing or identifying phenomena

Description or identification of phenomena can be achieved through various descriptive research designs. The specific purposes of the study indicate the most appropriate design. When a specific purpose is to identify or describe concepts, investigators usually select a descriptive design.

An investigator who is concerned about the concept of "suffering" may describe the concept based on existing literature and thus derive a definition of suffering. Using this definition, Battenfield (1984) interviewed suffering persons to refine further the concept and to determine if the information gathered from existing literature was in agreement with suffering individuals' descriptions of their experiences. In this type of study design the investigator sought to describe the experiences of individuals selected because of their particular experiences. Through informal open-ended interviews she found that clients' experiences ranged from turmoil to contentment and that their descriptions of suffering

resembled categories derived from the literature, including turmoil without resolution, coping, finding meaning, and accepting-understanding. The application of a descriptive design allowed this investigator to identify multiple dimensions of suffering that were in agreement with definitions from earlier literature (see boxes below and on p. 122).

A *descriptive survey* can be used when the purpose of the study is to describe the prevalence or incidence of a phenomenon or to estimate the value of a phenomenon for a population. The descriptive survey is a research design that involves collecting information from a variety of persons who resemble the total population of interest to the investigator. When estimating how common a phenomenon is or the average value of the phenomenon for a defined population is important, a descriptive survey that involves participants who resemble the population of interest is appropriate. Feldman, Voda, and Gronseth (1985) conducted a telephone survey of a random sample of 594 perimenopausal women to study the prevalence of menopausal hot flashes, their frequency, and the number of years women experienced hot flashes. Women between 35 and 60 years of age participated in the study. They found that 88% of women experienced hot flashes. Most women who had hot flashes experienced fewer than five per day.

SAMPLE INTERVIEW OF SUFFERING PERSON

Female, 104 years of age, had been in nursing home for two years. Mentally alert, vision poor, hearing adequate. Mobile without help.

When I first came here I cried for a month. I was lonely, so unhappy. I never thought it would happen to me. Then one day I heard a preacher say that Christians had to be happy and content so they could help others be happy and content. I tried it. It works. I go to other peoples' rooms and when they see I'm happy it helps them be happy.

Interview: Turmoil-contentment rating = 5.
Panel: Content-analysis = finding meaning.

From Battenfield, B. (1984). *Image: The Journal of Nursing Scholarship, 16*(2), 41.

RANGE OF EXPERIENCES AMONG SUFFERING PERSONS

Initial impact
 Immobility, shock, dulled senses
 Hurt, agony
 Disbelief, denial, evasion
Turmoil without resolution
 Fear
 Anger, striking-out, revolt
 Depression
 Shame
 Guilt
 Hopelessness, helplessness, despair
  Feeling of abandonment, separation
Recovery
 Coping
  Changing attitude
  Altering course
  Finding courage through others
 Accepting/understanding
  Nonresistive acknowledgment
  Facing limitations
  Resignation
  Stoicism
 Finding meaning
  Expanding self-awareness, growth
  Developing unity of existence with
  nature
  Developing and strengthening interpersonal relationships
  Reappraising and strengthening values
  Developing creative activities
  Finding joy in suffering

From Battenfield, B. (1984). *Image: The Journal of Nursing Scholarship, 16*(2), 38.

Although 26% said the hot flashes were too infrequent to count, 10% experienced four or more per day. The hot flashes persisted from 1 year to more than 11 years. This application of a descriptive design was one element of an extensive research program directed at understanding women's experiences of the menopausal hot flash.

Another variation in descriptive design is the *descriptive longitudinal study,* which is designed to observe stability or change over time and involves repeated observations. Its aim is to characterize the course of a phenomenon such as human develop-

ment or adaptation. Updike, Accurso, and Jones (1985) studied evidence of a circadian rhythm in pulse, respiratory rate, transcutaneous oxygen level, frequency of respiratory pauses, and skin temperature in six 34- to 37-week preterm infants. They observed each variable every 30 minutes for 24 hours. Five of the six infants demonstrated a rhythm in skin temperature. Lowest temperatures were found between 11 PM and 4:30 AM. Two or three infants demonstrated circadian rhythms for other variables. Respiratory pauses and lowest transcutaneous oxygen levels were seen in the early morning hours (Fig. 8-4). In this example the descriptive longitudinal design spanned a 24-hour period rather than a period of weeks or years. Nevertheless, this design is important for charting the course of phenomena to determine if they remain stable or change over time.

Case studies also can be used to describe concepts. Case studies are intensive, systematic investigations of a single individual, group, community, or some other unit. The case study is typically conducted under naturalistic conditions; the investigator examines in depth data related to background, current status, environmental characteristics, and interactions of individuals, groups, and communities. Case studies may be applied for multiple purposes of theory building, but usually they are used to describe phenomena and their relationships. Case studies are used to investigate a contemporary phenomenon within its real-life context, especially when the boundaries between the phenomenon and the context are not clearly evident and in which multiple sources of evidence are used (Yin, 1984).

Other approaches to describing phenomena include grounded theory and ethnographic and phenomenologic inquiry. These are discussed in greater detail in Chapter 9.

Exploring relationships or differences

Exploring relationships and differences between phenomena is a second aim of theory-generating research. Exploratory work usually proceeds after the concepts have been identified and described. Having identified the phenomenon of interest, the investigator begins to explore how the phenomenon might be related to other factors.

Exploring relationships or differences between phenomena can be achieved by using a variety of exploratory research designs, most commonly corre-

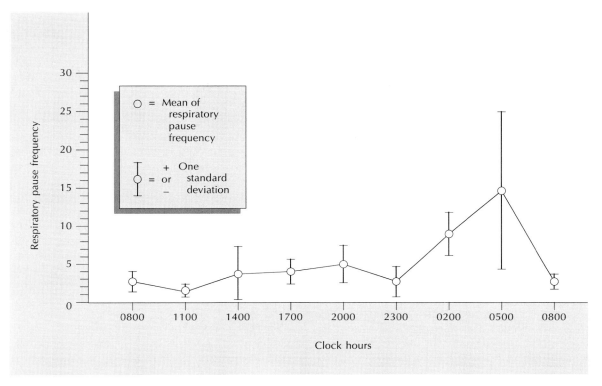

Fig. 8-4. Frequency of respiratory pauses as a function of clock time over a 24-hour period in six preterm infants. (From Updike, P., Accurso, F., and Jones, R. [1985]. Reprinted with permission from *Nursing Research, 34,* 163. ©, 1985, American Journal of Nursing Company.)

lational and comparative surveys. Case studies also can be used to explore relationships and differences.

Comparative surveys contrast the experiences of two or more groups of individuals. The groups usually are selected through sampling procedures (see Chapter 7) so they resemble one another as much as possible but yet differ with regard to the particular variable(s) being studied. Ideally, groups being compared represent the populations of interest to the investigator. Often, random sampling procedures are used.

Basing their work on earlier descriptions of the concept of hope, Stoner and Keampfer (1985) explored two research questions: (1) What is the relationship between recalled life expectancy information and hope in cancer patients? (2) What effect does phase of illness have on the level of hope in cancer patients? The investigators included participants who were experiencing different phases of cancer progression and treatment, including 11 patients with no evidence of disease, 11 cancer patients in the terminal phase of their illnesses and enrolled in a hospice program, and 33 inpatients and outpatients who were undergoing treatment for various types of cancer. Participants were asked what they remembered being told about their chances for recovery from this illness and how long they expected to live. They also completed a scale to measure hope (Stoner Hope Scale). Results of the study indicated that the phase of the illness had no effect on hope, but recalled life expectancy information did influence hope. Individuals who had no recollection of receiving information regarding their prognosis were more hopeful than those who did recall information regarding prognosis. Individuals in treatment were slightly less hopeful than those who were terminally ill; those who had no evidence of disease were most hopeful.

This exploratory comparative survey demonstrated some differences in the experiences of groups of cancer patients, including those who had no active disease, those who were still in treatment, and those who were terminally ill, relative to the type of information they recalled receiving about their prognosis. Theory-generating research of this nature suggests hypotheses for testing in further research. For example, the investigators might test the hypothesis that patients suppress recall of prognoses regarding their life expectancies as one means of maintaining hope. Alternatively, the investigators could hypothesize that those individuals who recall information about their prognoses have more realistic appraisals of their disease progression and therefore demonstrate levels of hope that correspond to the seriousness of their prognoses. Studies that test hypothesized relationships similar to these could culminate in a theory about fostering hope in cancer patients and even could be extended to other populations of patients.

Correlational descriptive surveys allow the investigator to assess the extent to which levels of one phenomenon correspond to levels of another. A major difference exists between a comparative survey and a correlational survey. In a correlational survey a sample representing a cross-section of a single population of interest is studied; in the comparative survey samples from two or more populations are compared. Because variability in each of the study factors is essential to allow associations to be seen in the data, a wide cross-section of experience is sought in the sample.

The study of hope in cancer patients also could have been designed as a correlational descriptive survey. Had this been the design choice, the investigators would have sought a population of cancer patients—perhaps through the registry of all persons diagnosed with cancer within a certain geographical region—and randomly sampled from that population. They would have assumed that within the population they would find patients who did not have active disease, patients who were in treatment, and patients who were terminally ill and enrolled in hos-

pice care. In addition they probably would have included patients who were terminally ill and not in hospice care, patients who had completed treatment but who were experiencing recurrences, and so forth. By sampling from the broader population, the investigators would have included a wider range of cancer-patient experiences. Similarly, they might have discovered a wider range of hope within the sample. Both design choices would have been appropriate for conducting the study of hope in cancer patients, but the design choice could produce slightly different results.

Case study designs also can be used to identify relationships or differences for further testing. In this application of case study design the focus is on the relationship between concepts or differences in concepts, not merely on describing a single concept. (See Chapter 10 for further discussion of application of the case study in testing relationships between phenomena.)

Predicting and explaining phenomena

Once investigators understand how one phenomenon of interest is related to others, they can propose specific relationships between them. These proposed relationships take the form of hypotheses. Hypothesis-testing studies are theory-testing studies; each study tests one or more hypothesized relationship that is part of the theory being tested.

A hypothesis-testing study generates a theory that may explain or predict. *Predictive theory* is a set of statements that interrelates necessary and sufficient variables so that a specific outcome can be expected when the theory is applied (Chinn & Jacobs, 1987). One can anticipate what will happen if the theory is applied. Predictive theory allows the researcher to predict what will happen even though the reason it happens is not known. *Explanatory theory* is a set of statements that provides a reasoned argument for *why* certain events happen (Chinn & Jacobs, 1987). The researcher can explain why the outcome occurred.

Many phenomena can be predicted reasonably well, although why they occur cannot be explained well. For example, a large volume of literature on social support contains much evidence for the protective effect of social support on health. People who lack a good basis of support experience more complications of pregnancy when they are exposed to a stressful environment (Norbeck & Tilden, 1983; Nuckolls Cassel, & Kaplan, 1972). Although predicting the relationship between social support and health is possible, explaining why it occurs is not. Currently, many hypotheses do exist about why social support protects health. Although prediction does not allow us to understand why a phenomenon such as pregnancy complication occurs, it does allow scientists and clinicians to develop control measures in the absence of this understanding. For example, clinicians can foster social support for their clients by helping them identify sources of support in their own networks or helping them complement or supplement their existing networks. These control measures should effectively lower pregnancy complication rates, although we do not understand how they work.

Many study designs allow the investigator to test hypotheses, leading to the generation of predictive and explanatory theory. These designs have been created to test causal hypotheses in which a cause, *A*, is proposed to produce an effect, *B*. In our example, social support, *A*, is predicted to have an effect on pregnancy complications, *B*. Designs such as these include the naturalistic survey, as well as the experimental designs. Investigators using naturalistic designs test hypotheses based on observation of phenomena as they naturally occur. Naturalistic designs for hypothesis testing include several types of survey research designs. Experimental studies involve changing the phenomenon in some way. Usually the intent is to produce a change in a phenomenon of interest to nursing, such as human health.

Naturalistic designs for testing hypotheses include prospective, retrospective, and cross-sectional designs. These designs can be applied to test predictive and explanatory theory. *Cross-sectional designs* involve selecting a representative sample from the population of interest and observing all the phenomena (including the putative cause and effect) of interest at the same point in time. For example, Woods (1985) hypothesized that women who performed multiple life roles (e.g., wife, mother, and employee) would experience symptoms of poor mental health only if their roles were performed in a social context that was itself associated with poor mental health. She studied a sample of 140 married women who were randomly selected from registrants at a family health clinic. Women responded on a single occasion to an interview about their roles, sources of support, and mental health. Women who performed more roles reported no more symptoms than women who performed fewer roles. Women who were spouse, parent, and employee had poor mental health when they had traditional attitudes about women's place in society, had low levels of sharing of household tasks with their spouses, and had little opportunity to confide their concerns in a significant other person.

In addition to cross-sectional designs, prospective and retrospective designs can be employed to test hypotheses, contributing to the development of predictive and explanatory theory. *Prospective designs* involve sampling from a population of interest to obtain a representative group and observing the sample on at least two occasions. The key difference between cross-sectional and prospective designs is that prospective designs follow the participants into the future for a designated period of time. The investigator is particularly interested in learning who will experience the effect during the period of the study. Woods could have used a prospective design to test the hypothesis relating women's roles to their mental health. Women could have been interviewed initially about their roles and sources of support. Those who already had poor mental health could have been eliminated from the study. The remaining women who were at risk of developing poor mental health could have been studied for several years to determine who developed poor mental health.

Another option for hypothesis testing is the retrospective design. *Retrospective designs* begin with the selection of representative samples from at least two groups. Usually one group has the effect that is being studied, and the other does not. The participants are studied regarding the putative causes. Using a retrospective design to test the hypothesis linking women's roles to their mental health, the investigator could have selected a random sample of women who exhibited poor mental health and a random sample of women who exhibited good mental health. The investigator would have interviewed both groups about their roles and sources of support and then compared the groups to determine whether their combinations of roles and support differed.

Clearly, several design options exist for testing the same hypothesis. Each of these designs will be discussed in greater detail; considerations for choosing these designs are explored in Chapter 11.

Experimental designs, quasiexperimental designs, and many variations on experimental designs also can be used to test hypotheses. Experiments are studies in which the investigator manipulates a putative cause and measures an effect. Typically, researchers refer to the variable they manipulate as an *independent, treatment,* or *causal variable.* The variable the investigator measures in response to the causal (treatment or independent) variable is called the *dependent variable* or *outcome variable.* Initially, the investigator randomly selects participants for the study and then randomly assigns them to two or more groups. The investigator administers the causal (treatment or independent) variable to one or more groups (usually termed the *treatment group*) and does not administer it to the other group (usually termed the *control group*). The investigator then compares the outcome variable for the participants who received the causal variable to those who did not. The three critical features of experiments are: (1) random allocation of participants to the treatment and control groups, (2) manipulation of the causal variable, and (3) control through comparison of participants who did and did not receive the treatment or causal variable.

Byers (1985) used a type of experimental design to test the hypothesis that exercise immediately before evening bedtime would reduce morning stiffness and increase joint mobility among persons with rheumatoid conditions. She randomly selected 30 patients from those receiving treatment at an outpatient rheumatology clinic who met criteria for inclusion in the study. The investigator obtained measures of stiffness and joint mobility on two consecutive mornings, one of which was preceded by evening exercise. Each morning elastic stiffness and mobility were measured before and after morning exercise. After the final measurements of elastic stiffness and mobility on the second day of the study, the patients compared stiffness on the two days. The elastic stiffness and subjective ratings of stiffness were less and mobility was greater when evening exercises were performed. In this application of experimental design the investigator randomly assigned the participants to one of two groups: the first exercised on evening 1 but did not exercise on evening 2; the second did not exercise on evening 1 but did exercise on evening 2. The investigator

manipulated the causal variable, exercise, by having the participants perform the evening exercises at designated times. The investigator also used a control or comparison condition, that of not exercising. This example illustrates only one type of experimental design; many variations exist. Several types of experimental design are discussed in greater detail in Chapters 11 and 12.

Quasiexperiments have the features of manipulation and control, but participants are not randomly assigned to the treatment and control groups. A study of the effects of progressive muscle relaxation training on blood pressure of clients with essential hypertension illustrates the components of an experiment. Pender (1984) studied persons in a hypertension monitoring program. Eligible participants had blood pressures above 140 mm Hg systolic and/or above 90 mm Hg diastolic, when averaged over three successive readings in the previous 3 to 5 months, and met other study criteria related to physician supervision and sodium-restricted diet. Pender randomly selected 30 persons for participation in the relaxation training (RT) program. A second group of 30 persons who met the study criteria served as a comparison group and was matched with the RT group on sex, age, number of medications, and systolic blood pressure. Instead of randomly allocating participants selected from the same population to the treatment and control conditions, Pender matched the members of the comparison group to the individuals in the treatment group.

After the participants gave their informed consent, three baseline blood pressure measurements were obtained from both groups. In addition, throughout the study Pender monitored medication regimen, medication and nutrition adherence, and level of physical activity. Participants in the treatment group received three 2½-hour sessions of relaxation training in groups of five to nine. Participants in the RT group also used a home practice cassette tape and were encouraged to practice daily. The RT participants were seen individually for 6 weeks after the group training to see if they had developed skill in relaxation training. To provide health monitoring and counseling, public health nurses saw those in the nontrained groups throughout the study. The nontrained group received individual attention, blood pressure and weight measurement, dietary review, and a discussion of medication compliance. The comparison group also received educational materials. For 4 months after relaxation training and individual monitoring, health department nurses, unaware of which clients were in the RT group versus the nontrained comparison group, monitored those in the RT group and the comparison group.

Pender's design differs slightly from an experimental design, because it does not contain the element of randomization of participants to treatment and control groups. Participants in the RT group were selected randomly from one population, and the comparison group members were individually matched to the participants in the RT group.

Pender's study contains the components of manipulation and control characteristic of experimental designs. She manipulated the treatment in the RT group by providing the relaxation training sessions for the participants and the follow-up sessions to assess what the participants had learned of the relaxation training methods. The follow-up sessions to assess learning in the RT group were a check that the manipulation of the treatment variable was effective; such a session is called a *manipulation check*. Pender also used several design elements to control effects not attributable to RT, including the comparison group that did not receive the experimental treatment. She matched the comparison group participants with the RT participants to control for the effects of age, sex, and other variables on the outcome. In addition, Pender provided a similar amount of attention to the nontreated group to ensure that the RT group response was not attributable simply to the increased attention they received. Likewise, the comparison group received information regarding diet, hypertension, and weight control.

The preceding examples illustrate the use of naturalistic and experimental designs for hypothesis-testing purposes. The outcome of application of these designs is the testing of components of nursing theory.

Testing prescriptive theory

Because nursing is a practice discipline, concerned with the delivery of caring services to humans, it has a professional obligation to contribute to prescriptive theory. Describing phenomena and their relationships to other phenomena of interest is not sufficient, nor is explaining or predicting phenomena. Dickoff, James, and Wiedenbach (1968) wrote of the importance of "situation-producing" theory. Because this type of theory contains prescriptions for practice, it has also become known as prescriptive theory. Prescriptive theories address nursing therapeutics and systems of care. *Prescriptive theories* are developed to control, promote, and change phenomena (Meleis, 1985).

Prescriptive theory is a type of practice theory. As such, it presupposes the development of normative theory, which conceptualizes the goal to be achieved, and scientific-empirical theory, which explains how to achieve the goal. *Normative theory* is developed to describe, explain, or predict values as opposed to empirical phenomena. Its adequacy is judged by consistency of logic against the underlying value assumptions on which the theory is based. *Scientific-empirical theory* seeks to describe, explain, and predict the empirical world and is evaluated through empirical testing. *Practice theory* is validated in natural practice settings (Chinn & Jacobs, 1987).

A significant difference between prescriptive theory and other types of theory is the commitment to a goal. Essential elements of prescriptive theory as described by Dickoff, James, and Wiedenbach (1968) include the aim or goal, prescriptions to bring about the desired goal, and a survey list. The goal states the explicit purpose of the theory, whereas the survey list provides the answers to six essential questions to be addressed as part of the theory. These include the following:

1. Who performs the activity (agency)?
2. Who is the recipient of the activity (patiency)?
3. In what context is the activity performed (framework)?
4. What is the end point of the activity (terminus)?
5. What is the guiding procedure, technique, or protocol of the activity (procedure)?
6. What is the energy source for the activity (dynamics)?

The answers to these questions are aspects of prescription to achieve the goals.

Agency includes not only the professional performing the prescription to bring about the desired aim but also all those who have the internal and external resources to do so, including family members, visitors, and other professionals. *Patiency* specifies the recipients of the prescriptions. Context, called the *framework* by Dickoff, James, and Wiedenbach (1968), includes all the variables that influence progress toward the goal, including sociopolitical realities. The *terminus* is the product of the activity. *Procedure* includes steps that must be taken to achieve the goal. Finally, *dynamics* refers to motivating factors in performing and sustaining the activities that produce the goal.

Diers used a simplified example to illustrate the elements of a survey list:

"Suppose you have a headache. You want to be comfortable (the goal) because pain is interfering with your composure and concentration. You (agency) give yourself (patiency) two aspirin (procedure) to relieve the pain (dynamics). You do this activity within a certain context in time and space (framework) and pretty soon your headache goes away (terminus). You then feel better and can get back to work (goal achieved). [Diers, 1979, p. 48]

In Diers's view, (1979, p. 203) prescriptive theory addresses *systems of care,* which includes a "set of agents, doing work with patients, in a given sociopolitical context, using certain processes or procedures with certain sources of motivation or energy, toward measurable end points, all in the service of achieving some desired goal." A system of care is not simply procedures, processes, or specific agents. Moreover, every element has some influence on every other element, often influencing one another in highly complex ways. Diers said that one way to visualize prescriptive theory is as a giant spider web in which the radii of the web are the elements (e.g., agency, patiency) of the theory. The threads that connect the radii are the hypotheses about the relationships among aspects of the theory. The whole web constitutes the theory, and all the elements are interconnected and interdependent (Fig. 8-5).

Prescriptive theory is testable only in practice. The prescription must be put into action, its aspects theoretically and operationally defined, and its effect measured by how well the system of care is able to actualize the goal (Diers, 1979, p. 204).

Testing prescriptive theory begins by formulating the prescription and goal. Prescriptive theory should designate the prescription and its components, the type of client who should receive the prescriptions, the conditions under which the prescription should occur, and the consequences of applying the pre-

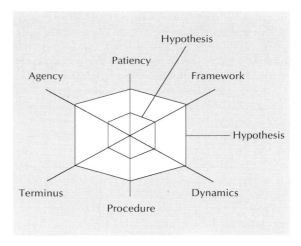

Fig. 8-5. Interrelationships of elements in prescriptive theory. (Based on Diers, D. [1985]. *Research in nursing practice.* Philadelphia: Lippincott.)

scriptions (Meleis, 1985). The prescription is introduced, measured, and tested. The goal of testing prescriptive theory is generalizing from a specific situation to the larger class of situations (Diers, 1979). A prescription is like a hypothesis in the sense that it relates concepts of interest. Unlike a hypothesis, it contains an explicit statement that the goal is a desirable one and the prescription is the way to achieve the goal. In testing prescriptive theory, nursing as agency is not the independent variable and patiency is not the dependent variable. Instead, the entire system of care is recognized as the entity to be tested.

Despite the fact that nursing is a practice discipline, relatively little discussion about designs for testing prescriptive theory appears in our literature, with the exception of Diers's proposals (1979). Moreover, designs for testing elements of prescriptive theory, such as the relationships between procedure and terminus, or therapeutics and outcomes, have received little attention. In the following pages we will explore some designs that may help to test prescriptive theory and propose designs that are necessary to fully test prescriptive theory as Diers has defined it.

Barnard, Booth, Mitchell, and Telzrow (1982) tested prescriptive theory that addressed nursing services to promote parenting and child development in families of high-risk, doubly vulnerable infants. The goal of the prescription was to improve health and development for the infant and more optimum parent-child interaction. The goal prompted the development of three models of care:

1. Nursing Parent and Child Environment (NPACE) emphasized assessment of the infant, parent, and environment for planning individualized nursing care.
2. Nursing Support for Infant BioBehavioral (NSIBB) included a structured curriculum for facilitating mother and infant adaptation.
3. Nursing Standard Approach to Care (NSTAC) included a traditional public health nursing approach, was problem oriented, and emphasized physical health.

The models were tested in 185 families who were vulnerable because they had demonstrated social and physical health problems. Each model included 3 months of intervention that began after birth. The investigators implemented the three nursing models (NPACE, NSIBB, NSTAC), described the models, and experimentally evaluated their effectiveness.

Mothers and infants were assigned randomly to one of the three programs at the time of birth. Nursing intervention began at discharge from the hospital. Data were collected about the mother, infant, parent-child interaction, and family when the infant was a newborn, 3 months, and 10 months of age. Based on the three models, no significant differences existed in the child and family outcomes. Children of families with no significant family problems other than initial pregnancy complications and social risk demonstrated normal outcomes at 3, 10, and 24 months. Mother-child interaction and mother's stimulation of the child improved over time. For children whose families demonstrated multiple or chronic family problems, the interaction scores were low and interaction declined further after the end of the intervention period. These infants demonstrated decline in mental performance from 10 to 14 months.

Nursing care delivered with the three different models differed in breadth of its focus, in the frequency of contact, and the specific topics addressed by the nurses. The least use of nursing resources was documented in the NSTAC program, with the NPACE program providing the fullest nursing approach in frequency of contact and attention to physical, emotional, and prevention needs. Nurses delivering NSIBB were most satisfied with their roles. The investigators concluded that when there were no related family problems, such as the lack of support for the caregiver, history of child abuse, multiple problems, any of the three models tested is appropriate. When the family has many other family problems, the models tested did not provide enough intervention during the first year to improve the mother-child interaction and the mother's stimulation of the infant. The investigators recommend more intense infant-oriented models for infants in multiple-problem or chronic-problem families. (Barnard, Booth, Mitchell, & Telzrow, 1982). Studies to test prescriptive theory are discussed in further detail in Chapter 13.

CONSIDERATIONS IN SELECTING A RESEARCH DESIGN

Investigators weigh many considerations when selecting a research design. Of paramount importance is the purpose and the theory development aim of the study. Theory development usually reflects the current level of knowledge about the phenomenon and thus has guided determination of the specific research purpose. Additional influences on the study design include ethical issues related to the phenomenon; feasibility, validity, and availability of data; precision; and cost. In the following pages we will explore each of these considerations in more detail.

Level of knowledge

Our level of knowledge about the phenomenon affects our design choices. When little is known about a phenomenon, the investigator may undertake a careful description of a single concept rather than attempt to determine the relationship of several factors. In early work on premature infants careful description of such behavior as sleep patterns was important before designing intervention trials to promote infant development. Likewise, early work describing what life was like for people with cancer was necessary before support protocols for cancer patients and their families could be developed. In nursing, many topics exist on which only a single study or a few studies have been conducted. At this stage of our scientific development careful description of the phenomena of concern to nursing practice—human responses to health problems—is as important as is work designed to enhance our understanding of the many factors that influence human health. The relationships among the theory-development aim, purpose of the study, and design options are outlined in Table 8-1.

Nature of the research phenomenon

The nature of the research phenomenon is an important concern in choosing how to study it. Investigators consider whether the phenomenon can be studied in a naturalistic or nonnaturalistic way. For example, certain disasters have helped health scientists to gain better understanding of how humans respond to crises. Events such as fires, volcanic eruptions, and wars can be studied only as they naturally occur.

Nature of the research purpose

Some research purposes imply the choice of a specific design. For example, when the purpose is to answer the question, "What is the effect of learning self-hypnosis on the pain experiences of children having bone marrow aspiration?" the investigator will probably manipulate the use of self-hypnosis. Another

question, "What are the experiences of children having bone marrow aspirations?" implies that the investigator will observe and describe the experiences of the children without purposively altering the perceptions in any way. In a program of research consisting of a series of studies, the investigator may raise a series of questions and over time incorporate a number of research design options, each building on the other.

Ethical considerations

Many phenomena are inappropriate to study in a nonnaturalistic way. Studies that would deprive humans of necessary health care or of essential nutrients would be inappropriate under most circumstances. Most would agree that depriving women of prenatal care that ordinarily would be available to them is unethical, as would be depriving them of nutrition. Thus these phenomena would be inappropriate for human experimentation and could be studied in animal models or in humans in the situations in which they naturally occur. Chapter 6 contains a discussion of a wide range of ethical and other human considerations that underlie the choice of research design.

TABLE 8-1. **Relationship between theory development, purpose of the study, and design options**

THEORY DEVELOPMENT AIM AND PURPOSE	DESIGN OPTIONS
Identification or description of phenomenon (concept)	
Identification of relevant concepts	Descriptive design, grounded-theory study, ethnography, phenomenologic inquiry, case study
Description of prevalence or incidence of a phenomenon	Descriptive survey
Estimation of the value of a phenomenon	Descriptive survey
Description of patterns (stability or change) of phenomena over time	Descriptive longitudinal design, time series design
Exploration of differences or relationships between phenomena	Exploratory designs, correlational or comparative survey, case study

Explanation and prediction of phenomena	Explanatory survey
	  Cross-sectional
	  Retrospective
	  Prospective
	Experiment, including single case, small N designs, case study, quasiexperiments

Prescription and control	Clinical trial, evaluation research designs

Feasibility

In some instances feasibility is a key concern in selecting a research design. Many research designs are elegant but not feasible. For example, randomly placing inpatients in different physical units in a hospital would not be feasible in institutions in which patients require specialized nursing care. In this case randomization could result in obstetrical patients being sent to coronary care, surgical patients to a psychiatry unit, and so on, making difficult access to the type of care the patients need. Therefore a design that did not require random placement of patients in various inpatient units would be feasible.

Another feasibility consideration is the amount of time the investigator can devote to the study. When the investigator has a limited period of time to conduct the research, such as in a graduate program, choosing a longitudinal design that spans several years is not likely to be feasible. Moreover, access to support for a longitudinal study may make this design choice infeasible for many investigators.

Validity and availability of data

Other important concerns in selecting a research design are the validity and availability of data. A major goal in selecting a research design is maximizing the validity of the data. This issue is discussed in greater detail in Chapters 11 and 15. Briefly, for a given topic different designs maximize or minimize validity. For example, when studying minor symptoms, a design that requires participants to recall retrospectively the types of symptoms they experienced 6 months ago would probably produce inaccurate information, whereas a design employing daily prospective recordings of symptoms would maximize accurate recording of minor symptoms. Sometimes the availability of data influences the design choice. In some instances the only data source available is archival data. When the investigator must rely on data sources such as historical documents or health records of patients, research designs are usually restricted to those that do not require the investigator to manipulate any variables.

Precision

An additional dimension investigators consider when choosing a research design is precision. *Precision* refers to the ability to obtain the most accurate estimate of a single variable or of the effect of a treatment variable on an outcome variable. A design that allows the investigator to account for or to control many other factors known to influence the variable of interest maximizes the precision of the estimates. For example, when investigators can account for the influence of children's past experience with hospitalization, they can predict more precisely the influence of an orientation program on children's subsequent adaptation to hospitalization.

Cost

A final concern in selection of a research design is cost. Typically, designs that have a longitudinal component (extending over months or years) are considerably more expensive than those designs that require a much shorter data-collection period. Although it is not the only consideration, cost is a major deterrent to selection of longitudinal designs, particularly for researchers who must complete their research within a finite time frame. In some instances, fulfilling the research purpose may be impossible without using some longitudinal component, for example, when studying child development or the aging process. In these instances several investigators might collaborate to enhance the productivity of the research effort and to share the cost across several research questions.

SUMMARY

A research design specifies the phenomenon (or phenomena) that will be studied, when and how often it will be studied, whether the investigator will manipulate the phenomenon, and whether and how participants will be grouped. Some research designs also enable investigators to control or hold constant the influence of phenomena that are extraneous to the focus of the study, thus limiting alternative influences on the phenomenon under study. Other research designs facilitate identifying the most important phenomena in a field of study.

Table 8-1 illustrates the relationship between theory-development aim, purpose of the study, and design options. For theory generation, purposes usually include identification of relevant concepts, description of prevalence or incidence of a phenomenon, estimation of the value of a phenomenon, and description of patterns of phenomena over time. Research design options for achieving these purposes include descriptive designs, descriptive surveys, descriptive longitudinal designs, and time series designs. Theory generation is supported also by research purposes directed toward exploration of differences or relationships between phenomena. Exploratory designs such as correlational or comparative surveys and case studies meet these research purposes.

Theory testing involves research purposes of explanation and prediction of phenomena, as well as prescription and control of phenomena. Explanatory surveys, including cross-sectional, retrospective, and prospective surveys, experimental designs, quasiexperimental designs, case studies, and small N designs permit testing hypotheses; their outcomes contribute to explanation and prediction of phenomena. Clinical trials and evaluation research designs provide beginning approaches to testing prescriptive theory. Each design will be described in greater detail in the chapters that follow.

References

Baltes, P., Reese, H., & Nesselroade, J. (1977). Life-span developmental psychology: *Introduction to research methods*. Monterey, CA: Brooks/Cole.

Barnard, K., Booth, C., Mitchell, S., & Telzrow, R. (1982). *Newborn nursing models: Final report of project to the division of nursing*, USPHS.

Battenfield, B. (1984). Suffering: A conceptual description and content analysis of an operational schema. *Image: The Journal of Nursing Scholarship, 16*(2), 36-41.

Brink, P., & Wood, M. (1983). *Basic steps in planning nursing research: From question to proposal*. Monterey, CA: Wadsworth.

Byers, P. (1985). Effect of exercise on morning stiffness and mobility in patients with rheumatoid arthritis. *Research in Nursing and Health, 8,* 275-282.

Campbell, D., & Stanley, J. (1963). *Experimental and quasi-experimental design for researchers*. Chicago: Rand McNally.

Chinn, P., & Jacobs, M. (1983). *Theory and nursing: A systematic approach*. St. Louis: Mosby.

Cook, T., & Campbell, D. (1979). *Quasi-experimentation*. Chicago: Rand McNally.

Dickoff, J., James, P., & Wiedenbach, E. (1968). Theory in a practice discipline: Practice oriented theory (Pt. 1). *Nursing research, 17,* 415-435.

Diers, D. (1979). *Research in nursing practice*. Philadelphia: Lippincott.

Feldman, B., Voda, A., & Gronseth, E. (1985). The prevalence of hot flash and associate variables among perimenopausal women. *Research in Nursing and Health 8,* 261-268.

Kazdin, A. (1980). *Research design in clinical psychology*. New York: Harper & Row.

Kerlinger, F. (1973). *Foundations of behavioral research*. New York: Holt, Rinehart & Winston.

Kleinbaum, D., & Kupper, L. (1978). *Applied regression analysis and other multivariable methods*. Belmont, CA: Wadsworth.

Meleis, A. (1985). *Theoretical nursing: Development and progress*. Philadelphia: Lippincott.

Norbeck, J., & Tilden, V. (1983). Life stress, social support, and emotional disequilibrium in complications of pregnancy: A prospective multivariate study, *Journal of Health and Social Behavior, 24,* 30-46.

Nuckolls, K., Cassel, J., & Kaplan, B. (1972). Psychosocial assets, life crises and the prognosis of pregnancy. *American Journal of Epidemiology, 95,* 431-441.

Pender, N. (1984). Physiologic responses of clients with essential hypertension to progressive muscle relaxation training. *Research in Nursing and Health, 7,* 197-204.

Selltiz, C. (1976). *Research methods in social relations*. New York: Holt, Rinehart & Winston.

Smith, H. (1975). *Strategies of social research: The methodological imagination*. Englewood Cliffs, N. J.: Prentice-Hall.

Stoner, M., & Keampfer, S. (1985). Recalled life expectancy information, phase of illness, & hope in cancer patients. *Research in Nursing and Health, 8,* 269-274.

Updike, P., Accurso, F., & Jones, R. (1985). Physiologic circadian rhythmicity in preterm infants. *Nursing Research, 34,* 160-163.

Waltz, C., & Bausell, R. (1981). *Nursing research: Design, statistics, and computer analysis*. Philadelphia: F. A. Davis.

Woods, N. (1985). Employment, family roles, and mental ill health in young married women. *Nursing Research, 34,* 4-10.

Woods, N., Most, A., & Dery, G. (1982). Toward a construct of perimenstrual distress. *Research in Nursing and Health, 5,* 123-136.

Woolridge, P., Leonard, R., & Skipper, J. (1978). *Methods of clinical experimentation to improve patient care*. St Louis: Mosby.

Yin, R. (1984). *Case study research: Design & methods*. Beverly Hills, CA: Sage.

9

DESIGNING STUDIES TO DESCRIBE PHENOMENA

NANCY FUGATE WOODS AND MARCI CATANZARO

Investigators who are studying new topics in nursing frequently confront the challenge of identifying and describing new phenomena. The investigator concerned with an escalating prevalence of suicide attempts among a population of young women appropriately asks, "What is going on here?" Answering these questions often involves identifying a concept or concepts. In the case of escalating suicide rates, hopelessness, escape, unmet expectations, and constrained aspirations might be some of the concepts that reflect the phenomena of central interest to nursing. Without clear understanding and description of these phenomena, future studies to identify and test therapeutic measures will be built on an incomplete knowledge base.

This chapter will address several types of research designs that are useful in identifying and describing significant phenomena in nursing. Ethnography, phenomenology, and grounded-theory studies will be described, and approaches to conducting studies in these traditions will be discussed. In addition, designs for describing the prevalence, incidence, and patterns of stability or change of phenomena and estimating the value of a parameter for a population will be addressed.

RESEARCH DESIGNS TO IDENTIFY AND DESCRIBE PHENOMENA

Designs that identify and describe significant concepts in nursing often have been neglected or oversimplified, yet their application is pivotal to building a science that addresses nursing phenomena. To date, much of the work on concept description and analysis has proceeded independently of empirical research, with much of the effort derived from clinical anecdotal data.

Several approaches to designing studies are aimed at identifying and describing concepts. Most of these approaches rely on qualitative methods. Ethnography, phenomenology, and grounded theory are examples of qualitative methods that are used to describe phenomena of interest to nursing.

Ethnography is a broad, detailed study of the lifestyles of persons of a particular cultural or subcultural group. "The ethnographer documents, describes, and analyzes physical, cultural, social, and environmental features as these factors influence people's patterns of living" (Leininger, 1985, p. 36). The focus of ethnographic studies is to understand the participants' view. Many nurses who have attained doctorates in anthropology have used ethnographic methods to study the health beliefs and practices of people in different cultures. For example, Boyle (1983) used ethnography to study the illness experiences and the role of women in Guatemala, and Dougherty (1978) investigated the process of becoming a woman in rural black culture. Other nurse researchers have used ethnography to study nurses. Field (1983) studied the way the perspectives of community health nurses influenced their judgment and decision making, whereas Leininger (1980) and others used an ethnographic approach to study the phenomenon of caring.

Broadly speaking, *phenomenology* attempts to understand human experience through analysis of the participant's description. As a structured method of study phenomenology is a recent entry into nursing research design, and nurse scientists have not used it extensively. Phenomenology attempts to understand the basic structures of phenomena as humanly experienced. Phenomenologists reach this understanding by analyzing explanations of such experiences as having a baby, having a chronic illness, or being in the hospital. Parse, Coyne, and Smith (1985) reported a phenomenological study designed to uncover ". . . a structural definition of health as it is experienced in everyday life" (p. 26). A group of 400 individuals ranging in age from 7 years to over 66 years wrote descriptions of a personal situation in which they experienced a feeling of health. These writings resulted in 762 descriptive expressions that were categorized into three general elements: energy, plentitude, and harmony. From these elements, a synthesized definition of health was derived: "Health is harmony sparked by energy leading to plentitude" (Parse, Coyne, & Smyth, 1985, p. 30).

Glaser and Strauss (1967) coined the term *grounded theory* to describe a methodology in which constructs or theories are generated from data and remain grounded in the real world. In their classic work on *Awareness of Dying* (1965), they uncovered a mutual deception operating when a dying patient was hospitalized. Although the patients knew they were dying, no one acknowledged that fact or allowed them to talk about their impending death. Similarly, the experience of pain is as old as humankind, and nurses and other care providers devote a significant portion of their time and energy to helping patients manage their pain. Fagerhaugh and Strauss (1977) explored the criteria hospital personnel used for controlling a patient's pain. Their study showed that the value system of the nurses and doctors, not the degree of pain the patient felt, determined when and how pain-relieving medications were administered.

Ethnography, phenomenology, and grounded theory are examples of qualitative research methods used to describe phenomena. These methods share similar characteristics, which include the following:

1. Being inductive and process oriented
2. Occurring in controlled observations in a naturalistic setting
3. Describing and explaining phenomena
4. Focusing on dynamic reality and interchange in social situations

An investigator using descriptive research observes, documents, analyzes, and interprets data to achieve a holistic understanding of the patterns, characteristics, and meanings of the phenomena under study.

The design of qualitative research directed toward description encompasses four basic elements: (1) concepts of the study, (2) methods for data generation, (3) plans for data analysis, and (4) methods of presenting findings. Ethnographic, phenomenologic and grounded-theory studies proceed in a cycle. Data are analyzed both informally and formally while data collection is in process. As new ideas emerge, further review of the literature is required. Data collection may be modified according to the advancing knowledge as false leads are identified or more penetrating questions seem necessary.

The study concept

The research problem. Factor-isolating studies ask, "What is this?" The phenomena of interest to nurses are the human circumstances related to health. The research problem is concerned with understanding the meaning and pattern of human responses in conditions of biopsychosocial health or illness. The context of the research question directs the researcher to the most appropriate research design. An ethnographic study is most appropriate to answer questions that are concerned with the cultural context in which meaning is derived. Grounded-theory studies are useful when the social context is of importance; a phenomenologic approach is used when the question is focused on intrapersonal experience of the phenomenon.

One of the most difficult tasks in stating the research question for a descriptive study is to limit the scope of the question. For example, Catanzaro (1980) was interested in the effects of chronic disease on the ill person's life. The literature clearly indicated that the majority of persons with deviations from the definition of "normal" in their society perceived themselves as stigmatized in at least some social situations. A study of stigmatization in chronic illness was too broad an undertaking. Exploration with chronically ill individuals, discussion with colleagues, and practical considerations of access to participants led the investigator to focus the study on persons with symptoms of urinary bladder dysfunction. Were people with problems of urinary frequency and incontinence stigmatized in North American culture? If so, how and under what circumstances did stigmatization occur? How was stigmatization communicated to them? How did they respond? Did their response to stigmatization in any way affect the quality of their lives? The study was concerned with the process in the social situation. The investigator was studying urinary bladder dysfunction, not in terms of its signs, symptoms, diagnosis, treatment, and so forth, but in terms of the social processes that affected the quality of life for the person with these symptoms.

Reviewing the literature. As discussed earlier, a literature search provides direction for the study. The literature is reviewed often and for different purposes throughout a research study. The primary literature search in a qualitative study is focused on the broad area of concern. In the study of urinary bladder dysfunction the literature that was initially reviewed was on the psychosocial aspects of disability. However, the researcher must be careful not to use the literature to prejudge the research inquiry. The investigator who learned from the literature that persons with a disability were stigmatized may have spent enough time in the research setting to confirm that those with urinary frequency and incontinence were stigmatized and thus conclude the research long before he or she understood the social situation that makes this stigmatization a reality. The researcher subsequently may learn that the initial literature search was misdirected and had little relationship to the actual social situation under study. For example, a considerable portion of the disability literature is a result of laboratory experiments in which able-bodied people reported how they respond to persons with various disabilities. The literature may also reveal information that is wholly or partially incorrect. Some disability literature implied that stigma is a problem only when the disability is visible to others. This could have led the investigator to focus on only one portion of the population of interest.

The research purpose in a proposal can be stated in terms of determining the factors involved in a particular situation. In the study of bladder dysfunction the investigator initially questioned whether people with urinary frequency and incontinence were stigmatized in North American culture, the process by

which stigmatization occurred, and the effect it had on the individuals. As the study progressed, the research question that served as the study's purpose changed to, "What processes are involved in attributing shame to persons with urinary frequency and incontinence?"

Sampling. In a descriptive study sampling should include as much information as possible. Maximum variation of sampling will not allow the investigator to generalize findings, but it will provide detail about the many specifics that give the phenomenon under study its unique flavor. The study sample in an ethnographic study consists of a *cultural group*. Spradley (1979) defined a cultural group as those who share knowledge, customs, objects, events, and activities. A cultural group may be a native tribe in a foreign country or nurses practicing in an operating room. Informants from the cultural group who are thoroughly familiar with and currently involved in the culture are chosen. In phenomenologic and grounded-theory studies a sample is drawn from a population of individuals, families, or groups who are experiencing the phenomenon under investigation. Purposive sampling of the study participants is used to obtain maximum information and a full array of responses. Purposive sampling is discussed in Chapter 7.

The number of informants or participants in a descriptive qualitative study is difficult to determine in advance. Data are generated until the researcher experiences repetition of statements that describe the phenomenon under study. Stern (1985) suggested that the best the investigator can do at the beginning of the study is to suggest a number that seems reasonable—enough but not too many. This estimate may be based on the scope of study. A master's candidate might study five people over a relatively short period of time, whereas a doctoral candidate may study five times as many participants. A funded study could include several hundred informants and extend over 5 or more years.

Methods for data generation

Data for a qualitative descriptive study are generated from individuals who possess expertise in living the phenomenon of interest. Data may be in the form of interviews, participant observation, documents, artifacts, pictures, and informal interaction with informants. Each of these methods is discussed in Unit

Three. Initially, general observations and questions are used. As the study progresses, more specific observations and questions become possible. Data may be obtained from a participant at one point in time, or repeated contacts may be made with the same informant over an extended period. Information is sought about the experiences of participants that shaped their current perceptions. Open-ended questions that are answered orally or in writing allow the informant to share the meaning of the lived experience under study. The participants in the study of bladder dysfunction were asked to "Tell me about a situation in which you were embarassed by your incontinence. Consider where you were, who was around, how you felt, and how those who were with you responded." A broad question such as this communicates to the participant that the investigator has no preset categories of interest and provides an opportunity for the informant to become a teacher and to share important feelings and beliefs. Participant observation involves more than just participating in the activities of the group under study. Addi-

TABLE 9-1. Reliability of qualitative studies

THREAT	SPECIFIC EXAMPLES	CONTROL
Researcher's status position	Investigator may be well known to the participants	Clearly identify the researcher's role in the research setting
	The gender of the investigator may influence the openness with which participants share information	Describe the content and development of the researcher's role as the study evolves
Participant choice	Intermediary may approach only those judged "good" participants	Encourage intermediaries to recruit participants nonselectively
	Those who elect to participate may possess characteristics that differ from nonparticipants	Describe characteristics of participants and the decision processes involved in their choice to participate
Social situation conditions	Participants may judge the appropriateness of information in relation to the context	Delineate the context (social, physical, and interpersonal) in which data are generated
		Record field notes immediately after data collection to ensure accurate recall of the structure and function of the context
Methods of procedure	Replicability of qualitative studies not possible	Report precisely and thoroughly the strategies used to collect, analyze, and report data
	Constant comparative analysis may result in lack of agreement on description or composition of events	Transcribe tape-recorded interviews verbatim
		At least two coders perform theoretical coding
		Phrase low inference descriptors in concrete, precise terms
		Seek reaction to working analysis from selected participants
		Compare findings with published studies and other investigators pursuing similar work

tionally, the researcher observes all that is happening to analyze and record what is going on. Observations that are recorded are called field notes.

Reliability and validity of qualitative research

The reliability of qualitative studies is judged by whether an independent researcher would generate the same constructs in a similar situation or would place the data in the same previously generated constructs. The influences on reliability of qualitative studies conducted in field settings include (1) the researcher's status position, (2) the participant choice, (3) the social situation and conditions under which data are collected, and (4) the methods of procedures (LeCompte & Goetz, 1982). Table 9-1 lists these threats to reliability and some specific proce-

TABLE 9-2. Validity of qualitative research

THREAT	SPECIFIC EXAMPLES	CONTROL
History and maturation	Particular problem when data are generated over time, (e.g., longitudinal studies)	Identify those changes that are recurrent, progressive, and cyclical as the sources of change Distinguish maturation from effects of intervening phenomena by use of constant comparative analysis and discrepant-case analysis
Observer effects	Participants may become dependent on researchers for status enhancement or satisfaction of psychological needs Participants may behave abnormally to put self in best light, lie, omit relevant data, or misrepresent their claims Researchers may see and report data as a function of their position	Independent corroboration from multiple participants, discrepant-case analysis, and observation Substantive and theoretical coding likely to elicit contrived responses Comparison of data to theories and analytical models derived from literature Presentation of data in relation to researcher's position and relationships Constant comparative analysis and validity checks with participants
Selection and regression	Possible distortion of data by selection of participants (see above)	Recruit participants who meet purposive sampling criteria Question commonly assumed meanings, utilize discrepant-case analysis, compare data across sampling categories
Mortality	Longitudinal study requiring hours of commitment	Remind participants often that they are experts in topic of study (input valued) Provide consistent follow-up to participants in the form of information about the ongoing study Make it easy for participants to notify the investigator of address changes, (e.g., provide return postcards)

dures for overcoming them. Examples of strategies used include random assignment of interviewers, nonselective recruitment of participants, and use of field notes and verbatim data.

A major strength of qualitative research is the validity of the data. Data are continually analyzed and compared to refined constructs to ensure the match between scientific categories and the participant's reality. The interview tends to be phrased more closely to the empirical world of the participants than are the instruments used in other research designs. Participant observation is conducted in natural settings that reflect the participant's reality to a greater extent than contrived settings.

Threats to validity include (1) history and maturation, (2) observer effects, (3) selection and regression, and (4) mortality (LeCompte & Goetz, 1982). The procedures that can reduce these threats are summarized in Table 9-2 and include discrepant-case analysis, time-sampled data, and verification of coding with participants and experts. Chapter 28 contains a more detailed discussion of these topics.

Plans for data analysis

Miles (1983) referred to qualitative data as an attractive nuisance. It will not take the qualitative researcher long to appreciate the truth of this statement. Reams of data begin rolling in much like tidal waves; the investigator who is unprepared will quickly drown.

The first issue to be resolved is how interview data will be captured. Whether interviews should be tape recorded is still questioned. If tape recorded, are verbatim transcriptions done? These issues are discussed in Chapter 19. Qualitative analysis is concerned with the nature rather than the amount of a phenomenon. Consequently, during the design phase of the study strategies such as coding and memos must be planned for reducing and displaying data. Techniques for qualitative data analysis are discussed in Chapter 28.

Presenting the findings

Qualitative research uses a variety of techniques for data generation and analysis that are implemented according to the phenomenon under study, the nature of the participants, and the investigator's analytic skills. When quantitative research findings are reported in statistical terms (e.g., chi square, correla-

tion coefficient), other researchers know exactly what was done. Qualitative researchers have neither standardized analytical techniques nor a common vocabulary. For this reason a qualitative research report must include the presentation of each activity performed in the process of analysis so the reader can understand how conclusions were reached. The purpose of the study was to answer the question, "What is this?" The presentation of findings includes the answer to this question in a phenomenologic definition, a taxonomy, a hypothetical proposition, or a proposed theory. Additionally, the researcher presents an integrated reconstruction of the data, often with direct quotations from the participants, that relates the outcome of the study to the context in which the study took place.

DESCRIBING THE INCIDENCE OR PREVALENCE OF A PHENOMENON

Designing studies to describe the incidence or prevalence of a phenomenon in a designated population requires an approach different from the qualitative approaches described earlier. The questions addressed in prevalence or incidence studies are: How common is the phenomenon? What is the magnitude of the problem? These questions require quantification of the phenomenon or estimation of its frequency. The design employed in studies conducted for this purpose is the descriptive survey.

Designing a descriptive survey

The design of a prevalence (or incidence) study involves sampling from a known population and classifying each individual selected according to whether each demonstrates the characteristic (concept or phenomenon) being studied. The prevalence of the phenomenon refers to the proportion of individuals who have ever experienced the phenomenon, whereas the incidence refers to the proportion of individuals who experience the phenomenon during the course of the study.

Sampling. Persons who are representative of a designated population are selected. The population might be adolescent mothers, elderly nursing home residents, or individuals seeking care at a mental health center. The aggregate of individuals selected for the study must truly represent the population from which they were selected. Individuals who are

T = Time
P = Participant
V = Variables

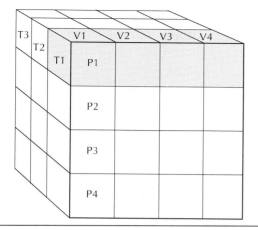

Fig. 9-1. Matrix of participants, variables, and time for a descriptive survey. Shaded area indicates data matrix.

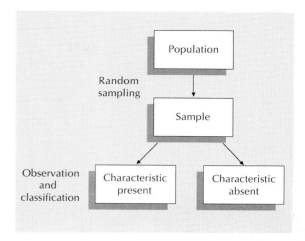

Fig. 9-2. Descriptive survey design. A sample of participants is randomly selected from the population, then observed and classified with respect to the variable(s) of interest.

selected from the population of adolescent mothers must be representative of that population. Individuals selected to represent elderly nursing home residents, as an aggregate, must be representative of the population of elderly nursing home residents.

Another approach to sampling for a descriptive survey is complete ascertainment and study of all eligible participants within a specific geographical area. With this approach all eligible participants are identified through contact with each household or through an existing enumeration list.

Variables and timing. The investigator using a descriptive survey design usually measures one or more variables at a single point in time. Fig. 9-1 shows the matrix of participants, variables, and time for a descriptive survey. Participants (*Pl* to *Pn*) are included on the horizontal axis, variables (*Vl* to *Vn*) on the vertical axis, and time point (*Tl* to *Tn*) on the third axis. Note that observations of the variables are made at a single time point.

The sampling, observations, and classification procedures for a descriptive survey are shown in Fig. 9-2. Note that a sample is drawn from a single population, observed, and classified with respect to the variables of interest to the investigator.

Woods, Most, and Dery (1982), concerned about lack of data on the prevalence of perimenstrual symptoms among women, designed a descriptive survey to estimate the proportion of women experiencing symptoms around the time of menstruation. To determine if a woman in the household met the study criteria, a trained interviewer contacted each household from five neighborhoods selected to represent black and white women ranging from lower-middle to upper-middle income. Women were eligible if they were between 18 and 35 years of age. From the 650 households identified from neighborhood census listings and contacted by an interviewer, 240 women were eligible and 193 participated in the study. Women were asked to rate the severity of 47 symptoms from the Moos Menstrual Distress Questionnaire for their last menstrual cycle, including the menstruum (days of flow), premenstrual week, and the remainder of the cycle. Each woman was classified as having the symptom if she rated it as mild or moderate. As shown in Table 9-3, the incidence of

TABLE 9-3. Percentages of women with MDQ symptoms according to oral contraceptive use and cycle phase (*n* = 179)

	MENSTRUAL				PREMENSTRUAL				REMAINDER			
	NO ORAL CONTRA-CEPTIVES		ORAL CONTRA-CEPTIVES		NO ORAL CONTRA-CEPTIVES		ORAL CONTRA-CEPTIVES		NO ORAL CONTRA-CEPTIVES		ORAL CONTRA-CEPTIVES	
MDQ SYMPTOM*	M/M[†]	S/D[‡]	M/M	S/D	M/M	S/D	M/M	S/D	M/M	S/D	M/M	S/D
1. Weight gain	30.8	2.2	30.3	2.3	39.7	7.4	41.9	0.0	15.5	3.7	9.3	0.0
3. Crying	14.7	2.2	18.7	4.7	19.1	5.1	20.9	2.3	4.4	2.2	4.6	0.0
4. Lowered work or school performance	14.0	5.1	16.3	0.0	11.8	3.7	11.6	2.3	4.4	0.7	4.6	0.0
8. Takes naps	23.5	4.4	21.0	0.0	16.9	0.7	18.7	2.3	7.4	1.5	9.3	2.5
9. Headache	27.2	8.1	27.9	4.7	30.1	6.6	18.6	9.3	12.5	5.9	9.3	0.0
10. Skin disorders	32.4	4.4	23.3	0.0	34.5	8.8	25.6	0.0	18.4	2.2	13.9	0.0
16. Cramps	36.7	19.7	34.9	7.0	20.5	7.4	37.3	2.3	10.3	4.4	9.3	0.0
21. Anxiety	19.2	4.4	23.2	2.3	27.5	3.7	25.6	2.3	12.6	2.2	9.3	2.3
22. Backache	20.6	7.33	39.6	2.3	15.5	5.9	21.0	2.3	8.8	2.2	14.0	0.0
25. Fatigue	38.9	8.1	44.2	4.7	27.9	3.7	30.3	4.7	19.9	0.7	18.7	2.3
30. Painful breasts	24.6	6.1	26.8	0.0	27.4	9.2	29.3	2.4	8.4	2.3	7.3	0.0
34. Swelling	34.4	6.1	34.2	0.0	41.2	6.9	34.2	0.0	9.9	3.1	7.3	0.0
36. Irritability	35.1	10.7	46.3	12.2	42.7	11.5	48.8	14.7	10.7	3.8	24.4	2.4
38. Mood swings	41.2	3.9	48.8	2.4	44.2	6.1	53.6	0.0	21.4	1.5	24.4	2.4
40. Depression	25.9	6.1	41.5	2.4	26.0	9.2	41.5	0.0	18.4	2.3	12.2	0.0
45. Tension	38.1	6.9	36.6	2.4	32.8	9.2	39.0	2.4	19.1	3.8	24.4	2.4

From Woods, N., Most, A., & Dery, G. (1982). *Research in Nursing and Health, 5,* 128.
* Number corresponds to item number on the MDQ.
† Mild, moderate.
‡ Strong, disabling.

symptoms is high for women who rate their symptoms mild or moderate, but it is markedly lower when only those women rating their symptoms as severe were included in the prevalence estimate. Note also that the prevalence of symptoms differs for women who are using oral contraceptives and those who are not. The prevalence of menstrual cramps is nearly three times greater among women who do not use oral contraceptives than among those who do. Irritability and depression are more prevalent among contraceptive users than among women not using contraceptives.

In this study the estimate of incidence (displayed as a percentage) was calculated as follows:

$$\frac{\text{Number with symptoms}}{\text{Number with and without symptoms}}$$

The sampling, observation, and classification procedures for the example dealing with perimenstrual symptoms is given in Fig. 9-3 (p. 142).

Designing a study to estimate a parameter

The same descriptive survey design may be used to estimate the value of a *parameter* for a designated population. A parameter is one characteristic of a population. A descriptive survey design can be used to answer such questions as: What is the average duration of sleep among breast-fed infants during the first 2 weeks of life? What is the average duration of sleep among women hospitalized for delivery during the first 24 hours postpartum?

In the study of the incidence of perimenstrual symptoms women described the severity of their

TABLE 9-4. Mean scores for premenstrual and menstrual phase for 16 MDQ items according to oral contraceptive use

MDQ Symptom*	ALL WOMEN (n = 179)		NO ORAL CONTRACEPTIVES n = 136		ORAL CONTRACEPTIVE USERS (n = 43)	
	PRE-MENSTRUAL	MENSTRUAL	PRE-MENSTRUAL	MENSTRUAL	PRE-MENSTRUAL	MENSTRUAL
1. Weight gain	2.45	2.03[‡]	2.51	2.04[‡]	2.28	2.02
3. Crying	1.74	1.56[†]	1.74	1.55	1.74	1.65
4. Lowered work or school performance	1.57	1.72	1.58	1.73	1.53	1.67
8. Take naps or stays in bed	1.53	1.77[‡]	1.51	1.83[§]	1.60	1.58
9. Headache	2.11	2.12	2.12	2.12	2.09	2.09
10. Skin disorders	2.16	1.93[§]	2.31	2.05[§]	1.67	1.58
16. Cramps	1.93	2.75[§]	1.87	2.88[§]	2.09	2.37
21. Anxiety	1.93	1.77[†]	1.98[†]	1.81[§]	1.77	1.65
22. Backache	1.75	1.98	1.73	1.93	1.79	2.11[‡]
25. Fatigue	2.06	2.41[§]	2.04	2.40[§]	2.14	2.44
30. Painful or tender breasts	2.21	1.99[†]	2.29	2.05[†]	1.95	1.78
34. Swelling	2.33	2.14[†]	2.40	2.18[†]	2.07	2.00
36. Irritability	2.80	2.57[†]	2.71	2.53	3.07	2.68
38. Mood swings	2.47	2.33[†]	2.50	2.33	2.39	2.32
40. Depression	2.23	2.10	2.21	2.08	1.46	2.19[‡]
45. Tension	2.31	2.26	2.36	2.32	2.17	2.07

From Woods, N., Most, A., & Dery, G. (1982). *Research in Nursing and Health, 5,* 129.
*Number corresponds to item number on the MDQ.
[†]$p < .05$.
[‡]$p < .01$.
[§]$p < .001$.

symptoms, as well as their prevalence. Estimates of average symptom severity are given in Table 9-4. Because the observations came from a designated population, it is possible to consider them estimates of the average experience for that entire population. The severity levels of the symptoms in Table 9-4 are consistent with the descriptors "barely noticeable to mild." Thus we could conclude that on the basis of this sample the severity of perimenstrual symptoms was mild.

DESCRIBING PATTERNS OVER TIME

Patterns: change and persistence

Pattern refers to the configuration of a phenomenon, that is, repetitive and regular occurrences of a phe-

nomenon. Patterns may increase, decrease, or maintain a stable state by oscillating up and down in degree of frequency. For example, body temperature fluctuates predictably over a 24-hour period. The concepts of change and persistence are important considerations in designing studies to describe patterns over time. *Change* refers to a transformation, a change in state. Watzlawick, Weakland, and Fisch (1974) describe two types of change. (1) *First order change* occurs in a given system that itself does not change. For example, an individual having a nightmare can run, scream, and try to escape, but nothing will change the course of the nightmare. (2) *Second order change* is a change of state, a change whose occurrence changes the system. Waking up from the nightmare is an example of second order change, a

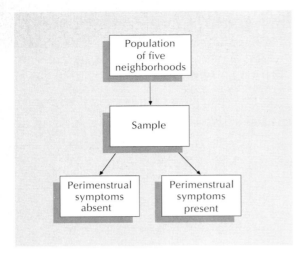

Fig. 9-3. From a population of five neighborhoods, a sample of women was selected and the presence of perimenstrual symptoms was assessed.

change in state. *Persistence* refers to dynamic equilibrium seen in living systems and does not imply inertia or stagnation. Instead, persistence implies an ongoing series of first order changes. Families who are experiencing the life-threatening illness of a member undergo many individual changes but demonstrate remarkable stability as a family throughout the experience. The family persists; it endures over time. Some families who experience a member's life-threatening illness are transformed in the process. They may change their rules for functioning as a family, becoming religious converts, or they may become reconstituted, losing a member through separation or divorce. In either instance the family is transformed.

Studying change over time requires consideration of both first and second order changes. In the case of first order change, or persistence, the investigator will focus on the oscillation of values of some parameter such as body temperature over time. In the case of the second order change, or transformation, the investigator will focus on changes of state.

Description of patterns of phenomena over time is important to the study of many nursing research topics. Most of the health-related phenomena of interest to nursing science are dynamic in nature,

such as feelings of well-being, moods, family coping, and the nature of the social environment for health. The processes of recovery from life-threatening illness, adaptation to parenthood, or transition to nursing home life all require a dynamic approach to investigation. In studying these phenomena a single measurement is likely to be uninformative—if not erroneous—and investigators may find remarkable stability rather than dramatic change.

Investigators in nursing frequently address such questions as the following:
1. What is the developmental course of premature infants who were cared for in a neonatal intensive care unit? At what age do the infants first sleep for more than 2 hours? More than 4 hours?
2. How do women experience menopause? How do their moods change from the time their periods become irregular until they stop? How long does menopause take?
3. How do men adapt to chronic illness in their lives? What demands do they experience over the first year after diagnosis?

Study designs that address these questions are *longitudinal* in nature. They involve obtaining repeated measures over time. Many types of designs have longitudinal elements. A time series design involves multiple repeated observations on a single entity or a small number of entities at a relatively large number of time points. A panel design involves observations on many entities but at relatively few times. For the time series design the time point is the unit of analysis. For the panel design the individual is the unit of analysis. A comparison of two kinds of longitudinal designs is given in Fig. 9-4. Both designs are important for characterizing change or stability of a phenomenon over time.

Panel design

Sampling. The sampling approach for a panel design resembles those described earlier for descriptive surveys. The sample must be representative of the designated population to allow the investigator to generalize findings to the population of interest. However, a longitudinal study requires the observation of participants over an extended period of time, often for years. The collective of individuals enrolled in a longitudinal study is termed a *cohort*. The same cohort of individuals will be followed for the duration of the study.

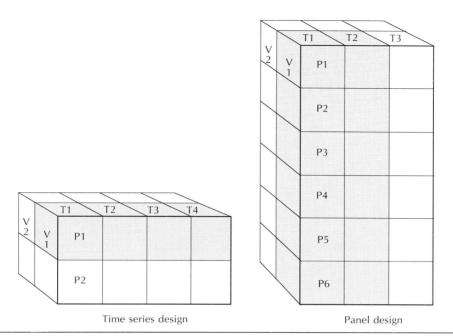

Fig. 9-4. A comparison of a time-series design and a panel design. Shaded area in time-series design shows one variable measured for one individual over four times, shaded area in panel design shows one variable measured for six individuals over two times.

A longitudinal study may involve single or multiple cohorts. A single cohort enters the study within a limited time period; for example, a cohort of men recovering from myocardial infarction could enter a study during 1985. Alternatively, cohorts can enter a study at different time points, for example, 1980, 1985, 1990. Because the cohorts live during different time periods, they may have very different life experiences. Suppose women participants in a longitudinal study of health and aging entered the study in 1940, 1950, 1960, and 1970 (Fig. 9-5). Each cohort was 30 years old at the time of entry. The dramatic changes in women's roles in western countries illustrate how these cohorts are likely to differ. With multiple cohorts investigators can differentiate the effects of aging per se from the variations in life context for each cohort. At 50 years of age women born in 1920 and women born in 1940 could differ significantly on health status largely as an effect of their cohort and not their age. The cohort effect is analogous to a generational effect (the effect of being born in a particular generation) and is likely to be most noticeable when cohorts enter the study during very different times.

Variables and timing. Panel studies require multiple observations, often with repeated measures of the same concept. In some instances the same measurement instruments are used repeatedly (e.g., measures of weight, height, and blood pressure are likely to be made under precisely the same conditions). In other circumstances, to reflect the concept accurately, the measures must be different. For example, measures of intelligence in a child differ with the child's age. An appropriate indicator for the 3-year-old is inappropriate for a 7-year-old. For infants, indicators of motor development change rapidly from measures of gross motor movement to those of finely coordinated motor skills. Likewise, measurement of parent-child interaction would differ for parent-infant pairs versus parent-adolescent pairs, even though the same construct, parental nurturance, is studied.

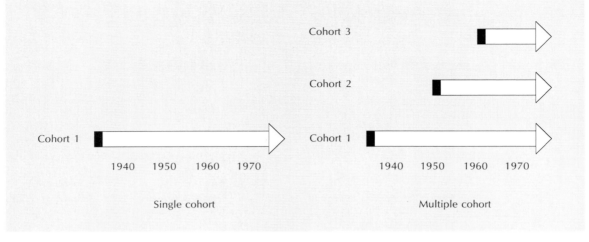

Fig. 9-5. Single-cohort studies versus multiple-cohort studies.

Another issue to consider when designing longitudinal studies is timing of the measures. The measures need to be made at times that reflect the aims of the study. For example, if the aims include characterizing a rapidly changing phenomenon such as motor development in infants, the measures must be made at frequent intervals (i.e., monthly or every 6 weeks) rather than every 6 months. When the phenomenon changes less rapidly, such as the transition to menarche, measures can be made at less frequent intervals. Another concern is how many measures to make or over what span of time to make the measures. This decision is concerned with the speed of the process being studied. Does the process require months or years for its occurrence? Is it a relatively rapid process requiring a few hours or days? For example, helping processes may take place over a very short or lengthy period. In inpatient care settings nurses develop helping relationships with clients that may be limited to a few days, whereas in outpatient community mental health settings, relationships may extend over periods of years.

Woods, Most, and Longenecker (1985) used a panel design to study women's experiences of daily stressors over the menstrual cycle. They identified and interviewed all women between 18 and 35 years of age from five neighborhoods that varied in racial and socioeconomic composition. After completing the interview, 100 of the women were randomly selected to complete a daily health diary for 2 months. Each day the women recorded whether they had experienced a stressor in the areas of work, friends, relatives or husband, children, or some other area. They also recorded whether positive events had occurred each day. Data for one complete menstrual cycle were available for 71 of the 74 women who completed the diary. The percentage of days with a stressor related to work, friends, relatives, and husband, and other sources was slightly higher for the premenstrual week than during menstruation or the remainder of the cycle. The percentage of days with a positive event was also highest during the premenstrual week. (See Table 9-5.)

In this study sampling was achieved in two stages. First, all eligible women were invited to participate in an interview. Second, a subset from those women was selected randomly to complete the daily diary for 2 months. The cohort consisted of the women asked to complete diaries. Only 74 of the 100 women in this cohort completed the diaries. Those who did complete the diaries were slightly better educated than their counterparts. The discrepancy between the number of women who completed the diaries and those who did not illustrates a significant problem in longitudinal studies: loss of participants. Payment is one means to increase participation. Of those

TABLE 9-5. Stressors experienced by participants ($n = 71$)	
VARIABLES	$\overline{X} \pm SD$
Days with work stressor (%)	
Premenstruum	13 ± 20
Menstruum	11 ± 17
Remainder	11 ± 17
Days with friends, relatives, or husband stressor (%)	
Premenstruum	12 ± 19
Menstruum	10 ± 18
Remainder	10 ± 12
Days with children stressor (%)	
Premenstruum	3 ± 7
Menstruum	3 ± 9
Remainder	4 ± 13
Days with other stressors (%)	
Premenstruum	20 ± 26
Menstruum	18 ± 23
Remainder	17 ± 18
Days with positive events (%)	
Premenstruum	48 ± 33
Menstruum	45 ± 36
Remainder	47 ± 33

From Woods, N., Most, A., & Longenecker, G. (1985). Reprinted with permission from *Nursing Research, 34,* 263-267. ©, 1985, American Journal of Nursing Company.

women who were paid, 66% completed diaries. Of those who were not paid, 32% completed the diaries.

The study of stressors and the menstrual cycle also illustrates the value of longitudinal measures. Because many stressors were minor, the likelihood of their being recalled is low. Moreover, the timing of events might have been telescoped. The time period of 2 months for data collection allowed the investigators to capture at least one complete menstrual cycle. The interval for data collection was daily, because the events were minor and not likely to be recalled as clearly as major life events or birthdays.

Measurements in this study were identical for the 2-month period. One problem associated with this approach to measurement is boredom when the measures are repeated over long periods. The net effect of boredom is usually noncompletion of the measures. The researcher must balance this risk with the demand placed on participants when different measures are completed on a frequent basis.

Time series designs

A second type of longitudinal design is the *time series design*. Time series designs involve multiple repeated observations on a single entity or on a small number of entities at a relatively large number of points in time. The time point, for example, the day or month, is the unit of analysis. In contrast, the person or participant is the unit of analysis in panel designs. Time series designs permit investigators to characterize a pattern over time, analyze unique fluctuations of a variable through time, and provide a framework for predicting further changes in the variable for that individual. Time series designs also allow prediction from one individual to that same individual on subsequent observations. These designs permit the investigator to assess change, not only as a deviation from a group mean, but also as a departure from an individual pattern. These designs are useful for forecasting clinical parameters; for example, temperature patterns for an individual can be forecast from one measurement period to subsequent time periods (Metzger & Schultz, 1981).

Sampling. Sampling for time series designs differs from that for panel designs in several ways. First, a major concern in time series studies is description of a pattern for one or only a few individuals for a unit of time, not a description of a large aggregate of individuals. An individual or a few individuals are selected because of some characteristic. To study temperature patterns of elderly men, Lentz (1984) selected elderly men because little was known about their temperature and sleep patterns. Updike, Accurso, and Jones (1985) selected infants from the neonatal intensive care unit who were between 34 and 37 weeks' gestational age. Sometimes investigators will select an individual because of some special characteristic, that is, they may want to characterize a pattern unique to that individual or a group of individuals. In this instance they may select someone who they believe exhibits an unusual pattern. Second, the sampling used in time series is a sample of observations over time, not a sample of individuals per se. Sampling in the Updike, Accurso, and Jones study (1985) of preterm infants occurred every 30 minutes. Their sample consisted of 48 measures taken over a 24-hour period for each of the infants.

Lentz (1984) monitored temperature continuously in her study of sleep and body temperature rhythms.

Variables and timing. Usually one or a few variables of interest are studied in a time series design. The variable is some parameter such as temperature that is selected because it varies over time. An investigator may select a second parameter that is also known to vary over time to relate it to the variables of interest. For example, when studying sleep-wakefulness, investigators often study temperature, as well as electroencephalographic indicators of sleep.

Time and timing are special concerns in time series studies. The field of *chronobiology* emphasizes the dimension of time for understanding human biology and has contributed several new concepts for characterizing the time dimension of human health. Many biological phenomena such as temperature occur in rhythmic patterns, having a cyclical, recurrent order of events. *Circadian* patterns refer to 24-hour patterns in contrast to rhythms occurring over shorter periods of time, such as ultradian rhythms. Three characteristics define a circadian rhythm: acrophase, amplitude, and mesor. The term *acrophase* designates the clock time at which a peak value occurs. *Amplitude* refers to the extent of change between the peak and trough value of the parameter, and the *mesor* refers to the average value of the parameter whose rhythm is being studied (Fig. 9-6).

Investigators designing time series studies are concerned with time and timing. First, it is important to consider how rapidly the rhythmical phenomenon or change occurs. Circamensual rhythms characterize the menstrual cycle and require approximately 28 days, whereas circadian rhythms require approximately 24 hours. Collecting data for a sufficiently long time period is important to capture the rhythm or change. Moreover, collecting data at sufficiently frequent intervals is important to detect change. For example, an investigator could obtain data at the points shown in Fig. 9-7 and conclude that no rhythmical change occurred, when in reality the sampling occurred too infrequently to detect the rhythmical change.

Lentz (1984) described the body temperature rhythm for nine healthy elderly men who maintained their usual patterns of activity, social interaction, and sleep-wake cycles during the course of the study. She monitored their rectal temperature continuously over a 24-hour period and sampled their temperature records at 10-minute intervals. Lentz found that the elderly men experienced their temperature acrophase earlier than the younger men studied previously.

Lentz's study illustrates several important aspects of time series designs. First, she obtained many data points from a small number of individuals and initially analyzed the data from each individual to determine the rhythmical pattern of body temperature. Next, time and timing of the presumed rhythmical pattern influenced the data collection procedure. Assuming a circadian pattern in temperature rhythm, Lentz collected data continuously for a 24-hour period. She sampled data at 10-minute intervals, assuming that this interval would permit identification of any significant changes in the temperature rhythm.

Time series designs can be used to describe a single parameter such as temperature or to study the relationship between two or more patterns. Lentz also collected data regarding sleep, allowing her to examine the relationship between temperature rhythms and sleep-wakefulness patterns.

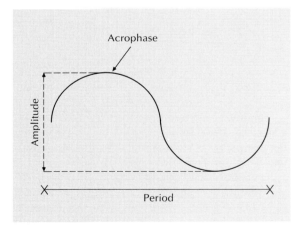

Fig. 9-6. Idealized fitted curve. *Amplitude,* peak-to-trough difference; *acrophase,* time of maximum value; *period,* time a defined event reoccurs. (Redrawn from Lentz, M. [1984]. Circadian phase relationships of sleep-wake cycle and body temperature rhythm in aging. Unpublished doctoral dissertation. University of Washington, Seattle.)

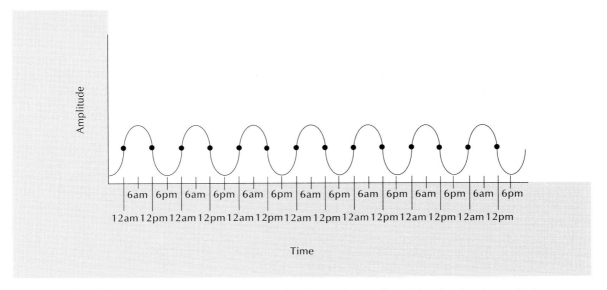

Fig. 9-7. If data were collected only at the time points indicated by the dot, it would be impossible to detect the rhythmical pattern in this variable.

VALIDITY OF DESCRIPTIVE STUDIES

Several factors influence the validity of a descriptive study. *External validity* of the study concerns generalizing from findings observed in one set of data to other potential samples or to the entire population. The investigator considers to what populations, settings, and observations the research findings should be generalized (Baltes, Reese, & Nesselroade, 1977). Investigators consider three dimensions when designing an externally valid descriptive study: (1) the participants or units being studied, (2) the settings for the study, and (3) the observations being made.

Participants who are selected for a descriptive survey to estimate prevalence or incidence of a phenomenon, to estimate a parameter, or to describe change over time in a parameter must be representative of the population to which the investigator wishes to apply the research findings. Studying hospitalized patients is inappropriate when the investigator's intent is to learn about the experiences of all adults. Typically, hospitalized individuals are ill; thus they do not resemble the total population of adults.

The setting of a study is a second important dimension to consider in relation to external validity.

Individuals may respond differently when studied in a laboratory setting than when studied in their own homes. For example, studying blood pressure in a strange setting that is associated with elevated anxiety may produce results that do not resemble typical blood pressure measurements taken in a familiar surrounding.

A third dimension that is related to external validity is the nature of the observations being made. When individuals are asked to recall their experiences with minor illnesses over the last 2 months, they may forget some, exaggerate some, and recall others accurately. When they are asked to complete a daily record of their illness experiences, the likelihood of valid observations increases. Issues that are related to the external validity of the study need to be considered when the study is designed, not after the study is completed.

Internal validity permits the investigator to reach unambiguous conclusions about the phenomenon being studied. Usually internal validity is related to the relationships among the variables being studied. In descriptive studies that address a single variable, internal validity may be considered as it relates to that single variable and its measurement on one or more occasions. Internal validity issues that apply to a descriptive survey include history, maturation, instrumentation, and selection.

History refers to the effects of secular trends or events external to the study on the observations made in the study. Prevalence estimates of the frequency of self breast examination have been influenced by historical events such as the media coverage devoted to famous women who diagnosed their own breast cancer.

Maturation refers to changes in the individuals being studied that are expected to occur with age. These changes, such as development of motor ability in young children, are expected to occur regardless of the study. The effect of maturation is often the focus of a longitudinal descriptive study. An important concern related to maturation is whether the timing of measurement—or in repeated observation studies the frequency of measurement—is adequate to allow appropriate description of the phenomenon. For example, making measurements on infants' motor development every 3 months is clearly inadequate to allow observation of a rapidly changing phenomenon.

Testing is another internal validity issue and refers to the influence of the observation itself on the phenomenon being observed. Testing effects can be seen in studies of children, some of whom are comfortable with the observer in the home and some of whom are uncomfortable with the observer's presence, and object strenuously, thus making it difficult to obtain valid observations of the child's typical behavior.

Instrumentation is another issue related to internal validity. Changes in the calibration of an instrument as it is applied to individuals in a sample can cause invalid measurements. For example, differences in blood pressures obtained from a large sample can be a function of sphygmomanometers that are not recalibrated over the course of the study.

Selection of participants is another issue affecting internal validity. Selecting only those participants who are extremely healthy will not be informative about the total population of chronically ill adults. An estimate of the morale of all the chronically ill that is based on a subset of persons with less severe illness will be deceptive.

Mortality, the loss of participants from the study, constitutes another validity issue. Loss of participants over time is a special threat to validity of longitudinal studies. Loss of participants affects the generalizability of the findings, as well as the ability to accurately understand change over time.

SUMMARY

This chapter describes the relationship between theory development aims and several types of descriptive designs, including grounded-theory studies, descriptive surveys, panel designs, and time series designs. Table 9-6 compares the sampling approaches, observations, and timing associated with

TABLE 9-6. A comparison of designs for description of phenomena

THEORY DEVELOPMENT AIM DESIGN	SAMPLE	OBSERVATIONS AND TIMING
Identify, describe concept: Grounded-theory study Ethnography Phenomenologic inquiry	Purposive sampling	Multiple variables measured at single or multiple time points
Estimate prevalence of phenomenon, estimate parameter: Descriptive survey	Random sample from designated population	One or more variables measured at single time point
Describe patterns of change or stability of phenomenon over time: Panel design	Random sample from designated population	One or more variables measured at multiple time points
Time series design	Purposive sample or single case	One or more variables measured at multiple time points

each design. When the theory development aim is to identify or describe concepts, a grounded-theory, ethnographic, or phenomenologic inquiry approach can be used. These designs incorporate purposive sampling and require multiple variables to be measured at one or more time points. When the theory development aim is to describe quantitatively the prevalence of a phenomenon or to estimate a parameter for a population, a descriptive survey can be used. The descriptive survey incorporates random sampling from a designated population and measurement of one or more variables at a single point in time. When the theory development aim is to describe patterns of change over time, panel designs and time series designs can be used. Panel designs incorporate random sampling from a population and measurement of one or more variables at multiple points in time. Time series designs incorporate purposive sampling of one or a few cases and measurement of one or more variables at multiple time points. Each design serves a specific purpose; together they provide a rich repertoire for building nursing studies to describe phenomena.

References

Baltes, P., Reese, H., & Nesselroade, J. (1977). *Life span developmental psychology: Introduction to research methods.* Monterey, CA: Brooks/Cole.

Boyle, J. (1983). Illness experiences and the role of women in Guatemala. In J. Uhl (Ed.), *Proceedings of the eighth annual transcultural nursing conference* (pp. 52-71). Salt Lake City: University of Utah College of Nursing and Transcultural Nursing Society.

Catanzaro, M. (1980). Shamefully different: A personal meaning of urinary bladder dysfunction. *Dissertation Abstracts International, 42,* 4166A. (University Microfilms No. DEO 82-04984).

Crawford, G. (1982). The concept of pattern in nursing: Conceptual development and measurement. *Advances in Nursing Science, 5*(1), 1-6.

Dougherty, M. C. (1978). *Becoming a woman in rural black culture.* New York: Holt, Reinhart, & Winston.

Fagerhaugh, S., & Strauss, A. (1977). *The politics of pain management.* New York: Addison-Wesley.

Field, P. A. (1983). An ethnography: Four public health nurses' perspectives of nursing. *Journal of Advanced Nursing, 8*(1), 3-12.

Glaser, B., & Strauss, A. (1965). *Awareness of dying.* Chicago: Aldine.

Glaser, B., & Strauss, A. (1967). *The discovery of grounded theory.* Chicago: Aldine.

Gottmann, J. (1981). *Time-series analysis: A comprehensive introduction for social scientists.* New York: Cambridge University Press.

Hall, B. (1983). Toward an understanding of stability in nursing phenomena. *Advances in Nursing Science, 5*(3), 15-20.

LeCompte, M. D., & Goetz, J. P. (1982). Problems of reliability and validity in ethnographic research. *Review of Educational Research, 52*(1), 31-60.

Leininger, M. M. (1980). Caring: A central focus for nursing and health care services. *Nursing and Health Care, 1*(3), 135-143, 176.

Leininger, M. M. (Ed.). (1985). *Qualitative research methods in nursing.* Orlando: Grune & Stratton.

Lentz, M. (1984). Circadian phase relationships of sleep-wake cycle and body temperature rhythm in aging. Unpublished doctoral dissertation: University of Washington, Seattle.

Metzger, B., & Schultz, S. (1982). Time series analysis: An alternative for nursing research. *Nursing Research, 31* 375-378.

Miles, M. B. (1983). Qualitative data as an attractive nuisance: The problem of analysis. In J. VanMaanen (Ed.), *Qualitative methodology.* Beverly Hills, CA: Sage.

Parse, R. R., Coyne, A. B., & Smith, M. J. (1985). *Nursing research: Qualitative methods.* Bovie, MD: Brady Communications.

Patton, M. Q. (1980). *Qualitative evaluation methods.* Beverly Hills, CA: Sage.

Spradley, J. P. (1979). *The ethnographic interview.* New York: Holt, Rinehart & Winston.

Stern, P. N. (1985). Using grounded theory method in nursing research. In M. M. Leininger (Ed.), *Qualitative research methods in nursing.* Orlando: Grune & Stratton.

Updike, P., Accurso, F., & Jones, R. (1985). Physiologic circadian rhythmicity in preterm infants. *Nursing Research, 34,* 160-163.

Watzlawick, P., Weakland, J., & Fisch, R. (1974). *Change: Principles of problem formation and problem resolution.* New York: Norton.

Woods, N., Most, A., & Dery, G. (1982). Towards a construct of perimenstrual distress. *Research in Nursing and Health, 5,* 123-136.

Woods, N., Most, A., & Longenecker, G. (1985). Major life events, daily stressors, and perimenstrual symptoms. *Nursing Research, 34,* 263-267.

10

DESIGNING STUDIES TO EXPLORE ASSOCIATION AND DIFFERENCE

NANCY FUGATE WOODS AND PAMELA HOLSCLAW MITCHELL

Exploring association and difference is an important mode for theory generation. The word "explore" implies scrutinizing unknown regions for the purpose of discovery. Indeed, exploratory studies serve this purpose and are particularly useful during the early stages of investigating the relationships between phenomena about which not much is known. Consider the human responses to new techniques in medicine or surgery. The recipients of artificial heart implantations are a case in point. No one could have predicted how the individuals and their families would respond to the application of this technology. What personal factors would influence the individual's perception of changes in body image? What factors would influence the family's acceptance of the intrusion of technology into their homes? How would the family influence the person's response to the implant? Instances such as these invite exploration for purposes of discovery instead of imposition of hypotheses. Exploratory studies provide a means for investigators to contribute to understanding about the relationships between phenomena—to discover relevant connections or differences.

Exploratory studies presuppose identification of the phenomenon and its description. Ideally, the exploratory study follows work that not only includes description of a phenomenon but also includes identification of ways of measuring it. These notions are explored more fully in chapters dealing with measurement issues (Chapters 14 and 15).

The focus of an exploratory study is identification of factors related to the primary phenomenon of interest. In nursing, these studies frequently address health-related phenomena such as pain, anxiety, or well-being. The investigative strategy attempts to identify factors related to those phenomena. For example, an investigator might address the influence of gender, age, education, ethnicity, access to support, type of surgical procedure, and past experience with surgery on reports of pain and the use of pain medication following abdominal surgery.

The results of exploratory studies are often the generation of hypotheses to be tested in subsequent studies. Thus exploratory studies provide an important link between identification and description of phenomena and hypothesis-testing studies. For example, an investigator conducting an exploratory study of adolescent parenting might observe that adolescent mothers experience an unusually high rate of parenting problems. This discovery could lead to a second study to test the hypothesis that parenting problems are related to the support available to the adolescent mother and to her own developmental level.

Several designs are particularly useful for exploration. These include correlational surveys, comparative surveys, panel designs, and case studies.

CORRELATIONAL SURVEYS

A *correlational survey* is a research design that relates multiple variables measured at a single time point in a sample from a designated population. This design enables the investigator to relate several variables to one another, allowing the investigator to address questions such as: What factors are associated with recovery from coronary artery bypass graft (CABG) surgery? Are the patient's gender, family constellation, marital relationship, past health history, health practices, and health goals related to recovery? Are the dimensions of recovery from surgery related to one another? Are improvements in physical function, mood, and social activity related to one another?

Sampling

The sample for a correlational survey should represent the designated population of interest. Ideally, random sampling approaches are employed to generate a sample; however, nonprobability sampling frequently is used, limiting the generalizability of the relationships beyond the sample studied. For example, an investigator studying recovery following CABG surgery could use systematic random sampling in hospitals in several regions of the country, selecting every third patient having the surgery for participation in the study. Alternatively, an investigator might elect to study all patients having CABG surgery in a single hospital during 1 year. Although the former plan enhances the generalizability of the study results, the latter approach often has the advantages of feasibility and lower cost.

Observations and timing

The correlational survey includes measures of multiple variables obtained on a single occasion. The variables are related to one another but not in a causal way. Instead, the analytical strategy emphasizes exploration of relationships as associations. For example, in a study of people's recovery from CABG surgery, an investigator might collect data with respect to physical and psychosocial indicators of recovery (e.g., activity level, mood, and interaction outside the home), as well as age, gender, marital quality, family constellation, past experience with surgery, health practices, and health goals. The relationships being studied are shown in Fig. 10-1. Notice that the arrows between family factors, personal factors, and recovery are pointing in two directions, implying that the direction of the relationship is unknown or perhaps reciprocal. At this stage in knowledge development, knowing which way the arrow should point may not be possible; finding that direction is one function served by this type of study. Also note that many of the factors thought to influence recovery can be grouped into larger categories. For example, marital quality and family constellation are both related to family and are called "family factors." Grouping individual factors helps to guide the data-collection process and analysis, because the investigator is prompted to think about how the individual factors relate to one another.

Ferrans and Powers (1985) used a correlational survey to examine the relationship of several factors that may influence employment potential of patients receiving hemodialysis. They explored three broad categories of factors: illness-related factors, occupational factors, and psychosocial factors. Illness-related factors included biophysiological parameters, subjective health appraisal, and physical impairments to job performance. Occupational factors included job satisfaction and performance, employment decision factors, and job discrimination as a result of illness. Psychosocial factors included life goal changes, overall life satisfaction, and dependency.

Hemodialysis patients, ranging in age from 21 to 59, who had been employed before dialysis and who were judged physically able to work by their physicians were eligible for the study. Of 195 patients, 44 met the criteria for the study, and 40 participated. Participants were interviewed during dialysis, and laboratory and illness-related data were obtained from their patient records. Of the 40 participants, 20 patients were employed currently. Job satisfaction and job importance before starting hemodialysis, biophysiological status, perceived health status, life satisfaction, and dependence were not different for the employed and unemployed groups. A greater proportion of those who were unemployed had held jobs requiring heavy physical labor, and the unemployed reported that symptoms of uremia prevented them from working. Job discrimination because of illness and a greater loss of career and life goals were found among the unemployed.

The study by Ferrans and Powers (1985) explores the relationships among four sets of variables as shown in Fig. 10-2. Data about all four sets of variables were obtained at a single point in time. Three

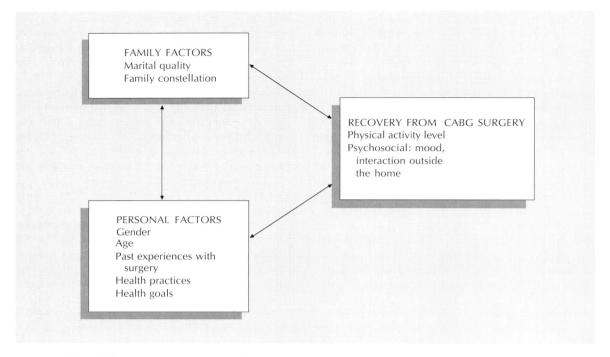

Fig. 10-1. Relationships between family factors, personal factors, and recovery from coronary artery bypass graft (CABG) surgery.

sets of factors were analyzed with respect to their relationships to one another and to employment status. In this example, use of the correlational survey made it possible to study associations between several variables thought to be related to people's return to work after hemodialysis treatment. Future study could include both testing hypotheses that allow prediction of return to work after dialysis and clinical programs of symptom control and physical conditioning to improve people's likelihood of returning to work.

COMPARATIVE SURVEYS

A *comparative survey* is a research design that involves comparing and contrasting two or more samples on one or more variables, often at a single point in time. Through comparative surveys researchers can address questions such as: Do people with diagnoses of lung cancer experience more symptom distress than those surviving myocardial infarction? Do they experience different concerns? Are their patterns of mood different? A comparative survey differs from a correlational survey in two ways. Because the aims of the two types of studies differ, different sampling approaches and different plans for observations and timing are used.

Sampling

The sample for a correlational survey is drawn from a single population, and the samples for a comparative survey are drawn from two or more underlying populations that are being contrasted (Fig. 10-3). In the correlational survey of hemodialysis patients, the sample was drawn from a population of all hemodialysis patients and then classified into employed and unemployed patients after their selection. In contrast, two samples could have been obtained, one from a population of employed hemodialysis patients and one from a population of unemployed

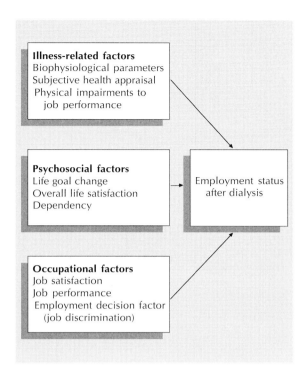

Fig. 10-2. Design for an exploratory study to identify factors related to employment status after dialysis.

hemodialysis patients. Note that this difference in sampling procedures might have resulted in the inclusion of different participants in the study.

Observations and timing

In the comparative survey, the emphasis is on how two or more populations differ with respect to factors of interest, whereas in the correlational survey the emphasis is on how a number of factors are associated with one another.

Both designs are also referred to as ex post facto designs from the Latin "after the fact." The term "ex post facto" indicates that the research was conducted after the variability in the independent variable occurred.

A comparative survey typically involves measurement of one or more variables in two or more groups at one or more points in time. Had the study of the employment experiences of patients receiving hemodialysis been conducted as a comparative survey, the

data collection procedures could have been essentially the same. The observations and timing simply would have been applied to two different samples, and the findings compared.

McCorkle and Benoliel (1983), interested in how patients cope with life-threatening disease and its consequences, sought to describe the levels of symptom distress, current concerns, and mood disturbance in persons with one of two life-threatening diseases. Because they were concerned about whether patients with cancer experience more distress than patients with different life-threatening illnesses, the investigators compared a sample of patients with lung cancer to a sample of patients who had had a myocardial infarction. They measured the degree of distress associated with 13 symptoms (e.g., nausea, loss of appetite, insomnia, pain, fatigue, and disturbances in bowel patterns, concentration, and breathing) and current concerns about health, self-appraisal, work and finances, family, religion, friends, existential issues, and mood states such as tension-anxiety, depression-dejection, and vigor-activity. They found that patients with lung cancer had more symptom distress than patients who had experienced myocardial infarction. Moreover, the patients with lung cancer reported more concerns, especially those related to health and existential concerns, and more mood disturbances than did the patients with myocardial infarction.

The McCorkle and Benoliel study (1983) departed from the definition of a comparative survey design because the measurements were made on two occasions (1 and 2 months after diagnosis). Technically, the measurements obtained on the first occasion would have satisfied the requirements for a comparative survey design. The extension of the comparative survey design used by the investigators permitted them to compare the patients with myocardial infarction and lung cancer on two different occasions. As seen in Table 10-1, the investigators found that the patients with lung cancer had more symptom distress at both interviews (note scores of 26.7 versus 19.3 on occasion one and 26.1 versus 19.2 on occasion two) than did the patients with myocardial infarction. Symptom distress remained the same on both occasions, but fewer concerns and mood disturbances were reported over time.

Use of multiple occasions of measurement is an important adaptation of the comparative survey and

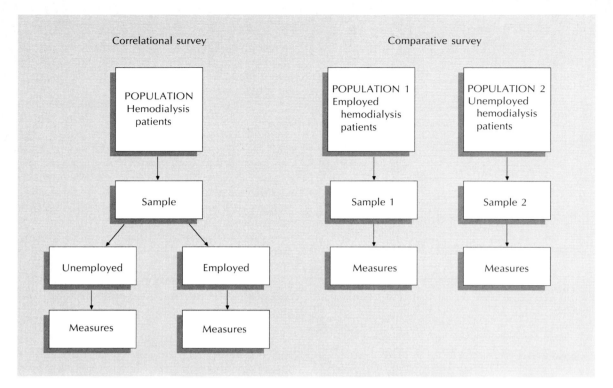

Fig. 10-3. A comparison of the sampling approaches for a correlational survey and a comparative survey. Notice that the comparative survey requires sampling from two or more different populations, whereas the correlational survey involves sampling from a single population.

TABLE 10-1. Normative data on scales for study sample at two interviews

SCALE	MEAN CA*	MEAN MI*	MEDIAN CA	MEDIAN MI	SD CA	SD MI	POTENTIAL RANGE OF SCORES
INTERVIEW ONE							
Symptom distress scale	26.7	19.3	24.5	18.7	8.4	4.9	13-65
Inventory current concerns	26.4	22.1	25.9	19.1	19.3	15.3	0-144
Profile mood states	32.2	17.8	27.5	17.1	29.9	25.6	−32-204
INTERVIEW TWO							
Symptom distress scale	26.1	19.2	25.5	18.2	8.4	4.9	13-65
Inventory current concerns	24.0	19.5	22.0	17.3	18.9	17.0	0-144
Profile mood states	22.2	14.1	26.9	11.3	24.2	27.3	−32-204

From McCorkle, R., and Benoliel, J. (1983). Reprinted with permission from *Social Science and Medicine 17* (Symptom distress), 431-438. © 1983, Pergamon Journals, Ltd.
*CA, participants with lung cancer; *MI, participants who have had a myocardial infarction.

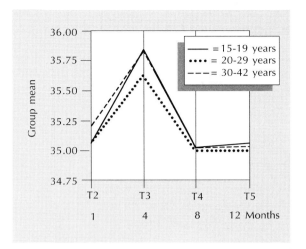

Fig. 10-4. Positive feelings expressed by mothers about their babies; group means over time. (From Mercer, R. [1985]. Reprinted with permission from *Nursing Research, 34,* 198-204. ©, 1985, American Journal of Nursing Company.)

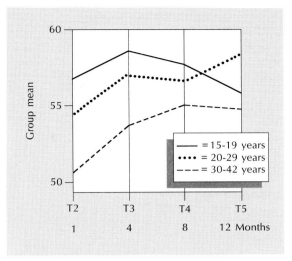

Fig. 10-5. Gratification in the maternal role; group means over time. (From Mercer, R. [1985]. Reprinted with permission from *Nursing Research, 34,* 198-204. ©, 1985, American Journal of Nursing Company.)

especially is appropriate when there is good reason to believe that the phenomenon being studied changes over time. The extension of the comparative survey to multiple occasions of measurement produces the panel design introduced in Chapter 9 and discussed below. The panel design, when extended to the study of multiple variables, enables the investigator to assess not only change over time but also the differences and similarities in two or more *cohorts* over time. An increasing use of multiple occasions of measurement to better understand people's experiences is an important trend in nursing research literature. These designs enable investigators to see dynamic processes such as recovery as they naturally occur.

PANEL DESIGNS

The comparative survey was extended to include two occasions of measurement in the McCorkle and Benoliel example (1983). Another design variation that allows investigators to study differences over time is the *panel design* with multiple cohorts. This design allows investigators to address questions such as: Do differences exist in maternal role attainment at 1, 4, 8, and 12 months after birth between mothers of different ages? At what point do mothers' feelings

about their babies reach a peak? When do mothers achieve optimum gratification in their maternal roles? When does maternal competency reach its peak?

Mercer (1985) studied the process of maternal role attainment in three age-groups of mothers (15 to 19, 20 to 29, and 30 to 42) throughout the first year of motherhood. All women who delivered their first normal live-born infant at 37 or more weeks' gestation during a 16-month period were invited to participate. Each woman was interviewed at 1, 4, 8, and 12 months after the birth. Mercer found that positive feelings about the baby peaked at 4 months and did not differ significantly among mothers in the three age-groups (Fig. 10-4). Gratification in the maternal role differed over time and across age-groups. Mothers in the first two age-groups experienced decreasing gratification after 4 months, while gratification increased among mothers 30 to 42 years old (Fig. 10-5).

Use of the repeated measures over 1 year to study three age cohorts combines elements of the comparative survey and panel design. This approach makes it possible to assess changes in maternal role dimensions over time and simultaneously to differentiate patterns of maternal role attainment for the three age-groups of women. On the basis of this study an investigator can generate several hypotheses about age and development of the maternal role. For example, one might hypothesize that younger women experience more gratification in the maternal role over time because they are not yet deeply committed to careers or to work outside their homes, whereas older women experience gratification both from mothering and their careers outside the home. The same panel design could be used for purposes of testing these hypotheses in future studies.

CASE STUDIES

A *case study* is an in-depth investigation of an individual, family, group, or organization of a larger social unit. A case study investigates a contemporary phenomenon within its real-life context and is especially useful when the boundaries between the phenomenon and its context are not clearly evident (Yin, 1984). Generally, multiple sources of evidence are used. The purposes of a case study may include description, exploration of relationships between phenomena, and sometimes explanation of the relationships between two or more phenomena. Our particular focus in this chapter is the use of case studies for exploration.

Case studies are not easy to describe because they are not identified with a single design, unlike the panel design. Instead, they are often combinations of designs. The term *case study* does not denote a single specific technique, but rather a general strategy for research. Typically, a case study involves one or several cases that are studied over time using multiple data-gathering methods. Case studies have a contemporary, rather than historical, focus. Instead of relying on past events, they emphasize the contemporary experience. They are naturalistic studies, conducted in a setting that is not controlled by the investigator.

It is helpful to think of a case study design as an action plan or blueprint for conducting a study in which the design is determined by the question posed. The unit of analysis and the observations and their timing are part of this plan.

Unit of analysis

The *unit of analysis* for a case study may be the observation, individual, family, group, organization, community, or some larger social unit. In nursing the case study has been applied most frequently to individuals and families or groups. Most of the published case studies in nursing research focus on individuals with particular health problems as the unit of analysis. Titles of case studies in the recent pediatric nursing literature illustrate their potential focuses:

"One five-year-old boy's use of play" (Accord, 1980)

"Manifestations of guilt in an immobilized school-aged child" (Ebmeier, 1982)

"Body-image concerns of a four-year-old boy with meningitis" (Griffiths, 1980)

"Coping strategies of a two-year-old girl hospitalized for cardiac catheterization" (Hinz, 1980)

These studies, each in the area of children coping with hospitalization, identify the individual's responses as the unit of analysis. While other studies have emphasized the family or small group as the unit of analysis, Bauder (1981a, 1982b) studied institutions as her unit of analysis. She used a case study approach to identify recurring themes of powerlessness and management-by-crisis in schools of nursing.

The distinction between the unit of analysis and the context for the unit of analysis is important to prevent blurring of the emphasis in data collection. Clarifying the central focus of the study by carefully describing the unit of analysis is an important element of design. In the studies of hospitalized children, the unit of analysis was the individual child, although data collection within the context of hospitalization was an important part of each study.

Selection of the case(s) for a case study may be based on several considerations. The investigator may want to identify a typical case, an extreme or unique case, or a revelatory case (Yin, 1984). A typical case provides knowledge about how most people, families, or groups experience a phenomenon. For example, a typical case for analysis might be a hospitalized adult who resembles most hospitalized adults, for instance, a middle-aged male with some form of cardiac disease. An extreme or unique case might be an individual who survived a massive injury that, under most circumstances, would have resulted in death. One focus of this case study could be the factors associated with the individual's unusual experience of survival. A *revelatory case* is one that provides an investigator with the opportunity to observe and analyze a phenomenon previously inaccessible to scientific investigation. As the first American woman in space, Sally Ride is an example of a revelatory case whose study will enlighten us about the health of women as they are exposed to life outside the earth's atmosphere.

Observations and timing

No single pattern of observations and timing exists for a case study. Instead, the observations and timing of the observations flow from the purpose of the study. In general, case studies address multiple variables that are measured at several points in time. In this sense, case studies resemble other longitudinal designs. A major difference between case studies and longitudinal designs is in the sampling approach and the fact that the same measure is not always repeated at each occasion of measurement. Investigators typically use multiple data sources in a case study, with some sources being used on only a single occasion and others used repeatedly throughout the study. For example, an investigator may use a medical record as a data source at the beginning and use both observation and interview techniques to produce data throughout the remainder of the study. Data sources for a case study might include documentation (such as correspondence or journals), archival data (such as clinical records), interviews, participant and nonparticipant observation, physiological recordings, and physical artifacts (such as children's toys or other possessions) (Yin, 1984).

Duration of study and timing of observations for case studies typically are directed by the purpose. For studies of hospitalized children, the duration of the study may span only a few days or several months. The timing of observations may be established at the onset of the study or may follow the progress of the child throughout the hospitalization, with data collection being initiated at significant milestones in the hospital stay (e.g., admission, the first time the parent leaves the hospital, preoperative morning, and return to the recovery room). The duration of the observations may be the same throughout the study or may vary, depending on the events happening at that point in time. For example, a child experiencing panic after anesthesia may be observed throughout the duration of the event, whereas an episode of the child's play may be observed for a preset period of time (e.g., 15 minutes).

Planning a case study involves developing a protocol for data collection. From the objectives for the case study, a review of relevant literature, and an outline of the issues to be explored in the case study, the investigator identifies appropriate sites and data sources. For example, nurses studying the adaptation of children who are respirator dependent and their families to discharge to home care might select both the hospital and home for study in order to understand fully the relationships between family factors, professional factors, and family and child health factors. Data sources might include hospital records, interviews with family members and staff, journals kept by the mother, and nonparticipant observation of the child and family. The protocol for the study might involve the administration of questions in interview form, an observation guide for the nonparticipant observation, and a questionnaire for the hospital staff (Thomas, 1986).

Commonly used analytical strategies include content analysis, constant comparative analysis, and the accumulation and comparison of cases. Case studies can be reported as a single case report or as a compilation of a series of cases.

Generalizability

The issue of generalizability is almost a nonissue given the purpose of case study research, but it is raised so often that it should be addressed. The point of the case study is not to discover what holds true for all people but to identify important factors in a given phenomenon. When such factors are identified, one can proceed to determine how often they occur and under what circumstances. Such questions about frequency are answered legitimately by survey design. The circumstances under which factors occur might be asked in a large survey, but they could also be discovered by the accumulation of representative and extreme cases.

Case study design option

To this point we have discussed case studies as if they involved a single case with data collection using only one unit of analysis. Yin (1984) offered a matrix to illustrate the variety of case study designs (Fig. 10-6). One dimension of the matrix differentiates single from multiple case designs; whereas the other differentiates holistic from embedded designs. A *single case design* refers to a design in which only one case (a family) will be studied; whereas a *multiple case design* refers to a study of more than one case (several families).

A single case design may use the unitary unit of

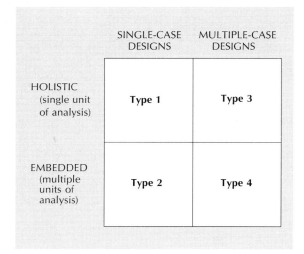

	SINGLE-CASE DESIGNS	MULTIPLE-CASE DESIGNS
HOLISTIC (single unit of analysis)	Type 1	Type 3
EMBEDDED (multiple units of analysis)	Type 2	Type 4

Fig. 10-6. Matrix of four basic types of designs for case studies. (From Yin, R. [1984]. Case study research: Design and methods. Beverly Hills, CA: Sage. Copyright © 1984. Reprinted by permission of Sage Publications, Inc.)

analysis, implying that analysis of the case study data will be at a holistic level. The holistic unit of analysis cannot or will not be divided into components. For example, when an investigator studies a family as a unit of analysis, collecting data at the level of the total family exemplifies the holistic case study design. Alternatively, in an embedded case study, the investigator uses multiple units of analysis. An investigator studying the family may employ an embedded design, studying each individual within the family, dyads in the family (e.g., mother-child, wife-husband), and the family as a totality.

The two dimensions may be crossed, producing single case–holistic designs, single case–embedded designs, multiple case–holistic designs, and multiple case–embedded designs. Thus it is possible to identify an array of four case study designs, each with a particular application.

Reporting case studies

Lincoln and Guba (1985) recommended a general format for the reporting of case studies that could be adapted easily to reporting case phenomena of interest to nursing. The format is useful for both single persons and organized groups as the case unit. The authors proposed a two-part report, part one being the substantive report suitable for publication and part two being the methodological appendix. A final report of a research project would contain complete information for both the substantive and methodological sections, whereas a journal publication would be prepared primarily from the substantive report. Lincoln and Guba outlined the following sections for inclusion in the substantive report.

1. Problem or phenomenon of interest
2. Context or setting in which the case study occurred
3. Transactions by which data were obtained and interpreted
4. Salient elements identified
5. Outcomes or conclusions that are drawn

Using this format to describe coping behaviors in hospitalized children, for example, the investigator would use the problem section for a description of the phenomenon of coping as it guides observations for the study, followed by a description of the setting or context in which data were gathered (home, hospital, clinic), and how data were obtained (chart review, interview of nurses who cared for the child, field notes, or parental interview). The discussion of salient elements is comparable to the results section of a standard report and in this example would include the behaviors or observations that are key indicators of the kind of coping. Of necessity, interpretation of the elements in light of what is already known also occurs in this section. Conclusions and hypotheses about the nature of coping in a child in this context would be reported in the outcomes or conclusions section.

Lincoln and Guba (1985) recommend adding methodological detail as a separate appendix. Methodological detail refers to such aspects as the identification of the investigators and their relationship to the subject, a detailed description of the training processes, the validity and reliability measures used during data collection, and a discussion of data analysis. Because much case reporting methodology is interactive and involves interpretation and transaction between subject and investigator, it is difficult to know from a summary of methods (e.g., "data were obtained by interview") how likely it would be that several different interviewers would come to the same conclusions. A detailed methodological appendix is one way to provide enough information about data collection to establish the trustworthiness of that data and a rational basis for determining if any two observers would come to the same conclusion.

Rubin's application (1984) of the case study has contributed to the understanding of the concept of maternal identity and the maternal experience. She has employed studies in the clinical field to discover aspects of the maternal experience and their relationships to other personal characteristics. Nurse observers collect data because they are able to "relegate medical, nursing, and hospital procedures into contextual background . . . as a given, against which the subject's behavior and responses can be foreground . . ." (Rubin, 1984, p. 147).

Data from individual case studies can be used in several ways: analyzed as individual cases, analyzed as an aggregate of cases, and analyzed from the perspective of units of behavior within the individual. Thus Rubin has incorporated multiple cases and embedded analyses into her studies.

The case study that follows illustrates a single case, analyzed from the perspective of cognitive dissonance, and suggests the relationship between a woman's experience with a diagnosis of pregnancy and her image of herself (see box on pp. 159-163). The recorded observation was the database.

Text continued on p. 164.

A CASE OF COGNITIVE DISSONANCE

Patient: Dorothy M.
Age 22, Black, Married
5th month, 2nd trimester
Gravida V, Para IV

L.M.P. August, E.D.C. ?
Nurse: Ruth Hrizo

I couldn't decide if Mrs. M. was wearing an uncombed wig or if her hair had been straightened and needed combing, badly. She wore an old camel colored coat—one bad tear near the pocket, cuffs frayed, buttons missing. She also wore loafers with gray wool socks, but they were in much better condition. I can't remember her dress except that it was a maternity dress. She wore no rings.

Except for maternity dress, body (? self) image is one to be neglected

Mrs. M. and another patient were sitting together in the waiting room. Mrs. M. looked very familiar, so I approached her. I soon found out that she had been here in the clinic earlier this week—reason for being familiar.

I was surprised at how easily she talked. She got right to the core of problems. (A crisis situation.) She had come to Planned Parenthood recently. She had been examined and told she was pregnant and given an appointment. "Oh, no, was my first reaction. It took me about a month—no, I mean a week to get used to the idea." "How will I manage?" seemed to be the major concern.

Surprise

She talked quickly with little concern about my comments. She needed a listener. Her husband had left her two months ago after seven years. "He got tired of babies, I guess."

During the course of her conversation, I learned about Terry, a boy, aged 4, and Randy, a girl aged 2, and another boy, Tyrone, who died at the age of 2. I couldn't place Tyrone because she would refer to him and then quickly drop the subject to go on. She had "given all my baby clothes away, except a bunting of Randy's and a snow-suit of Terry's which were never used." Diapers had been torn up. "All except two which I used for dust rags. I was so glad to get rid of them. I had a ceremony."

Finished

Continued.

A Case of Cognitive Dissonance—cont'd

*Conditional acceptance
Note change in time
frame from past self to
future self*

The crib had been sold to a sister-in-law a couple of months ago. "I guess I will have to buy it back." Her mother was "on welfare like me, so you know she can't help me. My father is dead." I suggested that perhaps she would receive gifts that would help. She said that her brother James said that he would pay for it, if it was a boy and was named James for him. "But I don't trust him, he don't buy anything for his own kid. He has a baby named for him already." Another brother would pay for a girl if it was named Raymie Lynn for him. "I like boys' names for girls."

She said she dressed her little girl in slacks. "She can wear dresses when she goes to school." She talked proudly about her children then. She told about them trying to make her breakfast and breaking a whole dozen of eggs to get them into the skillet. "When I came downstairs, there was egg everywhere. Boy, did I whip! They cried and said that they 'were only trying to make you breakfast, Mommy,' but I sent them upstairs."

She then told me the problem that she was having with Terry refusing to let his sister Randy use his little potty. She then went on to tell me that Terry wants anything but another baby. "He said he wants a horse or a kitty or a puppy, 'Bring home a puppy, Mommy.'"

For some reason, Mrs. M. then told me about one of the nurses that she "hated." She identified her as the tall nurse who usually worked in Dental Clinic. She was in the Emergency Room when Mrs. M. came in by Police Ambulance with her mother during her first pregnancy. "I told her that it was coming and she said that she was a nurse and it wasn't coming. I had one bad pain and it was born. She said that she was real sorry afterwards but that didn't help. My mother doesn't get mad but she was swearing at her." This story was repeated with the added information that she was fifteen at the time and that this was about a five month gestation that died at the time.

"Like"/model, self

*The depletion syndrome
in a multip with premies.
—And "like"/model, her
children*

Mrs. M. told me that all her babies had been born on the seventh of March. I think she was telling me that this baby would be born then also. One baby weighed 4 pounds, one baby weighed 3 pounds, and one baby weighed 2 pounds.

The last baby, Randy, stayed in the hospital four months. "It didn't seem like I had a baby. I never saw them until the day I went home and then I didn't see them again until I came to get them. I called everyday, but it seemed like I was calling about a girl friend's baby. When Randy came home, I heard her crying and I thought, I wish that baby's mother would get that baby and change its diaper and give it a bottle. Then I thought, 'That's mine!'"

When she was in on Monday, she had been examined by a medical student and "a man in a suit." She said that her sister-in-law ("well, I call her my sister-in-law, she goes with my brother") worked at the clinic. She had been in the room with her on Monday and they had "laughed and carried on so that she said that we were going to get her fired."

She was called into the office at this time. After I weighed her and found that she had gained two pounds since Monday, the conversation quickly moved to food. She laughingly told me that she loved chocolate sundaes and bacon rinds. She said that she and a girl friend had stayed up until midnight the night before and had played with one of the kid's games, Uncle Wiggley, and they had eaten peanut butter crackers and Pepsi. At this time I moved her into the examining room.

A kid's food and a mother's food

She continued to talk about food. She said that she loved pork, but it was hard to imagine such good meat coming from those beasts that ate garbage. Seeing I wasn't shocked, she continued. She told about wringing the neck of a chicken when she was five. She got to the part where she should have given a hard snap but got sick, dropped the chicken and ran into the woods. Her mother was mad at her but "I was only five, imagine?" I asked if she had been living on a farm then. She said that she had been living on a farm in Alabama. She and her family had come north when she was seven. Besides wringing the necks of chickens and saving the dishwater and garbage for the hogs, she remembers "there was nothing to do." They never celebrated Halloween and for Christmas, they received fruit and nuts. "We never got toys. Our first Christmas up here, my brother got a bike and I got a doll. We were wondering about all those fruit and nuts when we were little. Old Santa got mixed up."

I said she liked it better up here, then. She certainly did. "Down there you lay in bed and looked up at the stars. The chickens ran under the house. There were snakes everywhere. I wouldn't go to the bathroom at night; I had my little pottie right under my bed. There were cotton snakes in the cotton fields. There was a big snake that lived in a tree beside the house. We used to feed him. Our mother yelled at us, but there was nothing to do. You fed snakes."

Her mother wants her to return (to Alabama). They had been back once for a visit. She told about telling her cousins about the Christmases up here, about wringing chickens' necks and about nothing to do. She said that if her mother wanted to go back, she could but she wasn't going.

Dr. Dym came into the room at this time. I was startled by the change in her. She was extremely quiet. He looked at the chart. As I helped her onto the bed and was getting the sheet fixed, she told me that one doctor had told her that she wasn't pregnant. Before I could find out more, Dr. Dym started the routines. He felt for the height of the fundus, measured, listened for fetal heart sounds. He had a perplexed look. He questioned her. Yes, the dates were right—she had the last normal period in August but had been spotting monthly. That's why she had thought she wasn't pregnant and had gone to Planned Parenthood. The doctor there had told her she was pregnant and had told her to come to regular clinic. She had felt life, she thought, about Christmas but she had thought at the time that it was her nerves. She got sick just the night before—like morning sickness.

"Like"/model, general other

Continued.

A CASE OF COGNITIVE DISSONANCE—cont'd

Dr. Dym did a pelvic exam and said something to me about a long cervix and then to both of us, "Just what I thought. Have her get a pregnancy test. I don't think she's pregnant."

Dissonance

Her expression was one of total bewilderment. I told her to dress and then wait for me. When I came back with the instructions for a pregnancy test, she was sitting on the chair in the office saying, "I don't understand, I just don't understand." I explained slowly what she was to do for the pregnancy test. She looked up and said, "What? Another one?" At that I asked her to come out to the front desk and wait for me. We called to the lab and got back a report of a pregnancy test that had been run on the 9th of January. It was negative.

After some difficulty, I got Dr. Dym's attention and told him about the negative test. His answer was to tell her to come to a Gyn Clinic. (He was very involved with another situation at the time.) I hesitated then I decided that it wasn't helping anything by letting her sit. I told her that the test had been found and that it was negative. I told her the doctor would check her on Monday. She shook her head and said, "I don't understand. I don't know what to do."

I decided that maybe she needed to hear it from the doctor. I asked Dr. Dym to tell her what had been found and what he wanted her to do. Although obviously busy, he came out and told her, "Well, Dorothy, seems you had a test and it was negative. We'll want you to come back to the Gynie Clinic and we'll see if we can get your periods regulated for you." Then he was gone.

Dissonance

Her first question was what was Gynie Clinic? I told her it was the Monday afternoon clinic for nonpregnant patients. She asked for her appointment book. I looked for it. It had been thrown out. I couldn't even find it in the waste basket. I had to return to her without it.

Dissonance

I told her how hard it must be to think pregnant and then to think non-pregnant. It must be hard shifting so fast and often, that I felt confused, myself. She asked me what to do. Whatever I said, I don't think she heard me. She had just remembered that she had even had a note written by the Monday's doctors to tell her welfare worker that she was pregnant.

Dissonance

That reminded her that she would not receive her check until the following Friday and that she could not come into the clinic until after it came. She started over to the desk to make an appointment when her "sister-in-law" came up. Mrs. M. told her that the doctor had said that she wasn't pregnant. "That's good!" she said. Mrs. M. repeated "That's good?" I was startled at the glibness of the statement myself. Mrs. M. wavered between me and her sister-in-law. "What should I do?"

Dissonance

Before I could answer, the sister-in-law started to talk to her and to walk away with all indications for Mrs. M. to follow. They left together.

Discussion

This unusual case highlights the distress of cognitive dissonance (Festinger, 1957). The surprise diagnosis of pregnancy some two or three months ago is still the presenting crisis situation today. Nevertheless, she has done and is doing a lot of work in preparation for becoming a mother and having another child. She puts away the concept of her being finished with babies and begins to face anew how it will be, that she will need the crib again. She has sought acceptance for her becoming a mother again, received outright rejection from her husband and a permissive acceptance from her family of origin. This young woman is poor financially but rich in familial attachments. She has pinpointed the financial problem and has already taken the initiative of getting a note from her doctor to her welfare worker that will increase her income to accommodate a baby. She has backfiled in memory to find her last normal menstrual period ignoring, as one does in cognitive dissonance resolution, the intervening and atypical menses since then. This makes her five months pregnant and from her own experience of premature labors, she has little time left. This may be why she is pressured in having her four-year-old son learn to share and why his preference for a pet to a baby is a bit less amusing. This may also be why she rejects the idea of moving back to Alabama at this time.

Note that there is no experience of a child within. She may have felt fetal movement at Christmas, but none since. She may have had morning sickness the night before last. She is fishing for signs, as one does in the first trimester. Despite her expectations of a premature, she is loading in food treats such as chocolate sundaes, peanut butter crackers, and Pepsi as for a school child, not a premie. There is an idea of a baby, but no experience of a baby. There is a wish, preferably a girl, and a psychosocial binding-in at the level of a two to three month pregnancy.

The diagnosis of not-pregnant is a shock in expectations and orientation of self in a world. "What should I do?" In some ways her experience is like those women who have a spontaneous abortion in the first trimester. But she lacks the experience of body image involvement and the anticipatory feelings of anxiety and fear. She is less prepared, more destabilized. She has not accepted the not-pregnant idea or self-image. How could she? Each doctor has a different story and one doctor gave her an official note saying she was pregnant. Anger at the doctors who gave her such a costly run around would be a normal summary of the feeling. But she is not summarizing an incomplete experience. She is making another appointment. She needs more information to support, refute, or substitute in a cognitive mapping and an orientation of self in a world to know what she "should do."

VALIDITY OF EXPLORATORY DESIGNS

External validity of research designs is related to the ability to generalize findings from the study to a population. The correlational survey and the comparative survey in which random sampling is used have high potential generalizability if the investigator has used probability sampling approaches, whereas the use of nonprobability sampling procedures limits generalizability. The findings of a case study, based on one or a few cases, lack generalizability without replication across other cases. As discussed in Chapter 8, the external validity of a study also is influenced by the setting for the study and the nature of the observations being made.

Internal validity of research designs relates to the accuracy of the relationships between the variables being studied. Because exploratory designs are meant to be hypothesis generating instead of confirming, the investigator does not exert great control. As a result, history, maturation, testing, instrumentation, selection, and loss of participants may be operative. History refers to the secular trends or events external to the study that affect observations of relationships made during the study. Historical events interfere with the validity of the observed relationships when they alter the nature of these relationships. For example, the discovery of limitations of new technology, such as an artificial heart, may influence how the family supports the patient, and in turn may change the nature of the relationship between family support and patient outcomes. Maturation refers to changes in the individuals being studied that affect the observations of relationships made during the study. In the study described earlier of the development of maternal role, maturation of the women who were very young mothers may have been occurring at a rate different from that for the older mothers. As a result, the relationship between age and maternal role attainment may have been a function of the maturational processes of late adolescence and not merely a function of the biological age of the mother.

The effects of testing are most likely to be seen in studies employing repeated measures over several occasions, such as in the panel study. Likewise, instrumentation problems are most likely to occur with repeated measures in which the calibration of the instrument may change over time. Selection of the participants also can influence internal validity. Individuals who participated in the study of coping with a diagnosis of lung cancer or with myocardial infarction may have been healthier than those who did not. The observed relationships between diagnosis and symptom distress may have been different had individuals with more severe disability been included in the study. Loss of participants is an important concern for studies involving repeated measures. The nature of the relationships between variables may change dramatically depending on whether a systematic difference exists between those

---

TABLE 10-2. A comparison of designs for exploration of relationships and differences

DESIGN	SAMPLE	OBSERVATIONS AND TIMING
Correlational survey	Random sample from designated population	Multiple variables measured at a single time point
Comparative survey	Random sample from two or more designated populations or purposive samples from two or more designated populations	Multiple variables measured at a single time point
Panel design	Random sample(s) from one or more populations	Multiple variables measured at multiple time points
Case study	Single case or small sample, purposive sampling	Multiple variables measured at one or more time points

who drop out of a study and those who remain in it. Loss of participants can affect both the generalizability of the findings and the validity of the relationships seen in the data.

SUMMARY

This chapter has included a discussion of designs to explore relationships and differences between phenomena. The correlational survey, comparative survey, panel design, and case study provide rich design alternatives to investigators whose work is directed toward generating hypotheses. Table 10-2 compares and contrasts the sample, observations, and timing dimensions for the correlational survey, comparative survey, panel design, and case study. Together these designs constitute an important complement for nursing research and theory generation.

REFERENCES

Accord, L. (1980). One five-year-old boy's use of play. *Maternal-Child Nursing Journal, 9,* 29-35.

Barnard, K. (1983). The case study method: A research tool. *MCN: American Journal of Maternal Child Nursing, 8,* 327.

Bauder, L. (1982a). Balancing organizational demands with human needs: The ironic emphasis in schools of nursing. *Western Journal of Nursing Research, 4,* 153-165.

Bauder, L. (1982b). Discontent and crisis at schools of nursing: The consequences of unmet human needs. *Western Journal of Nursing Research, 4,* 35-38.

Ebmeier, C. (1982). Manifestations of guilt in an immobilized school-aged child. *MCN: American Journal of Maternal Child Nursing, 11,* 109-115.

Ferrans, C., & Powers, M. (1985). Employment potential of hemodialysis patients. *Nursing Research 34,* 273-277.

Griffiths, S. (1980). Body-image concerns of a four-year-old boy with meningitis. *MCN: American Journal of Maternal Child Nursing, 9,* 127-136.

Hinz, E. (1980). Coping strategies of a two-year-old girl hospitalized for cardiac catheterization. *MCN: American Journal of Maternal Child Nursing, 9,* 1-11.

Lincoln, Y., & Guba, E. (1985). Case reporting. In Y. Lincoln & E. Guba (Eds.), *Naturalistic inquiry.* Beverly Hills, CA: Sage.

McCorkle, R., & Benoliel, J. (1983). Symptom distress, current concerns, and mood disturbance after diagnosis of life-threatening disease. *Social Science and Medicine, 17,* 431-438.

Meier, P., & Pugh, E. (1986). A case study: A viable approach to clinical research. *Research in Nursing and Health, 9,* 195-202.

Mercer, R. (1985). The process of maternal role attainment over the first year. *Nursing Research, 34,* 198-204.

Mitchell, P., Ozuna, J., & Lipe, H. (1981). Moving the patient in bed: Effects on intracranial pressure. *Nursing Research, 30,* 212-218.

Neale, J., & Liebert, R. (1986). *Science and behavior: An introduction to methods of research.* Englewood Cliffs, NJ: Prentice-Hall.

Rubin, R. (1984). *Maternal identity and the maternal experience.* New York: Springer.

Schultz, P., & Kerr, B. (1986). Comparative case study as a strategy. In P. Chinn, (Ed.), *Methodological issues in nursing,* Rockville, MD: Aspen.

Thomas, R. (1986). *Ventilator dependency consequences for child and family.* Unpublished doctoral dissertation, University of Washington, Seattle.

Yin, R. (1984). *Case study research: Design and methods.* Beverly Hills, CA: Sage.

11

DESIGNING STUDIES TO TEST HYPOTHESES: TOWARD EXPLANATION AND PREDICTION

NANCY FUGATE WOODS

In earlier chapters we have considered the relationship between theory development and research design. In particular, we have discussed research designs whose theory-generation aims encompassed the identification and description of phenomena, as well as exploration of relationships between phenomena. We turn now to consideration of research designs that support testing of theory. *Theory-testing research* enables investigators to determine how accurately the theory accounts for the empirical world. The investigator translates abstract theoretical relationships into hypotheses, or statements of relationship that can be tested empirically. Through hypothesis-testing research, the investigator can contribute to explanatory and predictive theory. *Explanation* refers to specification of how or why phenomena are related to one another, whereas *prediction* refers to specification of the necessary and sufficient variables that will produce a desired outcome. It may be possible to predict the occurrence of a phenomenon when it is not possible to explain why a phenomenon occurs. For example, it is possible to predict that individuals who are exposed to many stressors and have little social support will become ill, but the mechanism responsible for the protective effect of social support remains unknown.

Theory-testing research presupposes description of the phenomena being studied and exploration of relationships between them. Theory-testing research begins with an abstract relational statement, a *proposition*. From the theoretical proposition, the investigator derives a hypothesis specific to a particular empirical situation. For example, from the theoretical proposition

$$\text{Social support} \rightarrow \text{Health}$$

the investigator could derive the hypothesis that

$$\begin{array}{c}\textbf{Spouse support behaviors}\\\textbf{during pregnancy}\end{array} \rightarrow \begin{array}{c}\textbf{Fewer}\\\textbf{pregnancy symptoms}\end{array}$$

The hypothesis linking spouse support to pregnancy symptoms can be tested empirically to determine its validity. Over time, evidence accumulates to support the proposition that social support influences health through some protective mechanism, and as research evidence accumulates, aspects of the theory are refined and revised. Theory-testing research is an essential element in the cyclical relationship between theory development and theory validation.

Many designs are employed in theory-testing research. The best known is the experiment and its many variations, including quasiexperimental designs. In addition, naturalistic designs can be used to test hypotheses that contribute to explanatory and predictive theory. Testing hypotheses that contribute to explanatory and predictive theory involves testing causal hypotheses in which some cause (X) is proposed to produce an effect *(Y)*. In this chapter we first will discuss the concept of causal relationships and procedures for establishing causal relationships. We then will turn to consideration of experimental and naturalistic designs for testing causal hypotheses.

CAUSAL RELATIONSHIPS

Much of our knowledge about designing research emanates from investigators' desire to identify cause-effect relationships. A causal hypothesis asserts that *X* causes *Y*, or whenever *X* occurs, *Y* will follow.

The notions of causality that humans have held reflect our desire to control the environment and perhaps ourselves. Early notions of causality in the health sciences emphasized seeking a single cause for each disease, for example, identifying the organism that causes tuberculosis. More recently the influences of multiple causes and factors modifying human susceptibility to disease have been recognized; current hypotheses address the multiple factors involved in premature births or depression. Moreover, contemporary notions of causality are not limited to deterministic notions of *X* compelling *Y* to happen. Instead, investigators now recognize the importance of partial causation and multiple causation, in which events are thought of in a probabilistic rather than in a deterministic way.

Criteria for causal relationships

Several criteria help an investigator assert that a causal relationship exists. The first is *covariation* between the presumed cause and effect. In short, when *X* changes, so does *Y*. Unless different values of *X* can be studied, covariation cannot be established. Therefore more than a single value of *X* must be studied; for example, *X* and not *X*, or multiple levels of *X*. To observe covariation between exercise *(X)* and cardiovascular fitness *(Y)*, variation in exercise levels must occur: several levels of exercise can be studied, or exercise and no exercise conditions can be compared.

The second criterion is *causal direction*. We must observe that changes in *X* precede those in *Y*: the cause must precede the effect. In some instances the investigator can manipulate the order of occurrence (time ordering) of *X* and *Y*. For example, the investigator can provide an exercise program *(X)* and

measure its effects *(Y)* later. In some studies where manipulating *X* is impossible, time ordering of the variables can be inferred logically. For example, an exercise history for the past 5 years *(X)* could be obtained and linked to current cardiovascular fitness *(Y)*. In this instance the investigator infers that *X* preceded *Y*.

The third criterion is *nonspuriousness*. We must be certain that other variables that cause changes in *Y* are not really responsible for the effect of *X* on *Y*. Eliminating plausible alternative explanations for the observed relationship is an important strategy in establishing causality. For example, an investigator studying effects of exercise on cardiovascular fitness would consider the participants' ages, because age has known effects on fitness measures.

Causal relationships may be direct or indirect. A *direct association* occurs when the cause *(X)* produces the effect or outcome *(Y)* without the influence of any intermediate variable.

$$X \rightarrow Y$$

For example, changing the patient's position directly produces a change in blood pressure. An *indirect association* occurs when the cause *(X)* is encompassed by another variable. For example, smoking is associated with longer hospital stays after surgery. Smoking does not directly produce a longer hospital stay; it does so indirectly by producing poor pulmonary function before surgery, which is, in turn, associated with poor pulmonary function and increased pulmonary complications after surgery.

Spurious associations occur when two variables are associated, but the association exists because of the influence of a third variable. An example of a spurious association would be that between race and infant mortality. Studies of infant mortality show that nonwhite infants have higher mortality rates than white infants in the United States. However, race does not cause the higher mortality rates; it is a confounding variable. Instead, low income and aspects of low-income lifestyle, such as poor nutrition and low access to prenatal care, are linked to infant mortality. Race is confounded with income.

Noncausal relationships

Many types of noncausal relationships exist, and some are particularly relevant to nursing research. Relationships between *X* and *Y* sometimes occur simply as a result of chance. Through replication (repetition) of the study, evidence from several investigations can be examined to determine whether the relationship observed in a particular study was merely happenstance, or indeed was characteristic of the relationships found in other studies.

Artifactual associations result from limitations in initial conceptualization of the research problem, problems in research design, measurement approaches, peculiarities of the sample under study, and from confounding variables. Many sources of artifactual associations exist, and these will be discussed in greater detail as we consider validity and experimental designs.

Establishing causal relationships

Much of the ingenuity required for designing research is directed toward creating optimum conditions for observing covariation, establishing causal direction, and establishing nonspuriousness. Observing covariation is achieved through experimental manipulation: the investigator changes the value of X. In nonexperimental studies the investigator observes the natural variation of both X and Y.

Investigators can establish causal direction by manipulating X. If a change in Y occurs consequent to a change in X, one has evidence to infer causal direction. If the investigator creates a change in Y, X should not change. In nonexperimental studies the occurrence of X can sometimes be dated, thus allowing the investigator to believe that X preceded Y. In addition to these techniques, the investigator can rely on what is known about X and Y—and other variables likely to be associated with X and Y—to infer causal direction.

An investigator can establish nonspuriousness in several ways. First, the values of the possible spurious variables can be controlled in an experimental design by holding them constant. For example, the ambient temperature can be controlled in a study of responses to warmed versus room temperature–tube feedings. Second, the investigator can disperse the spurious effects by randomly allocating persons to different groups in an experiment. Ideally, this procedure produces groups that are similar in some value such as age or social class, so that no systematic differences exist between the group that receives the manipulation and the group that does not. Next, the

investigator may guarantee homogeneity of the potentially spurious variables by making the group under study as similar as possible, for example, by restricting the focus of the study to a very homogeneous group, such as a narrow age-group. Finally, the investigator can measure the potentially spurious variables and take into account their influence on Y in the analysis of data. For example, a person's gender might affect the influence of a stress-reduction measure. The investigator could take gender into account in analyzing the results of the study. This is sometimes referred to as "partialling out" the effects of a variable. This strategy for controlling potentially spurious variables is only effective when the factor under study is not totally confounded with the potentially spurious variable, that is, when the two variables are not highly correlated with one another. Each of these strategies is discussed in greater detail as we consider alternative research designs.

DESIGNING EXPERIMENTS

Features of experimental designs

Experimental designs have three critical features: manipulation, control, and randomization. In experimental studies the investigator manipulates or changes the phenomenon in some way. The phenomenon that is manipulated is labeled the independent, treatment, or causal variable. The variable the investigator measures in response to the independent variable is labeled the dependent, outcome, or effect variable. The investigator attempts to discern whether X influences Y.

$$\text{Independent} \rightarrow \text{Dependent}$$
$$\text{Cause} \rightarrow \text{Effect}$$
$$\text{Treatment} \rightarrow \text{Outcome}$$
$$X \rightarrow Y$$

Initially, the investigator randomly selects participants from a population and then randomly assigns them to one of two or more groups. An experiment has at least one (but can have more) experimental group and at least one control group. The investigator administers the treatment or manipulation to the experimental group and does not administer the manipulation to the control group. The most basic strategy of the experimenter is to compare the measures of the dependent variable for the experimental group and the control group to discern if the measures differ.

The MAX-MIN-CON principle

The MAX-MIN-CON principle (Kerlinger, 1986) guides the design of experiments. The abbreviations stand for the following:

MAX   Maximize experimental variance
MIN   Minimize error variance
CON   Control extraneous variance

To comprehend this principle, it is essential to understand the concept of variance. *Variance* refers to the variability in the dependent (outcome, effect, or Y) variable. *Experimental variance,* sometimes called systematic variance, refers to the variance or variation in the dependent variable attributable to the manipulation of the experimental treatment (X). *Extraneous variance* refers to variance in the dependent variable caused by some unwanted influence other than X; the factor usually is one that is not of primary interest to the investigator, but it may compete with X to influence Y. Finally, *error variance* (random variance) refers to variance in Y that is attributable to measurement error.

Maximizing experimental variance

Because the investigator's objective is to see the optimum effect of the experimental treatment, the variance attributable to the independent variable must manifest itself. If little difference exists between the treatment (the independent variable) and the control or no-treatment conditions, the chance of separating the effect of the treatment from all the other factors influencing the dependent variable is minimal. The wise investigator designs, plans, and conducts the study so that the experimental conditions are as different as possible from the nonexperimental ones, that is, so that a great difference exists between the treatment and no-treatment conditions. A great difference in the values of the independent variable provides reasonable assurance of seeing some difference in the dependent, or outcome, variable if the treatment truly makes a difference. The independent variable must make an impact on the dependent variable. For example, if preoperative teaching consists of only 5-minute visits from a nurse on the morning of surgery, the teaching may not make a major impact

on the person's well-being after surgery unless the intervention is particularly potent.

Controlling extraneous variance

Controlling extraneous variance implies minimizing, nullifying, or isolating the effects of any independent variables that are extraneous to the purpose of the study. The investigator tries to reduce the effects of the extraneous variables or at least to separate their effects from those of the experimental treatment. The investigator can eliminate the variable by restricting its value to a very narrow range. Choosing study participants who are as homogeneous as possible with respect to the extraneous variable is one way to minimize its potential impact. For example, in a smoking cessation intervention trial one might study only those persons with no past experiences in which they tried to quit smoking. The disadvantage of this strategy is that the application of the results of the study is subsequently restricted to a very homogeneous group, such as those who have never before tried to quit smoking.

A second way to control extraneous variance is by randomly allocating participants to treatment groups and no-treatment groups. In theory, randomization should make the groups equal in all possible ways. In reality, this technique does not guarantee equality, but it does work well in studies with large numbers of participants.

An investigator can also build variance into the design as an independent variable. This strategy makes it possible to extract from the total variance of the dependent variable that portion of the variance attributable to the extraneous factor. In this case the investigator would measure the extraneous variable along with the independent and dependent variables. An investigator studying smoking cessation could purposefully include those who had tried to quit smoking before and those who had not. Building variance into the design provides additional information about the effect of the extraneous variable and its possible joint effects with other independent variables. Building variance into the design as an independent variable becomes problematic when the extraneous variable is highly related to the independent variable. In this case differentiating the effects of the two variables—the independent and the extraneous variables—may be impossible.

An investigator also may use a technique called *matching* to control extraneous variance. In this case each participant in the treatment group is matched to one or more participants in a no-treatment group on the basis of one or more variables. For example, the investigator could match prospective patients for gall-bladder surgery on their previous history of surgery. For each person who has had surgery in the experimental group, one person who has had surgery would be placed in the control group. Each person who had not had surgery before would be matched with another person with a similar history. Matching participants on more than one variable (e.g., age and surgical history) is often difficult. Unless the matched variable is moderately related to the dependent variable, this procedure often is not feasible because of the small amount of control it yields. However, when the investigator knows from previous research that the correlation between the matching variable and the treatment variable is greater than .5, matching usually reduces error variance and maximizes experimental variance. When participants are matched, they should be assigned at random to a treatment group or no-treatment group. That is, some means should be used to randomize the members of the matched pair to the treatment group and the control group. During data analysis, matching requires that the investigator use special matched analytical tests, because matched pairs, rather than the individual, become the unit of analysis.

A final technique for controlling extraneous variance involves comparing the participant's original set of values with the participant's own subsequent values on repeated measurements over time. This technique allows the participant to serve as his or her own control and is referred to as an *ipsative* control. The investigator studying smoking-cessation treatment could measure the number of cigarettes each participant smoked before the treatment and compare the pretreatment values to the posttreatment values.

Minimizing error variance

Error variance is the variability of measures due to random fluctuation. When the sample is not unduly small, these fluctuations cancel out one another so that their mean is zero, that is, they are self-compensating. Some measures are randomly higher and some are randomly lower than the true measure. Error variance is unpredictable and includes variance associated with errors of measurement; these might be due to respondent fatigue, guessing or inattention, or random fluctuations in an instrumentation system.

Investigators can minimize error variance in two ways:
1. Using controlled conditions
2. Increasing the reliability of measurement

Investigators can reduce errors of measurement by using controlled conditions such as carefully specified protocols that must be followed by everyone working on the study. Precisely duplicating the conditions of a nursing approach that is being tested is both extremely difficult and extremely important. Unless the protocol is specified precisely, factors that cause error variance will probably influence the outcome variable. The protocol at right (see box) describes how measurements were obtained in a study of effects of passive range of motion, turning, and head rotation on intracranial pressure. Investigators also can reduce error variance by increasing the reliability of the measures they employ. This strategy increases the measurement accuracy of the dependent variable. Reliability is a concern both in the interpersonal approaches to data collection and in the use of instrumentation systems. These issues are discussed more fully in Chapters 14 and 15.

The total variance in the dependent variable can be regarded as the sum of the variance attributable to treatment and to error. Note that as the amount of error in the measurement of the dependent variable becomes greater, the proportion of the total variance attributable to the treatment becomes smaller. In other words, a great degree of measurement error makes it difficult to see the effect of the treatment.

Validity and experimental design

Validity refers to truth. Well-founded and sound conclusions have validity. Investigators worry about two types of validity when designing experiments: internal validity and external validity. *Internal validity* refers to the relationship between the independent and dependent variables. Simply stated, did the independent variable really have an effect on the dependent variable, or was the effect attributable to something else? If the independent variable did not have an effect on the dependent variable, was the lack of effect due to interference from another variable? That is, do alternate explanations exist that can

PROTOCOL

Research assistants used the following time sequence in collecting data for each procedure:

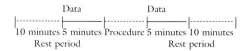

At least 15 minutes elapsed between arm extension and hip flexion and between head left and head right. In addition, 15 minutes elapsed between hip flexion and the first turn; approximately 1 hour elapsed between turns. The entire process took about 5 hours with about 4 hours (in separated segments) in actual contact with the patient.

Measurements were taken for correction formulas for true pressure before the baseline period of the first procedure. The angle of the head of the bed was measured with a protractor. The distances from the external auditory meatus to midbrow and to manometer and from midbrow to manometer were measured with a centimeter ruler and carpenter's level. On some occasions the physician positioned the drainage burette sufficiently low that cerebrospinal fluid (CSF) did not reach the manometer secured to the head of the bed. Pressure still could be measured, however, by securing a centimeter tape to the drainage tubing, measuring fluctuations in the tubing, and applying the correction formula.

The preintervention and postintervention rest periods were 15 minutes long. Data were collected during the last 5 minutes of the preintervention period and the first 5 minutes of the postintervention period. The conscious patient was asked to lie quietly; the person with altered level of consciousness had no activities performed by investigators or nursing staff. Spontaneous patient activity or unavoidable nurse activity was noted and the rest period begun again. Relatively continuous spontaneous patient activity was accepted as baseline in patients with altered levels of consciousness. The observer recorded the level of CSF in the manometer every 15 seconds during data-collection periods. The following standardized procedures were used in the order described earlier.

Arm extension
1. Inform patient of rest period: "I want you to rest as quietly as you can for 15 minutes."
2. Inform patient of activity: "I am going to exercise your arm."
3. Raise arm 180 degrees over head.
4. Return arm to side.
5. Repeat five times each arm within 1 minute.

Hip flexion
1. Inform patient of rest period.
2. Inform patient of activity: "I am going to exercise your leg."
3. Hold leg by knee and ankle; flex hip 90 degrees.
4. Hold flexion 1 second.
5. Return leg to bed.
6. Repeat five times each leg within 1 minute.

Turns:
1. Inform patient of rest period.
2. Inform patient of activity: "I am going to turn you on your right side; let me do the turning for you."
3. Position arm across midline away from nurse.
4. Position leg across midline away from nurse.
5. Walk to opposite side of bed.
6. Grasping shoulder and hip, turn patient toward nurse.
7. Stabilize leg in 90-degree angle with pillow.

Reverse all steps to achieve supine from lateral position. For the last 6 patients, a third person held the head in midline during each turn to prevent head rotation.

From Mitchell, P. (1982).

explain the findings other than the hypothesis being tested? *External validity* refers to the representativeness or generalizability of the study results. In short, can the results of the study be applied to other populations or in other contexts? Was the finding simply a function of the particular population being studied? However, an investigator first must be concerned with internal validity. If internal validity cannot be supported, there are no results that can be generalized beyond the study.

Threats to internal validity

Maturation. Investigators consider several threats to internal validity when designing an experiment. Events occurring between the first and second measurements of a variable can distort the influence of the independent variable on the dependent variable. These events can be related to the maturation of the participants and occur as a function of the passage of time. Maturation can be a problem in a study involving children who are learning new skills rapidly or in a study of a population of ill individuals where the time course of the illness itself could affect the dependent variable.

Contemporaneous events. The influence of contemporaneous events on the outcome variable is another threat to internal validity. Suppose an investigator was testing the impact of a patient-education program on breast self-examination behavior. Suppose also that the program began before several prominent women in the community discovered small, curable breast cancers as a result of self-breast examination. Massive publicity in local newspapers and television talk shows about the usefulness of self-breast examination would follow. Under these circumstances it would be especially difficult to ascertain whether the experimental treatment had affected women's own breast-examination practices or whether the change in behavior was simply due to the publicity.

Testing. Testing on one occasion often influences scores on subsequent tests. Individuals who have been asked to examine their health habits on one occasion may have the opportunity to reflect on their health and, by the time of the subsequent administration of the test, may have initiated different health behaviors. Testing effects present a special problem in studies that incorporate multiple repeated measures.

Instrumentation error. Instrumentation error also may interfere with internal validity. Changes in

the calibration of a measuring instrument or changes in observers' performance both induce invalid changes in the values of the dependent variable. Investigators working with instrumentation systems, such as temperature or blood pressure monitoring systems, must recalibrate their instruments at several points during data collection. Observers may take time to rest during a study or plan for a limited period of data collection to prevent fatigue and erroneous measurement. Observers also can "recalibrate" themselves by repeating checks of their reliability during the course of a study.

Statistical regression. In groups that have been selected because they are extreme, for example, critically ill or extremely precocious children, statistical regression is likely to occur. *Statistical regression* implies that participants' scores on an instrument are likely to change in the direction of the mean simply because extreme scores are unstable. The change would not reflect any effect of the independent variable; it simply would be expected because of the instability of the initial scores.

Differential selection. Differential selection of participants into the study groups refers to systematic differences in the allocation of participants to study groups.

To avoid major differences between the groups (except for those attributable to treatment), the investigator usually uses randomization of participants across study groups or sometimes matches individuals in the treatment group with those in the no-treatment group on some characteristic. Unfortunately, these techniques do not always work. Getting an uneven distribution of some characteristic such as age or gender in the study groups is possible. When this occurs, the characteristic may influence the dependent variable by exaggerating or attenuating the treatment effect. Suppose an investigator who was studying the effects of preoperative preparation for pulmonary therapy discovered that 80% of the individuals in the treatment group had a history of chronic lung disease and only 20% of those in the no-treatment group had a similar history. Under these circumstances pulmonary function measures obtained after the treatment was instituted might look much worse for the group that had the special intervention. The investigator rightfully would be concerned that the treatment appeared to have a deleterious effect on pulmonary function rather than the intended positive effect, when in reality poor pulmonary function was attributed to the chronic obstructive lung disease.

Differential loss of participants. Differential loss of participants from a study group (sometimes referred to as experimental mortality) also presents problems in interpreting the relationship between the independent variable and the dependent variable. Suppose that participants in the treatment group were so satisfied with the preoperative preparation and postoperative care they received that they continued to participate in the study for the 2-week study period. Suppose on the other hand that participants in the no-treatment group became so disenchanted with their care that 30% of them left the hospital early and refused to participate in the remainder of the study. If these disgruntled participants were really much less healthy postoperatively than those in the treatment group, loss of these participants would lead the investigator to underestimate the effectiveness of the treatment under study, because only the healthiest people would remain in the no-treatment group.

Some threats to internal validity operate jointly, such as the effects of maturation and selection. Their joint effects may either potentiate the effect of the treatment or dilute it. In a study of preoperative preparation for the elderly, those who were at greatest risk for pulmonary complications might be selected for the treatment group. Because those in the treatment group also were experiencing circulatory problems due to aging, they had compounded risk for poor outcomes. Should this situation occur, the joint effects of selection and maturation mitigate against finding a positive effect of the treatment on postoperative complications.

Threats to external validity

Several factors compromise external validity, including reactivity, novelty effects, testing effects, joint effects of history and manipulation, and effects of multiple treatments.

Reactivity. *Reactivity* refers to participants' responses to being studied. Of particular concern is their response to the attention of being studied. One classic instance of reactivity is termed the "Hawthorne effect." Employees of the Hawthorne plant of Western Electric Corporation were involved in an experiment in which working conditions such as lighting and work hours were manipulated. They improved their production rates significantly simply as a consequence of being involved in a study: being

part of a special group led to increased morale. Other types of reactivity occur when the participants guess the purpose of the study and try to please (or perhaps outwit or displease) the investigator. In these instances the participants are responding more to exposure to the study than to the independent variables being studied. For example, some literature suggests that when women are aware that the menstrual cycle is the focus of a study, they report more stereotypical patterns of symptoms than is the case when they are not aware of the specific focus.

Novelty. The novelty of being involved in a study can reduce the generalizability of the results to other populations and may produce behavior that is unrelated to the independent variable. Individuals who had never before participated in a study in a university teaching hospital might feel compelled to report their experiences more positively than if they were not being studied, thus presenting an invalid picture of typical experience.

To account for the influence of mere involvement in a study, many investigators use a control procedure rather than no treatment at all for the control group. One example is placing people on a waiting list during the early phases of a study and subsequently including them in the experimental treatment. Data obtained from these individuals during the waiting-list period then can be compared with data obtained from those individuals who did take part in the experimental treatment. The individuals who were on the waiting list also are exposed to the novelty or the hope of being studied.

Testing. Pretesting for a study makes the results less generalizable to the population that has not been pretested. Persons exposed to an instrument such as an inventory of health beliefs will have had cause to reflect on their own beliefs; their performance on a subsequent testing occasion may differ from those who have never seen the inventory before.

Joint effects of reactivity and manipulation. The joint effects of being selected for a particular study group and the treatment variable may operate to decrease the generalizability of the study findings. Suppose healthier individuals are selected for the treatment group in which an exercise regimen is the experimental treatment. If the comparison group consists of individuals who have poorer health and who do not get the exercise training, their performance on an outcome measure of aerobic fitness probably would be considerably worse than the treatment group's performance. The results of this study would be difficult to generalize to the population at large, because it would be difficult to know whether the treatment would have worked equally well for individuals who were in poorer health.

Multiple treatments. A special problem for clinical studies is the effect of multiple treatments. Often, patients are involved in many protocols within a relatively short period of time, or they may be engaging in self-care, as well as medically prescribed therapy. If the current investigator is unaware of previous treatments, the experimental effect may be attributed wrongly to the experimental treatment or perhaps the other protocols may attenuate the treatment effect. In addition, when certain populations are overstudied, they may receive treatments in connection with more than one study at a time. For example, if a patient is receiving medication that the investigator is not aware of, an effect may be attributed to a nursing therapy that is really due to the medication the person is being given. Collaborating with other investigators who are studying the same patient populations and obtaining complete health histories from the participants can prevent this occurrence.

Selection. A special type of selection bias occurs when participants seeking health care are entered into the experimental group and compared to controls who are not seeking health care. On one hand, those seeking health care may be socioeconomically advantaged: they can afford care. On the other hand, those not seeking care may be in better health and have no need of treatment. In either case this situation produces problems in generalizing results of the study to other populations.

EXPERIMENTAL DESIGN OPTIONS

The investigator planning an experiment has many experimental design options from which to choose. We will discuss those most commonly used in nursing studies and will use the nomenclature and definitions developed by Campbell and Stanley (1963).

Notation

The use of standard notation is helpful in understanding alternative experimental designs. We will use X to denote the experimental manipulation (treatment or intervention), O to denote observation or measurement, and R to denote randomization. To denote time we will say, for example, $O1$ for the first observation and $O2$ for the second observation.

Pretest posttest control-group design

As we noted earlier, the classical experimental design has the components of randomization, manipulation, and control. These components are illustrated in the pretest posttest control-group design shown in Fig. 11-1. The two lines of notation in this design represent two separate groups. The investigator initially randomly (R) assigns participants selected from one population into one of the two groups. The investigator then observes both groups on one occasion $(O1)$ and subsequently administers the experimental treatment (X) to only the first group. The investigator then observes both groups again on a second occasion $(O2)$.

This design has several advantages. First, the investigator is able to account for events occurring between time 1 and time 2 through observation of the control group. If the investigator were studying the influence of a health-teaching program for preschoolers on their health habits and if a children's television program addressed the same topic during the study, the effect of the television program could be seen in the control group, allowing the investigator to attribute the effect correctly either to the teaching program or to the television program.

Because participants are being studied over time, controlling for maturation is possible by examining the change over time in the control group. Changing scores in the control group over time are not a function of the experimental treatment, because this

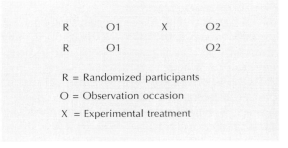

$$R \qquad O1 \qquad X \qquad O2$$
$$R \qquad O1 \qquad \qquad O2$$

R = Randomized participants
O = Observation occasion
X = Experimental treatment

Fig. 11-1. Pretest posttest control-group design. *R,* Randomly selected participants; *O,* observation occasion; *X,* experimental treatment.

group does not receive the treatment; the changes are instead a function of maturation. Since both groups are observed or tested at times 1 and 2, the influence of testing is equalized. This design also allows the investigator to control for changes in instrumentation, since changes or drifts in measurement should affect both groups equally.

Because the participants are randomly assigned to the study groups, extreme scores and regression of the extreme scores to the mean are unlikely to trouble only one group. Randomization of participants to the study groups also should decrease the likelihood of selection bias. Although this design will not prevent loss of subjects, it allows the determination of whether differential losses occurred between the two study groups. The randomization process should control the joint influence of selection and maturation. In addition, the investigator can assess differences in the control group on the observations at time 1 and time 2. When analyzing the data from a study using this design, the investigator wants to know how much change occurred between time 1 and time 2 for both of the groups and whether the change was greater in the treatment group or the control group.

Dixon's study (1984) of the effects of nursing interventions on the nutrition and performance status of cancer patients illustrates an extension of the pretest posttest control-group design to multiple experimental groups. Dixon randomly assigned persons with cancer who were nutritionally at risk to one of five groups: four experimental groups and one control group. Before treatment began, measures $(O1)$ of weight, arm-muscle circumference, triceps skinfold, and performance status were made. Each experimental group received one of the following treatments: nutrition supplements and relaxation training $(X1)$, relaxation training $(X2)$, nutritional supplements $(X3)$, or biweekly nurse visits with discussion of nutrition and eating problems $(X4)$. The control group received no visits, relaxation training, or nutrition counseling until after the study was completed. The premeasures were repeated at the end of the study 4 months later $(O2)$ (Fig. 11-2). The greatest gains in weight, arm-muscle circumference, and triceps skinfold were seen in the relaxation group, and the most severe losses occurred in the control group.

Four-group design

The Solomon four-group design, a second experimental design option, is complex but particularly useful in studies of developmental phenomena and permits the investigator to differentiate many effects (Fig. 11-3). This design employs two experimental groups and two control groups. Initially, the investigator randomly assigns participants to the four groups. Those in the first experimental group are observed on occasion 1, given the experimental treatment, and observed again on occasion 2. Those in experimental group 2 also receive the treatment but are observed only after the treatment, not before. Those in control group 1 are observed on occasions 1 and 2, but they are not given the experimental treatment. Those in control group 2 are observed only on the second occasion, without previous observation or treatment.

R	O1	X1	O2
R	O1	X2	O2
R	O1	X3	O2
R	O1	X4	O2
R	O1		O2

Fig. 11-2. Experimental design for a study of nursing interventions on nutrition and performance status of cancer patients. *X1,* Nutrition supplements and relaxation training; *X2,* relaxation training; *X3,* nutrition supplements; *X4,* nurse visits with nutrition discussion.

Experimental group 1	R	O1	X	O2
Control group 1	R	O1		O2
Experimental group 2	R		X	O2
Control group 2	R			O2

Fig. 11-3. Solomon four-group design.

The usefulness of this design rests on the assumption that if those in experimental and control groups 2 were observed on occasion 1, their scores would be similar to the averaged scores of those in experimental and control groups 1. To estimate the amount of change in experimental and control groups 2, the averaged pretest scores of experimental and control groups 1 are used as a baseline.

This design offers several advantages and has great potential for generating information about differential sources of effect on the dependent variable. Because all four groups are studied at the same time, both the effects of events occurring between time 1 and time 2 and the maturation of the participants are controlled. One can examine the scores of control group 2 for a measure of maturation without the influence of treatment.

The Solomon four-group design could be used to study the use of relaxation by children who are experiencing bone marrow aspiration. Two groups (experimental group 1 and control group 1) would be pretested for anxiety and pain perception. Two groups (experimental group 1 and experimental group 2) would be instructed in the relaxation technique. All four groups would complete the measures of anxiety and pain perception after the treatment. One could also examine the scores of the second experimental group to assess the effects of maturation and the experimental treatment.

The four-group design allows the investigator to assess the effects of observation 1 by comparing the scores at time 2 for control groups 1 and 2. If the scores for these groups were different, pretesting the participants would have had some effect on their subsequent scores. Changes in the scores for experimental group 1 would indicate the influence of both the pretest and the experimental treatment.

Comparing the scores $(O2)$ for experimental group 1 and control group 1 shows the effect of the experimental treatment. If a great difference exists between the posttest scores for the two groups, then the experimental treatment has had an effect on the outcome.

The investigator also can compare the differences in the experimental group 1 and control group 1 posttest scores with the differences in the experimental group 2 and control group 2 scores to determine the joint effects of the pretest and the experimental treatment. If the experimental treatment is effective,

then the $O2$ score for experimental group 1 should be greater than that for control group 1 and greater than the experimental group's scores on the pretest $(O1)$. In addition, one would expect to see that the $O2$ scores for experimental group 2 are greater than those for control group 2 and that the $O2$ scores are also greater than the pretest scores for control group 1.

No difference is expected in the $O2$ measures between the experimental groups or between the control groups when the differences between the experimental groups and control groups are due to the manipulation and not to some other factor.

Posttest only control-group design

Another option is the posttest only control-group design. Pretesting can be eliminated as nonessential as long as the participants have been randomly selected for the study group and the investigator can assume randomization to be an effective way of equalizing the differences between the treatment group and control group. In this design participants are randomly assigned to a treatment group or control group. No pretest is given, but both groups are observed after the treatment. The use of relaxation training during bone marrow aspiration could be evaluated using two groups. Both the treatment and the control groups would complete ratings of anxiety and pain after the procedure. A weakness in the design is that equalization before the test is not always certain and is merely assumed. This design can be useful in situations where it is not possible to pretest the participants (Fig. 11-4).

Factorial design

Another design option is the *factorial experiment*, in which the investigator simultaneously manipulates two or more independent variables. This design permits simultaneous analysis of two or more factors

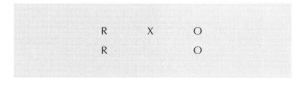

Fig. 11-4. Posttest only control-group design.

and provides information on whether the factors interact with one another. An *interaction effect* is the effect of two or more independent variables acting in combination rather than independently. The factorial design allows the investigators to determine whether the two factors acting jointly (interaction effect) produce an effect different from the sum of the individual effects (additive effects) of each of the factors.

Rice and Johnson's study (1984) of the influence of preadmission self-instructional information on levels of performance and time to achieve mastery of exercise behaviors illustrates use of a factorial design. The investigators randomly assigned clients to one of three levels of preadmission instruction for coughing, deep breathing, ambulation, and leg movements: (1) specific exercise instruction, (2) nonspecific exercise instruction, and (3) no exercise instruction. A 3 × 2 factorial design was used in which three levels of preadmission exercise and two types of surgery (cholecystectomy and herniorrhaphy) were included. Regardless of type of surgery, patients in the specific exercise group performed more of the exercise behaviors than those in the nonspecific exercise group. Both groups who received preadmission booklets required significantly less teaching time in the hospital (Fig. 11-5).

To assess whether the factors (type of surgery and type of instruction) had an interactive effect, Rice and Johnson compared the results for the groups receiving specific or nonspecific instruction according to the type of surgery they had experienced. They found that type of surgery and type of instruction did not have a joint effect on the teaching outcomes.

Extending this design to accommodate a larger number of factors is also possible. For example, one could study the influence of the type of information, the medium in which it is presented, and the characteristics of the clients having surgery. Sime and Libera (1985) looked at the interaction effects of presurgery anxiety and two intervention strategies (sensation information, self-instruction information, combined sensation and self-instruction information, and control group) on adjustment during dental surgery. They found that anxiety and type of instruction produced joint effects. Those individuals who had high-state anxiety reported less tension and distress after receiving sensation information, less tension after receiving self-instruction information, and increased positive self-statements after receiving the combined information. Individuals with low-state anxiety showed negative effects of treatment, including a reduced number of positive self-statements with sensation information or with the combined types of information.

Counterbalanced design

Another design option is the *counterbalanced* design. In this design all respondents or participants have all treatments or "cross over" to the other treatment groups. Suppose an investigator was attempting to discover whether measurement of cardiac output

	TYPE OF SURGERY	
TREATMENT	Cholecystectomy	Herniorrhaphy
Specific booklet		
Nonspecific booklet		
No preadmission booklet		

Fig. 11-5. Factorial design used in Rice and Johnson (1984). Three levels of treatment are crossed with two types of surgery.

varied as a function of patient position. The investigator could select two clinically relevant positions: supine and head elevated to 20 degrees. To ascertain whether the changes in cardiac output were not merely a function of the earlier positions, the investigator could control for the carryover effects by systematically ordering the positions. This approach would allow the investigator to determine whether the difference across the positions was greater than the difference attributable to the order of the positions. In the protocol given in the box below, the investigator has counterbalanced the order of the positions. Beginning with the flip of a coin to allocate people randomly to the first condition, she has selected which of the position sequences to test first. Each successive patient then is positioned according to the listing on the protocol.

QUASIEXPERIMENTAL DESIGNS

Quasiexperimental designs are designs in which the investigator does not randomly assign the participants to treatment conditions but does manipulate the experimental condition and incorporates various types of control to enhance the internal validity of the findings. Some designs lack either a control group or randomization. In others both the control group and randomization are absent.

Nonequivalent control-group design

In the *nonequivalent control-group* design the groups are natural collectives, for example, the patients on two different wards, women who gave birth in June versus women who gave birth in July, or men or women. The one important distinction between the pretest posttest control-group design and the nonequivalent control-group design is that the control and experimental groups are not drawn from the same population in the nonequivalent design. The nonequivalent control-group design is illustrated in Fig. 11-6.

The dotted line separating the experimental and control groups implies that the participants were not allocated randomly to the treatment or control groups at the same point in time. As a result the investigator cannot assume the equivalence of the two groups. This design may be useful, however,

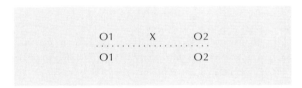

Fig. 11-6. Nonequivalent control-group design.

COUNTERBALANCING POSITIONS

The flip of a coin indicates which position the person will assume first. If heads, the person is supine first. If tails, the person has the backrest of the bed elevated 20 degrees. The following sequences will be observed:

Heads

   1. Record the position in which the person was found. Position person supine for 10 minutes, then obtain the first cardiac output measurement.

   2. Reposition the person so that the backrest of the bed is elevated 20 degrees. After 10 minutes obtain the second cardiac output measurement.

Tails

   1. Record the position in which the person was found. Position the person so that the backrest of the bed is elevated 20 degrees. After 10 minutes obtain the first cardiac output measurement.

   2. Reposition the person to the supine position. After 10 minutes obtain the second cardiac output measurement.

when studying questions for which randomization is not feasible. For example, an investigator interested in the influence of exercise programs on chronically ill persons may find it impossible to offer the program to some individuals within a clinic and withhold it from others.

To conduct the study, the investigator may need to identify and select participants for the control group from another clinic in the same area. In this case the two groups could not be considered as coming from the same underlying population; they would be nonequivalent. However, as with the pretest posttest control-group design the investigator would be able to determine whether the same amount of change would have occurred in the dependent variable in the treatment and experimental groups.

Weiss's study (1984) of transition modules for new graduates illustrates the use of a nonequivalent control-group design. She studied all nurses in eight hospitals who had graduated during the first or second year of the study. To avoid influencing the control group through their nonintended exposure to the experimental modules, she included nurses graduating in the first year of the study as the control group and those graduating in the second year of the study as the experimental group. The experimental group used the modules designed to prepare them for transition to practice, including a clinical competency module, an adjustment module, and a module dealing with pragmatics of the hospital system. Graduates using the module experienced less discrepancy between their desired and existing level of clinical skill, greater orientation to bureaucratic expectations, greater job satisfaction, and less role deprivation than the graduates in the control group. Weiss's use of a nonequivalent group design allowed her to conclude that the transition modules were effective. Moreover, the design enabled her to limit influence of the modules on the contrast group, a potential problem had both groups been tested similarly.

One-group pretest, posttest design

The one-group pretest and posttest design is a second type of quasiexperimental design in which the investigator pretests the sample, introduces the experimental manipulation to everyone in the study,

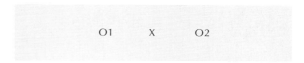

Fig. 11-7. One-group pretest, posttest design.

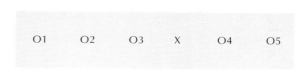

Fig. 11-8. Interrupted time series design.

and then obtains posttest measures. The design is illustrated in Fig. 11-7. Had Weiss (1984) not included a control group, the design would have been a one-group pretest, posttest design.

This design enables the investigator to determine the influence of the treatment variable on the dependent variable by using ipsative controls: each participant serves as his or her own control. Scores on the premeasure can be compared with scores on the postmeasure. Because participants in this study all receive the experimental manipulation, it is impossible to ascertain whether the same amount of change between $O1$ and $O2$ would have occurred without the experimental condition. Thus Weiss's use of the control groups increased the likelihood that her conclusions regarding effectiveness of the transition modules were accurate.

Interrupted time series design

A third commonly used quasiexperimental design is the interrupted time series design. This design is similar to the time series design explored in Chapter 9, with the single exception that the time series is "interrupted" by an experimental manipulation. The interrupted time series design is illustrated in Fig. 11-8.

The interrupted time series design involves collection of data over an extended period of time during which an intervention is interspersed. In some studies use of a control group would be impossible or inappropriate, for example, in studying the impact

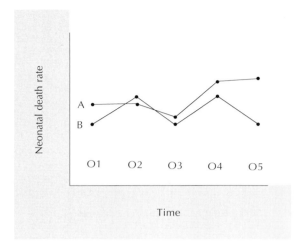

Fig. 11-9. Interrupted time series design. Note the discontinuity in the pattern of the death rate in line *A* after occasion 3 in contrast to the random fluctuation in line *B. O,* Observation occasion.

X   O

Fig. 11-10. One-time case study.

on the health of pregnant women and their infants of deleting a nutrition supplement program. Suppose that a policy were introduced in a state health department to cancel all prenatal nutrition supplementation. The concerned investigator might monitor the incidence of neonatal deaths and morbidity for 3 consecutive years before cancellation of the program *(O1, O2, O3)* and for 2 or more years after the program has been canceled *(O4, O5)*. These data would allow an assessment of the impact of cancellation on neonatal death rate and morbidity through comparison of the death rates while the program was operational with those after cancellation. If the data resembled those in Fig. 11-9, line *A,* the investigator would conclude that the cancellation of the program had devastating effects on neonatal health, whereas if the data resembled those in Fig. 11-9, line *B,* the investigator would have no evidence of impact. Indeed, it would appear that the data in Fig. 11-9, line *B,* merely reflect fluctuation over time.

One time–case study design

The one time–case study design involves an experimental manipulation and observation of the outcome on a single occasion. This design, illustrated in Fig. 11-10, enables the investigator to measure the outcome of an experimental treatment. However, since the investigator does not have the opportunity to obtain measures of the outcome variable before the treatment, internal validity cannot be ensured. Because the participants are not randomly allocated to the treatment, the threats to external validity are not controlled. This design is termed "preexperimental" by Campbell and Stanley (1963), because of its inherent limitations. A major dilemma is the inability to ascertain whether the outcome would occur without the treatment condition. Nevertheless, this design is useful in studying naturally occurring events that could not be manipulated by the investigator, such as the impact of natural disasters on human health.

Murphy's study (1984) of people who experienced losses ranging from death of a close relative or friend to property loss in conjunction with a natural disaster illustrates the value of the one-time case study. On May 18, 1980, the volcano Mt. St. Helens erupted, resulting in the presumed or confirmed deaths of 60 persons. Murphy examined the influence of the presumed bereavement, confirmed bereavement, loss of a permanent residence, and loss of a leisure residence on life stress, depression, somatization, and physical health. Because of the nature of the event Murphy studied, a one time–case study design enabled her to study the effects of this devastating natural experience.

DESIGNING NATURALISTIC STUDIES

In addition to using experimental designs to test hypotheses, investigators can employ naturalistic designs for these purposes. These designs resemble the panel design, cross-sectional designs, and comparative survey designs discussed in earlier chapters. The major difference between designing hypothesis-testing studies and exploratory studies is the emphasis on controlling for or accounting for factors that would distort the evidence bearing on the causal hypothesis being tested. Investigators establish causal relationships through designing studies that incorporate three aims: to maximize covariation; to clarify time ordering of the cause-and-effect variables; and to prevent spurious findings. The designs discussed in the following pages vary in the degree to which they allow the investigator to meet these aims.

Importance of naturalistic designs

Despite the advantages experimental designs have for the study of causal relationships, many occasions arise when the investigator must consider naturalistic designs. Some variables cannot or should not be manipulated, controlled, or randomized. For example, age and gender cannot be manipulated. For ethical reasons variables such as prenatal care or malnourishment should not be manipulated because of the hazardous consequences to participants deprived of care or food. It may be impractical (and hazardous) to manipulate a variable that affects treatment, such as changing the assignment of patients with myocardial infarctions from an intensive care unit designed for cardiac patients to an intensive care unit designed for an entirely different patient population.

When the purpose of the study requires description of phenomena as they naturally occur, it is illogical for the investigator to consider a true experimental design. By definition, the investigator must allow the phenomenon to occur at its own pace and under circumstances not determined by the investigator.

Types of naturalistic designs

Naturalistic designs can be described as futuristic, historical, or concurrent. In a *futuristic* design (also referred to as longitudinal, panel, or prospective) the researcher measures the antecedent and consequent variables in their order of occurrence, for example, the antecedent variable at *T1* and the consequent variable at *T2* and *T3*, and so on. For example, a population of women would be studied over 40 years to identify what aspects of lifestyle contribute to their health. In a *historical* design (sometimes referred to as retrospective or case-referent), the researcher measures the consequent or outcome variable first and then looks backward in time to antecedent events. For example, elderly women who have remained unusually healthy would be asked to reflect on earlier life events that the researcher

assumes are important to health. In a *concurrent (or cross-sectional)* design, the researcher measures the antecedent and consequent variables simultaneously. Elderly women would be studied at a single point in time at which their health and antecedent conditions that possibly affected their health in previous years would be assessed simultaneously.

Futuristic designs

Futuristic designs involve looking forward in time. The investigator is usually interested in studying change over time within the individual (intraindividual change) or between groups of individuals (interindividual change) and factors that cause or influence that change. Futuristic designs involve the measurement of the causal variable(s) at one point in time and the effect variable(s) at another, later point in time. Participants are assessed at least twice, once at the beginning and again at the end of the study; some studies involve multiple repeated measures. Futuristic designs include the panel design, discussed in Chapter 10, and the prospective or longitudinal design. Futuristic designs are useful in planning investigations that span a period of time from weeks to years. They are sometimes intended to describe the influence of one variable on another in the natural evolution of a life process, as is often the case in studies of human development, and at other times to allow the passage of time necessary for a process to occur, such as recovery from an illness. Futuristic designs enable the investigator to consider intraindividual change over time, as well as changes in a study group.

Sometimes the primary emphasis of a futuristic design is on what effect a characteristic such as health behavior has on a health outcome. Epidemiological studies of the development of poor health or death commonly take this approach; a variation of a panel design called a *prospective design* is employed. In this type of study investigators select the participants from a population that is known to be free of the health outcome under study and classify the participants according to whether they have one or more factors (independent variables) presumably related to the outcome. These participants, who are often referred to as a cohort, then are studied for a period of time, ranging from months to years, to determine who develops the health outcome.

In a study to predict acute confusional states in

TABLE 11-1. Prospective design employed in a study of the development of confusion in elderly hospitalized patients

TIME	1 ADM	2 OD	3 PO$_1$	4 PO$_2$	5 PO$_3$	6 PO$_4$	7 PO$_5$
Background data*	X						
Laboratory data[†]	X						
Clinical data[‡]	X	X	X	X	X	X	X
Confusion rating	X	X	X	X	X	X	X

ADM, Admission; OD, operative day; PO, postoperative day.

* Includes age, sex, hours from injury to admission, mental status examination, etc.
[†] Includes hemoglobin, sodium, potassium, etc.
[‡] Includes pain ratings, quality of sleep, etc.

elderly hospitalized patients, Williams and her colleagues (1985) used a prospective design. The investigators recruited all persons admitted to four hospitals for surgical treatment of hip fractures. On the first observation patients with mental impairment or delirium tremens present before the injury were eliminated from the cohort. In all cases surgery occurred within 2 days of admission. Each person was observed each day from admission to the fifth postoperative day. Table 11-1 illustrates the prospective design employed in the study of confusion. Those individuals who were older, had a low level of preinjury activity, and more errors on the mental status examination given on admission were most likely to develop confusion.

Selecting the sample. The initial cohort is selected for various reasons. First, they may be particularly likely to have one or more of the characteristics related to the health outcome under study. Confusion is likely to occur when elderly people are immobile, so a cohort at risk of confusion is elderly people who are immobilized for a hip fracture. Second, the cohort may belong to a group such as a health maintenance organization or a nursing alumni organization where follow-up is facilitated. Third, they may be as appropriate as any other group and convenient to the investigator.

Observations and timing. Once the cohort has

been identified, the investigator collects data regarding the independent and dependent variables. During the first observation obtaining data regarding the potential causes of the phenomenon being studied is emphasized so that the data reflect the evidence for the time ordering of the hypothesized cause and effect. Williams and her colleagues incorporated seven measurements into their study of confusion, allowing the investigators to link background data, laboratory data, and clinical data with the subsequent occurrence of confusion in elderly hospitalized patients. This is a strong design element for establishing time ordering of the cause-and-effect variables.

Data sources for information about the independent variables are diverse; they may include self-report, records of the individual's health, physical examination reports, or other sources of information. Williams and her colleagues (1985) used multiple data sources.

One of the most difficult aspects of obtaining data from individual members of a cohort is nonresponse. When some persons with the cause being investigated do not respond, the investigator has an underestimate of the causal variable in the population and the results become biased. In Williams's study if a proportion of individuals with a low level of preinjury activity did not respond to the study, then the proportion of those individuals in the population of elderly hospitalized patients would be underestimated. When the nonresponse is related to the effect, as for example, when those who are most ill do not respond, then the health-effect rate for the cohort will be underestimated, with the cohort appearing healthier. In Williams's study if the individuals most likely to develop confusion refused to participate, then the rate of confusion would be underestimated. When people who do not respond to the study have both the cause and effect being studied, then the association between the hypothesized cause and effect also will be biased.

When individuals refuse to participate in a study, the investigator can do little to estimate the type of bias that is operating. Some investigators request that the individual complete a short refusal interview that provides basic demographic data. This allows the investigator to assess the nonresponse bias with respect to demography of the sample. Another approach is to examine group data for the total population, comparing the sample to the data for a population. When these data are available, the investigator can assess the extent to which those who participated in the study resemble the total population. For example, individuals who participate in surveys typically are better educated than the population as a whole.

Some approaches that investigators use to decrease the problem of nonresponse during the follow-up period include sending out a second questionnaire, attempting to reschedule interviews, or attempting to obtain data from another source such as records. The investigator also can compare the dropouts from the cohort to the respondents on other variables to assess the extent to which nonresponse was likely to have biased the conclusions.

One problem peculiar to the prospective study is that over time people may be involved in different experiences that alter their exposure to characteristics under study. Williams and her colleagues (1985) considered the need for repeated measures of the hypothesized causal variables throughout their study. They anticipated that such information as laboratory and clinical data would be changing constantly, thus repeated assessment of these variables throughout the study was essential.

In a prospective study several problems must be considered in assessing outcomes. For example, during even a short follow-up period of a few months loss of participants caused by migration is a major concern. In a study of confusion in the elderly some of the participants are likely to die during the duration of the study. In other studies participants' moving away from the area of the study interferes with accurate assessment of the effect variable. When the proportion of participants who move away from the study area is large and when follow-up efforts are unsuccessful, the investigator is faced with concerns regarding bias in the independent variables, dependent variables, and the relationship between them. When the proportion of participants lost from the study to those who initially were enrolled is large, it may be necessary to terminate the study in view of the biased results that would be obtained were it to continue.

Another difficulty encountered in prospective studies is misclassification. When the outcome under study is misclassified, as for example, if a person in Williams's study (1985) who is confused is rated as not confused, the findings will be spurious. Changes in criteria for diagnosis or measurement over time may be responsible for misclassification and, in turn, may produce spurious findings. For example, if the methods used to assess the health outcome under study are greatly improved, then it would be more likely that the investigator will identify individuals with that outcome. If raters' ability to diagnose confusion improved during the course of the Williams's study (1985), the net effect would be an apparent increased incidence of confusion and perhaps an altered relationship between the independent variables and the outcome.

Measurement equivalence refers to the conceptual similarity of measurements made at one point in time to measurements made at other times. It is particularly challenging to studies of developmental processes. For example, children's concepts of health differ with age. Does an instrument measuring definitions of health mean the same thing to a child 6 years old versus the same child at 12 years of age? Does the instrument reflect a change in the definition of health or a change in the child's ability to conceptualize? A related problem is the effect of testing and instrumentation in repeated measures. *Testing effects* refer to changes in people as a consequence of repeated testing. People who are asked repeatedly to record their symptoms either often improve through the consciousness-raising effects of self-monitoring or in some cases record increased symptoms because of increased attention to them.

A final problem in assessing health-related outcomes is that the individual collecting outcome data may introduce bias through awareness of the participants' status with respect to the independent variables. For example, if the raters in Williams's study (1985) were aware of the participants who had marginal mental status on admission, they might have been more inclined to rate them as confused than if they were unaware of their mental status on admission.

Analysis. The basic strategy involved in analyzing data from a prospective study is assessing the degree of association between the hypothesized causes and effects. In the study of confusion in elderly hospitalized patients the investigators were concerned with the prediction of individuals most likely to experience confusion. The investigators used a data analysis technique that allowed them to develop an equation to help predict confusion. Another important analytical strategy involves considering the effects of confounding variables on the relationship being studied. In Williams's study (1985) the investigators considered age as an important cause of confusion, and their results indicated they were correct. In future work other investigators would need to consider age as a variable of primary interest or as a variable likely to confound the relationship between other variables related to both age and confusion.

In addition to the analytical strategies noted, specific adjustments may be made in the analyses because of the nature of the prospective design. In long-term studies the cohort is aging over time, so it is useful to calculate measures of association or rates for specific age-groups. Procedures for adjusting rates for these age-groups are described in detail elsewhere (Kleinbaum, Kupper, & Morgenstern, 1982). In addition, when participants are lost to follow-up, the investigator can attempt to estimate the distortion in the results. For example, the investigator might assume that persons lost to follow-up all had the cause or the effect under study (e.g., were very old and developed confusion). Measures of association could be calculated using the assumption that varying proportions of the lost participants had either the cause or the effect. By comparing the findings of these calculations with those based on the participants who completed the entire study, the investigator can determine how different the actual findings are from the possible alternatives.

Advantages. The prospective design has several advantages. Often, the participants in the cohort are drawn from a reference population, thus enabling the investigator to generalize from the sample studied to the population with some degree of certainty. In Williams's study (1985) the population represented elderly people hospitalized for surgical correction of hip fractures. In addition the causal variable under study clearly preceded the development of the effect, one of the necessary criteria for a causal inference.

The investigator can estimate from the cohort the actual prevalence of the cause-and-effect variables under study. For example, based on data from Williams's study, the proportion of elderly expected to experience confusion when hospitalized for a hip fracture could be estimated at slightly more than one half. Because the hypothesized cause is measured before the effect is ascertained, the likelihood of bias in reporting the relationship between the cause and effect is reduced.

Disadvantages. Prospective studies are very costly in time, personnel, and follow-up and are not feasible when the outcome being studied is rare. Attrition of persons in the cohort (or even among the investigators over many years) constitutes a considerable problem in the interpretation of results. Finally, other changes may occur over time in the environment or in the cohort, and these may affect the outcomes of the study.

Historical designs

Historical designs involve looking into history. A commonly used type of historical design is the *retrospective design*. The basic strategy of a retrospective design involves comparison of one or more groups of individuals with respect to a hypothesized cause that occurred at some time in the past. Not to be confused with historiography, which will be discussed in Chapter 21, the historical or retrospective design is commonly used in epidemiological studies, in which the groups usually include at least one with a health-related condition and another without that condition. Individuals with the health condition are referred to as cases, and those without the condition are referred to as controls or referents. In nursing a similar design strategy can be applied to test causal hypotheses when a prospective study is not feasible.

Worcester and Quayhagen (1983) used a retrospective design in their study of caregivers for elderly family members. The investigators initially identified two groups of caregivers: 19 persons who were currently providing care for an individual 60 years of age or older who was perceived to need too much care to live alone and 29 persons who had cared for an individual 60 years of age or older in the past, with the client now living in a nursing home. The two groups of caregivers were interviewed regarding hypothesized causes of success in the caregiving role: medical-physical, psychological-behavioral, and environmental-personal aspects of caregiver stress, caregiver satisfaction, and background and demographic data regarding the client. Comparison of current and past caregivers showed past caregivers had more stress in psychological and environmental areas and significantly lower satisfaction than did their counterparts who were current caregivers.

Selecting the cases. In selecting the cases for a retrospective study the criteria for the definition of the health state under study, the source of the cases, and the inclusion of incident or prevalent cases are extremely important considerations. Worcester and Quayhagen (1983) used specific criteria for defining who was a past or current caregiver, so the groups were comparable in most ways except their current caregiving status. When health status is the outcome, valid and reliable definitions of the health state are essential. Often the investigator must decide whether to include borderline cases or how to cope with differences in raters' application of criteria.

Cases may be obtained from persons being treated for specific illnesses or identified as having the particular health condition through another source. It is important for the investigator to ascertain that the cases do indeed meet the study criteria for inclusion; those criteria may differ from clinical criteria.

Inclusion of incident or prevalent cases is another important consideration. Prevalent cases would be those individuals who had the health outcome or outcome variable at some point in time, whereas incident cases would be those individuals who are experiencing the health outcome during the time of the study. Whether an individual has ever experienced caretaking or is currently experiencing caretaking would be an important concern.

Selecting the controls. Decisions about the source of controls are also important in the conduct of retrospective studies. Controls may be obtained from the general population, hospitalized clients, or relatives or associates of the cases. In Worcester and Quayhagen's study (1983) all the participants were obtained from home health-care agencies. In general, if the cases represent all the affected persons in a population, then controls should be selected from the same population. Some of the concerns in the selection of controls relate to whether information on the study variables can be obtained from the control group in a manner similar to that by which it was obtained from the case group, whether to match the controls with the cases to control for a certain confounding factor, whether the controls are similar to the cases in general, and whether controls can be found practically and in a financially feasible way. One particular concern relevant to nursing studies is the selection of cases who have entered the medical care system and comparison of these cases with controls who have been selected from another sampling frame, such as the community at large. An immediate difference in the cases and controls is likely to be their access to medical care.

Sampling. Once the source of controls is identified, the investigator must decide whether to study the entire population or a sample from the population. Because of the difficulty in enumerating everyone who is a case and everyone who is a control to draw a random sample from a large population, paired sampling is often used. This means that for each case one or more controls is selected. This may be accomplished by asking the cases to identify someone in the same neighborhood of the same age or by asking someone in a health-services agency to help in the identification of controls.

Information about the independent variables. Sources of data about independent variables may include self-report, report from a relative, records such as hospital charts, employment records, and other archives. If the data on the independent variables differ systematically in completeness or accuracy between cases and controls, the association between the independent variables and the outcome will be spurious. The validity of the data on the independent variables is extremely important; where possible, information about these variables recorded before discovery of the health outcome is desirable to limit the effect of recall bias in reporting. Using similar procedures for cases and controls will also help to ensure validity.

Analysis. The analysis of a retrospective study consists of a comparison between cases and controls with respect to the frequency of the causal variables believed to be related to the health outcome being studied. The investigator considers whether the presumed causal variables occur more frequently among those who experience the health outcome than among those who do not. Worcester and Quayhagen (1983) compared the incidence of stress in current and past caregivers, finding the greater experience of stress among those who were no longer caregivers. An estimate of the association between the hypothesized cause(s) and effect(s) is the primary focus of the analysis.

Concurrent designs

Concurrent designs involve simultaneously measuring the experience of hypothesized cause-and-effect variables. Individuals are identified from a reference population, and the independent and dependent variables are ascertained concurrently. Note that this design is essentially the same as the cross-sectional survey discussed in Chapter 10.

Brandt's study (1984) of social support and maternal discipline of children aged 6 months to 3 years with developmental delays illustrates a concurrent design. She asked mothers of children attending a developmental preschool/clinic to complete a mailed questionnaire dealing with social support, stress, discipline, and demographic information. All measures were administered simultaneously. Brandt found that for mothers with high stress, social support reduced the use of restrictive discipline. Social support was most influential for mothers who had children with three to five developmental delays as contrasted with one to two delays. Use of negative methods of maternal discipline decreased when mothers felt supported.

Advantages. When concurrent designs involve sampling from a reference population, the investigator can estimate the prevalence of a phenomenon relative to the underlying population, for example, the proportion of persons in a census tract who need home care after early discharge from the hospital. The investigator can also estimate associations between variables that can be generalized to the reference population.

Disadvantages. The investigator cannot sort out age versus cohort effects, that is, whether age or having lived during a certain era was more important. The investigator also cannot be sure about the antecedent-consequent relationships. For example, in Brandt's study the social support available to the woman may have decreased after she gave birth to a child with multiple developmental delays or may have decreased as her social network became alienated by her disciplinary style, rather than being unavailable to her before her developing negative discipline patterns.

Case study

Although the case study usually is used for exploratory studies as the basis for hypothesis generation, case studies can also be used to test hypotheses (Schultz & Kerr, 1986). One particular application is the multiple case–comparison design, in which the investigator systematically compares patterns of findings across several single case studies. This approach is especially useful when the entire single case involves multiple levels of interaction and causation. The strategy involves comparing two or more cases systematically to determine if hypothesized explanations hold across the cases. The most similar cases and the most different cases can be compared to determine whether the hypothesized relationships occur. Alternatively, the investigator can discover an explanation in the first case and then test it in subsequent cases. Schultz and Kerr (1986) used a comparative case-study design in studying rural primary health-care services. They compared three underserved communities with one community not so designated, addressing the following questions:

1. What is the health status of the populations in those areas designated as underserved?
2. Do certain types of interorganizational relationships facilitate access to appropriate care?
3. What is the organizational context of such relationships?
4. What is the community context of such relationships?

They collected data permitting four levels of analysis: the individual, the organization, interorganizational links, and the community. These data were used to test hypothesized relationships between community factors such as lifestyle and environment, interorganizational relationships, organizational factors such as the nature of primary health-care organizations, and health systems outcomes such as health status. At the individual level of analysis, screening measures and health habits could not be predicted by the independent variables. Moreover, neither access to local health-care services nor personal attributes of biological endowment or lifestyle explained the variance in health outcome dependent variables. Analysis at the level of the community revealed that underserved communities differed from the better-served community with respect to several variables as Schultz and Kerr had predicted. For example, they found that in small, rural underserved communities, the older the population, the fewer the early diagnostic screening tests, resulting in higher death rates from selected diseases.

Comparison of nonexperimental designs: internal and external validity

As seen in Table 11-2, prospective designs allow investigators to be more certain of antecedent-conse-

TABLE 11-2. **A comparison of nonexperimental designs: internal and external validity**

	PROSPECTIVE	RETROSPECTIVE	CONCURRENT
INTERNAL VALIDITY PROBLEMS			
Antecedent consequent relationship	−	+	+
Secular trends (history)	+	−	−
Recall bias	−	+	+
Selective survival (attrition)	+	±	−
EXTERNAL VALIDITY PROBLEMS			
Selection bias	±	+	+
Estimation of association	−	±	−
Generalization to reference population	−	+	−

Note +, present; −, absent.

quent relationships than the other designs, but their long-term course introduces the possible effects of secular trends. Recall problems are greatest with retrospective and concurrent designs, whereas attrition of study participants is most problematic with a prospective design. Attrition may also be problematic for retrospective designs. Selection bias is a problem with every type of design, but it is most likely to distort findings when the design is retrospective. Both prospective and concurrent designs allow the investigator to estimate directly an association between the independent and dependent variables, but indirect estimates of association can be inferred from retrospective designs. The prospective and concurrent designs allow the investigator to generalize results to a reference population, provided such a population was used in selecting the sample for the study. In some instances retrospective designs can enable the investigator to generalize to a reference population, but the sampling strategy must be applied to a known reference population.

SUMMARY

Through hypothesis-testing studies investigators can contribute to explanatory and predictive theory. Explanatory and predictive theory rests on the study of causal relationships.

Much of the effort of designing research studies has been directed at testing hypotheses about causal relationships. Criteria that support an assertion of a causal relationship include covariation, causal direction, and nonspuriousness. Causal relationships may

be direct, as well as indirect. Spurious associations occur when two variables are associated, but the association exists because of the influence of a third variable.

Experimental designs have three critical features: manipulation, control, and randomization. The MAX-MIN-CON principle guides the design of experiments: maximize experimental variance, minimize error variance, and control extraneous variance.

Study designs have both internal and external validity. Internal validity refers to the relationship between the independent and dependent variables, whereas external validity refers to the representativeness or generalizability of the study results. Threats to internal validity include maturation, contemporaneous events, testing, instrumentation error, statistical regression, differential selection, differential loss of participants, and combinations of these. Threats to external validity include reactivity, novelty effects, testing effects, joint effects of history and manipulation, and effects of multiple treatments.

There are several experimental design options, including the pretest posttest control-group design, the four-group design, posttest only control-group design, factorial design, and counterbalanced design. Quasiexperimental designs are those in which the investigator does not randomly assign the participants to treatment conditions but does manipulate the experimental condition and incorporates varying types of control to enhance the internal validity of the findings. Quasiexperimental designs include the nonequivalent control-group design, one-group pretest, posttest design, interrupted time series design, and the one-time case study.

Naturalistic designs are those in which investigators observe the occurrence of the independent and dependent variables but do not manipulate the independent variable. Moreover, they do not randomly assign individual participants to a treatment or control group but randomly select individuals from specified populations; they do not create a control group but use naturally occurring controls as a basis of comparison. They establish causal relationships by incorporating three aims: maximizing covariation, clarifying time ordering of the hypothesized cause-and-effect variables, and preventing spurious findings. Naturalistic study designs for testing hypotheses include futuristic, historical, concurrent, and case study designs.

───────REFERENCES

Baltes, P., Reese, H., & Nesselroade, J. (1977). *Life-span developmental psychology: Introduction to research methods.* Monterey, CA: Brooks/Cole.

Barnard, K., Magyary, D., Booth, C., & Eyres, S. (in press). Longitudinal design: Considerations and application to nursing research. In M. Cahoon (Ed.), *Recent advances in nursing: Research methodology.* Edinburgh: Churchill Livingstone.

Brandt, P. (1984). Stress-buffering effects of social support on maternal discipline. *Nursing Research, 33,* 229-234.

Campbell, D., & Stanley, J. (1963). *Experimental and quasi-experimental designs for research.* Chicago: Rand McNally.

Dixon, J. (1984). Effects of nursing intervention on nutritional and performance status in cancer patients. *Nursing Research, 33,* 330-335.

Grose, B., Woods, S., & Laurent, D. (1981). Effect of backrest position on cardiac output measured by the thermodilution method in acutely ill patients. *Heart and Lung 10*(4), 661-665.

Kerlinger, F. (1986). *Foundations of behavioral research.* New York: Holt, Rinehart, & Winston.

Kleinbaum, D., Kupper, G., & Morgenstern, H. (1982). *Epidemiologic research: Principles and quantitative methods.* Belmont, CA: Lifetime Learning.

Mitchell, P. (1982). Relationship of selected nurse-patient activities and intracranial pressure variations: Passive range of motion, turning, and head rotation. Final report to the *American Nurse Foundation,* Kansas City, Mo.

Murphy, S. (1984). Stress levels and health status of victims of a natural disaster. *Research in Nursing and Health, 7,* 205-216.

Rice, V., & Johnson, J. (1984). Preadmission self-instruction booklets, postadmission exercise performance and teaching time. *Nursing Research, 33,* 147-151.

Schultz, P., & Kerr, B. (1986). Comparative case study as a strategy. In P. Chinn (Ed.), *Methodological issues in nursing,* Rockville, MD: Aspen.

Selltiz, C., Wrightsman, L., & Cook, S. (1976). *Research methods in social relations.* New York: Holt, Rinehart, & Winston.

Sime, M., & Libera, M. (1985). Sensation information, self-instructure, and responses to dental surgery. *Research in Nursing and Health, 8,* 41-48.

Thomas, R. (1986). *Ventilator dependency consequences for child and family.* Unpublished doctoral dissertation, University of Washington, Seattle.

Weiss, S. (1984). The effect of transition modules on new graduate adaptation. *Research in Nursing and Health, 7,* 51-59.

Williams, M., Campbell, E., Raynor, W., Musholt, M., Mlynarczyk, S., & Crane, L. (1985). Predictors of acute confusional states in hospitalized elderly patients. *Research in Nursing and Health, 8,* 31-40.

Worcester, M., & Quayhagen, M. (1983). Correlates of caregiving satisfaction: Prerequisites to elder home care. *Research in Nursing and Health, 6,* 61-67.

12

DESIGNING SMALL SAMPLE STUDIES

PAMELA HOLSCLAW MITCHELL

Many studies reported in the nursing literature have relatively small samples of subjects (fewer than 10 to 15). General research design texts recommend larger samples for experimental studies. Are these small sample studies poorly designed? Does nursing research compromise important principles because subjects are hard to come by? Does small sample experimental and nonexperimental research have a legitimate place? The purpose of this chapter is to validate the small sample design, discuss appropriate and inappropriate uses of small samples, and to relate the small sample design to evaluation strategies in clinical nursing.

Early research or systematic inquiry was based on careful observations of one or a few persons or objects of interest. The nineteenth century naturalists developed science from accumulations of detailed observations of individual animals, plants, or objects. Freud's highly influential theories regarding the origins of human neuroses stemmed from case studies of his patients. Koch's famous experimental postulates regarding causation of disease by microscopic organisms could be demonstrated with one animal, as well as many. It was only with the advent of R. A. Fisher's development of statistical techniques for evaluation of agricultural experiments that the validity of experimentation with small numbers of subjects began to be questioned. By the early twentieth century most biological sciences and many social sciences had adopted the position that the only truly scientific method was the experimental design with a randomly selected sample that was large enough to detect experimental effects statistically.

Although the dominant paradigm in many sciences became the large random-sample controlled experiment, some social scientists, particularly in psychology, contended that valid experiments could be performed with single subjects. Most notable of these was B. F. Skinner, from whose "experimental analysis of behavior" came the principles of single subject or small sample experimentation.

A number of terms have arisen over the years to describe or name small sample research. Among these are single case design, intensive research, N = 1 design, ideographic research, experimental analysis of behavior, applied analysis of behavior, and case study designs. The principles of small sample design appear in such large sample designs as repeated measures, within-subject control, and time series. Although these are all legitimate designs for small sample research, the latter terms convey frequent sampling of criterion measures over time rather than describe anything about the number of subjects sampled.

Limiting ourselves to the dominant paradigm for inquiry limits science and thus limits the many ways in which we can know and understand our world. The large-sample experimental study is only one way to understand phenomena of interest to any given discipline. To understand those ways in which people share or differ in cultural aspects, anthropologists study the single culture or the single group. Clinicians in human services continue to try to help people one at a time and to keep careful records of patterns of response to intervention. From these traditions derives the case study as a method of small sample research.

Many of the terms traditionally used to describe small sample research, such as "N = 1" and "single-case design," tend to be identified with experimental design. However, legitimate research with one or a few participants can be both nonexperimental and experimental. Therefore the term *small sample research* will be used to refer to the whole class of research involving small numbers of participants. *Small N experimental design* will be used to refer to the principles of designing valid experiments with one or a few participants.

NONEXPERIMENTAL SMALL SAMPLE DESIGN

Factor-searching or factor-relating questions usually lend themselves well to small sample nonexperimental design. When we know little about a phenomenon, the single case or small sample approach is useful to identify and describe phenomena (see Chapter 9) and to describe patterns over time (see Chapters 9 and 10). Small N designs are not appropriate to describe the incidence or prevalence of a phenomenon, because parameter estimation cannot be done from one or a few cases.

Case study

The case study approach is useful for in-depth examination of a phenomenon of interest (see Chapters 10 and 11). Many ways are available to examine a phenomenon via the case method. When little is known about the phenomenon, the intensive case study approach may be useful to document every known aspect to understand how an occurrence of the phenomenon differs from a nonoccurrence. For example, one might be interested in understanding the effects of biomedical technology on quality of life. One approach might be to administer a quality-of-life survey to a large number of families or individuals whose illness problems require a specific biotechnological device. Although this large survey approach can tell us about the frequency with which the device affects some aspect of living, it cannot give much of the same sense of the experience and adjustments people make in adapting their lives to the demands of technology. Thus a large survey study

may not help us to learn factors most relevant to nursing intervention, that is, how persons cope with biotechnological devices. A case study approach to the same problem could entail taking either extreme or representative cases and identifying what those individuals experience in response to high technology care. As noted in Chapter 11, the case study can be useful for generating hypotheses. By creating specific contrasts across case studies and by accumulating information across studies, the case study can also be useful in testing hypotheses.

Within-subject analysis over time

Single subjects or small samples also can be used to help us describe the patterns in a phenomenon over time or how that phenomenon changes in relation to the environment or other phenomena over time. Within-subject analysis focuses on analysis of variation within data obtained from the same participant. For example, our current knowledge about the architecture of sleep—the patterns of sleep stages—has been derived from relatively small samples of people of a variety of ages, whose brain waves and other physiological indexes were monitored over several nights of sleep. Similarly, our knowledge of changes in these patterns in relation to age is derived from studies of a small number of people of various ages during sleep.

Updike, Accurso, and Jones (1985) used both behavioral indexes of sleep and physiological indexes of temperature and ventilation to determine if circadian rhythm patterns existed in biologically immature infants. They found a circadian pattern for skin temperature in each of six infants and detectable rhythms for respiratory rate of oxygenation in some subjects but not all. Thus they extended our knowledge of developmentally related patterns of biological function and formed the basis for hypotheses regarding interventions to create an environment that may promote more normal rhythms.

Mitchell and Mauss (1978) described the relationship between variations in intracranial pressure (ICP) and bedside-care activities in a small sample. Using minute-by-minute observations of ICP and all ongoing activities at the bedside, they established that increases in ICP occurred in relation to activity in general and identified specific activities that consistently were associated with increases in ICP both within and among subjects. These observations have formed the basis for a variety of studies confirming and extending the original findings.

Both the Updike and Mitchell and Mauss examples exhibit several characteristics of small N studies over time. To establish patterns and associations, measurements are taken frequently over an extended period of time and are dependent upon instrumentation. In other words, the design usually repeats measures over time and depends on sophisticated behavioral or physiological instrumentation. Both the previous examples used clinically available technology that measured a physiological variable continuously or sampled it at regular intervals. Behavioral observation studies, for example, children in a play situation or women interacting with their infants, can include mechanical devices to code ongoing observations or to signal the observer to encode activity at given times. Such studies generate large amounts of data, which lend themselves to both simple graphic and complex time series analysis strategies. Analysis of time series data is discussed later in this chapter under general considerations for analysis of repeated measures data.

EXPERIMENTAL SMALL SAMPLE DESIGN

Experimentation with one subject or a small number of subjects may sound like a contradiction in terms if we accept the dictum that randomization of subjects must occur for there to be a "true" experiment (Campbell & Stanley, 1963). However, if we return to the purpose of an experiment, we will see that randomization is not an inherent component but is one means to ensure the equivalency of control groups or conditions.

Recall from Chapter 11 that experiments are used when we want to explain relationships or to understand and verify the direction of the relationship. For example, apparently *A* (or perhaps *A*, given *C*, *D*, and *E*) explains why *B* happens. To have confidence that *A* actually explains *B*, we need to control or eliminate all the other things that also could explain the occurrence of *B*. Thus to say that introducing a predébridement relaxation technique in burned patients explains the decrease in pain and need for medication, it is necessary to eliminate, control, or equally distribute the effects of the other variables that also could influence experienced pain and need for medication (e.g., previous experience with relax-

ation therapy, extent of burn, cultural style of pain expression). The most commonly recommended way to do this is to randomly assign subjects to an experimental group and a control group.

Randomization

The purpose of randomization is to *reduce the variability due to extraneous variables* by distributing them randomly between the two groups. An extraneous variable is a variable other than the independent variable that influences the dependent variable. In theory, each extraneous variable has an equal chance to be in either group. However, this even distribution actually occurs only when the group of subjects is large enough. To visualize why randomization requires a large sample, consider the occurrence of "heads" or "tails" in coin flipping. An ordinary coin has an equal chance of landing heads or tails when flipped. We might consider the coin to represent our extraneous variable (e.g., previous use of relaxation therapy) and that it will influence the outcome in the experimental group if it comes up heads and the control group if it comes up tails. Based on the equal chance of heads or tails, we use the coin flip to achieve random assignment of subjects possessing prior relaxation experience to the control group and the experimental group. If we flip a coin often enough (about 100 times), one half of our flips will yield heads and one half will yield tails; we will have achieved even distribution of the extraneous variable and equalized its effect between the groups. However, if we flip the coin only 10 times, it is entirely possible to have eight heads and two tails, resulting in a markedly uneven distribution of the extraneous variable. If we translate coin flips into numbers of subjects, it becomes clear why having large numbers of subjects is necessary to achieve the aims of randomization in controlling variability attributable to extraneous variables.

Randomization, however, is not the only method by which one can reduce or control variability. One can minimize variability due to nonexperimental variables by:

1. Eliminating the extraneous variables
2. Holding the effect constant in both experimental and control conditions
3. Distributing the effect evenly in both conditions

Randomization is intended to achieve aim *3* and thus

represents only one means of control. If one can achieve aim *1* or *2*, it is not necessary to distribute the effect of extraneous variables. It stands to reason that if one can control extraneous variables adequately, one can make strong explanatory statements regarding change in the behavior of a single individual after the introduction of some event or act. For example, if we choose to study only individuals with the same extent of burn, we have eliminated the variability caused by the varying extent of burns. When we study the effect of relaxation therapy within an individual, we automatically hold constant the effect of prior experience, since that is present both before and after the pain-relieving intervention.

Methods of control in small sample experimental design

In large sample research we are concerned with the variability across subjects and in reducing that variability caused by nonexperimental variables. In small sample research we are concerned with the variability of data within each subject and with means to reduce variability that is unrelated to the independent variable.

When only one or a few subjects are available for study, we clearly cannot assign subjects randomly into experimental and control groups to control the variability caused by nonexperimental variables. How then can one deal with the problems of internal

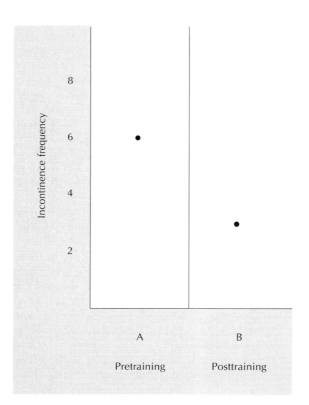

Fig. 12-1. Hypothetical data showing a reduction in frequency of incontinence after bladder training. Posttraining rate (phase *B*) is a 50% reduction from the rate before the intervention. However, without more data points in phase *A*, we cannot know if the postintervention response is related to the intervention or if it is a natural fluctuation in frequency of incontinence.

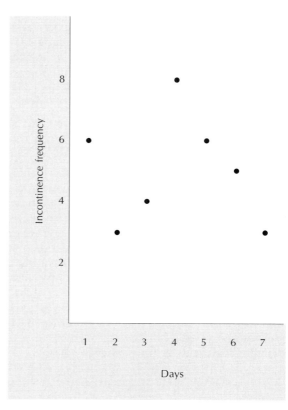

Fig. 12-2. Hypothetical data showing regular pattern of alternating high and low frequency of incontinence over time. If bladder training was instituted on day 2 (as was the case in the example in Fig. 12-1), it would appear that the low frequency on day 3 was a result of the intervention, when it is actually a part of a recurring pattern.

validity in small sample research? The best answer is to eliminate or hold constant the extraneous variables and to achieve a long and stable baseline set of measures before introducing the independent variable. Figs. 12-1 through 12-3 illustrate the importance of a stable baseline with repeated observations in making a causal inference about the relationship of the independent variable (hypothetical bladder-training intervention) to the target behavior (frequency of incontinence). In Fig. 12-1 we have measured the frequency of incontinence for 1 day, instituted a bladder-training regimen, and taken a 1-day posttraining measure of incidence of incontinence. Although clearly a change in level of incontinence

has occurred, one cannot be confident that it is related to the intervention. It is equally possible that we have simply tapped into a natural pattern of variability in incontinence, as shown in Fig. 12-2. Suppose, however, that we have 2 weeks of data with a stable and high incidence of incontinence (Fig. 12-3). Taken against that baseline, the postintervention level for an equivalent time period provides a much stronger case for inferring that the bladder-training program caused the change in incontinence. When all nonexperimental variables have been controlled or eliminated, this simple pretest posttest design with a long and stable baseline can provide the basis for a defensible causal inference. This simple design illus-

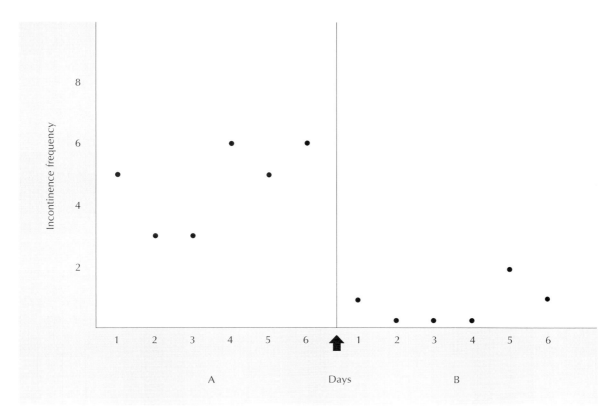

Fig. 12-3. Hypothetical data showing clear difference in frequency of incontinence before and after a bladder-training intervention *(arrow)*. The presence of a long enough baseline to capture the natural pattern of behavior is the key to interpreting the effect of the intervention in this A-B design.

trates three important principles of small sample experimental design:

1. The importance of the baseline period in determining patterns against which to compare postintervention data
2. The importance of using a number of data points to establish the degree of variability within the subject's data
3. The importance of stability of the baseline data to identify a clear difference in the experimental condition data

Interestingly, there are no generally accepted criteria for determining that stability indeed exists. Most commonly, investigators report using visual criteria for stability of baseline data, but the nature of those criteria is not reported. When questioned, investigators report that they are looking for absence of variability and trend (Kazdin, 1982; Killeen, 1978). The amount of variability or trend tolerated depends on the behavior being monitored. For example, Baltes and Zerbe (1976) determined the number of sessions in each phase (baseline and treatment) by the stability of the target behavior. The target behavior for their study was self-feeding in a nursing home resident. Only 1 week of observation was required to establish that baseline frequency of self-feeding (defined as one mouthful) for all meals that week was nearly zero. Had the self-feeding frequency fluctuated markedly during the week, the investigators would have been obliged to extend the baseline period until some pattern emerged against which to test the treatment program.

With behaviors that change in absolute values (such as weight gain in maturing mammals), one can transform the data to examine stability of rates. DeSomery and Hansen (1978) monitored caloric intake and weight gain for several months in rhesus monkeys to calculate an average baseline rate and introduced the experimental condition (parenteral feeding) when the rate of weight gain and caloric intake were stable. They do not define their critera for stability in quantitative terms, however. Thus we do not know if any variability occurred in the rate or number of calories.

Finally, one can set specific stability criteria before the investigation. For example, with physiological variables such as heart rate or blood pressure, one might set a stability criterion of "no greater than five beats per minute deviation from the mean rate for X

minutes." This approach is most likely to ensure a reproducible and clearly stable baseline. However, considerable prior knowledge of the phenomenon is required to determine the feasibility of the criterion. For example, is it reasonable to expect a fluctuating variable such as blood pressure to remain within a narrow range of variability? If that is not feasible, one can attempt to stabilize the behavior by additional means that do not interact with the experimental condition. For example, the use of nonnutritive sucking (pacifier) in infants can stabilize externally observable behavior (sucking) and internal behaviors such as heart rate, blood pressure, and transcutaneous oxygen tension (Anderson, McBride, Dahm, Ellis, & Vidyasugar, 1982).

Parallel comparison designs

Large sample designs typically collect data at two time points—once before and once after introducing the independent variable—and collect data about both experimental subjects and control subjects in parallel, or simultaneously. The possibility that the postintervention data represent a naturally occurring pattern is somewhat offset by the large number of subjects (all of whom would not be likely to have the same pattern of behavior) and by use of a control group (a similar group that does not get the experimental treatment).

In small sample research one generally uses a *control condition* rather than a control group. The control condition is generally the subject's baseline period and is measured sequentially, rather than simultaneously, with the experimental condition. However, it is possible to design a control condition to occur simultaneously with the experimental condition within a single subject. Gill and Atwood (1981) report an ingenious design in which they tested the relationship of mouse epidermal growth factor (mEGF) to wound healing. In a single pig, one of three strengths of mEGF was applied to each of three wounds, with three additional wounds serving as a control for each strength of mEGF. Rates of healing then were compared among the three strengths of the independent variable and the three control wounds.

One could envision other examples of using a simultaneous within-subject control. For example, a method of reducing postpartum breast engorgement could be tested, using one breast as a control and the other for the treatment. This type of simultaneous within-subject control design is appropriate whenever the effect expected will remain localized. It would not be appropriate, for example, to test two methods of local pain relief, because one expects generalized or systemic response to pain and pain relief from local remedies.

Sequential comparison designs

In many situations it is impossible to provide the experimental intervention and a control condition simultaneously, because the effect of the intervention is on the whole person. Consequently, the experimental condition cannot be compared in parallel or simultaneously with the control condition. In such cases we must use the subject's baseline as the control condition and then, in sequence, introduce the experimental condition. Fig. 12-3 illustrates a sequential comparison design.

A-B design. The simplest sequential design is shown in Fig. 12-3. In small sample design notation this is called an A-B design. *A* stands for baseline before introducing the independent variable and *B* for an equivalent period after introduction of the independent variable. Even with a relatively long baseline, this design does not completely protect us from the internal validity threats of maturation, instrumentation, or statistical regression. For these reasons, Kazdin (1982) likens A-B designs to the "pre-experimental" category of Campbell and Stanley (1963). The best protection from these threats to internal validity is to use the A-B design only when one has a sufficiently long baseline to feel confident that it represents the preintervention pattern and to use it only when maturation (or state change) is not likely to occur.

Fig. 12-2 uses hypothesized rhythmical data to illustrate how inappropriate conclusions might be drawn from an A-B design when the baseline is not sufficiently long to capture naturally occurring variations. Obviously, an experimental condition introduced at the peak of the wave capitalizes on spontaneous patterns.

A-B-A and A-B-A-B design. The reversal, or A-B-A, design is one way to strengthen the causal inference in such situations. In the reversal design the independent variable is removed after the postintervention data collection period, in effect reestablishing the baseline condition (A-B-A). If the target

behavior reverts to baseline level, one's confidence in the causal relationship of the independent variable to the change in behavior is strengthened. The causal argument is even stronger if one can reestablish the experimental condition and achieve the same change in behavior seen in the first instance of *B* (A-B-A-B design). Robinson and Foster (1979) called the A-B-A-B design intrainvestigatory affirmation, or confirmation of the experimental result within the same subject or study. Obviously, causal inference from a reversal design requires that the independent variable not have a carryover effect or that changes in the state of the subject do not alter the baseline behavior.

The A-B and A-B-A-B designs are analogous to the within-subject control designs of large sample research. The major difference between the within-subject control in small and large sample research is the degree to which the investigator is free to alter the protocol in light of the behavior of the subjects during the baseline or experimental conditions. Typically in large sample research, decisions regarding the duration of the control (baseline) and experimental (intervention) condition are made in advance of the study, applied equally to all subjects, and not altered during the course of the investigation. To do so would require "peeking" at the data, an activity that violates the assumptions on which the strength of the statistical analysis relies.

Small sample design, in contrast, does not rely heavily on typical statistical analysis of effects and thus is not constrained from examining the data (behavior) as it is occurring. Indeed, to make rational decisions regarding how long the baseline must be to capture the baseline pattern, monitoring the ongoing behavior being observed is essential. Decisions about when to change phase (from baseline to intervention) are usually made during the investigation, unless the investigator knows from experience how long the baseline usually must be for the particular phenomenon. Since evaluation of the intervention effect requires that the behavior be visibly different from the baseline, considerable baseline stability is important. Therefore the decision rule regarding baseline length is based on evidence of stability.

Baltes and Zerbe (1976) used the A-B-A design to evaluate the effect of a positive reinforcement program to increase the frequency of self-feeding in a nursing home resident. Feeding frequency (self-feed-

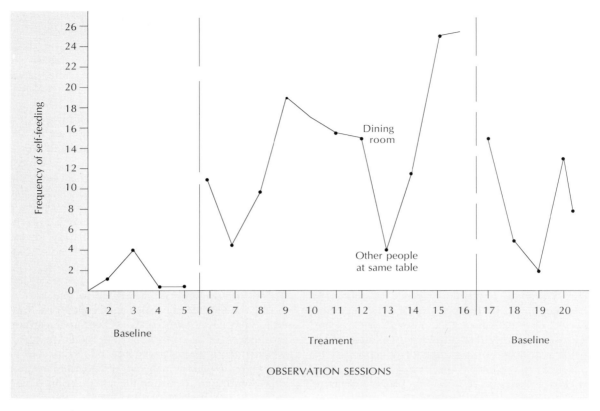

Fig. 12-4. Example of an A-B-A design. The dependent variable is the rate of self-feeding in a nursing home resident. (From Baltes M. M., & Zerbe, M. B. [1976]. *Nursing Research, 25,* 25. Copyrighted by the American Journal of Nursing Company.)

ing of one mouthful) rose from near zero in the baseline period to a range of 4 to 24 during the treatment period. Withdrawal of the treatment contingencies resulted in a drop from a high of 24 self-feedings at the end of the experimental phase to a range of 0 to 14 during the next few days. Although the authors termed this an A-B-A-B design, they did not present data resulting from reinstitution of the experimental condition. The conclusions would have been strengthened by such an addition in view of the fluctuations of behavior in both the treatment and second baseline phase (Fig. 12-4).

Incremental intervention phases. DeSomery and Hansen (1978) and Martyn, Hansen, and Jen (1984) used an A-B-A reversal design to evaluate the effect of total parenteral nutrition on a variety of measures of food intake and gastric function in rhe-

sus monkeys. Their basic interest was the extent to which varying levels of parenteral supplementation of food intake alters regulation of oral intake. Rather than perform many separate studies introducing varying percentages of oral baseline intake, they used an incremental design, successively adding varying strengths of parenteral feeding when a stable response had been established to the preceding strength of feeding. One might call this an A-B_1-B_2-B_3 . . . B_x-A design. *A* serves as baseline for all variants of *B* and the stability of B_1 serves as a baseline criterion for the introduction of B_2, etc. Finally, all interventions were withdrawn to determine the time necessary for oral feeding to return to a nonsupplemented baseline. The investigators chose the incremental design because it closely approximates clinical protocols for introduction of parenteral feeding. It is also an efficient design, because one can systematically test increments of an intervention without having to design several sequential studies.

When one suspects that an intervention has more than one mechanism of action, the incremental baseline design can be useful in separating components of the experimental condition. For example, Mitchell, Amos, and Astley (1986) used both reversal and incremental baseline designs to evaluate the influence of turning and lateral neck flexion on intracranial pressure and cardiovascular responses. Baboons were passively turned, and, after all variables had stabilized, the head was allowed to flex 45 degrees from midline. Response to turn *(B)* was measured against the baseline *(A);* that response then served as a baseline for the lateral head movement *(C).* The lateral head movement was reversed by returning the head to midline, and finally the turning process was reversed by returning the animal to a supine position. The design could be considered an A_1-B_1-A_2-C-A_3-B_2-A_1 design with three baselines.

Analysis of small sample experimental data

Statistical versus descriptive analysis. Large sample research is based on statistical analysis of the reliability of the results and, because of the use of statistical analysis, is designed to capture small effects. Small sample research began in a tradition of capitalizing on strategies to show large effects and thus did not rely on statistical analysis. It is argued that if one has a stable baseline and if the intervention has an effect, one should clearly see it in graphic display, thus obviating the need to search statistically for small effects. In the tradition of experimental analysis of behavior, many investigators use only visual analysis of data and consider only effects large enough to be evident to the eye as important (Kazdin, 1982; Robinson & Foster, 1979).

The basic principle of an experiment is to predict or hypothesize what will happen in the experimental condition. The baseline phase is used to establish a pattern of behavior that allows one to predict what reasonably would be expected to happen if the behavior continued undisturbed. Thus inspection of a graph of the data is essentially creating a mental projection of that data in time. When the intervention is applied, with control of other plausible explanatory variables, a discontinuity in the data line is reasonable evidence that the intervention was the best explanation for the change in pattern. Such a

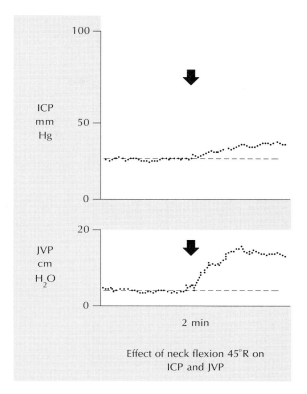

Fig. 12-5. Discontinuity in data from baseline to intervention phase. The arrow represents the point at which the subject's head is laterally flexed 45 degrees. Note the sharp rise in values of intracranial pressure (ICP) and jugular venous pressure (JVP) and the discontinuity with the projected data trend *(dashed lines).* (Data from Mitchell, Amos, & Astley [1986].)

discontinuity is shown in Fig. 12-5. Thus a primary method of analysis in small sample design is to visualize the data for projections of baseline continuity and evidence of postintervention discontinuity.

Reestablishing the baseline condition should reestablish the baseline visual pattern. Thus visual analysis should be sufficient to establish the validity of the effect of the experimental condition when the following exist:

1. A clear and stable baseline pattern
2. A clear break in the pattern with intervention
3. A clear return to baseline with withdrawal of the intervention

Size of effect is evident from the graphic presentation of the data; reliability is established by the ability to return to baseline or experimental conditions in the reversal design.

In general, visual analysis consists of judgments about magnitude and rate of the behaviors in question (Kazdin, 1982). Magnitude, or size, of the effect is inferred from changes in mean and level of the data. Change in rate is inferred from examination of trend and latency across phases.

Magnitude dimensions. When there are multiple data points in each phase of the experiment, one infers that a sizable effect has occurred by looking at changes in the mean or average data. In Fig. 12-5 the mean intracranial pressure of a baboon is indicated by the dashed line through the continuous recording of this variable. A clear difference from the projected mean occurs in the mean pressure several seconds after the experimental variable, displacement of the head 45 degrees from the midline, has occurred.

A change in level is defined as a discontinuity in the data from the end of one phase to the beginning of another. In Fig. 12-4 the discontinuity from baseline to treatment and again to baseline is evident.

Rate dimensions. Rate refers to frequency in a dimension of time. Therefore visual analysis of rate contributes to judgments about trends in rates and about latency of change. *Trend* is inferred from the slope of the data (increasing or decreasing) and is a useful dimension when one is dealing with a phenomenon in which frequency is not constant. Important change is inferred when the slope changes with

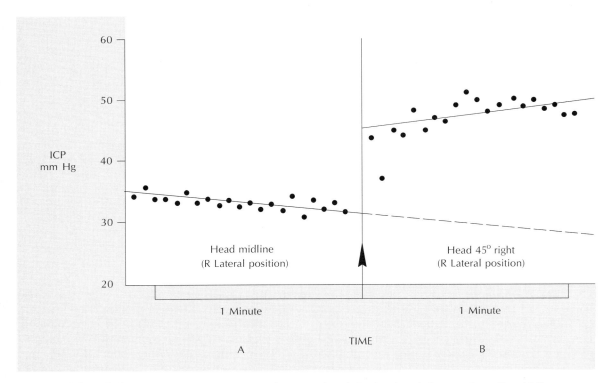

Fig. 12-6. Change in level and slope after lateral neck flexion in a baboon. The split-middle technique has been used to divide data points in phase *A* and *B* so that half are above and half are below the trend line. Change in level is indicated by the phase *B* line, whose values all lie above the projected phase *A* data line. Change in slope is evident because phase *A* data are on a decreasing slope and phase *B* data are on an increasing slope. (Data from Mitchell, Amos, & Astley [1986].)

the introduction of the experimental condition. Fig. 12-6 shows not only a change in level of performance (discontinuity at end of the phase) but also a change in trend (slope)—decreasing during baseline and increasing after intervention.

Latency refers to the time lapse between change of condition and change in behavior. In Fig. 12-5, a latency of several seconds occurs between the onset of the experimental condition (lateral head movement) and the change in mean and in trend of intracranial pressure response.

Statistical analysis. For a great many single case and small sample research designs, visual description of graphs of the data and presentation of the individual responses in small group within-subject designs is adequate for inference of experimental effect. However, in a number of circumstances considering statistical analysis of the reliability of the result is useful:

1. When the baseline is excessively variable
2. When the treatment condition is excessively variable
3. When the effect appears to be small
4. When the political environment requires statistical data

When the research environment (i.e., one's local or reviewing colleagues) seems to find only statistical results believable, it is tempting to adapt conventional *t* and *F* tests to single subject design. Some investigators have suggested that we simply treat each condition with the single subject design as if it were a group and then use the correlated *t* test or repeated measures analysis of variance to test the hypothesis that no difference in variability exists within or between conditions: A-B or A-B-A (Gentile, Roden, & Klein, 1972).

Unfortunately, such application of conventional *t* and *F* tests is likely to violate an important assumption of these statistical tests, namely, that the successive measures are independent of each other. Within an individual, repeated measures over time are likely to be highly correlated, or *serially dependent*, and thus would tend to violate the assumption of independence. Several investigators have shown that such a violation can produce both type I and type II errors (Hartmann, 1974; Kratochwill, 1974; Michael, 1974; Thoreson & Elsahoff, 1974). Therefore it is strongly recommended that conventional *t* and *F* tests be used *only* when one can demonstrate that

serial dependency or autocorrelation does not exist in the data (Kazdin, 1982).

Kazdin (1982) describes two nonparametric tests that are not influenced by serial dependency and are particularly useful in multiple-baseline or multiple-condition studies. The mechanics of the *randomization test* and the R_N *test of ranks* are well described in Kazdin (1982); only their use will be described here. The randomization test is particularly useful in A-B-A-B designs in which there are multiple applications of the conditions over time. The test determines whether the data in any condition (for example, all the *B* conditions) differ significantly from those of any other condition. The test assumes that the order of the conditions is assigned randomly and that there is an equal chance that any of the conditions will be in effect at a given time.

The R_N test of ranks is useful in a design with multiple baselines. The test evaluates the hypothesis that no difference in ranking of behavior change exists among the various baselines.

Time series analysis is predicated on autocorrelation, or serial dependency of data, and thus is ideal for many analyses of change in level and trend in single subject design. However, the various techniques for time series analysis require many data points and computer facilities for the computation required. Time series analysis is discussed further in Chapter 27.

One variant of time series analysis that does not require computer processing is the *split-middle technique* as described by White (1972, 1974). Kazdin (1982) provides clear directions for the use of this technique. The technique requires multiple data points in each condition but not nearly so many as other time series techniques. It further requires only a ruler and graph paper to plot a line that splits the data at the median of each condition and thus provides visual evidence of continuity or discontinuity across phases (see Fig. 12-6). The binomial test then can be applied to determine the probability that the proportion of data points falling above a trend line projected from phase *A* differs from chance.

GENERALIZABILITY

It is often asserted that small sample studies may be generalized only in a limited way. This is indeed the case when one develops a large sample design and then has only a few subjects. However, the appropriately designed small N study can have applicability beyond the individual in a variety of circumstances.

First, the goal of some research is to discover the properties of a phenomenon, as described in the section on case studies. In such cases generalization is not the primary aim of the research. If we wish to know the frequency of the properties of the phenomenon in the population, we might wish to design a large sample study for that purpose. Alternatively, one might choose to use systematic replication.

Systematic replication requires that one try to determine the enduring factors in the experiment by systematically altering some conditions to discover those circumstances under which similar findings among subjects occur. When Mitchell, Amos, and Astley (1986) found that 45-degree lateral neck flexion consistently produced increased intracranial pressure in three baboons, they systematically varied the degree of lateral neck flexion to discover the minimum angle that would produce the effect.

Interinvestigatory affirmation refers to the process of repeating the same investigation over many subjects. In essence it is a method to build a larger sample, one subject at a time. It is particularly effective in generalizing the findings of clinicians, who see patients one at a time.

Nursing is a clinical discipline: our science is a means to understand the nature of humans and of their responses to health problems or situations. Because we generally practice our discipline with human beings one at a time, or in small groups, research designs that preserve the uniqueness of the individual should be considered by both academic and clinical researchers. The small N experimental and nonexperimental methods are such designs.

SUMMARY

Small sample studies, those with fewer than 10 to 15 participants, incorporate nonexperimental and experimental study designs. Nonexperimental study designs such as the case study and within-subject analyses over time permit the investigator to obtain intensive information about a few individuals to characterize naturally occurring processes and to test hypotheses. Experimental small sample designs include the sequential comparison designs (such as

A-B, A-B-A, A-B-A-B) and the parallel comparison designs in which the experimental and control conditions are tested simultaneously. Methods of control in small sample design involve eliminating or holding constant the extraneous variables and achieving a long and stable baseline set of measures before introducing the independent variable.

REFERENCES

Anderson, G. C., McBride, M. R., Dahm, J., Ellis, M. K., & Vidyasugar, D. (1982). Development of sucking in term infants from birth to four hours prebirth. *Research in Nursing and Health, 5,* 21-27.

Baltes, M. M., & Zerbe, M. B. (1976). Reestablishing self-feeding in a nursing home resident. *Nursing Research, 25,* 24-26.

Barlow, D. H., Hayes, S. C., & Nelson, R. O. (1985). *The scientist practioner: Research and accountability in clinical and educational settings.* New York: Pergamon Press.

Campbell, D. T., & Stanley, J. C. (1963). *Experimental and quasi-experimental designs for research.* Chicago: Rand McNally.

Caty, S., Ellerton, M. L., & Ritchie, J. A. (1984). Coping in hospitalized children: An analysis of published case studies. *Nursing Research, 33,* 277-282.

DeSomery, C. H., & Hansen, B. W. (1978). Regulation of appetite during total parenteral nutrition. *Nursing Research, 27,* 19-24.

Gentile, J. R., Roden, A. H., & Klein, R. D. (1972). An analysis-of-variance model for the intrasubject replication design. *Journal of Applied Behavior Analysis, 5,* 193-198.

Gill, B. P., & Atwood, J. R. (1981). Reciprocy and helicy used to relate mEGF and wound healing. *Nursing Research, 30,* 68-72.

Gottman, J. M. (1973). N-of-one and n-of-two research in psychotherapy. *Psychological Bulletin, 80,* 93-105.

Gottman, J. M. (1981). *Time series analysis: A comprehensive introduction for social scientists.* Cambridge, England: Cambridge University Press.

Hartmann, D. P. (1974). Forcing square pegs into round holes: Some comments on "An analysis of variance model for the intrasubject replication design." *Journal of Applied Behavior Analysis, 7,* 635-638.

Kazdin, A. E. (1982). *Single-case research designs: Methods for clinical and applied settings.* New York: Oxford University Press.

Killeen, P. R. (1978). Stability criteria. *Journal of the Experimental Analysis of Behavior, 19,* 17-25.

Kratochwill, T., Alden, K., Demuth, D., Dawson, D., Panicucci, C., Arntson, P., McMurray, N., Hempstead, J., & Levin, J. (1974). A further consideration in the application of an analysis of variance model for the intrasubject replication design. *Journal of Applied Behavior Analysis, 7,* 629-633.

Martyn, P. A., Hansen, B. C., & Jen, K-L. C. (1984). The effects of parenteral nutrition on food intake and gastric motility. *Nursing Research, 33,* 336-337.

Metzger, B., & Schultz, S. (1982). Time series analysis: An alternative for nursing. *Nursing Research, 31,* 375-378.

Michael, J. (1974). Statistical inference for individual organism research: Some reactions to a suggestion by Gentile, Roden and Klein. *Journal of Applied Behavior Analysis, 7,* 627-628.

Mitchell, P. H., & Mauss, N. K. (1978). Relationship of patient-nurse activity to intracranial pressure variations: A pilot study. *Nursing Research, 27,* 4-10.

Mitchell, P. H., Amos, D., & Astley, C. (1986). Nursing and ICP: Two clinical studies. In J. D. Miller, G. M. Teasdale, J. D. Rowan, S. L. Galbraith, & A. D. Mendelon (Eds.). *Intracranial Pressure VI* (pp. 701-704). Berlin: Springer-Verlag.

Robinson, P. W., & Foster, D. F. (1979). *Experimental psychology: A small-N approach.* New York: Harper & Row.

Thoreson, C. E., & Elsahoff, J. D. (1974). An analysis of variance model for intrasubject replication design: Some additional comments. *Journal of Applied Behavior Analysis, 7,* 639-641.

Updike, P. A., Accurso, F. J., & Jones, R. H. (1985). Physiologic circadian rhythmicity in preterm infants. *Nursing Research, 34,* 160-163.

White, O. R. (1972). *A manual for the calculation and use of the median slope—a technique of progress estimation and prediction in the single case.* University of Oregon, Regional Resource Center for Handicapped Children, Eugene, OR.

White, O. R. (1974). *The "split-middle": A "quickie" method of trend estimation.* University of Washington, Experimental Education Unit. Child Development and Retardation Center, Seattle, WA.

13

DESIGNING
PRESCRIPTION-TESTING STUDIES

NANCY FUGATE WOODS

Nursing is a practice discipline, yet few contemporary nursing research reports focus on the effects of nursing practice on human health. Moreover, most of the nursing practice literature assesses the impact of a single procedure, process, or a specific therapeutic agent on health. Few published reports reflect the assessment of theoretically motivated systems of nursing care (Silva, 1986). During the past three decades, many nurse theorists have proposed conceptual models to guide nursing curricula and nursing practice, but validation of these models in practice settings lags far behind their development (Stevenson & Woods, 1986). The lag in empirical validation of prescriptive theory is attributable to several factors, including the broad orientation of the models and the difficulty in operationalizing them (Silva, 1986). Moreover, empirical validation of prescriptive theory requires commitment to complex and lengthy research pursuits. Programmatic research, involving multiple studies over a prolonged period of time, and innovative application of existing research designs are essential for the practical validation of prescriptive theory.

Diers (1978) proposed approaches for empirical validation of prescriptive theory. She suggested that evaluation research designs, because of their programmatic emphasis on assessing systems of care, could guide empirical testing of prescriptive theory, in particular the relationships between context, process, and outcomes. The clinical trial, long used in other health-science disciplines, provides another

important approach that investigators can use to test relationships between elements of prescriptive theory, specifically the relationship between therapy and outcome. This chapter includes a discussion of designs for clinical trials and for evaluation research. It concludes with proposals for extensions of the designs commonly used for clinical trials and evaluation research to stimulate testing of prescriptive theory.

AIMS OF PRESCRIPTIVE THEORY

The aims of *prescriptive theory* include controlling, promoting, and changing nursing phenomena. Essential elements of prescriptive theory, as proposed by Dickoff, James, and Wiedenbach (1968), include the aim or goal, prescriptions to bring about the desired goal, and a survey list. The goal specifies the purpose of the theory; the *survey list* specifies agency, patiency, framework, terminus, procedure, and dynamics. *Agency* is the person or group of people who perform the activity. Agency includes not only professionals but others who have the internal and external resources to perform the activity under study, including family members, visitors, and other professionals. *Patiency* is a theoretical construct specifying the recipients of the prescriptions, such as potential self-care agents. *Context,* labeled "framework" by Dickoff, James, and Wiedenbach (1968), includes all the variables that influence progress toward the goal, including sociopolitical and organizational realities. It includes but is not limited to the setting for care. *Terminus* is the product of the activity, and it reflects not only the outcomes of the procedures on health but also the effects on the cost of care, the caretakers, and the practices of other health professionals. Procedure includes steps that must be taken to achieve the goal. Finally, *dynamics* refers to motivating factors in performing and sustaining the activities that produce the goal, such as money or other reward systems in the organization.

In Dier's view (1978), prescriptive theory addresses systems of care. As defined by Diers, a "system of care" includes a "set of agents, doing work with patients, in a given sociopolitical context, using certain processes or procedures with certain sources of motivation or energy, toward measurable end points, all in the service of achieving some desired goal" (p. 203). Diers suggested that one way to view prescriptive theory is to compare it to a giant web in which the radii of the web are the elements of the theory, such as agency and patiency. Threads connecting the radii are the hypotheses about the relationships among various aspects of the theory. The entire web constitutes the theory, and the elements are interconnected and interdependent. Thus each element of the system affects every other element in complex ways (see Fig. 8-5).

TESTING PRESCRIPTIVE THEORY

Practice theory in nursing guides the delivery of nursing care. Prescriptive theory, a kind of practice theory, presupposes both normative theory, which conceptualizes the goal to be achieved, and scientific, empirically based theory, which explains how to achieve the goal. Practice theory is validated in natural, not artificial, settings, that is, the real settings in which nurses practice nursing.

Testing prescriptive theory requires its application in practice. The theory to be tested is the theory of the system of care, the prescription. The process begins with formulation of the goal and prescription, with the prescription often based on multiple theories. In a study of self-management training, Kogan and Betrus (1984) identified the goal in training as client self-regulation of behavior, cognitions, emotional responses, and physical signs associated with stress. The prescriptions included:

Self-monitoring or a self-observation period dur-

ing which the client is helped to identify the behavior to be measured and altered
Establishment of criteria by which success of the self-management program can be measured
Acquisition of self-awareness and discrimination of functioning levels based on feedback and documentation of changes in the behavior
Administration of self-reinforcement based on successful changes in behavior
Cognitive restructuring to link cognitive events to pathophysiological processes

To test prescriptive theory, the prescription is introduced theoretically and operationally defined; then its effect is measured and evaluated by how well the system of care is able to actualize the goal. Kogan and Betrus (1984) found that clients who participated in the management of stress-response protocol to teach self-management experienced significant improvement in symptoms, lower electromyograph (EMG) levels reflecting lower muscle tension, and increased skin temperature consistent with relaxation. Moreover, they retained the improved effects 6 months following treatment. A comparison of the results for the group that received the self-management training with other individuals who began the study at the same time but who received the training 8 weeks later (a delayed-treatment control group) revealed a different outcome. Although the treatment group experienced significant improvement, the delayed-treatment group experienced no significant changes during the control period.

The goal of testing prescriptive theory is to be able to generalize from a specific situation to a larger class of situations. Therefore, using research methods that permit inference to a reference population from a sample is essential. In addition to testing how well the prescriptions achieved the goals, investigators also need to test the coherency and feasibility aims of the theory. *Coherency* refers to the consistency between the theoretical specification of the prescription and its implementation. *Feasibility* is an assessment based on human and financial cost-benefit comparisons.

In the following sections we will consider designs for testing prescriptive theory. We will begin with a discussion of designs commonly used for clinical trials and evaluation research and conclude with proposals for application of these designs to test prescriptive theory.

Designing clinical trials

A *clinical trial* is a planned experiment involving participants, usually patients, for the purpose of determining the most appropriate therapy. The clinical trial is used in biomedical research to test the efficacy of a new therapeutic strategy, device, or intervention and is viewed as the principal method for obtaining reliable evaluation of treatment effects. The clinical trial does not refer to a single research design but instead to applications of a variety of experimental designs. Because the ability to generalize beyond the sample studied in the trial is important, single case or small sample experimental designs are not considered adequate clinical trials.

Clinical trials imply the experimental study of the comparison of effects of one therapeutic approach to another, usually standard care (Pocock, 1983). Although most biomedical clinical trials test the efficacy of new therapies for disease, often drugs, some trials are prophylactic or preventive in nature, such as field trials of such vaccines as the Salk vaccine for polio.

Elements of clinical trials

Essential elements of the clinical trial include specifying the purpose of the trial, designing the trial, implementing the trial, analyzing the data, and drawing conclusions about the results. We will discuss each of these in greater detail.

Specifying the purpose. Although the general purpose of the trial is to assess the effects of a therapeutic approach on some health outcome, specific hypotheses guide the trial. These hypotheses reflect the population to be studied, the therapeutic approach, end points for evaluating the outcomes, and the comparison or control group. With the exception of a comparison group, these elements resemble Diers' concepts (1978) of patiency, procedure, and terminus, respectively.

Designing the trial. The design of the trial is, by definition, an application of experimental design in which one group receives the therapeutic treatment being tested and another group receives standard care or a placebo. Unique to the clinical trial is the development of a very specific protocol, based on the theory and hypotheses about the therapeutic approach, that specifies how the therapeutic treatment should be administered. Another aspect of the protocol is the specification of procedures for selection and randomization of the participants into treat-

ment and control groups. The protocol also details whether the person administering the therapeutic treatment and the participant are aware of or not aware of (blinded to) the therapeutic treatment the participant is receiving. Finally, the protocol specifies the end point(s) for follow-up and measures to be taken before, during, and following the treatment.

The extensive detail of the protocol is essential to ensure the valid implementation of the trial during the sample selection phase and during each aspect of administering the therapeutic treatment. In instances involving the use of multiple sites or centers in the trial, a very specific statement of the protocol is essential.

Conducting the trial. Conducting the trial involves several essential processes that include obtaining participants, securing informed consent from the participants, dealing with violations of the protocol, accommodating withdrawal of participants, and monitoring interim results. Specific challenges encountered in each of these processes will be discussed in greater detail later in this chapter.

Analyzing the data. Data analysis includes both interim analyses conducted during the trial and hypothesis testing conducted after completion of the trial. Interim analyses are performed to detect untoward effects that would warrant stopping the trial, whereas hypothesis testing is conducted to determine the trial's final effects.

Drawing conclusions. Conclusions focus on the effectiveness of the therapeutic approach relative to the desired health outcomes compared to the standard care or placebo control group. They are based on the results of hypothesis testing with the goal of generalizing to the reference population for the sample studied.

Developing the protocol for clinical trials

A *study protocol* is a formal document specifying how the trial will be conducted. The protocol should contain detailed specifications of the trial procedure as it relates to each participant. A typical protocol contains background and specific aims for the trial, criteria for selection of participants, treatment schedules, methods of evaluation, the trial design, procedures for registration and randomization of participants, procedures for obtaining consent, sample size specifications, procedures for monitoring progress of the trial, procedures for handling data, protocol deviations and their management, plans for statistical analysis, and responsibilities of research staff. Each of these components will now be discussed in detail.

Background and specific aims. The background for the trial includes analysis of the theoretical and empirical work that guides the trial. In particular, specification of the nursing conceptual framework or model guiding the choice of therapeutic agent and the rationale for its predicted outcome are essential. Kogan and Betrus (1984) based their trial of self-management for stress response on the concepts of self-management, regulation, and disregulation. Self-management is a mode of nursing influence in which the locus of control rests with the client: self-assessment and self-awareness are emphasized; goals are negotiated between client and professional; client action produces change; knowledge is openly shared with the client; and feedback is essential to promoting change. Regulation implies a homeostatic state, and disregulation implies the breakdown of homeostatic or self-regulatory mechanisms. Kogan and Betrus justified their self-management approach on the basis of psychophysiological and cognitive-behavioral aspects of self-regulation and disregulation. They hypothesized that a self-management training program for individuals with stress-related disorders (including tension headache, chronic muscle tension, anxiety, insomnia, hypertension, and migraine) would produce a significant reduction in emotions, cognitions, behavior, and physiological signs associated with stress.

The specific aims of the Kogan and Betrus trial (1984) included determining effects of self-management training on the cost of stress, symptoms of stress, frontalis EMG, and peripheral skin temperature. The study also sought to determine retention of the effects of self-management training 6 months following treatment and to compare the results of individuals completing self-management training with those for individuals in the control group who were recipients of delayed treatment.

Selecting the participants. Selecting participants requires precise definition of those individuals who would be eligible for the trial. The goal of selection is to increase representativeness of the individuals who would be most likely to benefit from the therapeutic approach being tested. Therefore the selection criteria cannot be too restrictive. However, the researcher must avoid recruiting an atypical

group, such as an unusual group with respect to socioeconomic status or health. For example, medical centers associated with major universities tend to attract patients who are not representative of the universe of patients. Typical patients seen at university hospitals and clinics tend to be referred from other care providers and thus may have more advanced or unusual disease, or they may be socially advantaged or disadvantaged. For results to be relevant to practice needs, nursing clinical trials need to study typical populations of individuals requiring nursing services.

Usually the health phenomenon being studied is a central concern to the investigator in selecting inclusion criteria. Kogan and Betrus (1984) decided to include individuals who had certain stress-related disorders but who were without other major health problems. Exclusion criteria reflected factors that would confound treatment effects. For example, individuals who were being treated actively with medications for stress-related conditions would be excluded from the self-management trial. Often individuals, particularly those who are hospitalized, are receiving multiple types of treatment, including medications, surgery, and other therapies. Therefore investigators conducting nursing trials need to consider which concurrent or past treatments would make it impossible to discern the effects of the therapeutic approach being studied.

Treatment schedules. Most biomedical clinical trials involve assessment of drug therapy. Treatment schedules for these trials commonly deal with the drug route, dose, frequency of administration, duration of treatment, side effects, dose modifications and rules for withdrawal of patients from the trial, adherence to the treatment, influence of ancillary treatment, distribution and packaging of the drug, and provisions for adapting the drug regimen to the individual patient's needs (Pocock, 1983). Although not all these considerations apply to nondrug trials, many are relevant to the nursing therapeutic trial. In particular, the treatment schedule should specify the type, frequency, and duration of the therapy, anticipated untoward effects and procedures for their management, methods of facilitating client adherence to the trial, procedures for accounting for other ongoing therapies, and the extent to which the therapeutic program can be modified to fit the needs of the individual client. Fig. 13-1 includes a summary

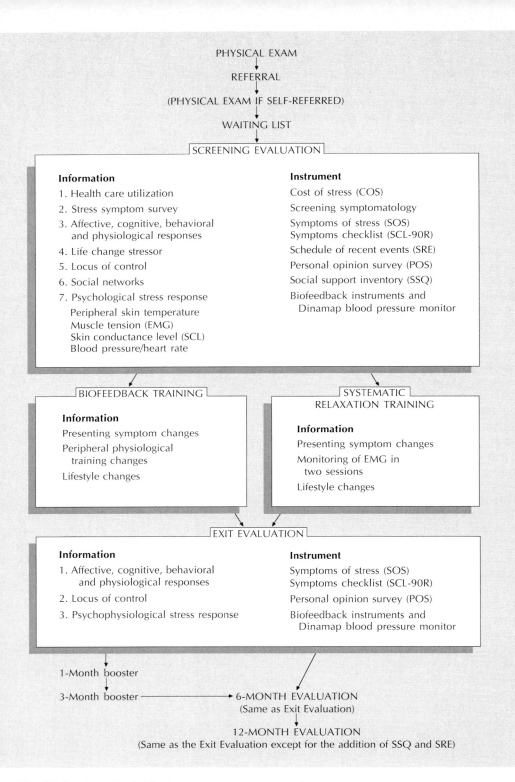

Fig. 13-1. Flow of activities in patients' management of stress response. (From Kogan, H., & Betrus, P. [1984]. *Advances in Nursing Science, 6* [4], 55-73. © 1984. Reprinted with permission of Aspen Publishers, Inc.)

of the treatment schedule used in the Kogan and Betrus study (1984) of self-management. A book-length manual provides detailed descriptions of the treatments and directions for their applications.

Yeaton and Sechrest (1981) advocate monitoring strength, integrity, and effectiveness for the duration of treatment. Strong treatment refers to treatment that is highly likely to have the intended outcome. Strength may be related to the amount and intensity of treatment, as well as to the strength of the theoretical links that can be made between treatment and outcome. Treatment that is too weak or too strong is wasteful and unacceptable. Decisions about complex therapy (treatments that include multiple elements) should take into account the problems associated with treatments that are too weak and thus ineffective or too strong and thus wasteful of resources. Identifying and using the weakest treatment that will work present significant challenges to researchers during the process of designing the protocol.

Integrity refers to the degree to which the treatment is delivered as it was intended. In field settings versus laboratory settings slippage may occur between the delivery of the treatment and the intent for its delivery. Data that monitor treatment variability are essential to assess the amount of variation between the intended and the actual treatment. Ease of administration facilitates delivery of the treatment as it was intended. Moreover, detection of errors in the delivery of the treatment permits correction during the conduct of the study. Degradability of the treatment, resulting in decreasing treatment effectiveness over time, is another problem that threatens the integrity of the treatment.

Effectiveness of treatment refers to the differences observed between the experimental and control groups or between the conditions and their success rates. Computing the proportion of successes and comparing the treatment results with norms for treatment effectiveness in terms of a similar problem and type of treatment provide the bases for assessing effectiveness of treatment. In addition, effectiveness can be evaluated by determining the extent of change necessary to solve problems or to achieve some standard, social validation of the utility of the treatment, assessment of cost-benefit ratios and risks associated with the treatment, and assessment of changes in response to the treatment over time.

Methods of evaluation. The investigator con-ducting a clinical trial specifies clearly the methods of evaluation of the therapeutic effect. The ideal methods produce accurate, objective, and consistent estimates of the outcome. Evaluation of the treatment requires the investigator to specify the procedures to be used for baseline assessment, primary criteria for response to the treatment, and other criteria important to achieve full evaluation. *Baseline assessment* refers to a description of the participant's initial status. Typically the baseline assessment includes a description of personal characteristics of the participants, such as age, gender, race, health-related characteristics, and prognostic factors that would influence the response to the trial. In the study by Kogan and Betrus (1984), extensive data were obtained from patients before they entered the trial, including patterns of health care, stress-related symptoms, affective, cognitive, behavioral, and physiological responses to stress, life-change stressors, locus of control, social-network composition, peripheral skin temperature, muscle tension, skin-conductance levels, blood pressure, and heart rate. As noted in Fig. 13-2, many of these same factors were used as indicators of treatment outcome at the completion of the trial and at 6 months and 12 months following completion of the therapy.

Specifying the criterion of response requires the investigator to indicate the most important outcome of the trial and its anticipated duration. Kogan and Betrus (1984) could have specified that either an increased sense of well-being, lowered blood pressure, decreased EMG level, or reduced stress was the most important outcome. Moreover, they could have indicated that effects at 6 or 12 months were the criteria for treatment success. Specification of the most important outcome is especially important when interim monitoring of trial results is ongoing. For instance, a new drug may cause symptoms to improve but may increase mortality. Thus it would be important for the investigator to identify the outcomes that would be most important to monitor, such as morbidity or mortality, and the time frame necessary to conclude that the treatment was effective.

Usually a researcher uses several outcome criteria for clinical trials. Although the emphasis is on efficacy of the therapeutic approach, its safety, side effects, and acceptability are also important concerns for the investigator. These criteria can be monitored routinely throughout the trial by using records of events, such as side effects or symptoms, kept by both the client and investigator.

Of paramount importance is the validity of the measures used to determine outcomes. Participants' reports, observations by the investigator, clinical assessments, and records can provide useful data about outcomes. Often using a blended approach to evaluation is helpful; the participant, treatment team members who actually provide the therapy, and the evaluators each contribute data. To prevent bias in measuring the outcomes an essential element of evaluation is that the evaluator remain unaware of the identity of the participant's treatment group throughout the study.

Frequency and duration of follow-up must reflect the study's purpose and the therapy's anticipated effects. Kogan and Betrus (1984) employed two follow-up periods, 6 and 12 months following the self-management training program.

Trial design: randomization. Random allocation of participants to treatment and control groups is an essential component of the controlled clinical trial. As with other experiments, the purpose of randomization is to prevent systematic bias that can lead to one treatment group receiving the most favorable conditions during the conduct of the trial. Random assignment of humans, particularly those with an illness, is not inherently appealing to clinicians. Indeed, any withholding of treatment is contrary to most clinicians' desire to give the best possible care to each of their clients.

Without randomization, however, obtaining valid assessment of treatment efficacy is difficult. Uncontrolled trials do not offer direct comparison with the standard therapeutic approach. Typically these trials start with less seriously ill individuals, exaggerate success, and omit reports of failure, thus giving a distorted view of the efficacy of the therapy. The laetrile studies illustrate problems associated with uncontrolled trials. When controlled trials were conducted, the drug proved ineffective despite popular claims to the contrary by those who had conducted uncontrolled trials (Pocock, 1983).

Use of *historical controls,* those individuals who have been treated with the standard treatment in the past, is also an inadequate alternative to randomization. Typically patient selection and the experimental environment are sources of bias. Patient selection bias occurs because the criteria for historical controls are likely to have been less clearly defined than the criteria for selection of participants in the trial of the new therapy being tested. Those individuals recruited previously were likely to be from different sources than the new volunteers and perhaps were also different types of patients. Also, the investigator is likely to be more restrictive in the selection of individuals for the new treatment than in the selection of individuals for the standard treatment. Probably the experimental environment also has changed over time, invalidating a comparison of the treatment and historical control groups. The quality of the recorded data for historical controls is probably poorer (less complete) than is the case for the newly recruited individuals. Criteria of response to treatment and other concurrent care may differ. Moreover, investigators are likely to invalidate more clients for participation in the trial of a new treatment than was the case for the historical controls. As a result of the bias of patient selection and changing experimental environment, studies with historical controls tend to exaggerate the value of the new treatment (Pocock, 1983).

Literature controls, participants from previously published studies, present some of the same problems with respect to patient selection and experimental environment as was the case for historical controls. Nonrandomized current controls, those individuals systematically or purposively assigned to the treatment or control group, also do not provide adequate control. Systematic assignment often results in the investigator knowing in advance which treatment the patient will get, thus tempting the investigator to exclude certain patients seen as vulnerable to side effects or to include patients seen as needy. Assignment of individuals in one clinical practice to the treatment group and individuals in another clinical practice to the control group is also ineffective because the experimental environment of the groups will differ. Purposive assignment also may result in the investigator assigning the favored treatment to the most seriously ill or needy patients.

Some question whether randomization is ethical. Pocock (1983) suggested that when the treatment is scarce, and when a reasonable possibility exists that the new treatment will be as good or better than the standard one, randomization is ethical. When not everyone can have access to the new treatment, randomization provides a nonbiased way of allocating the opportunity for the new treatment. However, it is controversial to conduct the trial after the treatment has become standard practice. When the new treatment has been accepted widely, it becomes standard treatment, and then patients must be deprived of it to test its effects. (For additional discussion, see Chapter 6.)

Trial design: blinding. In addition to randomization, *blinding* is an important component of designing clinical trials. Potential bias exists if everyone involved in a trial is aware of which treatment the participant is receiving. The patient is likely to perceive psychological benefit from being involved in the trial of a new therapeutic approach. Particularly with an experimental treatment, the treatment team is likely to modify the therapy if they are aware of the treatment the patient is receiving. Prior knowledge may cause the evaluator of the treatment outcome to be biased in ranking the outcome, probably favoring the new treatment. The goal of blinding is to make the conditions as similar as possible for both the treatment and control groups.

THE DOUBLE-BLIND TRIAL. In the *double-blind trial* neither the patients nor the persons responsible for care and evaluation of the trial outcome know which treatment the person is receiving. For drug trials, this anonymity is achieved with matched placebos that look like and mimic some of the side effects of the drug being tested. The assignment of the participants to the treatment group or the control group is unknown to the therapists and evaluators; instead, someone else keeps the randomization lists that identify each participant's corresponding treatment or control group assignment. A clinician who believes that blinded treatment is harmful to the patient because of side effects or failure to respond may break the code for that patient under these circumstances.

THE TRIPLE-BLIND TRIAL. Another strategy for blinding is the *triple-blind trial* in which the person interpreting the results of the trial and the therapist and evaluator are blind to the treatment group. Data analysts remain unaware of which is the treatment group and which the control group until after they have analyzed and interpreted the data.

Blinding is feasible under certain conditions such as drug trials in which it is possible to keep the patient, therapist, and evaluator unaware of the patient's assignment to a treatment or control group. Blinding both the participant and the therapist is not always practical, however. With surgery or an interpersonal intervention such as counseling, the partic-

ipant and the therapist know the nature of the therapy, although the evaluator can remain blind to the treatment. In these instances, using a no-treatment control group makes the assignment to either group obvious. Other control approaches, however, such as using a sham treatment, would enable the investigator to use blinding in such a trial. For example, clients receiving biofeedback training for self-management of stress could be assigned to one group that received accurate biofeedback or to a control group that received sham biofeedback. With this technique the same procedure is used, but the feedback to the control group is random and does not correspond to the actual level of the muscle tension or temperature parameter being measured. In this instance the client, therapist, and evaluator could all remain unaware of assignments to the study group. Because blinding helps avoid bias, it is useful even when the procedure must be compromised, such as by single-blinding the study so that only the participant is uninformed about the experimental or control status.

Of primary importance, blinding should produce no harm or undue risk to the patients who participate in the trial. Because it may involve deception of participants or withholding information from them, the technique of blinding raises important ethical issues regarding the protection of human subjects. When blinding is used, interim analyses that identify potentially hazardous conditions in either the treatment or control group become extremely important to safeguard the welfare of the participants.

THE CROSSOVER TRIAL. The *crossover trial* includes the same individuals in both the treatment and control groups in the same study. It offers an opportunity for within-person (ipsative) comparisons and is particularly useful for evaluating short-term outcomes, such as pain relief. Two or more treatments can be evaluated over separate and equal periods of time, providing evaluation of both treatments for each patient. The design for a crossover trial in which two treatments, A and B, are tested, is given below:

	TIME 1	TIME 2
Group 1	A	B
Group 2	B	A

Stability of the phenomenon and the cooperation of the participant are important issues to consider when weighing the possibility of using a crossover design. If the time for evaluating the treatment is too short, there will not be adequate time for the effects of treatment to appear. Insufficient opportunity for observing effects may produce spurious conclusions. Moreover, a carryover effect may exist with the effect of treatment A persisting during the period when treatment B is being evaluated. Carryover effect may be minimized through use of a withdrawal period (W) between A and B as follows:

	TIME 1		TIME 2
Group 1	A	W	B
Group 2	B	W	A

When the treatment time is too long, adherence to the protocol is likely to be inadequate, and a high proportion of participants will withdraw. Moreover, health may well be unstable over a long period of time, thereby producing spurious conclusions.

Data for a crossover trial are analyzed by using paired comparisons and assuming no time-effect and no time-treatment interaction. Use of paired tests is discussed in Chapter 26.

Registration and randomization. Registration and randomization are important aspects of implementing the clinical trial, and they require careful supervision. Registration involves recruiting appropriate, representative participants, checking their eligibility, obtaining agreement of the clinicians to allow randomization of trial participants, obtaining participants' consent, and formally entering them into the trial. It is important to identify formally those eligible individuals who consent to participate in the trial before randomization occurs. The necessity of obtaining consent to participate before randomization requires that individuals know they will be allocated to a treatment group, and they must agree to involvement in the study without knowledge of their randomization status. Otherwise, participants or clinicians may refuse to participate when they learn they are participants in the experimental or control group.

The randomization list is a record of consecutive random-treatment assignments maintained by a neutral person who neither treats the participants nor evaluates the treatment. The randomization list can be prepared in several ways. Simple randomization involves using random digits such as 0 to 9 and ruling that for two treatment groups, assignment to A group will be made if the number is 0 to 4 and assignment to B group will be made if the number is 5 to 9. Thus for the random sequence 1, 3, 7, 4, 5, 6 (obtained from a table of random numbers), the sequence for assignment would be A-A-B-A-B-B. A similar procedure can be used when there are more than two groups. Because having a similar or equal number of participants in each group is advantageous for certain data analysis approaches, it is useful to have a substitute randomization list prepared that can be used if the proportion of individuals assigned to one group is quite different from that assigned to another group under the conditions of the first randomization list. For example, under truly random conditions, it would be possible to assign 70% of the participants to the treatment group and 30% to the control group. Both the randomization list and its substitute are prepared and checked before randomization begins.

Another option that facilitates allocating equal numbers of participants to the treatment and control groups is the use of random permutated blocks so that a block of AB-BA-BA-AB is used as the randomization list. The first participants would be assigned to group A, the second to group B, the third to group B, the fourth to group A, and so forth. An approach such as this would ensure that equal numbers of participants are entered in both the treatment and control groups.

Obtaining consent from the participants. In the United States, written informed consent is required for participation in a clinical trial. Yet in other countries where attitudes about medical care and certain diseases differ, trials proceed without consent of the individual participants. The procedures for obtaining informed consent for participants and the guidelines for protecting the rights of human participants in research are detailed in Chapter 6.

One difficulty that may occur with clinical trials is that individuals may not consent to being assigned randomly to treatment or control groups. Zelen (1979) offered an alternative design called the "randomized consent design." Individuals are randomly assigned to two groups: group 1 consents to receive the standard treatment, A1, and is not asked for consent to participate in the experimental treatment, B. Group 2 is asked to consent to participate in treatment B, the new treatment. Those who accept are given treatment B, and those who decline receive the standard treatment, A2. Analysis of the results compares all three groups. With this approach one com-

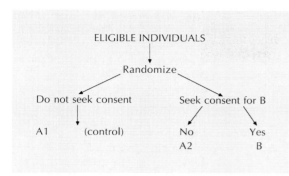

ELIGIBLE INDIVIDUALS

Randomize

Do not seek consent   Seek consent for B

A1   (control)   No   Yes
                                 A2   B

Fig. 13-2. Randomized consent design.

pares the policy of offering participants the opportunity of receiving the new treatment (A1 versus A2 and B) with the policy of giving everyone the standard treatment (A1 and A2 versus B) (Figure 13-2.).

Estimating sample size. Sample size estimation for the clinical trial and other study designs is discussed in Chapter 7. The danger of small trials is that type II error, the likelihood of missing small effects, will occur. Thus an effective therapeutic approach may be concluded to be ineffective when only a small number of individuals are studied.

In estimating the sample size for a clinical trial, several important considerations include:

The main purpose of the trial

The principal outcome measure and its reliability

Data analysis procedures to be used to detect treatment-effect differences

Type of results anticipated, including the anticipated size of the treatment effect and the degree of certainty with which the effect can be anticipated

When the purpose of the trial is testing a life-threatening or life-saving intervention, the results need to be compelling to support adoption of a new treatment. This situation requires statistically significant results and a large effect from the new treatment. A large sample size maximizes the likelihood of detecting significant effects. When the outcome measure is highly reliable and the effect size is anticipated to be large, the sample size can be smaller than when the outcome measure is unreliable and the effect size is small (Chapter 7). Finally, the sample size depends on the analytical strategy and the number of participants needed to make valid use of the statistical test.

The investigator also considers the accrual rate and the time period required for recruiting the participants. Often the ability to obtain participants is a limiting factor in achieving the desired sample size, and it may be necessary to secure additional sites for recruitment of participants.

Monitoring trial progress. During the conduct of a clinical trial, it is essential that someone who is not involved as a therapist, evaluator, or investigator monitor progress of the trial to determine effects of randomization, differential dropout rates from the treatment and control groups, protocol adherence, the presence of adverse effects, adequacy of data processing, and interim analysis of treatment effects. Randomization enhances the likelihood that treatment and control groups will be equivalent. Nevertheless, careful monitoring of the effects of randomization is essential to ensure the comparability of treatment and control groups. Moreover, once the trial has begun, it is essential to monitor dropout rates and reasons for dropouts. When differences in rates occur across the treatment and control groups, it is essential to assess whether the reasons for dropouts are similar across groups, such as occurs with a higher proportion of untoward effects in one group.

Monitoring adherence to the protocol on the part of therapists and clients is essential to ensure that the treatment is provided by the therapists as intended and that clients participate as intended. Investigators can monitor application of the treatment through videotaped or audiotaped sessions or client records.

Some trials involve the use of therapies that, when tested, have unanticipated hazardous effects. Others use new therapies that have dramatic positive effects, making the treatment of the control group with the standard therapies unacceptable.

Interim analysis is necessary for the trial to be ethically acceptable. Analysis of interim outcomes is important to determine if it is necessary to stop the trial. Guidelines for discontinuing a trial (a stopping rule) need to be established before the trial begins to ensure that no hazardous complications or outcomes, such as a disproportionate number of deaths in one group, will be allowed to continue. Usually, interim analysis is not as elaborate as the final data analysis but is directed toward detecting unanticipated effects that compromise the well-being of the participants. Unless the trial is stopped, the interim results are kept confidential to ensure the successful completion of the trial as planned.

Data handling and management. Data management for clinical trials requires procedures similar to those discussed in Chapter 24. Data handling and management must proceed throughout the trial to support interim analysis.

Protocol deviations. No matter how well-planned the trial, some participants' requirements will deviate from the protocol. Moreover, protocol violations will occur if the participants or the investigators fail to follow the procedure. Avoiding protocol deviations reduces the likelihood of biasing the therapeutic comparisons and can be accomplished by minimizing inclusion of ineligible participants, promoting adherence, and, failing these, clearly identifying each protocol violation. Minimizing the number of ineligible participants occurs through careful eligibility checks at the outset of the trial, following all individuals throughout the trial, and including in the analysis those with and without protocol violations. Nonadherence can be reduced through support for the participants, such as teaching about the protocol, reinforcing their efforts, and ceasing or modifying the therapeutic treatment, when necessary. Providing supplies such as recording forms for the participants facilitates their adherence to the protocol. When the data are collected, investigators carefully consider the results, taking into account those individuals who withdrew from the trial, those for whom the evaluation was incomplete, those who did not adhere completely to the protocol, and those who were eliminated because of clinical judgment. Omitting any of these groups from the analysis would probably bias the estimation of the therapeutic effect. Data analysis would include all groups of participants, those who withdrew, those for whom the evaluation was incomplete, those who did not adhere, and those who were eliminated; results obtained for the total sample would be compared to those that would have been obtained had each group been included.

Analysis plan. The analysis plan for a clinical trial is designed to test whether the new therapeutic treatment is significantly better than the standard one. Usually, it is not quite so simple. The typical major clinical trial contains multiple treatments, multiple end points, and several repeated measures. In addi-

tion, the data usually support analysis of differential effects across specific groups of participants, such as across age-groups; other risk factors that affect the outcome of the trial also should be considered in the analysis.

When the goal is to determine that the new therapeutic treatment is similar to the standard one, that is, they are equally effective, the analytical strategy differs from traditional tests of difference. An alternative to the t test, analysis of variance, or analysis of covariance involves specifying the overall percentage of successes the investigator anticipates as the basis for comparing the effectiveness of both treatments. Pocock (1983) describes this procedure in detail.

Using clinical trials to test prescriptive theory

The elements of prescriptive theory and corresponding components of clinical trials are compared in Table 13-1. The primary emphasis of a clinical trial is evaluation of the influence of the procedure (treatment) for a designated patiency (patient group) on the terminus (outcome). Agency corresponds to the therapist's role in the conduct of the protocol. Typically, agency is restricted to the professional, not to the family or other nonprofessionals in traditional clinical trials. Patiency is described usually in the participants' eligibility criteria listed explicitly in the protocol. Procedure is described in the section of the protocol that specifies elements of treatment. Finally, terminus is contained in the description of the treatment outcomes, that is, the dependent variables in the trial. Two elements of prescriptive theory that are

TABLE 13-1. Elements of prescriptive theory and corresponding components of clinical trials

PRESCRIPTIVE THEORY	CLINICAL TRIAL
Framework*	—
Agency	Therapist's role in administering the treatment
Patiency	Target population specified in eligibility criteria
Procedure	Treatment specified in the protocol
Dynamics*	—
Terminus	Outcome, dependent variable

*This element not addressed in clinical trials.

not addressed in the clinical trial are framework and dynamics.

Jacobsen and Meininger (1986) found that the clinical trials published in the nursing literature fell short of the criteria for such trials in other disciplines. Absence of justification of sample size, specific description of the methods used to allocate participants to groups, demonstration of pretreatment equivalence of groups, and explanation for withdrawal from the trials according to group assignment compromised the validity of conclusions from these trials. Unless these problems are corrected in the nursing literature, the contribution of the clinical trial to testing prescriptive theory will be limited.

Evaluation research

Although not designed to test relationships between all the elements of prescriptive theory as Diers (1978) defines it, evaluation research strategies and designs can contribute to testing elements of prescriptive theory. Evaluation research refers to studies in which a comparison is made to some standard of acceptability. The aim of evaluation research is to determine the ability of an intervention, such as a system of care, to achieve the intended effect.

Evaluation can be formative or summative in nature. *Formative evaluation* refers to the measurements and judgments that are made before or during implementation of an intervention to control, ensure, or improve the quality of the performance or delivery of the intervention. *Summative evaluation* refers to measurements and judgments that permit conclusions about the effects of a program. Both types of evaluation are significant in the testing of prescriptive theory.

Formative evaluation

An early step in testing prescriptive theory is implementing the prescription for the therapy. Formative evaluation informs the investigator about the delivery of the therapeutic approach being tested. Evaluation of implementation includes assessment of the integrity with which the therapeutic program is delivered, the response within the sites in which it is being tested, the response of participants in the therapeutic program, the response of clinicians implementing the program, and the competencies of the clinicians to deliver the program (Green & Lewis, 1986).

Integrity of the program. Evaluation studies, in contrast to clinical trials, require specification of a

standard against which the outcomes can be assessed. The standard relates to the quality of the program, that is, to the appropriateness of the intervention as it is performed in relation to the goals of the program. Quality is not determined by outcomes of the program but by assessment of the extent to which the standards previously established are met. The statement of standards is essential to determine the extent to which the intervention has been implemented (Green & Lewis, 1986).

Site response. Green and Lewis (1986) stipulate the importance of assessing responses in the sites in which health education programs are being tested. They suggest evaluating both supportive and nonsupportive responses of the staff of participating agencies and of consumers, community members, and professional groups.

Participant response. Green and Lewis (1986) also recommend assessing three aspects of participant response: progression through the program, quality of the progression, and satisfaction with the program. Progression is indicated by the numbers of participants entering and completing the program and reasons for attrition among those leaving the program. Quality of progression can be assessed by multiple performance measures including perceptions, behavior, skills, attitudes, perceptions about the experience, the meaning for the participant, and the participant's emotional response. Green and Lewis recommend using these assessments diagnostically to enhance the health education program. Similar application can be made to other nursing therapeutic programs. The assessment of recipient response is analogous to the manipulation check in an experiment. Through the use of focus groups of eight to ten people who are asked to discuss the program and their responses to it investigators can obtain qualitative feedback about the program.

Clinician response and competence. The clinicians implementing the therapeutic program can also contribute to the refinement of the program through identification of its strengths and weaknesses. The competency of the clinicians in delivering the intervention is critical and is assessed as a component of formative evaluation.

Summative evaluation

In contrast to formative evaluation, summative evaluation is concerned with the influence of the therapeutic program on the outcomes central to the study. These may include the immediate or long-term effects of the therapeutic program. Often multiple effects occur in nursing trials. For example, the Kogan and Betrus (1984) study of self-management for stress response included immediate outcomes of change in self-monitoring of symptoms, intermediate outcomes of learning relaxation through systematic relaxation or biofeedback techniques, and long-term outcomes such as reduced morbidity and mortality. Summative evaluation focuses on assessment of the effects of an intervention.

The structure-process-outcome model. The structure-process-outcome (SPO) model has been used for several decades to guide evaluation research in delivery of health services (Bloch, 1975; Donabedian, 1966; Suchman, 1967; Weiss, 1972). The model's three primary elements are structure, process, and outcome. Structure refers to the setting or system for care and to the attributes of the providers. It may include the physical structure for delivery of services, such as geographical proximity, or the social structure, such as the nature of the relationship between providers of care in the setting. Process refers to the care itself and how it is provided. Process might include particular approaches to assessment, intervention, and evaluation—elements of the nursing process. Outcome focuses on the client or patient and encompasses the range from mortality to high-level wellness. Although outcome traditionally has included measures of health status, Bloch (1975) pointed out the importance of including additional parameters such as cognitive outcomes (knowledge about health), psychosocial outcomes (attitudes toward care and participation in therapy), and behavioral outcomes (health-related behaviors). Bloch proposed that the SPO model could be modified to promote evaluation of nursing care in terms of structure, process, and outcome, making an analogy between structure and the nature of care providers and their environment, between process and nursing care, and between outcome and status of the care recipient.

The SPO model guides evaluation of nursing therapies, but it does not correspond to each element in Diers' concept (1978) of prescriptive theory. Structure in the SPO model is analogous to some aspects of Diers' use of framework in the sense that it includes information about the physical and social context in which care is provided. Framework, as Diers used it, is a more encompassing concept that includes all the variables that influence progress toward the goal. Moreover, structure contributes to the understanding of agency through emphasis on characteristics of providers of care. Agency, as Diers defined it, differs from the use of structure in evaluation research in that agency includes all those who have the resources to perform the care activity, such as family members. Process reflects the concepts of procedure and, to some extent, dynamics as Diers described them. Outcome reflects the element of terminus, the desired product of the caring activity.

The context-input-process-product model. Another model combining elements of formative and summative evaluation is the context-input-process-product (CIPP) model. Stufflebean (1973) advanced the CIPP model for judging decision alternatives regarding programs. Context evaluation defines the environment in which the program will operate, both the actual and desired conditions. Observation, interview, and archival data provide the basis for context evaluation.

Input evaluation involves assessing relevant capabilities of those involved in the program, strategies for achieving objectives, and ways of implementing the strategies. Typically the context and input evaluation begin before the program starts. Process evaluation is formative evaluation and, as such, provides feedback data to guide program modifications before implementation. Product evaluation measures program achievements.

Context in the CIPP model is analogous to framework in prescriptive theory, although Stufflebean's use of context (1973) is restricted to focusing on a need for the program in a particular environment. Input evaluation also relates to the concept of framework but is more inclusive, implying consideration for agency and dynamics as well. Process evaluation reflects dynamics, those factors that motivate and sustain efforts toward goal attainment and procedure. Product evaluation is analogous to terminus. Patiency is not considered explicitly in the CIPP model, although it might be construed to be part of context (Table 13-2).

Designs used in evaluation research

Green and Lewis (1986) recommend using a true experimental design for evaluation research. They suggest that, at minimum, the design should have at least five components: (1) representative samples, (2) one or more pretests, (3) a comparison group not exposed to the program being assessed, (4) random assignment of participants to the treatment and con-

TABLE 13-2. Elements of prescriptive theory and corresponding components of the SPO and CIPP models for evaluation research

PRESCRIPTIVE THEORY	CIPP MODEL	SPO MODEL
Framework	Context, input	Structure
Agency	Input	Structure
Patiency*	—	—
Dynamics	Input, process	Process
Procedure	Process	Process
Terminus	Product	Outcome

*This element of presciptive theory not specifically addressed in CIPP and SPO models.

trol groups, and (5) one or more posttests.

To maximize internal validity of evaluation studies, Green and Lewis (1986) recommend the following hierarchy of designs:

   True experimental design to include the five elements listed previously
   Experimental design in a convenience sample
   Experimental design with no pretests
   Experimental design in a convenience sample with no pretest
   Quasiexperimental design with matched comparison groups rather than random assignment to obtain a true control group
   Quasiexperimental design with matched comparison group without pretests
   Quasiexperimental design with pretest but no control group
   Quasiexperimental design in a convenience sample with pretest but no control group
   Quasiexperimental design with no pretests and no control group
   Quasiexperimental design in a convenience sample with no pretests and no control group

In addition, Green and Lewis (1986) recommend the following design hierarchy to maximize external validity:

   True experimental design with the five elements identified previously: representative samples, one or more pretests, a comparison group not exposed to the program being assessed, random assignment of participants to the treatment and control groups, and one or more posttests
   Experimental design with no pretests
   Quasiexperimental design with matched control groups

   Pretest-posttest design with no control group
   Quasiexperimental design with no pretest and no control group
   The designs described previously without representative samples of patients or target populations

TESTING PRESCRIPTIVE THEORY: PROPOSED STRATEGIES

As we have seen, clinical trials and evaluation research models alone are not adequate for testing prescriptive theory. Although the clinical trial and the CIPP model for evaluation research each highlight certain elements of prescriptive theory, none completely reflects the intent of prescriptive theory as Diers (1978) would operationally define it. Not only does a definitional mismatch exist between concepts and design elements as seen in Tables 13-1 and 13-2, but also the relationships tested commonly are causal and directional, unlike the weblike configuration of prescriptive theory proposed by Diers (see Fig. 8-5). Our analysis of clinical trials and models of evaluation research suggests that no single approach is adequate to test prescriptive theory. Instead, we propose several general strategies that incorporate elements of clinical trials and evaluation research, augmenting them with other research designs in a programmatic effort to test prescriptive theory. We advance the following approaches for consideration: specifying models that reflect the complexity inherent in theoretically based systems of nursing care, employing multiple designs to test relationships between the elements of prescriptive theory, and using multiple measures and data sources.

Models of theoretically based nursing-care systems

Models of theoretically based nursing-care systems must reflect the complex nature of nursing care. Typically, a nursing therapy is multifaceted, such as that described by Kogan and Betrus (1984). Nurses in the program for management of stress response applied either biofeedback or systematic relaxation training and counseling about lifestyle changes throughout the therapeutic encounters. Not unlike many other systems of nursing care, the management of stress-response protocols included physiological and interpersonal therapeutic agents. The effects of therapies such as biofeedback, which focuses on producing changes in a physiological parameter, were tested along with the effects of interpersonal relationships. Indeed, even in studies of physical therapies, the effects of caring interpersonal processes occur. These caring effects are often ignored or labeled as "placebo effects." Not only are the therapies themselves complex but their outcomes also are complex. Just as the management of stress-response protocol involved several therapies, it also included several outcome measures. Some of these were immediate and some were not observable until many years after the completion of the nursing-care program. The stress-management protocol included measurements over several occasions. Immediate effects included the individual client's altered physiological response produced by biofeedback or systematic relaxation. Intermediate effects involved the changes in mood and symptoms that were produced by stress. Changes in lifestyle to reduce stress constituted long-term outcomes that may have occurred after completion of the program. Because the investigator expects multidimensional therapies to produce multidimensional responses that occur within different time periods, it is necessary to include multiple-graded outcome measures that are repeated over many occasions.

Multiple designs

To test relationships between elements of prescriptive theory as illustrated in Fig. 8-5, investigators need multiple-design options. As we noted earlier in this chapter, the clinical trial is particularly well-suited to test relationships between therapies (procedure) and outcomes (terminus) for a designated population (patiency). Approaches to evaluation research, such as those guided by the CIPP model, extend the clinical trial to permit assessment of relationships between context, agency, procedure, and terminus for a designated population (patiency). Additional designs can be used to complement the contributions that result from application of clinical trials and designs for evaluation research to permit assessment of the relationships not otherwise addressed.

Testing prescriptive theory requires careful description of the concepts that are part of the theory and testing of relationships between concepts. Although it should be possible to hypothesize relationships between therapy and outcomes, some elements in Diers' web of prescriptive theory (1978) may require careful qualitative or quantitative description. Moreover, some of the relationships between elements cannot be predicted before the study but instead require careful description and exploration. Description in the tradition of ethnography or grounded theory may be particularly important for characterizing the framework or context for the theory and dynamics, two components of prescriptive theory that cannot be addressed typically with clinical trials and designs for evaluation research. Case study designs that permit intensive description of phenomena and relationships between elements of prescriptive theory, such as between framework and dynamics, may be particularly useful complements to the clinical trial or evaluation study design. In addition, intensive understanding of the complex relationships between agency, patiency, procedure, and terminus can be achieved through application of the small sample experimental design in which a variation of the aforementioned elements can be tested within a single individual or among a few individuals. Indeed, a comparative case study, in which multiple cases can be selected for their ability to serve as exemplars, may be particularly informative (Schultz & Kerr, 1986).

Multiple measures and data sources

Another strategy for complementing traditional applications of clinical trials and designs for evaluation research involves the use of multiple measures and data sources. Their use within a single study is termed *triangulation*, a word derived from navigation referring to a strategy of taking multiple reference points to locate an unknown position accurately (Campbell & Fiske, 1959; Denzin, 1970). Although the four types of triangulation include triangulation of multiple investigators, theories, data sources, and methods, the two types of triangulation most relevant to testing prescriptive theory are triangulation of data and methods.

Triangulation of data from different persons at various times and places, retrospectively and concurrently, are possible approaches to complement traditional evaluation research designs and clinical trials. To comprehend the relationship between framework, agency, patiency, and procedure, an investigator might use several approaches to study stress-mediated health problems: gathering observations from the client seeking help, family members, and nurses; repeating the observations under differing circumstances, such as at home, at work, and in the clinic; and following the client's progress over a period of years. Using multiple data sources over several occasions of measurement and under different circumstances could clarify the relationships such as those between framework, agency, patiency, and procedure. For example, the investigator might find that when the stress-management strategy was applied at home, the family members assumed more responsibility for agency than did the client, and the procedure was modified to accommodate these changes in responsibility. The investigator also might find that one procedure was tested in the context of the clinic, but another procedure was being tested in the context of the client's home and family. These differences might have occurred largely because of alternative models of agency and patiency held by the client and family members.

In addition to using triangulation of data sources, the investigator also could include triangulation of methods. Triangulation of methods might include use of qualitative and quantitative methods or a combination of interview, questionnaire, observation of performance, archival retrieval, and observation of physical evidence.

In particular, qualitative measures can be used in conjunction with quantitative measures to:

Develop and delineate elements of the prescription before its implementation

Assess implementation of therapeutic programs and their strength

Document actual versus intended effects of the prescriptions

Describe how, why, and under what conditions the prescription achieves (or does not achieve) intended outcomes

Generate theory to extend understanding of the dynamics of the prescription

Document effectiveness of prescriptions with broad aims that cannot be captured with existing measures

The use of multiple indicators of a construct is consistent with the use of multiple indicators to test causal models as discussed in greater detail in Chapter 14.

It is also possible to triangulate within and between methods. Triangulation within methods would be exemplified by use of several scales to measure anxiety within the same interview. Because all scales would be administered by interview, the approach would be considered triangulation within the interview method. Triangulation between methods would involve obtaining data by using more than one method. For example, the investigator would obtain data about the same concept through a combination of interview and observation rather than interview alone. A holistic design described by Jick (1979) involved triangulation both within and between methods.

Triangulation within methods is exemplified in the Kogan and Betrus study (1984) of stress management through their use of multiple indicators of the concept of stress, the symptoms of stress (SOS) questionnaire, and the symptoms checklist 90 (SCL-90). Between-method triangulation is also used in the same study. In addition to paper-and-pencil measures such as the SOS questionnaire and the SCL-90, the investigators have incorporated several physical indicators of stress response such as electromyography and skin conductance levels. All measures were repeated over several occasions. Moreover, both clinician and client ratings were obtained for certain measures.

SUMMARY

Use of multiple designs and triangulation of methods and data sources complement clinical trials and evaluation research designs for investigators attempting to test prescriptive theory. What is obvious is that no single existing design is adequate to test prescriptive theory in the way that Dickoff, James, and Wiedenbach (1968) and Diers (1978) conceived of it. Inherent in the challenge of testing prescriptive theory is the necessity for using a complex of multiple designs and methods, probably over a prolonged period of time. Testing prescriptive theory requires the commitment to a program of research, a complex of studies that, taken as a whole, inform the profession about the system of nursing care. Why? The nature of the research must parallel the complexity inherent in systems of contemporary nursing practice.

REFERENCES

Argyris, C., & Schon, D. (1976). *Theory in practice: Professional effectiveness.* San Francisco: Jossey Bass.

Berg, D., & Smith, K. (1985). The clinical demands of research methods. In D. Berg & K. Smith (Eds.). *Exploring clinical methods for social research* (pp. 21-34). Beverly Hills, CA: Sage.

Bloch, D. (1975). Evaluation of nursing care in terms of process and outcome: Issues in research and quality assurance. *Nursing Research, 24,* 256-263.

Bloch, D. (1980). Interrelated issues in evaluation and evaluation research: A researcher's perspective. *Nursing Research, 29,* 69-73.

Cammann, C. (1985). Action usable knowledge. In D. Berg & K. Smith (Eds.), *Exploring clinical methods for social research* (pp. 109-122). Beverly Hills, CA: Sage.

Campbell, D., & Fiske, D. (1959, March). Convergent and discriminant validation by the multitrait-multimethod matrix. *Psychological Bulletin, 56,* 81-105.

Chalmers, T., Smith, H., Blackburn, B., Silverman, B., Schroeder, B., Reitman, D., & Ambroz, A. (1981). A method for assessing quality of randomly controlled trials. *Controlled clinical trials, 2,* 31-49.

Chinn, P., & Jacobs, M. (1987). *Theory and nursing: A systematic approach,* (2nd ed.). St. Louis: Mosby.

Cook, T., & Reichardt, C. (1979). *Qualitative and quantitative methods in evaluation research.* Beverly Hills, CA: Sage.

Denzin, N. (1970). Strategies of multiple triangulation. In N. Denzin (Ed.). *The research act* (pp. 297-313). New York: McGraw-Hill.

Dickoff, J., James, P., & Wiedenbach, E. (1968). Theory in a practice discipline. *Nursing Research, 17,* 415-435, 545-554.

Diers, D. (1978). *Research in nursing practice.* Philadelphia: Lippincott.

Donabedian, A. (1966). Evaluating the quality of medical care. *Millbank Memorial Fund Quarterly, 44,* 166-206.

Feinstein, A. (1978). The scientific and clinical tribulations of randomized clinical trials. *Clinical Research, 26,* 241-244.

Green, L., & Lewis, F. (1986). *Measurement and evaluation in health education and health promotion.* Palo Alto, CA: Mayfield.

Hill, A. (1981). *Principles of medical statistics.* London: Lancet.

Huberman, A., & Miles, M. (1985). Assessing local causality in qualitative research. In D. Berg & K. Smith (Eds.), *Exploring clinical methods for social research* (pp. 351-380). Beverly Hills, CA: Sage.

Jacobsen, B., & Meininger, J. (1986). Randomized experiments in nursing: The quality of reporting. *Nursing Research, 35,* 379-382.

Jick, T. (1979). Mixing qualitative and quantitative methods: Triangulation in action. *Administrative Sciences Quarterly, 24,* 602-611.

Kogan, H., & Betrus, P. (1984). Self management: A nursing mode of therapeutic influence. *Advances in Nursing Science, 6* (4), 55-73.

Lowman, R. (1985). What is clinical method? In D. Berg & K. Smith (Eds.), *Exploring clinical methods for social research* (pp. 173-190). Beverly Hills, CA: Sage.

Meinert, C. (1986). *Clinical trials: Design, conduct, and analysis.* New York: Oxford.

Meleis, A. (1985). *Theoretical nursing: Development and progress.* Philadelphia: Lippincott.

Mitchell, E. (1986). Multiple triangulation: A methodology for nursing science. *Advances in Nursing Science, 8* (3),18-26.

Pocock, S. (1983). *Clinical trials: A practical approach.* New York: Wiley.

Schultz, P., & Kerr, B. (1986). Comparative case study as a strategy for nursing research. In P. Chinn, (Ed.). *Nursing research methodology: Issues and implementation* (pp. 195-220). Rockville, MD: Aspen.

Shapiro, S. (1983). *Clinical trials: Issues and approaches.* New York: Dekker.

Silva, M. (1986). Research testing nursing theory: State of the art. *Advances in Nursing Science, 9* (1), 1-11.

Stevenson, J., & Woods, N. (1986). Nursing science and contemporary science: Emerging paradigms. In American Academy of Nursing (Ed.). *Setting the agenda for the year 2000: Knowledge development in nursing.* Kansas City: Author.

Stufflebeam et al. (1971). *Educational evaluation and decision making.* Itasca, IL: Peacock.

Suchman, E. (1967). *Evaluative research: principles and practice in public service and social action programs.* New York: Russell Sage Foundation.

Thomson, M., & Kramer, M. (1984). Methodologic standards for controlled clinical trials of early contact and maternal-infant behavior. *Pediatrics, 73* (3), 294-300.

Weiss, C. (1972). *Evaluation research: Methods of assessing program effectiveness.* Englewood Cliffs, NJ: Prentice-Hall.

Wooldridge, P., Leonard, R., & Skipper, J. (1978). *Methods of clinical experimentation to improve patient care.* St. Louis: Mosby.

Yeaton, W., & Sechrest, L. (1981). Critical dimensions in the choice and maintenance of successful treatments: Strength, integrity, and effectiveness. *Journal of Consulting and Clinical Psychology, 49* (2), 156-167.

Zelen, M. (1979). A new design for randomized clinical trials. *New England Journal of Medicine, 300,* 1242-1245.

MEASUREMENT AND DATA PRODUCTION

14

MEASURING THE PHENOMENON

NANCY FUGATE WOODS

Once investigators have identified the research problem, analyzed existing knowledge about the problem, and specified a conceptual framework and purpose for the study, they confront the task of translating their abstract ideas about the problem into a plan for the study. Selecting the most appropriate design for the study, designing the sampling plan, and choosing appropriate measures of the phenomena are critical elements of this process. Measurement decisions, like design and sampling decisions, constitute important transition points from the conceptual to the empirical phase of research. Determining which indicators of the concepts will be of central importance to the study, that is, the way in which concepts will be measured directly influences the validity of the empirical findings and ultimately the validity of the theory under development. Unless the measures validly reflect the concepts that constitute the theory, conclusions drawn from the empirical phase of the research study will be invalid and will not advance the development of nursing theory.

In this and the following chapter we will consider several issues related to measurement. We will begin with an introduction to measuring nursing phenomena and then consider general measurement principles, characteristics of ideal measuring instruments, sources of variation in measurement results, and methods to cope with potential threats to valid measurement. Finally we will address two processes, one or the other of which nursing investigators consider in every study: choosing an instrument and developing a measurement instrument.

MEASUREMENT PRINCIPLES IN NURSING RESEARCH

Sources and types of information in nursing studies

In conducting nursing research, investigators measure many types of phenomena. To achieve an understanding of human responses in health and illness, nurses study people's thoughts, feelings, attitudes, experiences, sensations, skills, behaviors, and physiological functions. For example, Shannahan and Cottrell (1985) needed to measure maternal blood loss for a study of the effects of using the birth chair on second-stage labor, fetal outcomes, and maternal blood loss. They used the difference between admission and postdelivery hemoglobin and hematocrit as a measure of maternal blood loss. Lowery and Jacobsen (1985), investigating people's causal attributions for success or failure outcomes in chronic illness, used two questions as measures of causal attributions: "Why do you think things have been going well?" and "Why do you think you're having problems?" Lowery and Jacobsen, concerned about quality of life for people living with arthritis, used three indicators of quality of life, including two scales measuring life satisfaction and a single question that required a rating from the participant on the overall quality of life.

Because nurse researchers study a variety of phenomena, they use several different approaches to measurement, including norm-referenced and criterion-referenced approaches. *Norm-referenced measurement approaches* permit meaning to be assigned to scores through comparing one participant's performance to the performance of others, that is, through reference to a group norm. Norm-referenced measures are appropriate when the investigator is interested in evaluating the performance of an individual relative to other individuals in a group. Standardized tests are one type of norm-referenced measure. *Criterion-referenced measures* allow the investigator to determine whether the participant has reached a certain specific performance criterion or has mastered a specific task. Criterion-referenced testing is appropriate for determining whether or not an individual has acquired a set of behaviors. How well the individual performs when compared to others is irrelevant in this approach. Instead, whether or not the individual meets the specified criterion is important, and a criterion-referenced score is directly interpretable without reference to group norms.

In addition to using both norm-referenced and criterion-referenced measurement approaches, an investigator uses several sources of information in measuring nursing phenomena. An individual can be a data source for information ranging from physiological functioning to thoughts and feelings. Other information sources can be family members, health professionals, and other individuals who can provide information about the person's observable behavior. Archives such as written records can be used as sources of information. As one might anticipate, information obtained directly from the participant and that obtained from other sources provides the investigator with different types of data. For example, only the person with the illness can tell another person the concerns he or she has about an illness. Other family members can report what they believe are the patient's concerns, but evidence indicates that people do not always disclose concerns to other family members (Germino, 1984). On the other hand, family members could be accurate observers of certain behaviors such as smoking, eating, or adhering to a medication regimen. Considering the type of phenomenon being measured in relation to the type of information desired for the study is important when specifying the source of information for the study.

Types of concepts

In most nursing studies, investigators measure variables that are judged to represent the concepts central to the study. *Concepts* are abstractions, thoughts, notions, or ideas (Chapter 2). In the context of nursing science, most concepts relate to nursing, humankind, health, and the environment (Fawcett & Downs, 1986; Meleis, 1985).

Concepts can be classified on the basis of the extent to which they are observable. Kaplan (1964) proposed a continuum ranging from concrete to abstract. At one end of the continuum (Fig. 14-1) is the *observation term*, a property that is a directly observable, empirical referent. An example of a directly observable referent is a person's statement reporting pain: "I am in agony."

The *indirect observation term* refers to a property that must be inferred. The concept "pain" cannot be observed directly but can be inferred by a variety of signs and symptoms such as writhing, perspiring, crying, and guarding a body part.

A *construct* is neither directly nor indirectly observable. Invented for a special scientific purpose, the construct has theoretical meaning but no empirical meaning unless it is linked to an observational term. Social support is an example of a construct developed for the purpose of studying the social environment. As seen in Table 14-1, Cronenwett

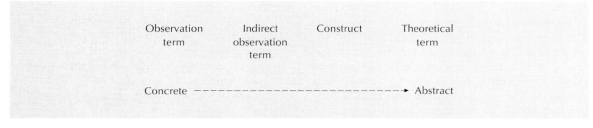

Fig. 14-1. Continuum of concepts.

TABLE 14-1. **Relationship between concept, constitutive definition, operational definition, and measures**

CONCEPT AND SOURCE	CONSTITUTIVE (THEORETICAL) DEFINITION	OPERATIONAL DEFINITION
Gastrointestinal function (Heitkemper & Marotta, 1985)	A balance of adrenergic (inhibitory) and cholinergic (excitatory) inputs to the gastrointestinal tract (acetylcholine and norepinephrine) is released by the autonomic nervous system and the enteric neurons of the intraneural plexus of the gut.	Choline acetyltransferase and tyrosine hydroxylase are involved in synthesis of acetylcholine and norepinephrine respectively; acetylcholinesterase and monoamine oxidase are involved in the degradation of acetylcholine and norepinephrine respectively. Acetylcholine, tyrosine hydroxylase, acetylcholinesterase, and monoamine oxidase are indicators of adrenergic and cholinergic components of gastrointestinal function. They are measured using assays specified in Heitkemper and Marotta (1985).
Social support (Cronenwett, 1985)	Social support includes four dimensions: Emotional support—person communicates love, caring, trust, or concern for you. Material support—person helps you directly, such as through gifts of money and help with house chores and work. Information support—person tells you things you need to know and helps you solve your problems by sharing information or finding out things for you. Comparison support—person helps you learn about yourself just by being someone in the same situation or someone with similar experiences; he or she is like you in some important way and you feel supported because you can share ideas and feelings with someone like yourself.	Network structure was assessed by: Network size—number of persons listed Frequency of contact Composition of network (kith and kin) Boundary density of network—degree to which an individual's network members overlapped with that of the spouse

(1985) specifies that within the theoretical framework for her study, the construct of social support has several dimensions: emotional, material, informational and comparison support. These dimensions cannot be directly observed, but they can be measured with indicators that are congruent with their meaning.

The *theoretical term* refers to a complex global property and is impossible to observe. Its meaning depends on its use in the theory. Nursing, as a theoretical term, has many meanings dependent on the context of the theory in which it is used (see box on p. 4 for a comparison of definitions of nursing).

Because most nursing concepts such as support, energy, well-being, and vulnerability are not directly observable, investigators measure *phenomena,* observable facts or events that reflect those concepts. Investigators translate nursing concepts into phenomena that can be measured in a process termed "operationalizing a concept."

Definitions

Definitions make the concepts of a theory empirically testable. Kerlinger (1986) differentiated between constitutive and operational definitions. *Constitutive definitions* define the construct with other constructs. As seen in Table 14-1, gastrointestinal function and social support can be defined with other concepts. Gastrointestinal function can be viewed as a balance of adrenergic and cholinergic inputs to the gastrointestinal tract. Social support is defined in terms of emotional, material, informational, and comparison support.

Operational definitions, in contrast, assign meaning to a construct by specifying the activities or operations necessary to measure it (Kerlinger, 1986). Operational definitions are also called "epistemic definitions," or "rules of correspondence or interpretation." Operational definitions describe how the construct will be measured. They are measurement-oriented interpretations of constitutive definitions. The *empirical indicators* are the instruments or experimental conditions used in a study. They are observables associated with a given concept that link constitutively defined concepts to the real world (Fawcett, 1986). Table 14-1 contains operational definitions of gastrointestinal function and social support. Note that these operational definitions specify the indicators of the concept.

Steps in operationalizing concepts

The first step in operationalizing concepts involves specifying the constitutive definition guiding measurement decisions. Investigators derive constitutive definitions from their own thinking, a thorough literature review of others' work in the area, processes of concept clarification, and concept mapping (Waltz, Strickland, & Lenz, 1984). Investigators typically begin this process by identifying their own preliminary definitions (i.e., specifying what they think the concept means). Analyzing literature often reveals several definitions of a concept. Selecting the theoretical or constitutive definition most appropriate to the study requires careful consideration of the framework guiding the study to ensure consistency between the definitions and the theoretical perspectives of the investigators. Investigators may use the technique of concept clarification as discussed in Chapter 2 for further refinement of the definition of the concept.

Another strategy for specifying the constitutive definition of the concept is mapping the meaning of the concept. Useful approaches in mapping the meaning of concepts include the following (Waltz, Strickland, & Lenz, 1984):

Listing the major elements in the schemes used by various authors who have written about the concept, and comparing and contrasting their elements

Constructing an outline with major headings representing key elements of meaning

Posing questions about the concept based on the theoretical framework and purpose of the study

Constructing diagrams to represent the concept meaning

An example of the process as applied to the constitutive definition of social support is given in Fig. 14-2. Cronenwett (1985) based her work on social support on dimensions described originally by Richardson and Kagan (1979), who identified emotional support and encouragement, cognitive guidance, and general socialization as important provisions of social networks. Moreover, Richardson and Kagan suggested that size and density of the network and number and type of network members were important dimensions. Barrera (1981) differentiated network members with whom the individual had conflicted and unconflicted relationships. From these

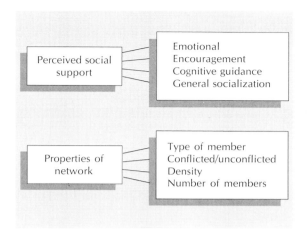

Fig. 14-2. Mapping the meaning of concepts. Perceived social support and properties of network.

sources, Cronenwett identified key elements of the meaning of the construct that could be mapped, as seen in Fig. 14-2.

The next step in operationalizing concepts involves specifying dimensions of the concept's meaning that can vary, that is, can assume different values, such as absent or present in some degree. Specifying the dimensions that can vary (i.e., identifying the variables) is related to the mapping procedure. Usually the theoretical definition provides clues to the important dimensions of the concept. From these, the investigator identifies those dimensions that can assume various values. For example, in the definition of social support used in Cronenwett's work (1985), the dimensions of emotional, material, informational, and comparison support emerge. Individuals can have variable amounts of each of these dimensions of support. The investigator may be able to identify several variables from the constitutive definition. Waltz, Strickland, and Lenz (1984) suggested that the investigator consider the following questions when deciding which of the variables to use in operationalizing the concept:

Which variables will provide the most useful information to nurses?

Which variables have others found to be most important in understanding the phenomenon?

Which variables have others found to be related to other concepts of interest or to help explain or predict occurrences of interest to nurses?

Which variables can be rendered observable and measurable, given our present state of knowledge?

The next step in operationalizing concepts involves identifying observable indicators. This process is guided by the theoretical (constitutive) definition of the concept, the mapping of the concept's meaning, and the variable dimensions identified earlier. Returning to the literature related to the concept is a good strategy for identifying possible indicators of the concept. Enumerating the indicators suggested by the literature and examining each to determine its consistency with the theoretical definition and purpose of the study are important processes. Often the literature will identify instruments used to measure the concept. However, the instruments or indicators suggested in earlier literature may not be congruent with the theoretical definition specified for the concept under study.

Williams and her colleagues (1985) developed an operational definition of an acute confusional state in their study of hospitalized elderly patients. The theoretical definition of an acute confusional state was "a disturbance in mental processes incorporating impaired memory, thinking, attention, and orientation to time and place" (p. 32). This disturbance could include a misperception of persons and objects, as well as hallucinations and accompanying hyperactivity or hypoactivity or emotional change. The state could be transient or prolonged (Williams et al., 1985). In earlier work the investigators had discovered that four categories of patient behaviors indicative of confusion and reported by the nursing staff correlated with tests of cognitive function performed on the same patients (Williams et al., 1979). The investigators used these four categories of behaviors as the empirical indicators of confusion. They included (1) verbal or nonverbal manifestations of disorientation to time, place, or persons in the environment, (2) inappropriate communication or communication unusual for the person, such as nonsensical speech, calling out, yelling, swearing, or unusual silence, (3) inappropriate behavior, such as attempting to get out of bed, pulling at tubes or dressings, or picking at the bedclothes, and (4) illusions or hallucinations. Each of the four categories of

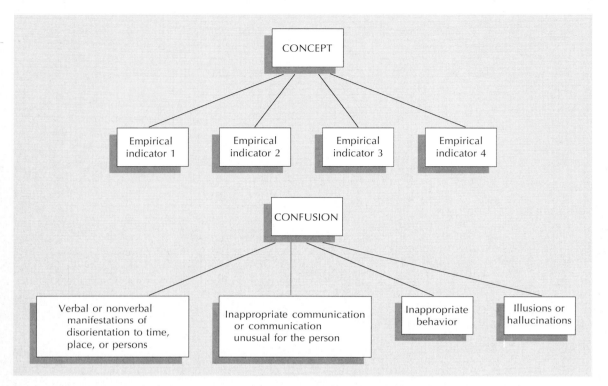

Fig. 14-3. Relationship between the concept of confusion and empirical indicators of confusion. (Based on Williams, M., et al., Nursing activities and acute confusional states in elderly hip-fractured patients. ©, 1979, American Journal of Nursing Company. Reprinted with permission from *Nursing Research,* Jan.-Feb., *28,* 25-35.)

behaviors was scored for each 8-hour shift, with *0* indicating not present at any time during the shift, *1* indicating present at some time but in mild form, and *2* indicating present at some time in marked form. Total scores could vary from 0 to 8. Fig. 14-3 illustrates the relationship between the concept of confusion and the four empirical indicators of confusion.

Having identified indicators of the concept, the investigator selects ways of measuring variables in a process called "instrumentation." Instrumentation may involve the development of devices or measures essential for the purpose of the study and the selection of an existing measure. In the example above, Williams and her colleagues (1979) identified as variables the four categories of behaviors that could change over time. In addition, they created rules for rating the behaviors according to whether they were

absent or present, mild or marked. In summary, Williams and colleagues specified the constitutive definition of confusion, and specified dimensions of the concept, identified empirical indicators, and selected ways of measuring the variables.

Criteria for evaluating the operationalization of a concept

Waltz, Strickland, and Lenz (1984) suggested several criteria for evaluating the adequacy of the operationalization of a concept. Clarity implies that the definition, indicators, and operationalization be understood easily. *Precision* is a criterion that provides that the description of the operationalization be explicit and specific. *Reliability* refers to reproducibility of the observations and operations. This criterion will be discussed further in Chapter 15. *Consistency* implies use of terms in a predictable manner

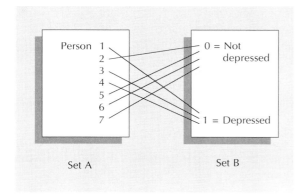 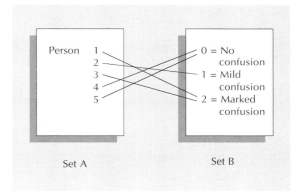

Fig. 14-4. Persons *1*, *3*, and *4* are depressed and are rated *1*. Persons *2*, *5*, *6*, and *7* are not depressed and are rated *0*.

Fig. 14-5. Persons *1* and *3* are markedly confused and are rated *2*, whereas person *2* is mildly confused and rated *1*. Persons *4* and *5* are not confused.

and also implies congruence between the meaning of the concept and observable reality. *Meaning adequacy* refers to the congruence that must exist between the meaning denoted by a concept and the indicators selected to represent the concept. *Feasibility* implies that indicators and operations should be able to be executed. *Utility* refers to the need for the operationalization to be useful within the context of the investigation and the discipline of nursing. *Validity* refers to the requirement that the observations selected to represent the concept do indeed represent it. Consensus refers to the acceptance of the operationalization by the scientific community.

Quantitative measurement

Measurement can be defined quantitatively and qualitatively. *Quantitative measurement* is the assignment of numerical values to objects or events to represent the kind or amount of a characteristic of those objects or events. The function that assigns each member of one set of objects to some value of another set is sometimes referred to as the "rule of correspondence." The function takes the form of

$$F = \{(x,y)\}$$

where *x* is any object and *y* is some numeral. Measurement as a quantitatively oriented activity assumes that characteristics of objects or events exist in some amount. The rule of correspondence is used to determine whether the characteristic is there and in what quantity it is present.

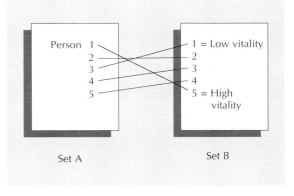

Fig. 14-6. Person *1* has the highest level of vitality and person *3* the lowest. The remainder have intermediate levels.

Suppose we have a set of individuals *(A)* and a set of depression scores *(B)* as illustrated in Fig. 14-4. Assume each individual in *set A* either is or is not depressed. Individuals who are depressed could be assigned the value *1* from *set B* and those who are not depressed the value *0*. If persons *1*, *3*, and *4* were depressed, the application of the rule of correspondence to *set A* would generate the relationships shown in Fig. 14-4. If we rated people on the confusion scale identified by Williams et al. (1985) in which the values could range from *0* to *2*, the results would resemble those in Fig. 14-5. Persons *1* and *3* have marked confusion, person *2* has mild confusion, and persons *4* and *5* are not confused. Suppose further that people are rated on a scale of vitality in which the values could range from *1* to *5*. Applying the rule of correspondence to the people in Fig. 14-6 might yield the relationship illustrated. Person *1* has the highest level of vitality, person *3* the lowest, and persons *2*, *4*, and *5* the intermediate levels.

These illustrations seem somewhat simplistic, but we will soon discover the complexity of measurement. Consider how complicated assignment of ranks of health would be. One must consider many factors in rating health and in discriminating levels of health from one another. Clearly the quality of the rule of correspondence is directly related to the quality of measurement. Precision in the specification of rules guarantees precision in measurement of the concept. Often this reality necessitates very complex rules for decisions, as we shall soon see.

Qualitative measurement

Qualitative measurement is a process of classification that involves assigning objects to categories (i.e., distributing phenomena into classes) that represent variations of the concept being studied. Several desirable characteristics of a classification system merit consideration in a discussion of qualitative measurement (Kerlinger, 1986; Murphy, 1978):

The classification system should be natural or relevant.

The set of categories should be exhaustive.

The individual categories should be mutually exclusive or disjoint.

The category system should be derived from and should develop a principle of ordering.

The individual categories should be formulated on the same level of abstraction or discourse.

The classification system should be useful.

The classification system should be constructable.

A classification system is natural if it corresponds to the nature or character of the objects or events being classified. It is relevant if it pertains to the phenomena being classified. Nursing diagnoses, in contrast to medical diagnoses, are natural and relevant to the phenomena of central concern to nursing.

The set of categories in a classification system is exhaustive when each member of the set of observations being classified fits in some category; that is,

the classification system can account for all the possible observations. It is disjoint or mutually exclusive when a single observation can fit into only one category. Being mutually exclusive implies that no overlap exists between categories. In the scheme below, note that the classification on the left is mutually exclusive whereas that on the right is not. Observations of *5*, *10*, and *15* could be included in either one of two classes in the scheme on the right.

CLASSIFICATION SCHEMES

0-4	0-5
5-9	5-10
10-14	10-15
15-19	15-20

Classifications schemes are derived from a principle of ordering and should develop that principle. The principle of ordering might differ from the conceptual framework used to guide the measurement decisions in a study. For example, some investigators might classify nursing phenomena according to the body system with which they are associated, and others might classify the same phenomena using concepts such as self, role, and environment.

Individual categories in a classification schema (sometimes referred to as a taxonomy) are formulated on the same level of abstraction or discourse. This implies that the classes and subclasses are parallel. The box below contains an illustration of parallel and nonparallel classification schemes.

The classification in the right column is nonparallel because light perception, sensation of heat, and proprioception could be subsumed as part of broader categories.

PARALLEL AND NONPARALLEL CLASSIFICATION SCHEMES

Parallel	*Nonparallel*
Sight	Sight
Smell	Light perception
Hearing	Smell
Touch	Hearing
Taste	Sensation of heat
	Touch
	Proprioception

Classification systems are useful when those who use them can understand the system and find it helpful rather than confusing. Users must recognize the terminology of the system and must be oriented to the system of classification. Researchers can construct a classification system when the sets of categories in the system are exhaustive and mutually exclusive.

Isomorphism

Isomorphism means identity or similarity of form. In measurement theory isomorphism relates to the correspondence of sets of objects to reality. Ideally, measurement is tied to reality. The definition of the sets of objects or events being measured, the definition of numerical sets from which we assign numbers to the objects being measured, and the rules of assignment (rules of correspondence) need to be tied to reality. The relationship of the objects being measured to the numerals in Figs. 14-4 through 14-6 can be said to be isomorphic when the person who is rated *1* in Fig. 14-4 really is depressed, and when the person rated *5* on the vitality scale in Fig. 14-6 really has the highest level of vitality.

LEVELS OF MEASUREMENT

The nature of the phenomena being measured influences the rules that can be applied to their measurement. For example, some phenomena, such as gender, can be described only qualitatively, that is, as one kind or another, whereas health can be a quantitative measure when it is said to be present in a greater or lesser degree. Levels of measurement refer to the classification of measurement according to whether the obtained scores reflect a category (quality) or a numerical value (quantity). The four levels of measurement are nominal, ordinal, interval, and ratio (Stevens, 1946).

Nominal measurement

Nominal measurement involves the assignment of numbers to represent categories or classes of things. The numbers represent the phenomenon's membership in a category that is mutually exclusive of other categories. The numbers have no quantitative value and are used only as labels. They cannot be ordered or added. The categories differ qualitatively, not quantitatively. One cannot describe the amount of the thing, only its characteristics. Participants in a study could be classified as male or female and assigned to a category labeled *1* or *2*. In an exhaustive system of categories, each person should belong to one category. The categories are also mutually exclusive in that any individual should belong to only one category. In this level of measurement, *1* is not less than *2*, but instead represents a different category. When more than two categories exist, more than two labels are used.

Ordinal measurement

Ordinal measurement requires that objects can be rank ordered on some operationally defined characteristic. On ordinal scale measures, numbers represent ordering of magnitude on some attribute. A number is assigned to represent membership in a mutually exclusive and exhaustive category, as in nominal measurement, but this number can also be ordered according to the amount of the attribute possessed. Rankings do not imply that intervals between scale categories are equal, only that *1* is less than *2*, which is less than *3*, and so on. Consider the educational level of participants in a study. We might use the measurement schema shown in Table 14-2 in which *1* indicates that the individual did not complete grade school, and *6* indicates that the individual completed graduate school. In this example, the level of education is ordered by rank; *6* indicates more education than *5*, *5* indicates more education than *4*, and so on. Note that the intervals between *1* and *2*, *2* and *3*, *3* and *4*, *4* and *5*, and *5* and *6* are not equal. Ordinal scale numbers indicate rank order, not absolute quantities.

Interval measurement

An *interval scale*, sometimes labeled an equal-interval scale, is one for which equal distances on the scale represent equal amounts of the phenomenon being measured. The numbers on the scale are spaced equally in relation to the magnitude of the phenomenon, but absolute amounts are not known. Absolute amounts can be measured only when the zero point for the interval scale is absolute, not arbitrary. Interval measurement permits categorization, ranking, and ordering according to relative size of differences between two measurements. For example, a temperature shift of 6° F is half as great as a temperature shift of 12° F, but 50° F is not twice as hot as

TABLE 14-2. Levels of measurement and examples of phenomena and values

LEVEL	PHENOMENON	VALUES
Nominal	Gender	1 = male
		2 = female
Ordinal	Education	1 = did not complete grade school
		2 = completed grade school
		3 = completed junior high school
		4 = completed high school
		5 = completed college
		6 = completed graduate school
Interval	Temperature (human)	87° F-106° F
Ratio	Height	0-nn inches

25° F because 0° F does not indicate absence of temperature.

Ratio level measurement

Ratio level measures have all the characteristics of nominal, ordinal, and interval scales, but also have absolute zero, meaning an absolute absence of the phenomenon. Thus magnitude from zero to some point on the scale is known. Height and weight are examples of ratio scales. An individual can be twice as tall or half as heavy as another individual. Some objects can have none of the properties being measured. The numbers on ratio scales indicate the actual amounts being measured.

Level of measurement is linked to permissible arithmetic operations, with some types of scales lending themselves to many more mathematical treatments than others. Fundamental algebraic operations, including addition, subtraction, multiplication, and division, can be applied to the ratio scale. These operations can be performed with ratio scales because they are invariant over all transformations where they are multiplied by a constant. If X represents all possible points on a ratio scale and c is a constant, the resulting scale X' is a ratio scale:

$$X' = c\,X$$

X' is the product of a constant (c) and X. Transforming a 5-point scale by a constant, such as $(c = 5)$

X	X'
0	0
1	5
2	10
3	15
4	20

preserves both the rank and ratios of the original scale. The zero point will also remain the same. For example, when one converts measurements in millimeters to centimeters, the transformation does not alter the ability of the scale to meet criteria for ratio-level measurement (Nunnally, 1978). With interval-level measurement, applications of the fundamental operations of algebra are limited. Addition, subtraction, multiplication, and division of intervals on the scales is appropriate, but forming ratios among the scale points on an interval scale is not permissible because of conditions of invariance. Invariance will be obtained when transforming one interval scale to another because the absolute magnitudes on an interval scale are irrelevant. When the scores (X) are transformed, they are invariant when multiplied by a constant (c) and when a constant is added to the score. Adding the constant does not change the ordinal positions of the points or the equality of the intervals. With ordinal scales, none of the fundamental operations of algebra is permissible.

Although some authors link level of measurement to the types of statistical tests that can be used (Chapter 26), this is currently a controversial issue. Nunnally (1978) argues that violations of the assumptions required for using inferential statistics usually have little effect on the indices or on the inferential statistics applied to the indices. For example, using an inferential statistical test with either ordinal or interval data should have little effect on the results. Nunnally suggested that the investigator consider whether the indices of the relationship, such as the ratios of two variances, should be computed and whether they can be meaningfully interpreted.

SCALING

Often results obtained with measuring instruments are expressed as a score on one or more dimensions. For example, the Williams et al. (1985) confusion scale could be scored with a total score ranging from

0 to 8 where the scores given patients on each of the four dimensions would be summed to give a total appraisal of the confusion level of each patient. The score an individual received on the confusion scale would facilitate distinctions among individuals regarding the degree to which they possess the characteristic (i.e., confusion).

A *scale* is a set of symbols or numerals constructed so that the symbols or numerals can be assigned by rule to characteristics of individuals to whom the scale is applied. The assignment of the symbols or numerals is indicated by the individual's possession of the characteristic the scale is supposed to measure. Scale scores permit comparison between individuals regarding the phenomenon of interest. Scales are composite measures of a phenomenon that consist of several items that have a logical or empirical relationship to one another. Scaling is the process of assigning a score to a participant to place her or him on a continuum relative to the phenomenon being studied. For example, if the rule of correspondence were properly applied, an individual who received an *8* on the confusion measure would be more confused than an individual who received a *3*.

Components of scales

Scales used to measure psychosocial constructs are comprised of a *stem statement* relating to the attitude or other phenomenon being rated, a series of scale steps, and *anchors* defining the scale steps. Table 14-3 illustrates the components of a scale. Scale steps are increments on the scale, denoted by numbers that remind participants of the meanings of the scale steps and facilitate data entry and analysis for the investigator. The anchors define the scale steps and are usually specified at the beginning of the scale and in some cases for each item.

Types of scales

Scales have been developed to measure intelligence, aptitude, achievement, personality, attitudes, and values. Most of the scaling techniques used in contemporary nursing research were developed originally to measure attitudes or sentiments, and they include summated scales, cumulative scales, and the semantic differential scale.

Summated rating scales

A *summated rating scale* contains a set of scales, each of which expresses some attitude or value. The participant's task is to respond with varying degrees of

TABLE 14-3. **Components of scales**

COMPONENT	EXAMPLE
Stem	There is someone I feel close to who makes me feel secure.
Scale steps	1 2 3 4 5 6 7
Anchors	Strongly agree Strongly disagree

intensity on a scale ranging between two extremes, such as "strongly agree" to "strongly disagree." Scores for all scales are summed or summed and averaged to yield each individual's score.

Several principles are used in constructing summated scales. First, the investigator generates items through brainstorming, reviewing the literature, and consulting with colleagues and experts on the topic. The constitutive and operational definitions provide the background for item construction. Of particular importance is generating items that reflect the many nuances of meaning of the concept being measured. All items in the item pool should address a single construct. In some instances, multiple dimensions are measured by a large item pool that contains several scales as part of a single instrument. Homogenous scales, that is, scales measuring only a single dimension, typically have fewer than 40 items.

Most items are stated moderately positively or moderately negatively. Extreme statements and neutral statements are ineffective in differentiating respondents on the concept being measured; that is, they do not produce much variance in response. Usually the item pool is divided so that about one half of the items are negative and one half are positive. This approach minimizes positive or negative response, inasmuch as it requires the individual to respond to items stated with different orientations.

Usually between five and nine scale steps are used, depending on the number of items. When there are many items, fewer scale steps are necessary to achieve high reliability. When there are only a few items, increasing the number of scale steps usually increases the reliability of the instrument. On the other hand, increasing the number of scale steps also places a burden on the participant to provide fine distinction in responses. Whether or not to use a category labeled "uncertain" or "undecided" is controversial. Some investigators insist that the participant select a response option. Others believe that providing a neutral or undecided option is preferable because a participant simply may be undecided or neutral and may be reluctant to provide a forced response to certain items.

An example of a summated scale is the Likert scale, named for Rensis Likert (1932) who developed it as a measurement device. It consists of several statements expressing viewpoints on a topic. Respondents indicate the degree to which they agree or disagree with each statement. The Likert scale usually contains ten to twenty items, although it may contain as few as four or five. It is scored by summing the numerical values attached to the scale anchors. Positive and negative items are scored differently. For example, when scoring a scale measuring the construct "satisfaction," the investigator sums all the scale values for the positively stated items. The scale values for the negatively stated items are reversed, so that the highest value reflects satisfaction rather than dissatisfaction. The scale values for the negative items are then summed and added to the score for the positive items. This process ensures that the total score on the scale reflects satisfaction. In theory, the higher the total score, the higher the degree of satisfaction.

Likert scales usually are unidimensional measures of the same concept, although it is not unusual for the same instrument to have several scales embedded in it. For example, a measure of social-support satisfaction could have three subscales that reflect satisfaction with three different dimensions of social support: affirmation, affect, and aid. In this event, each subscale is scored separately and is treated as a unidimensional scale.

The summated scaling technique has been applied to constructs other than attitudes in the nursing research literature. Some applications include anxiety, depression, and social-support satisfaction. Laffrey (1986) developed the Health Conception Scale to measure individual perceptions of the meaning of health. The instrument addresses four dimensions of health conceptions as described by Smith (1981): the clinical model, in which health is viewed as the absence of disease or symptoms; the functional model, in which health is viewed as the ability to fulfill socially defined roles; the adaptive model, in which health is viewed as flexibly adjusting to changing circumstances; and the eudaimonistic model, in which health is viewed as exuberant well-being. The scale includes 28 items such as "For me, health or being healthy means being able to adjust to changes in my surroundings" that are scored on a six-point Likert scale where 1 represents "strongly disagree" and 6 represents "strongly agree." Table 14-4 contains the final set of items included in the scale.

Because the Health Conception Scale is a multidimensional scale, scores for each dimension—clinical, functional, adaptive, and eudaimonistic—are important. The investigator scores the dimensions by summing the scores for each item representing that dimension.

Reliability and validity estimates are sample-specific. That is, they will vary across samples. For this reason, reliability and validity estimates for summated scales should be made under conditions that replicate those for their intended application. That is, the sample, conditions, and timing of the measure should resemble what is anticipated for the final sample.

Cumulative scales

Cumulative scales (also called Guttman scales) consist of items constructed so that the person who agrees with item 2 also agrees with item 1, but not necessarily with item 3. Cumulative scale construction requires developing a number of items of increasing intensity regarding some construct, usually an attitude. Cumulative scales contain a homogeneous set of items, that is, they are related to only one construct. Moreover, cumulative scales are hierarchical; that is, they contain items reflecting increasing intensity.

An example of a cumulative scale is the type initially developed by Louis Guttman (1949). Participants are asked to agree or disagree with a series of items (typically four or five items) representing a hierarchy. Individuals who endorse items that are higher in intensity should also endorse items of lower intensity. Consider an example of a Guttman scale representing attitudes about immunization administration. The items might include:

1. Immunizations should be available to infants whose parents request them.
2. Immunizations should be available to all infants whose parents consent.
3. Immunizations should be mandated for infants at greatest risk for disease.
4. Immunizations should be mandated for all infants.

TABLE 14-4. Loadings and factor structure of items in the Laffrey Health Conception Scale (N = 141)

ITEMS	DIMENSION			
	CLINICAL	FUNCTIONAL	ADAPTIVE	EUDAIMONISTIC
Free of symptoms	X			
Do not require doctor's services	X			
Not under doctor's care for illness	X			
Do not require pills for illness	X			
Not sick	X			
Do not require medication	X			
No physical/mental incapacities	X			
Fulfill daily responsibilities		X		
Able to do what I have to do		X		
Able to function as expected		X		
Adequately carry on daily responsibilities		X		
Carry out normal functions of daily living		X		
Fulfill role responsibilities		X		
Perform at expected level		X		
Adjust to changes in surroundings			X	
Adjust to life's changes			X	
Cope with stressful events			X	
Change air and adjust to demands of environment			X	
Adapt to things as they really are			X	
Cope with changes in surroundings			X	
Do not collapse under ordinary stress			X	
Feeling great				X
Creatively live life to fullest				X
Face day with zest and enthusiasm				X
Actualize highest and best aspirations				X
Live at top level				X
Realize full potential				X
Mind and body function at highest level				X

Modified from Laffrey, S. (1986). *Research in Nursing & Health, 9*(2), 107-113.

The person who endorses the fourth statement should agree with all the statements listed earlier. The cumulative scale, although originally developed to measure attitudes, is also useful for measuring capabilities.

Orem's systems of nursing care (1980) could constitute a cumulative scale:

1. Supportive-educative nursing system—nurse assists patient in decision making, behavior control, and the aquisition of knowledge and skill.
2. Partly compensatory nursing system—nurse assists patient in some self-care activities.
3. Wholly compensatory nursing system—nurse compensates for the patient's total inability to engage in self-care activities.

Individuals who require wholly compensatory care also require partly compensatory and supportive-educative care; those who require only a supportive-educative nursing care system do not require partly or wholly compensatory care.

Scalogram analysis is a procedure that investigators can use to determine if a cumulative scale is unidimensional and reproducible. The statistical procedure determines whether it is possible to reproduce a person's responses to specific items given the individual's score on the scale. Using the scale for attitudes toward immunizations a person whose final score is *1* should not endorse item *2, 3,* or *4.* If it is possible to reproduce the items that a subject would endorse from knowing the total score, then the scale is said to have a high degree of reproducibility. Reproducibility is similar to reliability of a measuring instrument, which will be discussed in Chapter 15.

Guttman scales rarely appear in the nursing literature, perhaps because of their limitations. Guttman scales do not yield fine discriminations between individuals because of the small number of items. Moreover, it is difficult to construct items that form a cumulative scale.

Semantic differential scales

The *semantic differential scale* is designed to measure attitudes toward concepts along dimensions such as evaluation, potency, and activity. Initially developed by Osgood, Suci, and Tannenbaum (1957), the semantic differential scale requires the respondent to rate a concept such as menopause on several 5- to 9-point scales anchored by bipolar adjectives such as kind-cruel, fast-slow, good-bad, and successful-unsuccessful. The semantic differential scale developed by Bowles (1985) to assess women's attitudes toward menopause uses a graphic response scale and is illustrated in Fig. 14-7. The investigator can select bipolar scales reflecting various dimensions to be used with the particular concept under study or can use those developed by other investigators. The adjectives reflect the dimensions; for example, in Fig. 14-7 important-unimportant reflects evaluation, strong-weak reflects potency, and alive-dead reflects activity.

The object or concept that a respondent is asked to rate can be a single word, phrase, sentence, or even a picture. Investigators constructing semantic differential scales typically choose contrasting concepts, that is, they ask participants to rate more than one concept. For example, Morgan (1984) asked respon-

DURING MENOPAUSE A WOMAN FEELS

Important	Unimportant
Passive	Active
Clean	Dirty
Fresh	Stale
Dumb	Intelligent
Sharp	Dull
Unsure	Confident
Worthless	Valuable
High	Low
Strong	Weak
Unattractive	Attractive
Pessimistic	Optimistic
Full	Empty
Pleasant	Unpleasant
Ugly	Beautiful
Needed	Unneeded
Useful	Useless
Interesting	Boring
Unsuccessful	Successful
Alive	Dead

Fig. 14-7. Example of a semantic differential scale. Attitudes toward menopause. (From Bowles, C. [1985]. Reprinted with permission from *Nursing Research, 35,* 81-85. ©, 1985, American Journal of Nursing Company.)

dents to rate black American patients, black Americans, white American patients, white Americans, and the ideal person. The adjective pairs used in the bipolar responses must be related to the concept, that is, they should make sense to the respondent.

Scoring the semantic differential scale may entail

factor analyzing the response and then computing subscale scores, one for each dimension, such as, evaluation, potency, and activity. The items are scored similarly to items on a Likert scale, taking into account the direction of positive and negative bipolar-adjective pairs. In addition to comparing respondents' scores for rating various concepts, investigators can also compare various groups of respondents' scores.

Visual analog scales

Visual analog scales represent a type of measurement technique designed to obtain interval-level data. Instead of requiring respondents to select a point on a Likert scale, the visual analog scale requires respondents to indicate a point on a linear scale that reflects the intensity of their feelings, opinions, or beliefs. Usually the respondent is instructed to read the items and place an *X* on the scale opposite the question at the point that best shows their intensity of feeling. Commonly a 100 mm line is used for the scale, with two anchor words to describe the end points of the scale. Scale values are obtained by measuring the point on the line (Aiken, 1969; Bond & Lader, 1974; Dixon & Bird, 1981; Maxwell, 1978; Revill, Robinson, Rosen, & Hogg, 1976).

Padilla and her associates (1983) used visual analog scaling in a study of the quality of life for cancer patients. The quality of life index focused on present quality of life. Fourteen items were used to reflect general physical condition, normal human activities, and personal attitudes related to general quality of life. Respondents were instructed as follows:

> Below are several questions pertaining to your physical well-being, normal activities, and general quality of life. To answer a question, place an *X* on the linear scale opposite the question at the point that best shows us what is happening to you at present. The description "normal for me" means what was normal prior to illness.

Patients were asked to respond on a 100 mm linear scale with no numbered markings. The end of the scale denoting the poorest quality of life was the *0* point. Scoring involved measuring from the *0* point to the *X* mark. An example of items from the quality of life index is given in Figure 14-8.

Magnitude estimation scales

Magnitude estimation is a measurement technique based on recent advances in psychophysics. Stevens (1957) first used the method by asking people to assign numbers to represent levels of light intensity, sound, and heaviness, for example. He found that people produced a series of ratio scales that were related in a curvilinear way to the corresponding physical stimuli. Since Stevens' initial work, the method has been applied in the social sciences.

Magnitude estimation requires participants to match numbers, lengths of lines, or pressure of hand grips to stimuli. For example, a person could be asked to squeeze a dynamometer so that his or her impression of the force exerted by squeezing the handgrip matched the intensity of a stimulus, such as an attitude about nursing care. The response modalities that could be used with magnitude estimation techniques include the brightness of light, intensity of sound, and strength of grip, to mention a few.

One feature of magnitude estimation that differs from other types of scaling procedures is that the method produces a score for the stimuli, or items, rather than generating a score from the items to yield a score for the participant. Scale items for magnitude estimation, like those for other scales, contain only one major cue; the stimulus (item) is stated clearly and concisely, and the stimuli vary on the major concept dimensions that are being scaled. Items are developed using the operational definition as a reference point. For example, Hinshaw and Schepp (1983) used the following definition of territorial intrusion: While you are a patient in the hospital, you may consider the room, bed, and chair as "your" room, "your" bed, and "your" chair. In other words the room becomes "your" territory. The nurse may do some things that annoy you or cause you to feel like she or he is more or less overstepping boundaries and intruding on your territory.

Usually the participants are told they will be presented with a series of stimuli in random order. They are instructed to indicate with the response modality how intensely they feel about the stimulus. Usually the first stimulus is a reference point. All further estimations are relative to the first response. Participants are trained to use the response modality and to estimate ratios before their actual rating of items. For example, they might be instructed to respond to the following instructions: Given the number 100, I'd like to have you give me a number that is one half as large, twice as large, or one third as large.

In Hinshaw and Schepp's study (1983), participants were instructed to use the same technique used in the training sessions to judge a set of nursing-care

With respect to your general physical condition please describe:

General physical condition:

1. How much PAIN you
   are feeling.   None _____ Excruciating

2. How much NAUSEA
   you experience.   None _____ Constant nausea

3. How frequently you
   VOMIT.   Not at all _____ Constantly vomiting
                                                                  or retching

4. How much STRENGTH
   you feel.   None _____ Normal for me

5. How much APPETITE
   you have.   None _____ Normal for me

Important human activities:

6. Are you able to WORK
   at your usual tasks
   (example: housework,   Not at all _____ Normal for me
   office work,
   gardening) ?

7. Are you able to EAT?
                             Not at all _____ Normal for me

8. Are you able to obtain
   SEXUAL satisfaction?   Not at all _____ Normal for me

9. Are you able to SLEEP
   well?   Not at all _____ Normal for me

General quality of life:

10. How good is your
    quality of life?   Extremely poor _____ Excellent
    (GENERAL QL)

11. Are you having FUN?
    (hobbies, recreation,   Not at all _____ Normal for me
    social activities)

12. Is your life
    SATISFYING?   Not at all _____ Normal for me

13. Do you feel USEFUL?
                             Not at all _____ Normal for me
14. Do you WORRY ABOUT
    THE COST of medical care? Not at all _____ A great deal

Fig. 14-8. Example using a visual analogue scale. Quality of life index. (From Padilla, G., et al. [1983]. *Research in Nursing & Health, 6,* 117-126.)

activities. They were instructed to select the nursing-care activity that produced the average amount of intrusiveness and to assign 100 points to that activity. Using that as a reference point, they were then requested to rate the other activities on the characteristic of intrusiveness. All the other stimuli were then judged relative to the average, not relative to the other stimuli.

Data from magnitude estimation scaling are analyzed by averaging the responses for each item. Reliability of the scales is usually determined by test-retest procedures.

Magnitude scaling offers the advantage of greater distinction than is possible when respondents are required to make choices on a scale with predetermined categories such as a Likert scale. In addition, magnitude scaling offers the advantage of ratio level measurement rather than the ordinal level measures obtained with Likert scales.

CHARACTERISTICS OF IDEAL MEASURING INSTRUMENTS

Several features are desirable in measuring instruments. Ideally, the measure is *valid*, meaning that it measures what it is supposed to measure. An instrument designed to measure anxiety in cancer patients must measure anxiety and not the side effects of the chemotherapy or pathophysiological changes that are part of the disease process (Lewis, Firsich, & Parsell, 1979).

Next, ideal instruments are *reliable*, meaning that measurements made with the instruments are reproducible. A thermometer should register the same temperature when repeatedly exposed to a water bath maintained at 98.6° F. Because of their importance, the characteristics of validity and reliability will be discussed in much greater detail in Chapter 15.

In addition to being valid and reliable, instruments should be sensitive, that is, capable of making sufficiently fine distinctions to suit the purpose of the measure. Instruments designed to assess health status in chronically ill persons often are not sufficiently sensitive to assess fine gradations in health in a primarily well population. The Sickness Impact Profile (SIP) consists of items grouped into 14 categories that describe an area of daily living or a type of activity that has been affected by illness, such as sleep and rest, home maintenance, eating, body care and movement, mobility, social interaction, ambulation, alertness behavior, communication, working, recreational pastimes, and emotional behavior (Bergner et al., 1976). If an individual were to endorse all SIP items, the maximum score would be 100%. When applied to a population of individuals recovering from a myocardial infarction, the scores on the SIP were quite low and did not vary greatly. Members of this population rarely endorse more than a few items on the SIP and a large percentage of the participants endorse none of the items. Because people recovering from myocardial infarction have very low scores on the profile even during their hospitalization, it is difficult through the use of the SIP to see improvement in their status over the 6 months following their hospitalization. The SIP is not sensitive to the more subtle changes seen in the status of the population with myocardial infarction, whereas it has been quite appropriate for studies of populations with chronic illnesses such as arthritis (Foley, 1982; Sivarajan et al., 1981).

Measurement instruments should be relevant to the population being studied. Investigators should consider particular characteristics of the population under study when selecting instruments. Investigators studying children must use measurements that are appropriate to children's developmental levels. Those studying children in a longitudinal way have the special challenge of selecting measures that reflect more than the child's maturational progress and that are reliable at different developmental stages.

The ideal instrument allows the community of investigators and clinicians to view phenomena in a similar way. Valid and reliable measures allow investigators to share information about a concept, such as anxiety, in a way that has the same meaning for each individual. Instruments that are valid, reliable, and sensitive also allow investigators and clinicians to share observations with precision. Blood pressure, for instance, can be described as 200/160 rather than merely as high. Finally, an individual interpreting the measures can trust that his or her interpretations will be the same as those of anyone else interpreting the measures.

CHOOSING A MEASURE

Concept of interest

Choosing a measure requires careful reflection about the concepts of interest to the researcher and the purposes for acquiring the information that the measure would yield. The first consideration should be the concept and its dimensions. Suppose an investigator is studying health in young adults. The concept "health" is abstract and multidimensional. Depending on the investigator's theoretical orientation, health could be defined on the basis of several dimensions including the ability to function, feelings of well-being, presence of symptoms, and ability to actualize one's potential in life. The model, theory, or conceptual framework guiding development of the measure should be consistent with that guiding the study. For example, a model of health that emphasizes self-actualization is not consistent with a measure of health status that emphasizes lack of symptoms as the only indicator of health (Smith, 1981; Tripp-Reimer, 1984).

Purpose of the study

The purpose of the investigation must also be considered. If the investigator is interested in studying health status in response to a health promotion intervention, then the measure must be capable of reflecting change in health status. A person whose health has improved should show improvement on the measure. If everyone in the population of interest obtains the highest possible scores on the pretest, the measure cannot adequately reflect any improvement in health. On the other hand, the same measure might be sufficient to find out what proportion of a given population met the norms established for the measure with another population. For example, the median scores on the SIP for people recovering from a myocardial infarction could be compared with the median scores of people who have diabetes or arthritis. When measures will guide policy decisions, the investigator must be certain that the measure will yield information necessary for a sound decision (Waltz, Strickland, & Lenz, 1984).

Content of the measure

The content of the measure under consideration may or may not be appropriate for its use. The item pool of a paper-and-pencil measure may need to be expanded to achieve the purpose of the study. For example, Norbeck (1984) added several items to a commonly used measure of stressful events that were important in adult women's lives but that were not included in the initial development of the instrument. The content of the measure should be appropriate for the age, literacy, and frame of reference of participants. Few paper-and-pencil measures are appropriate for adults with little formal education.

Psychometric properties

Psychometric properties of a measure refer to their technical quality. In particular, the investigator considers evidence of the reliability and validity of the instrument and procedures used in developing and testing the measure. Several references are cited in Appendix B that include technical specifications for instruments.

Measurement norms

Measurement norms refer to the values (e.g., mean, standard deviation, and range of values) obtained when using the instrument. Considering the norms in relation to the population of interest is important; considering the age and health status of the population is particularly important in nursing investigations. Instruments developed on populations of freshman psychology students are normed for that population, and the technical specifications are not always appropriate for older adults, populations of people who are ill, or even the general population. Using normative criteria from adolescents and young adults to determine the presence of a typical level of a phenomenon such as anxiety may be quite inappropriate for an elderly population of chronically ill individuals.

Procedures for administration

Procedures for administering the measure are important to minimize measurement error. Explicit instructions should be given for use of the instrument. Directions for use are equally important with biological instruments, observation guides, or paper-and-pencil measures.

Scoring directions

Directions for scoring or rating the results obtained with the instrument are also important. For example, access to a computer may be necessary to score the paper-and-pencil measure or to transform electronic signals obtained with a physiological instrument to a form that the investigator can interpret. The processes for generating results from the measure can be time consuming, and perhaps inappropriate, given the investigator's abilities, time constraints, and financial resources. Interpretation of the scores, that is, the data generated by the instrument, is extremely important. Usually guidelines for interpreting the results of the instrument are included with the instrument when it is purchased; sometimes guidelines are published in journals. Often critical reviews are available that summarize the strengths and problems associated with the measure and other investigators' experiences with the measure (Waltz, Strickland, & Lenz, 1984).

Investigators will find that considering the ease, time, and cost of using the measure is important. In some instances the ideal measure is prohibitively expensive, and in others the procedure is too cumbersome to allow use in clinical settings. The cost of an instrument includes not only the purchase price (when the instrument is not available free from the person who developed it) but also the cost of administration, scoring, and maintenance of equipment. Waltz, Strickland, and Lenz (1984) have discussed these issues in greater detail.

Resources useful in selecting measurement instruments and devices

Many resources are useful to the investigator selecting an instrument, including professional journals and instrument compendia. In nursing, some journal sources include *Heart and Lung, Image, Journal of Nursing Administration, Journal of Nursing Education, MCN: American Journal of Maternal Child Nursing, Nurse Educator, Nursing Research, Research in Nursing and Health,* and the *Western Journal of Nursing Research.* In addition to nursing publications, journals from related fields often contain the results of studies of instrument development. Some of these include *Advances in Psychological Assessment, American Journal of Psychology, American Journal of Public Health, American Journal of Sociology, Annals of Clinical Research, Annals of Internal Medicine, Child Development, Developmental Psychology, Educational and Psychological Measurement, Evaluation and the Health Care Professions, Family Process, Health Care Management Review, Hospital Administration, Journal*

of the American Medical Association, Journal of Educational Psychology, Journal of Educational Research, Journal of Marriage and the Family, Medical Care, New England Journal of Medicine, and *Pediatrics.* Journal articles typically will describe the measurement device or instrument, but they may or may not include the instrument in its totality; in the case of a biomedical device, they may not give the complete specifications. Usually communication with the author of the paper is the most efficient route to gain additional information about the instrument.

Additional major resources for investigators are compendia of instruments and resource books. Compendia and resource books range from those that include a compilation of instruments and detailed descriptions of instrument development to those that include only citations of instruments that have been classified according to topic. Two sources specific to nursing include Ward and Fetler's (1979) publication, *Instruments for Use in Nursing Education Research* and Ward and Lindeman's (1978) publication, *Instruments for Measuring Nursing Practice and Other Health Care Variables.* In both volumes, instruments are described and reproduced. For most instruments included in these volumes, psychometric information about the instrument and its applications is available.

Instruments developed in related fields are described in several compendia. Attitudinal measures are described in Robinson and Shaver (1973) and Shaw and Wright (1967); behavioral measures are described in Andrulis (1977) and Ciminero, Calhoun, and Adams (1970). Health-related measures are described in Comrey, Backer, and Glaser (1973), Lyerly (1973), and Reeder, Ramacher, and Gorelnik (1976). Other general compendia include Anastasi (1976), Buros (1974; 1978), Chun, Cobb, and French (1975), Goldman and Saunders (1974), and Miller (1977). Biological and physiological measures are described in Bauer (1982), Cromwell, Weibell, and Pfeiffer (1980), Ferris (1980), Geddes and Baker (1975), and Weiss (1973) (see also Appendix B).

APPLYING A MEASURE

Application of an instrument is as important to assuring the validity of the study findings as is the initial selection of the instrument. Consideration of sources of variation in measurement scores and strategies for minimizing measurement error are essential as investigators apply various measurement techniques in their research.

Sources of variation in measurement scores

Observed scores on any instrument can be considered to have two components: a true component and an error component. If X represents the individual's score, then

$$X_o = X_t \pm X_e$$

where X_o is the observed score, X_t is the true score, and X_e is the error component. The observed score (X_o) is the actual value the investigator obtains by using the instrument. The true component (X_t) is the hypothetical value that would be obtained in the absence of the error component (X_e). The error component (X_e) represents errors of measurement or distortion in X_t. For example, an observed score for weight might be 120 pounds, whereas the true score is really 119.6 pounds. The error component would be .4 pounds.

True difference in the characteristic one is attempting to measure is a valid and desirable source of variation. A measure of self-esteem should yield different scores when given to people who have high and low levels of self-esteem. Another source of variation in measurement is attributable to true differences in relatively stable characteristics of the individuals being studied, such as gender, education, and age; this variation results in a systematic influence within a group of scores. These systematic differences can be accounted for if their influence on the variable measured is considered when the results of the study are analyzed. For example, self-esteem varies systematically with gender in adults, thus self-esteem scores for men and women can be analyzed separately or gender can be included in the analysis when the investigator is considering the influence of other study variables on self-esteem.

Sources of measurement error

Sources of measurement error are many, including the participants, the context for measurement, and the instrument. We will discuss each of these in turn.

Errors related to participants

Errors of measurement induced by the participants include response sets and transitory factors affecting the person. In some studies investigators face the challenge of a socially desirable (or undesirable) response. In studies of very threatening topics, people may be too embarrassed to reveal information they believe is deviant or socially undesirable. Imagine the plight of hospitalized people who must rate their satisfaction with nursing care. Chances are the ratings will be good, particularly if the hospitalized person feels some risk of offending the caregivers. On the other hand, if people perceive that no great risk exists and they are very dissatisfied, they may rate the entire range of nursing care as poor, including those aspects that were not. Acquiescent response sets occur when people endorse every item on a measure such as those on a symptoms check list, perceiving that they are pleasing the investigator by doing so. Extreme response sets occur when people strongly agree or strongly disagree with every item on a questionnaire or scale. Transitory factors that affect participants include variation in attention span, mood, and state of health, for example, people simply have "bad days" when their test results do not reflect their normal levels of well-being.

Errors related to study context

Measurement error also is related to the context of the study. For example, being aware that responses are not private, as occurs when individuals are interviewed in the presence of other family members, may encourage participants to respond differently than they would if privacy and anonymity were guaranteed. Measurements of physiological values known to vary with time of day (diurnal variation) need to be scheduled at a similar time, if not at the same time, each day the measurement will occur. When the interviewer has difficulty establishing rapport with the respondent and the respondent seems suspicious, the measurement results will probably be distorted. Circumstances surrounding the administration of instruments may vary and thus may introduce variability in the results. For example, interviewers may change the way they ask questions so that some questions may be asked in different words, some may be embellished, and some even omitted. When this occurs, the participants are not responding to identical stimuli, and consequently their responses are likely to vary.

Errors related to the instrument and its use

Other sources of variability are related directly to the instrument. Paper-and-pencil measures related to a specific construct, such as "demands of illness," may not measure every indicant of the construct but measure only a sample of the indicants that could represent the construct's meaning, such as changes in family adaptation, integration, and decision-making. As a result, the picture of the demands experienced by families as a consequence of illness may be incomplete. Differences also may be attributable to a lack of clarity of items. People responding to the instrument may interpret the items differently from the investigator.

Mechanical factors such as poor layout of a questionnaire or poorly printed directions may contribute to response differences. Careful pretesting of instruments can help investigators identify these problems before the data collection begins. Differences caused by the format of instruments also may account for different responses. For example, a written questionnaire requires different levels of verbal fluency and reading ability than does an interview. When both methods are used interchangeably in a study, inconsistency in responses may be attributable to the use of different methods rather than to differences in true scores. Differences that result from errors in coding, scoring, and tabulation of results from instruments also can be responsible for the error components of scores.

When using an instrument to measure biological or physiological phenomena, such as blood pressure, the investigator must ascertain that the instrument is calibrated to yield accurate measurement. Recalibrating an instrument often is essential on many occasions throughout a study. The purpose of repeated calibration is to ensure that all measurements are accurate throughout the course of the study and that the measurements obtained at an early point in the study are directly comparable to those obtained at later points in the study.

Strategies for minimizing measurement error

Although the sources of measurement error are many, investigators can use many strategies for minimizing them. Providing privacy during interviews or experiments can attenuate the likelihood of measurement error related to study participants. For example, the people being interviewed can be given the most threatening items written on cards and asked to sort them into different piles according to the response format, obviating the need to discuss embarrassing items with the interviewer. Participants can also be given written questions and an envelope in which to seal the responses instead of telling the investigator the answers to the most threatening questions. Additionally the investigator can avoid inducing a socially desirable response set by "unloading the questions," a technique in which the investigator points out that a range of behaviors and beliefs exists, thus assuring participants that their responses are not highly unusual. The skill of the interviewer in eliciting accurate responses is paramount, and an interviewer who is capable of establishing rapport with participants often is amazed at the information that study participants are willing to share. Establishing rapport will be discussed in greater detail in Chapter 19.

The investigator also can identify and document the mood, fatigue level, or other obvious transient changes in the participants. A sensitive interviewer knows when rescheduling of interviews is preferable to continuing and learns to recognize participants' signals that warrant their returning on another occasion.

The investigator can manipulate the context of the study to decrease measurement error. Adhering to careful instructions regarding privacy for the parcipants and to the protocols for physiological measures and others, teaching interviewers how to develop rapport, and promoting emotional and physical comfort and safety for the participants also are essential elements for reducing error and maximizing validity and reliability of the data.

The investigator who has carefully screened the instrumentation for the study has already begun to minimize measurement error. The investigator has ensured that the instrument adequately samples the content domain; it contains clearly written directions and items; it has mechanical properties that meet the requirements of the study and is appropriate for the population; and it has technical specifications that assure its validity and reliability. The final step is screening completed measures for coding or scoring errors and checking data that have been entered into a computer file for accuracy. These steps are discussed in detail in Chapter 24.

Triangulation

Triangulation is a strategy that is useful to increase the precision of research measurement (Denzin, 1970; Mitchell, 1986; Smith, 1975). Many procedures for triangulation exist, but one type involves the triangulation of data collected by different measures. For example, an investigator may wish to use multiple measures of the same concept. In a study of well-being, it may be desirable to use physiological, observational, and paper-and-pencil measures of varying dimensions of health. In some studies investigators may choose a combination of methods, particularly when they wish to have perspectives about a topic from both the participants and the investigators. In a study of perimenstrual symptoms, women could be asked to record their symptoms and to rate symptom severity in a daily diary for several menstrual cycles. At the completion of the diary, the investigator could ask the women which symptoms they find most distressing. Some women might describe one set of symptoms as most depressing when they are interviewed despite the fact that they rated other symptoms most severe in the diary. Were the investigator to ask another person living in the household which symptoms were most severe, it is likely that yet another group of symptoms would be identified. This pattern of findings would indicate that different perceptions of women's experiences emerge when different measures are used. Using a combination of measures provides a more complete picture of the construct being studied than a single measure would convey (Denzin, 1970; Smith, 1975).

DEVELOPING AN INSTRUMENT

Once the investigator identifies the concept of interest, she or he searches existing literature for an appropriate measure. Because of the newness of nursing science, frequently there are no measures that appropriately reflect the concept of interest. When no appropriate measure is available, the investigtor faces the challenge of developing an instrument. The processes involved in developing an instrument are complex. We will consider these processes briefly. A more sophisticated discussion of instrument development can be found in Edwards (1957); Nunnally (1978); and Waltz, Strickland, and Lenz (1984) and in Chapter 18.

Many types of instruments are used in nursing research, including physiological measures, observation guides, interview guides, questionnaires, and scales. Regardless of the type of measure, the investigator begins by considering the concept or phenomenon to be measured. After carefully describing the concept, the investigator proceeds to specify possible indicators. In developing observational guides, interview measures, questionnaires, or scales, investigators usually begin by generating multiple indicators of the phenomenon, for example, a large item pool reflecting multiple dimensions of the concept. For physical, chemical, or biochemical and microbiological measures, the investigator also carefully specifies the phenomena to be measured, reviews the technical approaches possible for measuring them, and develops specific procedures to be used for the assay or physiological measurement. Once the item pool or procedure is developed, the investigator then must test the procedure for technical adequacy. The validity and reliability of biological measures or biochemical assays and questionnaires are determined in multiple ways. These will be discussed in detail in Chapter 16. In brief, the measure is typically tested on one or more populations to assess its technical adequacy. Instruments must meet the standards of the scientific community, including sufficient sampling of the domain with an adequate item pool of a scale or measuring the correct substance with a biochemical assay. Moreover, the technical qualities required by the scientific community need to be demonstrated; these technical qualities include factors such as the accuracy, sensitivity, and reproducibility of an assay for a hormone or the validity and reproducibility of results on a scale measuring a psychological construct such as anxiety. The investigator usually publishes norms obtained through the application of the instrument to one or more populations. These norms provide a reference point for future investigators. In addition, explicit guidelines for using the instrument are essential. These include protocols for calibration of biological instrumentation systems or directions for administration, scoring, and interpretation of questionnaires.

Let us consider the development of the uncertainty in illness scale as an example. Mishel (1981) proposed that uncertainty was one of the conditions producing a stress response in hospitalized patients. Uncertainty in the form of ambiguity, vagueness, unpredictability, and lack of information pervade hospitalization, but these conditions had not been studied systematically at the time Mishel began her work. Mishel's model of uncertainty in illness uses the process of appraisal to link the individual's perception of illness-related events to responses to the events. She reasoned that a high degree of uncertainty decreased the use of direct actions and information seeking and encouraged intrapsychic modes of coping such as vigilance and avoidance.

Mishel began constructing the uncertainty in illness scale through a exploratory study to identify events perceived as uncertain with interviews of 45 hospitalized patients. The interviews centered on illness-related tasks. A panel of judges determined 62 statements to reflect the concept of uncertainty. These statements were rewritten into 54 items such as:

I don't know what is wrong with me.
My treatment is too complex to figure out.
When I have pain I know what it means about my condition.
I can generally predict the course of my illness.

The early scale contained items worded both positively and negatively. The items were thought to reflect ambiguity, lack of information, unpredictability, and lack of clarity. The 54-item scale was constructed on a 5-point Likert scale and subsequently reviewed by nurses, physicians, and general medical and surgical patients to check the wording of the items. Rewording of the items and elimination of some items resulted from this review.

The scale was then administered to medical and surgical patients. Factor analysis (Chapter 27) was used to determine the clustering of items. Two factors, ambiguity and unpredictability, were identified. The reliability of the factors was assessed through the use of a measure of internal consistency. When the factor analysis was repeated on a second group of 100 patients, the items clustered similarly on the original factors of ambiguity and unpredictability. A series of validation studies revealed that the uncertainty in illness scale discriminated between a sample of patients who were having diagnostic workups and a sample of patients who had already been diagnosed. In addition, the uncertainty in illness scores were related to the degree of stress experienced by hospitalized patients. Finally, the uncertainty in illness scores were related to patients' scores on tests of comprehension.

SUMMARY

Measurement decisions constitute important transition points from the conceptual phase to the empirical phase of research. Because of the complexity of phenomena that nurses study, most investigators use several sources of information; for example, individuals provide information ranging from physiological phenomena to thoughts and feelings.

In most nursing studies, investigators measure variables that represent the concepts central to the study. Often the concepts studied by nurses are more abstract than concrete, necessitating careful identification of their empirical referents. Operationalizing concepts involves specifying the constitutive definition guiding measurement decisions, specifying the dimensions of the concept's meaning that can vary, identifying observable indicators, and selecting ways of measuring variables.

Both quantitative and qualitative measurement are used in nursing research. In both instances, the investigator must assign objects to values that represent variations of the concept being studied. Nominal, ordinal, interval, and ratio variables are common in nursing studies. The level of measurement used in a study influences the types of statistical analyses permissible.

Results obtained with measuring instruments often are expressed as a scale score on one or more dimensions of a concept. A scale is a set of symbols or numerals constructed so that the symbols or numerals can be assigned by rule to characteristics of individuals to whom the scale is applied. Scales consist of a stem statement relating to the attitude or other phenomenon to be rated, a series of scale steps, and anchors defining the scale steps. Several types of scales are used commonly in nursing research, including Likert scales, summated scales, cumulative scales, and semantic differential scales. Visual analog scaling and magnitude estimation techniques recently have been incorporated into nursing studies.

Ideal measuring instruments possess the characteristics of validity, reliability, sensitivity, and relevance to the population studied. Choosing a measure requires reflection about the purpose for acquiring the information the measure would yield. Investigators need to consider the concept and its definition and dimensions, the purpose of the investigation, the content of the measure, psychometric properties, measurement norms, the procedure for administration of the measure, directions for scoring or rating the results, and ease, time, and cost of using the measure. Resources useful in selecting measurement instruments and devices include professional journals and instrument compendia.

Application of the measure requires that investigators consider the sources of variation in measurement scores and strategies for minimizing measurement error. Sources of measurement error include the participants, the context for measurement, and the instrument. Strategies for minimizing measurement error include providing privacy to participants, enhancing comfort of the participants by establishing rapport, identifying and documenting the mood, fatigue level, or other transient changes in the participants, manipulating the context of the study by adhering to instructions for administration of the instrument, assuring that the instrument adequately samples the content domain and is appropriate for the population using triangulation with other measures, and maintaining the calibration of physiological instruments.

Development of an instrument is a complex process. After carefully describing the concept to be measured, the investigator specifies possible indicators, reviews the approaches for measuring them, and develops specific procedures for measurement. Next, the investigator tests the procedure for its adequacy by establishing reliability and validity. Pretesting the instrument with the intended population is essential before establishing the utility of the instrument.

The process of instrument development is complex and time-consuming, but essential if nursing concepts are to be studied accurately. In the following chapter we will consider issues related to validity and reliability of measurement in greater detail.

REFERENCES

Aiken, R. (1969). Measurement of feelings using analogue scales. *Proceedings of the Royal Society of Medicine, 62,* 989-996.

Anastasi, A. (1976). *Psychological testing.* New York: Macmillan.

Andrulis, R. (1977). *A source book of tests and measures of human behavior.* Springfield, IL: Charles C Thomas.

Barrera, M. (1981). Social support in the adjustment of pregnant adolescents: Assessment issues. In B. Gottlieb (Ed.) *Social networks and social support* (pp. 69-96). Beverly Hills, CA: Sage.

Bauer, J. (1982). *Clinical laboratory methods* (9th ed.). St. Louis: Mosby.

Bergner, M., Babbit, R., Kressel, S., Pollard, W., Gilson, B., & Morris, J. (1976). The sickness impact profile: Conceptual formulation and methodology for the development of a health status measure. *International Journal of Health Services, 6*(3), 393-415.

Bond, A., & Lader, M. (1974). The use of analogue scales in rating subjective feelings. *British Journal of Medical Psychology, 47,* 211-218.

Bowles, C. (1985). Measure of attitude toward menopause using the semantic differential model. *Nursing Research, 35,* 81-85.

Buros, O. (1974). *Tests in print two.* Highland Park, NJ: Gryphon Press.

Buros, O. (1978). *The eighth mental measurements yearbook.* Highland Park, NJ: Gryphon Press.

Chunn, K., Cobb, S., & French, J. (1975). *Measures for psychological assessment.* Ann Arbor, MI: Survey Research Center.

Ciminero, A., Calhoun, O., & Adams, J. (1970). *Handbook of behavioral assessment.* New York: Wiley.

Comrey, A., Bacher, T., & Glaser, E. (1973). *A sourcebook for mental health measures.* Los Angeles: Human Interaction Research Institute.

Cromwell, L., Weibell, F., & Pfeiffer, E. (1980). *Biomedical instrumentation and measurements,* (2nd ed.). Englewood Cliffs, NJ: Prentice-Hall.

Cronbach, L. (1970). *Essentials of psychological testing.* New York: Harper and Row.

Cronbach, L., & Snow, R. (1976). *Aptitudes and instructional methods.* New York: Irvington.

Cronenwett, L. (1985). Network structure, social support, and psychological outcomes of pregnancy. *Nursing Research, 34,* 93-99.

Cronenwett, L. (1985). Parental network structure and perceived support after birth of first child. *Nursing Research, 34,* 347-352.

Denzin, N. (1970). Strategies of multiple triangulation. In N. Denzin, (Ed.), *The research act.* Chicago: Aldine.

Dixon, J., & Bird, H. (1981). Reproducibility along a 10 cm vertical visual analogue scale. *Annals of the Rheumatic Diseases, 40,* 87-89.

Edwards, A. (1957). *Techniques of attitude scale construction.* New York: Appleton-Century-Crofts.

Edwards, A. (1981). *Techniques of attitude scale construction.* New York: Irvington.

Fawcett, J., & Downs, F. (1986). *The relationship of theory and research.* Appleton-Century-Crofts.

Ferris, C. (1980). *Guide to medical laboratory instruments.* Boston: Little, Brown.

Foley, J. (1982). *Sex differences in recovery from myocardial infarction.* Unpublished master's thesis. University of Washington, Seattle.

Geddes, L., & Baker, L. (1975). *Principles of applied biomedical instrumentation.* New York: John Wiley.

Germino, B. (1984). *Family members' concerns after cancer diagnosis.* Unpublished doctoral dissertation, University of Washington, Seattle.

Goldman, B., & Saunders, J. (1974). *Dictionary of unpublished experimental measures.* New York: Behavioral Publications.

Guttman, L. (1949). The basis for scalogram analysis. In *Studies in social psychology in World War II: Vol. 4. Measurement and prediction.* Princeton, NJ: Princeton University Press. (Reprinted from *Bobs Merrill Reprint* s-413.)

Heitkemper, M., & Marotta, S. (1985). Role of diets in modifying gastrointestinal neurotransmitter enzyme activity. *Nursing Research, 34,* 19-23.

Hinshaw, A., & Schepp, K. (1983). Territorial intrusion and client outcomes: The use of magnitude estimation. *Communicating Nursing Research, 16,* 77.

Kaplan, A. (1964). *The conduct of inquiry.* San Francisco: Chandler.

Kerlinger, F. (1986). *Foundations of behavioral research.* New York: Holt, Rinehart, & Winston.

Laffrey, S. (1986). Development of a health conception scale. *Research in Nursing & Health, 9*(2), 107-113.

Lewis, F., Firsich, S., & Parsell, S. (1979). Clinical tool development and accuracy for adult chemotherapy patients: Process and content. *Cancer Nursing, 2*(2), 99-108.

Likert, R. (1932). A technique for the measurement of attitudes. *Archives of Psychology, 22,* 5-55.

Lowery, B., & Jacobson, B. (1985). Attributional analysis of chronic illness outcomes. *Nursing Research, 34,* 82-88.

Lyerly, S. (1973). *Handbook of psychiatric rating scales.* Rockville, MD: National Institute of Mental Health.

Maxwell, C. (1978). Sensitivity and accuracy of the visual analogue scale: A psycho-physical classroom experiment. *British Journal of Clinical Pharmacology, 6,* 15-24.

Meleis, A. (1985). *Theoretical nursing.* Philadelphia: Lippincott.

Miller, D. (1977). *Handbook of research design and social measurement.* New York: David McKay.

Mishel, M. (1981). The measurement of uncertainty in illness. *Nursing Research, 30,* 258-263.

Mitchell, E. (1986). Multiple triangulation: A methodology for nursing science. *Advances in Nursing Science, 8*(3), 18-26.

Morgan, B. (1984). A semantic differential measure of attitudes toward black American patients. *Research in Nursing and Health, 7,* 155-162.

Murphy, E. (1978). *The logic of medicine.* Baltimore: Johns Hopkins University Press.

Norbeck, J. (1984). Modification of life-event questionnaire for use with female respondents. *Research in Nursing and Health, 7,* 61-71.

Nunnally, J. (1978). *Psychometric theory.* New York: McGraw-Hill.

Orem, D. (1985). *Nursing: Concepts of practice.* New York: McGraw-Hill.

Osgood, C., Suci, G., & Tannenbaum, P. (1957). *The measurement of meaning.* Urbana, IL: University of Illinois Press.

Padilla, G., Presant, C., Grant, M., Metter, G., Lipsett, J., & Heide, F. (1983). Quality of life index for patients with cancer. *Research in Nursing and Health, 6,* 117-126.

Reeder, L., Ramacher, L., & Gorelnik, S. (1976). *Handbook of scales and indices of health behavior.* Pacific Palisades, CA: Goodyear.

Revill, S., Robinson, J., Rosen, M., & Hogg, M. (1976). The reliability of a linear analogue for evaluating pain. *Anaesthesia, 31,* 1191-1198.

Richardson, M., & Kagan, L. (1979). Social support and the transition to parenthood. Presented at American Psychological Association, New York.

Robinson, J., & Shaver, P. (1973). *Measures of social psychological attitudes.* Ann Arbor, MI: Survey Research Center.

Selltiz, C., Wrightsman, L., & Cook, S. (1976). *Research methods in social relations.* New York: Holt, Rinehart, & Winston.

Sennott-Miller, L., Murdaugh, C., & Hinshaw, A. (in press). Magnitude estimation: Issues and practical applications. *Western Journal of Nursing Research.*

Shannahan, M., & Cottrell, B. (1985). Effect of the birth chair on duration of second labor, fetal outcome and maternal blood loss. *Nursing Research, 34,* 89-92.

Shaw, M., & Wright, M. (1967). *Scales for the measurement of attitudes.* New York: McGraw-Hill.

Sivarajan, E., Bruce, R., Almes, J., Green, B., Belanger, L., Lindskog, B., Newton, K., & Mansfield, L. (1981). In Hospital exercise after myocardial infarction does not improve treadmill performance. *New England Journal of Medicine, 305*(7), 357-362.

Smith, H. (1975). Triangulation: The necessity for multimethod approaches. In H. Smith, (Ed.), *Strategies of social research: The methodological imagination.* Englewood Cliffs, NJ: Prentice-Hall.

Smith, J. A. (1981). The idea of health: A philosophical inquiry. *Advances in Nursing Science, 3,* 43-50.

Stevens, S. (1946). On the theory of scales of measurement. *Science, 103,* 677-680.

Stevens, S. (1957). On the psychophysical law. *Psychological Review, 64,* 153-181.

Thorndike, R., & Hagen, E. (1969). *Measurement and evaluation in psychology and education.* New York: Wiley.

Tripp-Reimer, T. (1984). Reconceptualizing the construct of health: Integrating and perspectives. *RINAH, 7,* 101-110.

Waltz, C., Strickland, O., & Lenz, E. (1984). *Measurement in nursing research.* Philadelphia: F A Davis.

Ward, M., & Fetler, M. (1979). *Instruments for use in nursing education research.* Boulder, CO: Western Interstate Commission for Higher Education.

Ward, M., & Lindeman, C. (1978). *Instruments for measuring nursing practice and other health variables* (Vols. 1-2). Washington, DC: U. S. Government Printing Office.

Webb, E., Campbell, R., Schwartz, R., & Sechrest, L. (1966). *Unobtrusive measures: Nonreactive research in the social sciences.* Chicago: Rand McNally.

Weiss, M. (1973). *Biomedical instrumentation.* Philadelphia: Chelton.

Williams, M., Campbell, E., Raynor, W., Musholt, M., Mlynarczyk, S., & Crane, L. (1985). Predicators of acute confusional states in hospitalized elderly patients. *Research in Nursing and Health, 8,* 31-40.

Williams, M., Holloway, J., Winn, M., Wolanin, M., Lawler, M., Westwick, C., & Chin, M. (1979). Nursing activities and acute confusional states in elderly hip-fractured patients. *Nursing Research, 28,* 25-35.

15

ASSESSING NURSING RESEARCH MEASURES: RELIABILITY AND VALIDITY

NANCY FUGATE WOODS

Measurement of nursing phenomena is a major challenge to investigators. Because many new constructs are relevant to nursing theory and few established measuring instruments are available to researchers, investigators frequently face the challenge of developing new instruments. Reliability and validity are of great concern whether an investigator chooses to use an available instrument or must develop an appropriate measure.

In Chapter 14 we reviewed many characteristics of ideal measuring instruments, including reliability and validity. Ideally, all instruments would possess these characteristics, but in reality few if any instruments meet all of these criteria. Nevertheless, validity and reliability are characteristics so important to the quality of measurement that most investigators invariably rank them first among their considerations.

This chapter includes definitions of the reliability and validity of measurement instruments and a discussion of their relationship to measurement error. We will look at the many ways to operationally define reliability and validity and consider them with respect to instrument selection and development.

RELIABILITY

Although dependability, stability, consistency, predictability, and accuracy are often used synonymous-

ly with reliability these terms actually describe slightly different aspects of reliability. Stability, dependability, and predictability all refer to the instrument's ability to produce the same results on repeated measurement occasions. Accuracy implies a second aspect of reliability: the instrument's ability to reflect the true value being measured. This aspect of reliability relates to the amount of measurement error in measurements made with a particular instrument. The greater the amount of measurement error present in the application of a measuring instrument, the less reliable is the information the instrument provides. Indeed, reliability can be defined as the absence of errors of measurement. The performance of two thermometers to measure temperature illustrates reliability as precision. As seen in Table 15-1 the first thermometer produces scattered results about the true temperature values, whereas the second thermometer precisely and dependably reproduces similar values each time. In the case of a thermometer used in the same manner on repeated occasions, we would expect reproducible, dependable values on every occasion of its use, with only a small amount of random measurement error in each measure.

Reliability and measurement theory

Before looking more closely at ways to assess the stability and accuracy of a measure, we must consider

TABLE 15-1. Frequency of observations of temperature given by two thermometers in a water bath standardized at 97.8° F

TEMPERATURE	THERMOMETER 1	THERMOMETER 2
97.4	0	0
97.5	0	0
97.6	1	0
97.7	1	0
97.8	2	9
97.9	1	1
98.0	3	0
98.1	1	0
98.2	1	0
98.3	0	0

the relationship of reliability to measurement theory. In the discussion of measurement in Chapter 14 we noted the two types of measurement error, systematic and random. When considering the reliability of a measurement instrument, we focus on random error, which is due to temporary conditions in the individual, context, or instrument administration that vary over time. Random error interferes with reliability of measurement. Because of random error the measurement will show variation in the characteristic being measured when actually none exists. For example, in the measurement of temperature random error introduces distortion caused by temperature fluctuation in the room, thermometer placement, and the person's attempting to talk, despite the fact that the person's true body temperature remains stable over several occasions of measurement.

Recall that the observed score obtained from any instrument reflects the "true" score or value, as well as an "error" score. The *observed value,* in the case of temperature measurement, is the actual value the researcher obtains when using the particular instrument. The observed value contains not only the information reflecting the hypothetical "true" value of the person's temperature, but also the *random error* induced by, among other factors, slight differences in placement of the thermometer on each occasion of measurement.

When considering scores derived from instruments that contain several items, such as the scores from a Likert scale, the total variance in the score on the instrument is analogous to the observed score for

a measurement of a single parameter measure such as temperature. The *total variance* in the score from a scale contains information from the true values *(true variance),* as well as errors of measurement *(error variance).* True variance is obtained only under the ideal conditions of no measurement error. Reliability reflects the proportion of true variance to total variance in the measure. In other words,

$$\text{Reliability} = \frac{\text{True variance}}{\text{Total variance}}$$

The reliability of measurements is the proportion of the total variance that is true variance, what would have been obtained under the ideal conditions of no measurement error.

Reliability often is described as a coefficient ranging from 0 to 1. *Reliability coefficients* are obtained through variations on the relationship between true variance, error variance, and total variance. The relationship

$$\text{Reliability} = 1 - \frac{\text{Error variance}}{\text{Total variance}}$$

is used to estimate reliability of measures. The greater the error variance, the larger the part of the equation error variance/total variance will be. When this part of the equation is large, the reliability coefficient is small. Likewise, when error variance is small, the reliability coefficient is large. A reliability coefficient of zero would indicate that all of the variance is due to measurement error, whereas a coefficient of one would indicate that no measurement error exists.

Interpreting reliability coefficients

Interpreting reliability coefficients is based on the proposed purpose of the measure. Reliability coefficients are coefficients of determination; when reliability coefficients are squared, they represent the proportion of variance of a measured variable that is true variance. A reliability coefficient of .8 indicates that the measure reflects .64 of the true variance of the measured variable.

The instrument's intended application determines the range in which the coefficient must fall. Some studies require higher reliability than others. When the investigator is using the measure for group-level comparisons, the reliability coefficient typically must exceed .7 for new scales and .8 for mature scales (see Edwards [1981] and Nunnally [1978] for a more detailed discussion of this topic). A reliability coefficient of .7 indicates that 50% of the variance in the scores obtained with the instrument is error variance. When the measure is being used as the basis for a lifesaving decision such as an ECG interpretation, the reliability coefficient must be much higher, usually .9, or above.

Reliability estimates are population-dependent measures, meaning that use of the same instrument with vastly different populations probably will result in different reliability estimates. For example, a measure that is reliable for outpatients may be quite unreliable for hospitalized, critically ill patients. Stability of internal consistency measures across studies of various populations increases the investigator's confidence in the reliability of measurement of the construct.

Estimating reliability

Each of the several ways of estimating reliability reflects a different type of information about an instrument's performance. The investigator who is concerned with the stability of repeated measures over several occasions is most likely to be concerned with the stability or reproducibility dimension of reliability. The investigator who is concerned particularly with the accuracy of the instrument is likely to be concerned with the equivalence of the measure with some other form of measurement or with the extent to which the scale measures only a specific phenomenon. No single "correct" way of assessing reliability exists; what is important is the investigator's assessment of the critical features of reliability in the context of the specific investigation.

Stability. The investigator who is considering using serial measures of the same phenomenon over time often is concerned with the stability aspect of reliability. This form of reliability is extremely important when the same measure will be applied at two or more points in time, such as occurs in a panel study or time series design. Stability is also extremely important when the investigator plans to study an intervention that is designed to change the level of a specific phenomenon in the population. One way to establish stability is to administer the measurement once and then again later at a specified time. This type of reliability is termed *test-retest reliability*.

Determining the appropriate time interval involves several considerations. First, the interval between measurements may vary, but it should reflect the approximate interval intended for future applications of the measure. The investigator also should consider how quickly the phenomenon itself is likely to change when estimating the interval for measurement. It would be foolish to estimate test-retest reliability from measures taken over a span of time that exceeds the real change exhibited in the construct being measured. For example, some enduring traits such as anxiety change rather slowly, whereas state anxiety, the type of anxiety related to a specific situation, changes more quickly. The investigator assessing the stability of a state anxiety measure could consider a short period of time, perhaps only 1 or 2 days, adequate to assess the reliability of the measure, whereas the reliability of a measure of trait anxiety might be estimated over several months. Finally a longer time interval between testing usually results in a lower stability of the two measures. Shorter time intervals between testing increase the likelihood that participants simply remember the way they answered the test on the first occasion.

The test-retest approach is designed to yield similar findings on subsequent occasions and is most appropriate for assessing the reliability of relatively stable traits. Nevertheless, it is important for the investigator to remember that some phenomena do change between the testing occasions. In addition, some events do occur between the two measurement occasions that influence the "true" value of the phenomenon being measured. For example, some participants may remember their responses to the first administration of a test or questionnaire, and their memories may influence their responses on a subsequent occasion, thus inflating the reliability coefficient. Women who rate their knowledge about breast self-examination on one occasion may become extremely interested in the topic and become better informed before being assessed on a second occasion, thus changing their scores and decreasing the reliability estimate. Finally, some may find it boring to repeat the same measures several times and answer the items without thinking about them in the same way as they did on the first occasion, ultimately decreasing the reliability estimate.

The test-retest method of assessing reliability tells the investigator about the relative stability of the rank order of respondents over time. A high stability coefficient indicates that measurements (e.g., scores or responses) changed very little between the test and the retest. In addition, a high stability coefficient reveals that the instrument measures the same phenomenon on each occasion. Stability reliability is indicated by a simple zero-order correlation coefficient between the two sets of scores. The Pearson product-moment correlation, the Spearman rank correlation, or another parametric or nonparametric correlation coefficient may be used. The higher the correlation coefficient, the greater the stability of the measure.

Norbeck, Lindsey, and Carrieri (1983) assessed the stability of the Norbeck Social Support Questionnaire by asking 75 master's-degree nursing students to complete the questionnaire at admission to graduate school and 7 months later. They assumed the composition of the social-support network might change but that the level of affect, affirmation, and aid would not change. As seen in Table 15-2, only the number in the network and the duration of the relationships changed significantly over the 7 months. Each correlation for the subscales as measured on two occasions was large enough to be statistically significant.

Internal consistency. Internal consistency refers to the homogeneity of the measuring instrument. The greater the reliability coefficient reflecting internal consistency, the greater the likelihood that the scale measures the attribute of interest and nothing else. The assessment of internal consistency rests on the covariance or intercorrelations among all the items in an instrument. The greater the intercorrelations, the greater the instrument's internal consistency.

Internal consistency estimates rest on the assumption that the instrument is designed to be unidimensional, that is, to measure only one concept. The researcher should be able to add the individual items to obtain a total score, because all items would be intended to reflect the same concept. Internal consistency estimates are based on all the items in a unidimensional scale. However, some instruments are multidimensional, for example, the Patient Satisfaction Instrument developed by Risser (1975) and modified by Hinshaw and Atwood (1982) includes three dimensions: technical-professional factors, trusting relationship, and education relationship. Technical-professional factors refer to technical

TABLE 15-2. Means, standard deviations, and test-retest correlations for initial and 7-month follow-up measures for the Norbeck Social Support Questionnaire

SUBSCALE	TIME 1*	TIME 2*	CORRELATION (PEARSON'S r)
Affect	103 ± 43	96 ± 41	.78
Affirmation	96 ± 41	89 ± 38	.78
Aid	74 ± 28	68 ± 26	.58
Total scales			.76
Number in network	13 ± 5	11 ± 5	.75
Duration of relationships	54 ± 22	47 ± 19	.75

Data from Norbeck (1982).
N = 44. All correlations are statistically significant at $p < .0001$ level.
*Mean ± standard deviation.

TABLE 15-3. Internal consistency estimates for subscales of the patient satisfaction instrument

STUDY	TECHNICAL-PROFESSIONAL	EDUCATION	TRUSTING
1976	.97	.95	.98
1980	.82	.83	.87

Data from Hinshaw and Atwood (1982).

activities and the knowledge base required to competently complete the nursing-care tasks, whereas trusting relationship refers to nursing characteristics that allow for constructive and comfortable patient-nurse interaction and communication aspects of the interaction. Education relationship refers to nurses' ability to provide information for patients, including answering questions, explaining care, and demonstrating techniques. These three dimensions comprise the objects of patient satisfaction (Hinshaw & Atwood, 1982). Instruments that contain multiple dimensions require separate internal consistency—reliability estimates for each dimension, as is shown in Table 15-3 for the Patient Satisfaction Instrument.

ASSESSING INTERNAL-CONSISTENCY RELIABILITY. Investigators commonly use four methods to assess internal-consistency reliability. The most common approach to estimating internal consistency is *Cronbach's alpha,* which is based on the intercorrelation or covariance of all the items in a scale examined simultaneously. In theory, alpha varies from 0 to 1, with 1 denoting perfect internal consistency and 0 no internal consistency.* In the reliability assessment of the Patient Satisfaction Index, Hinshaw and Atwood (1982) found in two recent studies of patient satisfaction with inpatient care that the alpha coefficients for the three subscales ranged from .82 to 0.98.

The *Kuder-Richardson (KR-20) coefficient* is an-

other estimate of internal-consistency reliability of a scale; it is designed to be used for *dichotomous scales* (having only two responses, such as yes and no). KR-20 theoretically varies from 0 to 1 with the highest values denoting the highest internal-consistency reliability.

Item-total correlations are also a function of the degree of interrelatedness of all the items in a scale measuring only a single concept. The item-total correlation is not a single statistic like Cronbach's alpha or the Kuder-Richardson value, it is instead a group of single correlations between each item and the total score for the entire scale. The item-total correlations indicate the extent to which the individual items relate to the total score for the entire instrument. Item-total correlations are very useful in instrument development: the investigator can use the correlations when deciding which items to retain and which to discard when formulating the final item pool. Item-total correlations should be high enough to indicate internal consistency but low enough to indicate that the items are not redundant (see Scott, 1968).

Split-half reliability involves correlating the scores on two halves of an instrument. The items are divided into two groups, such as odd and even or randomly, and these halves are then correlated with one another. A correction formula for the shortened scales (each of the two halves is shorter than the total scale) called the Spearman-Brown correction formula* then is applied. This approach can yield slightly

---

*Occasionally, an investigator will obtain a negative alpha value for a scale, indicating that some of the scale values that were stated opposite to the scale's orientation should have been recoded and were not. For example, on a depression scale for which the highest score indicated the greatest degree of depression, the item "I felt on top of the world" would need to be recoded so that high values indicated depression, not happiness. Failure to recode similar items could produce a negative alpha value.

---

*Spearman-Brown correction formula:

$$r = \frac{2r'}{1 + r'}$$

r, estimate of reliability; r', correlation on split halves.

different estimates of internal consistency depending on the way in which the items are divided. For example, the correlation from an odd-even division may not be exactly the same as the correlation from two random groups of items.

Estimating internal-consistency reliability should be given high priority when accuracy and precision are important. An investigator who cannot be assured that the instrument really measures the concept of interest can only guess at the accuracy of the findings. When estimating the relationship between concepts or the size of the difference between groups or over time, internal-consistency reliability is extremely important. Unreliability (indicated by reliability coefficients lower than .7) decreases the likelihood of finding true differences and associations. However, when the internal consistency coefficients are unduly high (greater than .9) many of the items are probably redundant and thus unnecessary.

Equivalence. *Equivalence* refers to the degree of similarity between two or more forms of a measuring instrument. In an effort to decrease the participants' reaction to repeated administration of a measure, some investigators develop two or more alternative forms of the same instrument; thus equivalence of the two forms is important. Equivalence is determined by correlating the scores from the two forms of the test. Hoskins' measure (1983) of interpersonal conflict has been revised for repeated applications in studying couples. She developed six alternative forms of the instrument so participants would not experience boredom in responding to the identical item pool each day. She found that estimates of internal consistency were similar for each of the six versions of the scale.

Interrater reliability. *Interrater reliability* relates to the level of accuracy when two or more individuals are applying the measuring instruments, for example, in the case of rating observations of behavior. This reliability coefficient reflects the accuracy of those doing the rating rather than the accuracy of the instrument itself. Interrater reliability usually is estimated with a percent agreement or with a modification of a formula such as:

Percent agreement =

$$\frac{\text{Number of agreements}}{\text{Number of agreements and disagreements}}$$

Suppose that two raters agreed on 175 of 200 ratings; their percent agreement would be 87.5%. However, this approach doesn't account for the proportion of agreements that are simply attributable to chance. See Fleiss (1981) for a discussion of kappa, a statistical technique that does consider the proportion of chance agreements when estimating concordance in ratings.

Interrater reliability is especially important when more than one rater makes repeated measures over time. Investigators usually stipulate a high reliability level as a criterion for the study. In a comparative study of several models of newborn nursing, Barnard, Booth, Mitchell, and Telzrow (1982) observed mothers teaching their infants a simple task. The observers scored the mother-infant interaction using a checklist of 73 yes or no items that describe the interaction between the mother and her infant. An 85% interrater agreement between observers was required for this study.

Repeating interrater reliability assessments several times is typical in a study that uses observation as a major data-gathering method. Because the rater's fatigue, boredom, or facility in doing the rating changes over time, consistently sampling reliability and retraining the observers as necessary is important.

VALIDITY

Validity describes the degree to which a test or instrument measures what it purports to measure. When an instrument is said to be valid, it truly reflects the concept it was intended to measure. A valid instrument that is designed to measure satisfaction with nursing care does so; it does not measure some other construct such as social desirability. An assay that is designed to measure urinary catecholamines measures catecholamines and not some other biochemical substance. A reliable measure can consistently rank participants on a given construct, but a valid measure correctly measures the construct of interest. A measure can be reliable but not valid. However, a valid measurement instrument is reliable. Green and Lewis (1986) pointed out that, whereas reliability is concerned with random error, validity is concerned with systematic error. When systematic error is minimal, the instrument is valid.

Systematic error can occur for various reasons. The

error can be due to relatively stable characteristics of study participants that may bias their behavior. Therefore their responses to the measure may be biased and influence the validity. A socially desirable response set, acquiescence, education, or other characteristic may influence the validity of measures by altering measurement of the "true" responses in a systematic way. For example, a person who wants to please the investigator may consistently answer items in a socially desirable way, thus making the estimate of the construct invalid. Systematic error may also occur when the instrument is improperly calibrated. Consider a thermometer that consistently measures body temperature one half degree lower than the actual body temperature. The thermometer could be quite reliable, that is, capable of reproducing the precise measurement on repeated measures, but it is consistently invalid. Finally, sometimes the context of the study induces systematic error. Consider what may occur when two interviewers, one of whom is extremely cheerful and one of whom is typically sad, administer a questionnaire. Participants who are asked to rate their moods probably will respond differently to each of these interviewers. When the sad interviewer talks with half of the participants and the cheerful one with the other half, a systematic difference in the mean scores for mood states between the two groups of participants would not be surprising.

Earlier in this text we discussed validity associated with the study design, including internal and external validity. In this chapter validity refers to the measure. Measurement validity influences internal validity, because invalid measures of constructs produce invalid estimates of the relationships between variables. Moreover, measurement validity influences external validity, because invalid measurements produce inaccurate generalizations to the population being studied.

Estimating validity

To illustrate the process of assessing the validity of an instrument, we will use the measurement of social support described by Norbeck, Lindsey, and Carrieri (1981). The Norbeck Social Support Questionnaire is based on conceptual definitions of social support as "interpersonal transactions that include one or more of the following: the expression of positive affect of one person toward another; the affirmation

or endorsement of another person's behaviors, perceptions, or expressed views; the giving of symbolic or material aid to another" (Kahn, 1979, p. 85). Norbeck et al. were concerned with questions such as: How does one really measure social support? What aspects of social support are important in specific life circumstances? The investigators needed to be certain that what they were measuring was support and not some other construct.

Content validity

Content validity refers to the adequacy of the sampling of the domain being studied. When investigators consider content validity questions, they are concerned with whether the measure and the items it contains really are representative of the domain being studied. They typically address the issues related to content validity early in the instrument's development; these issues are especially important when considering the scope of items to be included in an instrument. The investigator maps the concept to be measured: its definition, boundaries, and the dimensions that are components of the concept. For example, Norbeck et al. developed two items to measure each of the functional properties of social support: affect, affirmation, and aid (Table 15-4). In addition, the Norbeck team included items dealing with the size of the network, the stability of the persons providing support (indicated by occurrence of recent losses from the person's network), and the duration of the relationships with the persons who were part of the network.

When constructing valid paper-and-pencil measures of concepts, investigators begin by considering the content domain of the instrument. Green and Lewis (1986) outlined five stages of establishing content validity: literature review, personal reflection, identification of components of the concept, identification of items, and empirical analysis of the items. The investigator typically begins with a thorough review of relevant literature in nursing and other disciplines. At this stage he or she may identify relevant work and existing measures of some aspect of the concept. Personal reflection requires the investigator's judgment about the concordance between the concept being studied and initial personal ideas about the concept. New insights emerge from both the literature and creative thinking. During this stage the investigator usually begins to identify the components of the concepts and their use in earlier work.

TABLE 15-4. Dimensions and items from the Norbeck Social Support Questionnaire

DIMENSION	ITEM
Affect	How much does this person make you feel liked or loved?
	How much does this person make you feel respected or admired?
Affirmation	How much can you confide in this person?
	How much does this person agree with or support your actions or thoughts?
Aid	If you needed to borrow $10, a ride to the doctor, or some other immediate help, how much could this person usually help?
	If you were confined to bed for several weeks, how much could this person help you?

Modified from Norbeck, J., Lindsey, A., and Carrieri, V. (1983). *Nursing Research, 32*, 4-9.

After identifying the relevant components of the concept, the investigator generates multiple items to reflect each component. Empirical analysis assumes that the investigator has actually administered the instrument and can examine the interrelationships between the items and how they cluster around the components of the concept.

Face validity and consensual validity. Two types of content validation are based on judgments of experts. Face validation is the process by which an expert judges the validity of the instrument. *Consensual validation* is the process by which a panel of experts judges the validity. Both approaches require consideration of the adequacy of the instrument for measuring the concept and its components. Investigators typically request that the judges indicate their agreement with the scope of the items and the extent to which the items reflect the concept of interest.

Criterion validity.

Criterion validity represents the relationship between one measure and another measure of the same phenomenon. The criterion is usually the second measure, which assesses the same concept under study. This approach to validation represents a challenge in nursing because of the newness of some concepts and the lack of instruments to measure them. Nevertheless, criterion validation represents an important avenue to assessing the adequacy of an instrument.

The two forms of criterion validity are concurrent and predictive. *Concurrent validity* represents the degree of correlation of two measures of the same concept administered at the same point in time. A high correlation coefficient indicates agreement between the two measures. *Predictive validity* represents the degree of correlation between the measure of the concept and some future measure of the same or similar concept. Because of the passage of time, the correlation coefficients are likely to be somewhat lower for predictive validation studies. Both types of validity are estimated with simple correlation coefficients. Norbeck, Lindsey, and Carrieri (1983) assessed concurrent validity of the Social Support Questionnaire by correlating scores with those from the Personal Resources Questionnaire (Brandt & Weinert, 1981), also designed to measure social support. They found that the scores on the affect, affirmation, and aid dimensions were significantly and positively correlated with the scores on the Personal Resources Questionnaire.

Construct validity

Construct validity involves attempting to validate a body of theory underlying the measure and testing hypothesized relationships. The major focus of construct validity is on the abstract concept that is being measured and its relationship to other concepts. Construct validation is a cyclical process that unites psychometric procedures with theory development. Constructs are specified and then interrelated with others in empirical testing. Empirical testing confirms or fails to confirm the relationships that would be predicted among the concepts. Construct validation is a complex process, often involving several studies.

The process of assessing construct validity entails several elements, as exemplified in Norbeck's developmental work with the Norbeck Social Support Questionnaire (NSSQ). Initially, an investigator asserts that an instrument measures a specific construct. In the case of the NSSQ, Norbeck et al. asserted that it measures social support. Next, the investigator specifies the constructs to which social support should be related. Norbeck et al. hypothesized that social support as measured by the NSSQ should be related to the constructs of need for inclusion and affection but not to the need for control as measured by the Fundamental Interpersonal Relations Orientation (FIRO-B) instrument. They found that affect and affirmation were modestly but significantly correlated with the need for inclusion and need for affection scales but not with the control scale. The empirical examination of the relationships between the constructs of interest typically is followed by a second review of the proposed relationships and sometimes an adjustment of the measure, the procedure for administering the measure, or a modification of the theory itself (Green & Lewis, 1986). After each adjustment empirical evidence is examined to determine the adequacy of the instrument.

Investigators commonly use two general strategies for assessing construct validity. Frequently investigators begin by searching for *convergence of evidence* from different sources, each of which should measure the same construct. For example, the convergence of the needs for inclusion and affection with the scores on a measure of social support indicates that both are related to the measure of social support in a way that is consistent with the proposed relationships. That both the need for inclusion and the need for affection are correlated consistently with social support is an indication of convergence. *Discriminance* describes the ability to differentiate the construct from others that may be similar. Norbeck et al. also correlated their social support scale scores with a measure of social desirability (Marlowe-Crowne Social Desirability Scale). None of the items on the social-support scale was correlated with the Social Desirability Scale, indicating that the new instrument did not measure only a socially desirable response set. Likewise, the social-support scores were not correlated with the Need for Control Scale of the FIRO-B.

Multitrait-multimethod approach. Campbell and Fiske (1959) proposed a specific method of assessing convergence and discriminance, referred to as the *multitrait-multimethod approach.* The multitrait-multimethod approach involves examining the relationship between indicators that should measure the same construct, between those that should measure a different construct, and between those measured by different methods. The basic assumptions underlying this approach are that different measures of the same construct should be highly correlated

with one another and that measures of different constructs should be poorly correlated with one another. Trait variance refers to the individual differences in the construct being measured, whereas method variance refers to the variance attributable to the type of measure used.

Hinshaw and Atwood (1982) examined the convergence and divergence in relationships between patient satisfaction, anxiety, and coping as measured by several indicators. They predicted that the three patient-satisfaction subscales would converge while diverging with low-to-moderate relationships from the other patient-outcome measures. They found that the three patient-satisfaction scales (technical-professional, education, and trusting) correlated with one another significantly (.80 to .90), whereas they were correlated with other constructs, including patient physical condition, direct quality of care as rated by the nurse, and direct quality of care as rated by the patient, between .06 to .63. This evidence suggests that patient satisfaction can be discriminated from the person's physical condition and the direct quality of care as rated by the nurse. As anticipated, dimensions of patient satisfaction are related to one another and also are related to the patient's perception of the quality of care.

As seen in Table 15-5, the multiple traits measured included patient satisfaction (education, trusting, technical-professional), patient physical condition, and direct-care quality. The multiple methods included patient rating of patient satisfaction, physical condition, and quality of care, as well as nurse rating of quality of care. In some instances it is possible to include multiple methods of assessing each construct, in this case the nurse's rating of the patient's physical condition and satisfaction.

Hinshaw and Atwood (1982) also examined the convergence and divergence in relationships between patient satisfaction, anxiety, and coping as measured by several indicators. They found that the three patient-satisfaction scales correlated with one another significantly, whereas they were unrelated to the patients' reports of anxiety preoperatively, immediately preoperatively, and postoperatively. Likewise, the satisfaction scales were unrelated to preoperative and postoperative coping. Measures of preoperative anxiety, immediate postoperative anxiety, and postoperative anxiety were significantly related, as were the coping measures. This evidence suggests that patient satisfaction can be discriminated from anxiety

TABLE 15-5. Validity estimation by convergent and discriminant strategy: RN staffing study correlation coefficients

| | PATIENT SATISFACTION | | | PATIENT PHYSICAL CONDITION | DIRECT-CARE QUALITY (NURSE) | DIRECT-CARE QUALITY (PATIENT) |
	EDUCATION $n = 43$	TRUSTING $n = 43$	TECHNICAL-PROFESSIONAL $n = 45$	$n = 13$	$n = 40$	$n = 13$
Patient satisfaction						
Education	(.95)					
Trusting	.80*	(.98)				
Technical-professional	.90*	.82*	(.97)			
Patient physical condition	.29*	.10	.26	(.79)		
Direct-care quality (Nurse perception)	.15	.07	.09	.06	(.61)	
Direct-care quality (Patient perception)	.63*	.62*	.44	.63*	−.19	(.53)

From Hinshaw, A., and Atwood, J. (1982). *Nursing Research, 31*, 170-175. ©, 1982, American Journal of Nursing Co. Reprinted with permission.
( ), Reliability coefficients for instruments.
*Correlation coefficients significant at the $p < .05$ level.

TABLE 15-6. Validity estimation by convergent and discriminant strategy operative trajectory study; $n = 88$; correlation coefficients

| | PATIENT SATISFACTION | | | PRE-OPERATIVE ANXIETY | IMMEDIATE ANXIETY | POST-OPERATIVE ANXIETY | PRE-OPERATIVE COPING | POST-OPERATIVE COPING |
	TECH-PROF	EDUCATION	TRUSTING					
Patient satisfaction								
Technical-professional	(.82)							
Education	.77	(.83)						
Trusting	.76	.73	(.87)					
Preoperative anxiety	−.05	−.08	−.12	(.86)				
Immediate preoperative anxiety	−.06	−.17	−.15	.73	(.89)			
Postoperative anxiety	.18	−.05	−.10	.28	.34	(.87)		
Preoperative coping	.01	.01	−.06	.17	.15	.00	(.63)	
Postoperative coping	.02	−.08	.00	.11	.16	.14	.55	(.66)

From Hinshaw, A., and Atwood, J. (1982). *Nursing Research, 31*, 170-175. ©, 1982, American Journal of Nursing Co. Reprinted with permission.
$r = ± .18$; $p < .05$.
( ), Reliability coefficients.

TABLE 15-7. Validity estimation by discriminance: comparison of means of patient-satisfaction instrument across two phases of care-comfort study

SUBSCALES	PHASE 1	PHASE 2
Technical-professional	3.04	4.02
Education	2.80	3.83
Trusting	3.01	4.06

Data from Hinshaw and Atwood (1982).

and coping and that the measures of the same construct converge (Table 15-6).

Known groups approach. Another method of assessing construct validity is the *known groups approach,* which involves administration of an instrument to groups who would be expected to differ on the construct being measured. Atwood and Hinshaw assessed the validity of the patient-satisfaction measure by comparing scores across two phases of implementation of care-comfort nursing standards. As predicted, the satisfaction scores improved from the first measurement 1 month before implementation

TABLE 15-8. Loadings and factor structure of items in the Laffrey Health Conception Scale (N = 141)

ITEMS	FACTOR 1 CLINICAL	FACTOR 2 FUNCTIONAL	FACTOR 3 ADAPTIVE	FACTOR 4 EUDAEMONISTIC
Free of symptoms	.65			
Don't require Dr.'s services	.70			
Not under Dr.'s care for illness	.87			
Don't require pills for illness	.82			
Not sick	.71			
Don't require medication	.73			
No physical/mental incapacities	.60			
Fulfill daily responsibilities		.56		
Able to do what I have to do		.73		
Able to function as expected		.68		
Adequately carry on daily responsibilities		.74	.37	
Carry out normal functions of daily living		.68	.39	
Fulfill role responsibilities		.63	.33	
Perform at expected level		.58		
Adjust to changes in surroundings			.59	
Adjust to life's changes			.75	
Cope with stressful events			.74	
Change and adjust to demands of environment			.69	
Adapt to things as they really are		.38	.55	
Cope with changes in surroundings		.39	.74	
Don't collapse under ordinary stress		.36	.45	
Feeling great				.73
Creatively live life to fullest				.66
Face day with zest and enthusiasm				.71
Actualize highest and best aspirations		.33		.62
Live at top level				.78
Realize full potential				.72
Mind and body function at highest level				.64

From Laffrey, S. (1986). *Research in Nursing & Health, 9,* 107-113.

of the standards (*phase 1*) to the second measure made 6 weeks after the change (*phase 2*) (Table 15-7).

Factor analysis. Another approach to assessing convergence and discriminance is the application of *factor analysis.* Factor analysis gives the investigator information about the extent to which a set of items measures the same underlying construct or a dimension of that construct. Factor analysis is a multivariate statistical procedure in which individual items on an instrument are correlated with a latent construct. Investigators can use factor analysis as a technique for assessing the extent to which the individual items on a scale truly cluster together (converge) around one or more dimensions. Items designed to measure the same dimension should load on the same factor, those designed to measure differing dimensions should load on different factors. For a further discussion of factor analysis, see Chapter 27 and references cited in that chapter.

Laffrey (1986) used factor analysis to assess the extent to which items on the Health Conceptions Scale converged on one of four dimensions of health conception: clinical, functional/role performance, adaptive, and eudaemonistic. Clinical health conception included the absence of disease, illness, or symptoms, whereas functional/role performance included the capacity to carry out usual roles in a satisfactory manner. Adaptive health conceptions included flexible adjustment to changing circumstances, such as the ability to adapt to environmental stresses, and eudaemonistic health conceptions included exuberant well-being. As seen in Table 15-8, items "Free of symptoms," "Don't require Dr.'s services," "Not under Dr.'s care for illness," "Don't require pills for illness," "Not sick," "Don't require medication," "No physical/mental incapacities" cluster on factor 1 and have factor loadings of .6 or greater. Items such as "Adequately carry on daily responsibilities" and "Carry out normal functions of daily living" load on both factor 2 and factor 3, suggesting that they contribute to both functional and adaptive dimensions of health conceptions. The results of the factor analysis confirm the existence of four dimensions of health conceptions in the Health Conceptions Scale, although there is some overlap in the measurement of the functional and adaptive dimensions. Factor analysis involves both mathematical operations and theoretical operations, because the investigator is challenged to interpret the fit between the items as they load on the factors and the theory that motivated the definitions of the dimensions of the instrument and the original development of the items.

Sensitivity and specificity. Another approach to assessing convergence and discriminance is evaluation of sensitivity and specificity of an instrument. This technique is particularly appropriate when developing a diagnostic instrument. *Sensitivity* refers to the ability of an instrument to detect true instances of the phenomenon (true positives) whereas *specificity* refers to the ability of the instrument to detect instances in which the phenomenon is not present (true negatives). Together, the sensitivity and specificity of a measure indicate how well an instrument can discriminate true from false instances of the phenomenon and how small a variation can be detected and measured.

Craig (1985) used the concepts of sensitivity and specificity to evaluate the accuracy of indirect measures of medication compliance in clients with hypertension. She collected data about compliance with medication regimens from interviews, blood pressure measurements, pill counts, urine analyses, and hospital record reviews. Using urine hydrochlorothiazide levels as a criterion, she found that patient interview had a sensitivity of 100% and a specificity of 40% (Table 15-9), whereas pill counts had a sensitivity of 70% and a specificity of 60% (Table 15-10).

TABLE 15-9. Sensitivity and specificity: Comparison of medication compliance rates in 40 hypertensives

PATIENT INTERVIEW*	URINE HYDROCHLOROTHIAZIDE		
	>−0.6 DEVIATION	≤−0.6 DEVIATION	TOTAL
>1 pill missed per week	4	0	4
≤1 pill missed per week	6	30	36
Total	10	30	40

From Craig, H. (1985). *Research in Nursing & Health, 8,* 61-66.
*Sensitivity of 30/30 = 100%; specificity of 4/10 = 40%; accuracy of 34/40 = 85%.

TABLE 15-10. Sensitivity and specificity: Comparison of medication compliance rates in 40 hypertensives

| PILL COUNT* | URINE HYDROCHLOROTHIAZIDE | | |
	>−0.6 DEVIATION	≤−0.6 DEVIATION	TOTAL
<80% consumption	6	9	15
≥80% consumption	4	21	25
Total	10	30	40

From Craig, H. (1985). *Research in Nursing & Health, 8*, 61-66.
*Sensitivity of 21/30 = 70%; specificity of 6/10 = 60%; accuracy of 27/40 = 68%.

TABLE 15-11. Reliability and validity assessment

TYPE	ASSESSMENT METHOD
RELIABILITY	
Stability	Test-retest correlations
Internal consistency	Coefficient alpha
	KR-20
	Item-total correlations
	Split-half correlations
Equivalence	Correlation between multiple forms
	Interrater reliability—% agreement, kappa
VALIDITY	
Content	Face validation by one expert
	Consensual validation by more than one expert
Criterion validity: predictive and concurrent	Correlation with criterion
Construct validity	Convergence and discriminance
	Multitrait-multimethod approach
	Known groups approach
	Factor analysis
	Sensitivity and specificity

SUMMARY

This chapter addresses two characteristics of an ideal measuring instrument: reliability and validity. Reliability can be defined as stability, internal consistency, or equivalence. Stability is assessed by means of test-retest correlations. Internal consistency is assessed in several ways, including coefficient alpha, KR-20, item-total correlations, and split-half correlations. Equivalence is assessed in two ways: correlating multiple forms of a measure and determining interrater correlations. Validity of an instrument also can be assessed in several ways. Content validity is assessed by face validation or consensual validation by experts. Criterion validity is assessed by correlations of the instrument with a criterion measure. Construct validity is determined by the degree of convergence or discriminance among measures. The multitrait-multimethod approach to assessing construct validity involves use of multiple measures of the same and different constructs, as well as multiple methods for measuring the same construct. The known groups approach involves contrasting groups that should differ on the construct being measured. Factor analysis is a technique of using an instrument to cluster items that reflect the same construct. Assessing sensitivity and specificity of an instrument reveals the extent to which application of an instrument yields accurate classification (see summary Table 15-11).

REFERENCES

Barnard, K., Booth, C., Mitchell, S., & Telzrow, R. (1982). *Newborn nursing models.* Washington, DC: Department of Health and Human Services, Division of Nursing, Bureau of Health Manpower, Health Resources Administration.

Blalock, H. (1982). *Conceptualization and measurement in the social sciences.* Beverly Hills, CA: Sage.

Brandt, P., & Weinert, C. (1981). The PRQ—a social support measure. *Nursing Research, 30*, 277-280.

Brinberg, D., & Kidder, L. (1982). *Forms of validity in research.* San Francisco: Jossey-Bass.

Campbell, D., & Fiske, D. (1959). Convergent and discriminant validation by the multi-trait–multimethod matrix. *Psychology Bulletin, 53*, 273-302.

Campbell, D., & O'Connell, E. (1982). Methods as diluting trait relationships rather than adding irrelevant systematic variance. In D. Brinberg and L. Kidder (Eds.), *Forms of validity in research* (pp. 93-112). San Francisco: Jossey-Bass.

Carmines, E., & Zeller, R. (1979). *Reliability and validity assessment*. In *Quantitative applications in the social sciences: No. 17*. Beverly Hills, CA: Sage.

Craig, H. (1985). Accuracy of indirect measures of medication compliance in hypertension. *Research in Nursing and Health, 8*, 61-66.

Cronbach, L., (1951). Coefficient alpha and the internal structure of tests. *Psychometrika, 16*, 297-334.

Cronbach, L., Gleser, G., Nanda, H., & Rajaratnam, N. (1972). *The dependability of behavioral measurements: Theory of generalizability for scores and profiles*. New York: Wiley.

Cronbach, L., & Meehl, P. (1955). Construct validity in psychological tests. *Psychological Bulletin, 52*, 281-302.

Crowne, D., & Marlow, D. (1960). A new sample of social desirability independent of psychopathology. *Journal of Consulting Psychology, 24*, 349-354.

Cupples, L. A., Heeren, T., Schatzkin, A., & Colton, T. (1984). Multiple testing of hypotheses in comparing two groups. *Annals of Internal Medicine, 100*, 122-129.

Dowling, G. A. (1985). Levels of cognitive functioning: Evaluation of interrater reliability. *Journal of Neurosurgical Nursing, 17*, 129-134.

Edwards, A. (1981). *The measurement of personality traits by scales and inventories*. New York: Holt, Rinehart & Winston.

Epstein, S. (1980). The stability of behavior: II: implications for psychological research. *American Psychologist, 35*, 790-806.

Fiske, D. (1982). Convergent-discriminant validation in measurements and research strategies. In D. Brinberg and L. Kidder (Eds.), *Forms of validity in research* (pp. 77-92). San Francisco: Jossey-Bass.

Fleiss, J. (1981). *Statistical methods for rates and proportions*. (2nd ed.) New York: Wiley.

Goodwin, L. D., & Prescott, P. A. (1981). Issues and approaches to estimating interrater reliability in nursing research. *Research in Nursing and Health, 4*, 323-337.

Green, L., & Lewis, F. (1986). *Measurement and evaluation in health education and health promotion*. Palo Alto, CA: Mayfield.

Hinshaw, A., & Atwood, J. (1982). A patient satisfaction instrument: Precision by replication. *Nursing Research, 31*, 170-175.

Hoskins, C. (1983). Psychometrics in nursing research: Further development of the interpersonal conflict scale. *Research in Nursing and Health, 6*, 75-83.

Kahn, R., & Antonucci, T. (1981). Convoys over the life course: Attachment, roles, and social support. In P. Baltes & O. Brim (Eds.), *Life-span development and behavior*. New York: Academic Press.

Kerlinger, F. (1973). *Foundations of behavioral research*. New York: Holt, Rinehart & Winston.

Knapp, T. (1985). Validity, reliability and neither. *Nursing Research, 34*, 189-192.

Laffrey, S. (1986). Development of a health conception scale. *Research in Nursing and Health, 9*, 107-113.

Likert, R. (1932). A technique for the measurement of attitudes. *Archives of Psychology, 140*, 252.

Norbeck, J., Lindsey, A., & Carrieri, V. (1981). The development of an instrument to measure social support. *Nursing Research, 30*, 264-269.

Norbeck, J., Lindsey, A., & Carrieri, V. (1983). Further development of the Norbeck Social Support Questionnaire: Normative data and validity testing. *Nursing Research, 32*, 4-9.

Nunnally, J. (1978). *Psychometric theory*. New York: McGraw-Hill.

Risser, N. (1975). Developing an instrument to measure patient satisfaction with nurses and nursing care in primary care settings. *Nursing Research, 24*, 45-52.

Scott, W. (1968). Attitude measurement. In G. Lindzey and E. Aronson (Eds.), *Handbook of social psychology* (vol. 2), (2nd ed.). Reading, MA: Addison-Wesley.

Waltz, C., Strickland, O., & Lenz, E. (1984). *Measurement in nursing research*. Philadelphia: F. A. Davis.

16

USING BIOLOGICAL MEASURES

JOAN F. SHAVER AND MARGARET M. HEITKEMPER

Human health status is determined by how well individuals function within their external environments. Sociocultural and physical information from within and outside of the individual is processed within individuals as they interact with the external environments. Such information processing is manifested as human behaviors (i.e., psychological and physiological functions), all of which depend on the aggregate action and integration of the output of groups of molecules, cells, organs, and organ systems.

Human physiological function generally is viewed according to body systems and cellular and subcellular subsystems. Human health status is at least partially assessed by observing separate components of such systems and making judgments about the normalcy of their function. These systems are commonly studied separately to explain what and how factors act on or affect the system (input or stimuli) to change function (output or response). The selection of systems for study can then occur on several levels (Fig. 16-1):

1. Integrated behaviors such as sleeping or eating that involve interaction of individuals with their external environments
2. Organ systems such as the cardiovascular system
3. Particular organs (e.g., the liver)
4. Particular tissues or cell types (e.g., epithelial cells)
5. Subcellular organelles (e.g., mitochondria)
6. Intracellular molecules (e.g., deoxyribonuclease)

The early study of physiological systems emphasized the physical behaviors of organ systems because measurement technology was not sufficiently developed to measure subsystems. With more recent technological development, organ systems have been divided into more particulate subsystems with descriptions of cellular and subcellular function increasingly pursued.

The goal of basic biological research usually is to determine how systems take in and process information and generate output. This knowledge then should make it possible to predict a precise output from a theoretical input and recognize deviation from normal. Clinical biological research often involves investigating abnormal output in response to perturbations of the system from either natural or contrived stimuli. Although systems often are defined and analyzed singly, the complexity of the interaction of biological systems makes such a task difficult.

This chapter reviews ideas related to studying systems relevant to human physiological function as a framework for considering measurement of those systems. Biological measurement then will be described according to the uses of animals in research, types of measurands, and characteristics of measurement. Biophysical measurement, including transduction of biological signals into physical or electronically interpretable information, is described, followed by biochemical measurement. Physiological or biopsychosocial human function commonly is described from a body system (e.g., cardiovascular

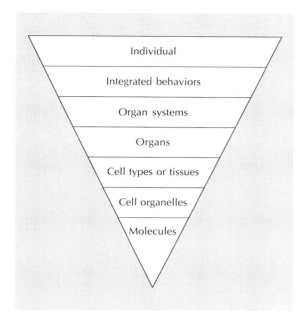

Fig. 16-1. Levels of systems and subsystems at which physiological function is investigated.

systems, respiratory systems) or a functional state phenomenon view (e.g., sleeping or eating behaviors). Therefore specific measurements of cardiovascular system and sleep variables are described as examples.

PHYSIOLOGICAL CONTROL SYSTEMS

Many physiological functions are seen as controlled or regulated by a series of events involving various physical components. Regulatory systems may be viewed as those regulating internal phenomena, such as extracellular fluid volume or external phenomena, such as the interaction of the individual with the external environment.

Internal regulatory systems

From a biological perspective, whether humans function in a healthy manner depends on how individual cells carry out (1) their maintenance functions (e.g., transport Na^+ out of the cells and K^+ into cells, and synthesize proteins) and (2) their specialized functions (e.g., generate tension, secrete chemi-

cals, conduct electrical messages, transport substances, or provide structure). Cells can do this only if the fluid environment in which they exist remains relatively constant. Human cells are healthy only in an environment that remains fairly constant relative to a number of characteristics, such as oxygen and carbon dioxide partial pressures, temperature, concentrations of ions, pH, and volume. These constant conditions are maintained by the operation of a number of internal regulatory systems, and the processes are said to maintain *homeostasis* or the *steady state* of the internal environment for cells.

Internal regulatory systems tend to be viewed as closed-loop systems in which the output partially determines the input. Part of the output is "fed back" and participates as input to the system. Three essential elements to such regulatory systems exist, including the following:

1. A sensor—to sense or detect the operative level of the characteristic that is regulated
2. A comparator or integrator—to compare the characteristic to some ideal or desired level
3. Effectors—to vary the characteristic that is being regulated

Fig. 16-2 shows the components of a closed-loop system that regulates osmolality of body fluids. Fluid osmolality is sensed by neurons acting as sensors in the brain. These neurons act as a comparator by firing at a certain rate when the osmolality is normal and firing differently if the body osmolality goes above or below a preferred level. If osmolality is increased, the change in patterns of nerve impulse output becomes a message to release antidiuretic hormone from the posterior pituitary gland. It circulates to the effector cells of the distal part of kidney tubule; these cells become more permeable to water. Water is reabsorbed back into plasma and reduces the osmolality of body fluids, returning it toward the normal level. As the osmolality returns to normal, the signals to the effector mechanisms disappear. A system in which an increase in the output (in this example, the rise or fall of osmolality) feeds back to cause a decrease in the output is called a *negative-feedback system*. Most of the characteristics of the internal cell environment are regulated at a fairly constant level by such feedback systems, including pH, body temperature, ion concentrations, substrate concentrations, and others.

To study closed-loop systems, a basic scientist

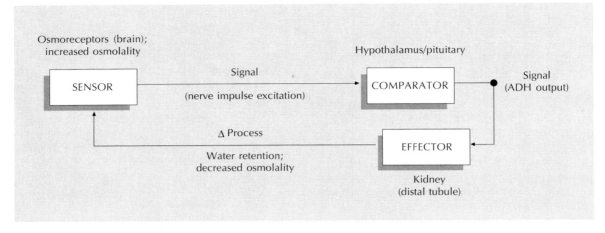

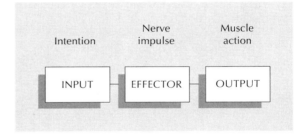

Fig. 16-2. Diagram of components of internal regulatory system (closed loop) negative-feedback system using regulation of serum osmolality as an example. *ADH*, Antidiuretic hormone.

manipulates the systems to open the loop. The scientist separates the part that is sensed from the variable that is fed back so that input can be controlled and quantified. In addition, certain components may be isolated to determine their role in the system operation. For example, if one were trying to demonstrate that low-pressure receptors in the right atria of the heart are part of the regulation of systemic blood pressure, procaine could be injected into the heart (in animal experiments) to incapacitate the receptors and the animal could be made to have low blood pressure. Information from sensors about low blood pressure is normally integrated in the brainstem and sent to effectors, one important effector being the activation of the renin-aldosterone system. If low blood pressure in the described experiment did not result in renin elevation, then the right atrial pressure receptors that had been blocked would be implicated as necessary in the regulatory system under study.

External equilibrium systems

Other systems for study of human function include systems that can be viewed as physical behaviors, these systems react to or act on the environment. Systems operating to lift a load or move the body in space are examples of external equilibrium systems. These systems are classified as *open-loop systems* in which the input to the system is not affected by the

Fig. 16-3. Diagram of components of external equilibrium system (open loop).

system output. The response of the system depends only on input and load. For example, the input to the system may be the intention (motivation) to lift a glass of water, while the output is skeletal muscle contraction to lift the glass. The muscle contraction is graded according to the weight of the glass (the load) (Fig. 16-3).

MEASUREMENT IN BIOLOGICAL SYSTEMS

Many aspects of the biological function of body systems remain obscure, and the complexity with which various subsystems interact remains a mystery. To probe beyond what is possible with intact humans, investigators use animals to study subsystems outside the body (i.e., in vitro).

Use of animals in research

Methodologically, a number of reasons exist for using subhuman animals in research. Besides the advantages of flexibility in scheduling studies, greater control is possible over intervening variables. A wider scope of measurements are available, including invasive modes; therefore mechanistic explanations for phenomena can be sought. New procedures or ideas can be tested more readily. The life span of many species is shorter than that of humans, so the effects of environment, social, physical and developmental variables, studied longitudinally are more realistic. Less variability tends to occur in the biological responses of subhuman animals compared to humans; thus interindividual comparison is sometimes more clearly informative.

However, problems in using subhuman animals for research include cost, decreased availability of some species, and care complexities. Housing, feeding, and overall care require appropriate animal care facilities. Animal models sometimes do not exist for certain phenomena of study, for example, dysmenorrhea or hot flash in female reproductive work. The validity of using animal results to deduce human function is naturally an issue, but many physiological mechanisms have been documented as comparable.

The majority of animal research is done to facilitate biomedical knowledge development, where the goal is to diagnose and treat disease or health problems. This model seeks to describe human function according to particulate subsystems. It might be argued that nursing seeks to diagnose and treat human responses to real or potential health problems on a more whole or integrated level; therefore the study of animals might be considered inappropriate. Although the study of small individual subsystems might be difficult to incorporate directly into nursing science, animal study of complex behaviors of direct interest to nursing such as sleep/wakefulness or appetite and eating behaviors may be immensely helpful. For example, if anorexia is a human response to cancer, valuable insight into possible therapeutic options could come from understanding what internal factors (e.g., hormonal or neuromodulator changes, taste changes, cognitive/affective factors) and what external factors (e.g., social milieu, food availability) contribute to the phenomenon.

Some of these aspects would be best studied in animals. Manipulation of various factors can be done humanely in animals to suggest logical intervention strategies. Psychosocial factors, as well as physical factors, can be manipulated in animals. Although not all nursing research problems (perhaps not even most) are appropriately studied using animal models, animal research has the potential to answer some questions in ways that are not possible in human research.

Measurands

The physical quantity, characteristic, or condition that is to be measured in a system or subsystem is called the *measurand*. In biological systems measurands may take various energy forms that must be converted into a form that is detectable and quantifiable to the researcher. Transduction refers to converting one form of energy to another form; the instruments that do this are called transducers.

Some of the phenomena of interest in body systems are assessed as physical events. The biopotentials generated in the electrical cells of the body (skeletal, cardiac, smooth muscle, and nerve) and other variables such as pressure in hollow structures, temperature of fluids and tissues, and volume and movements of fluids and gas are physical phenomena and can be converted into detectable signals for measurement. However, because much of the function of body systems is biochemical, the means for detecting such events requires conversion of a chemical event to a physical one. Such conversion might involve incorporating a physically detectable molecule (i.e., radioactive or fluorescent) into a given substance or making use of molecules that will react with an agent to change color, which in turn can be detected.

One major problem in measuring the function of living systems is gaining access to the event of interest. The measurand may be internal (cardiac output, gut motility) or on the body surface, such as a biopotential (muscle tension or contraction). Internal measurands are particularly difficult to measure in humans and usually require invasive procedures. For example, measuring cardiac output by thermodilution requires placement of a catheter in the pulmonary artery. Even in a model whereby invasive measurement is possible, the measurand may be difficult to access. For example, it is difficult to access the cell or to measure brain catecholamines. When a measurand is not accessible, an indirect means of measurement often is substituted. Probably the most difficult organ to study directly is the brain. To determine where in the brain a particular neurochemical is located, it may be necessary to react the neurochemical with an antibody that will fluoresce so that the physical energy of the fluorescence can be detected and monitored electronically. If the pattern of gut motility is to be monitored, a pressure transducer might be attached to a feeding tube, passed into the gut, and motility inferred from the pressure changes due to smooth muscle contraction. In using indirect measurements, one must be aware constantly of the limitations of the substitute variable in accurately reflecting the phenomenon of interest.

In addition to accessibility, other factors create problems of measurement. Most of the biological measurands have ranges of energy output that are low: most voltages are in the microvolt range; pressures are low; and concentrations are in the milligram, nanogram (10^{-9} gm), or even picogram (10^{-12} gm) range. These low ranges limit the choices for and design of detection instruments. Most measured quantities vary with time and vary widely between individuals, especially in humans. Interactions between many physiological systems through feedback loops create interference with the measurement of a particular event. The most common method of dealing with the inevitable variability is to generate outcome data on large groups of individuals under similar circumstances and derive empirical statistical and probabilistic functions of how the measurand behaves. Single measurements then are compared to these normative data.

Many measurement situations are affected in some way by the presence of a measurement transducer (e.g., the introduction of a microelectrode into a cell may damage or kill the cell). In the process of biological measurement some form of energy often is applied to tissue or occurs as a consequence of the measurement process (e.g., x-ray, ultrasound). Safe levels of these energies are difficult to establish, and measurement constraints, particularly in humans, thereby are present (Webster, 1978).

Measurement characteristics

Selection of the best measurement technique for biological events is based on several aspects of how the technique reproduces quantitative information about such events as the following:

1. The accuracy of a single measured quantity is the true value (V_T) minus the measured value (V_M), divided by the true value.

$$\frac{V_T - V_M}{V_T}$$

Since the true value is seldom available, a reference value should be traceable to the National Bureau of Standards Laboratory near Washington, D.C. These standards are derived from international standards maintained at the International Standards Laboratory at Sevres, France (Weiss, 1973). An instrument then can be calibrated against the standard. For example, urinary bladder thermistors, rectal probes, or esophageal thermistors must be calibrated before use in a stirred water bath using a National Bureau of Standards certified thermometer as standard for accurate research measurement. Accuracy is a measure of total error without regard for type or source of error. This aspect is similar to validity considerations in measuring psychosocial variables.

2. Precision expresses the number of distinguishable alternatives from which a given result is selected (e.g., the number of decimal places that can be read on a meter). High precision does not imply high accuracy.

3. Sensitivity of an instrument is the amount of change in output for a given change in the input measurand (e.g., the number of divisions that a pressure-gauge needle will move for 1 mm Hg change in the pressure in a blood pressure cuff). Sensitivity determines how small a variation in the variable or event can be detected reliably. The sensitivity of a biochemical assay refers to the smallest concentration of a hormone or chemical that can be detected by the assay. The sensitivity directly determines the resolution of the device. For example, basal body temperature thermometers have an expanded scale so that smaller changes in temperature can be detected by the mercury movement.

4. Resolution is the smallest incremental quantity that can be measured with certainty. It expresses the degree to which nearly equal values of a quantity can be discriminated.

5. *Reproducibility* is the ability of an instrument to give the same output for equal inputs applied over some period of time. This is similar to the concept of reliability in measuring psychosocial variables.

6. *Range* generally includes all the levels of input variation (intensity, amplitude, and frequency) over

which the device is expected to operate.

7. *Linearity* refers to the degree to which variation in the output of an instrument directly follows input variation. Linearity should be obtained at least over the most usual range of inputs, although it may not occur for the entire range of possible inputs.

8. *Frequency response* is the variation in sensitivity (amount of change in output for a given change in input) over the frequency range of the measurement. An instrument should be able to respond rapidly enough to reproduce all frequency components of the waveform with equal sensitivity.

9. Stability is the ability of a system to resume a steady-state condition after a disturbance of the input rather than be driven into uncontrollable oscillation. The overall system must be stable over the useful range. Baseline stability means that a constant baseline value can be maintained without drift.

10. *Specificity* refers to the ability of the measuring device to detect only those phenomena that represent the event of interest and ignore competing or extraneous phenomena. For example, a scintillation counter is set to detect energy photons only within the wavelength range of the isotope of interest, such as tritium (^{3}H). Specificity in a biochemical assay refers to the amount of cross reactivity or chemical interaction that occurs with substrates other than the one being measured.

Biophysical measurement

Biophysical phenomena are generally measured in three steps:

1. Usually a nonelectrical signal (e.g., body temperature, pressure, muscle tension) is converted into an electrical one. This is done by an input transducer.

2. After being sensed by a transducer, the event of interest will be modified or processed; it often will be amplified so that it can be quantified.

3. The signal then is displayed in some form of output by the output transducer (Fig. 16-4).

Input transducers

The biological signals that are sensed by the input transducer can take several forms, including displacement (velocity or acceleration), flow, pressure, force and torque, sound, electricity and magnetism, temperature, humidity, time and frequency, nuclear and penetrating radiation, chemical reactions or concentrations, properties of materials, and impedance (Goldstein & Free, 1979; Webster, 1978). The transducer senses the event and usually converts it into an electrical or mechanical (displacement or pressure) signal.

The measurand often can be interfaced directly to the transducer because the event is accessible directly (e.g., sphygmomanometer) or acceptable invasive procedures are present (e.g., direct arterial line with pressure transducer). When the event is not directly accessible, either another measurand is used that has a known relationship to the one of interest or some form of energy is used that interacts with the event of interest to generate a new measurand (e.g., blood flow to organs can be measured by injecting radioactive microspheres that lodge in blood vessels and then scanning for their presence or counting the tissue). Some measurands such as body temperature change slowly and can be sampled at low frequency, whereas others such as the electroencephalogram brain waves change so rapidly that they have to be sampled at high frequency. Some transducers produce their signal output from energy taken from

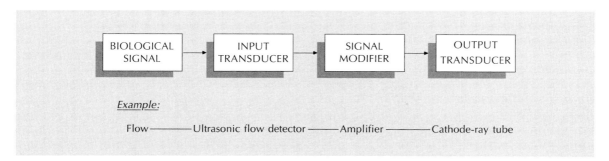

Fig. 16-4. Components of biophysical measurement.

TABLE 16-1. Biophysical measurement

AUTHORS	MEASURED VARIABLES	INSTRUMENTS OR METHODS	PURPOSE
PRESSURE TRANSDUCERS, STRAIN GAUGE			
Baun, M.M.	FRC	Helium dilution	Outcomes after endotracheal
	Exhaled V_T	Spirometer	suction
	Tracheal pressure	Harvard apparatus	
	Pa_{CO_2}	Pressure transducer	
Kirchhoff, K., et al.	MAP	Pressure transducer	Variations with positions and transducer level
Mitchell, P.	ICP	Pressure transducer	Effect of touch on critically ill children
Parsons, L.C., & Wilson, M.	HR MABP	ECG Pressure transducer	Effect of body position changes and hygienic interventions
Parsons, L.C., et al.	MICP Core temperature	Pressure transducer Rectal probe	Effect of hygiene interventions on cerebrovascular status
Perry, P.	Vascular smooth muscle contraction	Pressure transducer	Compared hypertensive to normotensive rats
Sitzman, J., et al.	V_T	Strain gauge of chest movement spirometer	Used to evaluate training for COPD
Wells, P., & Geden, E.	Tissue pressure	Pressure transducer	Effect of mattresses on paraplegics
Woods, S.	PAP	Pressure transducer	Effect of backrest position on critically ill patients
THERMISTORS			
Dressler, D.K., et al.	Oral and rectal temperature	Electronic IVAC-2000	Temperature during O_2 therapy by mask
Lancaster, L.	Core temperature	Bladder thermistor Esophageal thermistor	Determine evidence of hypothermia in emergency room patients
Neff, J.	Core temperature	Esophageal thermistor	Determine evidence of hypothermia in emergency room patients
Newport, M.A.	Axillary temperature	Electronic thermistor IVAC	Study of thermal energy in newborn

CAB, Coronary artery bypass; *ECG*, electrocardiogram; *EMG*, electromyogram; *EOG*, electrooculogram; *FRC*, functional residual capacity; *FSH*, follicle stimulating hormone; *GIT*, gastrointestinal tract; *HR*, heart rate; *ICP*, intracranial pressure; *LH*, luteinizing hormone; *MAP*, mean arterial pressure; *MICP*, mean intracranial pressure; *PAP*, pulmonary artery pressure; *RIA*, radioimmunoassay; *RR*, respiratory rate; V_T, tidal volume.

TABLE 16-1. Biophysical measurement—cont'd

AUTHORS	MEASURED VARIABLES	INSTRUMENTS OR METHODS	PURPOSE
BIOPOTENTIAL AND ELECTROCHEMICAL ELECTRODES			
Coyne, C.	Muscle tension	EMG	Relation to premenstrual symptoms
Hathaway, D.	RR	Pneumograph	Energy expenditure with leg exercises
Geden, E.	HR	ECG	
	O_2 consumption	Waters MRM/computer Polygraph (Grass)	
Heuther, S. & Jacobs, M.K.	Skin blood flow	Laser doppler flowmeter	Assessed in six sites in healthy adults
Lee, K.	Sleep temperature	EEG, EOG, EMG, thermistor	Compare follicular and luteal phases of menstrual cycle
Osborne, D.	Heart rhythm post-CAB	ECG	
Randolph, G.L.	Muscle tension	EMG	Effect of therapeutic and physical touch
	Skin conductance	Skin conductance electrode	
	Skin temperature	Peripheral skin electrode	
Shaver, J., et al.	Sleep	EEG, EOG, EMG	Measuring sleep in symptomatic and asymptomatic perimenopausal women
	Breathing	Impendance pneumograph	
	Body temperature	Thermistor	
BIOCHEMICAL MEASUREMENT			
Farr, L., et al.	Catecholamine met.	Fluorometry	Rhythmometric analysis after surgery
	17-OH ketosteroids	Colorimetry	
	Na^+, K^+	Flamephotometry	
	Creatinine	Colorimetry	
Felver, L.	Serum K^+, Na^+, Ca^{++}	Flamephotometry	Circadian rhythms in hypokalemic and normokalemic rats
Goosen, G.	Endorphine plasma	RIA	Levels postburn
Heitkemper, M.M., & Shaver, J.	Estrogen	RIA	Levels in dysmenorrheic and eumenorrheic women
	Progesterone		
Heitkemper, M.M., & Marotta, S.F.	Neurotransmitter enzymes in GIT: choline acetyl transferase, tyrosine hydroxylase, acetylcholinesterase, monoamine oxidase	Radiochemical scintillation spectrophotometer	Relation to diet
Miller, K.	Serum K^+	Flamephotometry	Serum levels after surgery
Shaver, J.	LH, FSH	RIA	Levels in perimenopausal women
Heitkemper, M.M.	Estrogen, progesterone, testosterone		

the measurand (generating transducers, e.g., photo-electrical cell), whereas others receive their energy from an external source and provide their output by varying this external energy according to input from the measurand (modulating transducers, e.g., photo-conductive cell). Signals that carry measurement information are either analog (continuous and can take on any value) or digital (discrete and able to take on only a finite number of different values) (Webster, 1978).

Examples of input transducers

Force of displacement transducers. A physical quantity can be used to cause the displacement of a component of a transducer. The displacement might be directly quantified on a scale or converted to electrical signals. Electrical properties that can be influenced by displacement include electrical resistance, inductance of a magnetic circuit, or capacitance. A common example of displacement being quantified on a scale is a mercury-column thermometer in which the volume of mercury is displaced proportional to temperature and the column containing the mercury is divided into divisions representing degrees. Another is a spirometer in which a movable bell is inverted over a chamber of water. Inside the bell and above the water is the gas to be breathed. The bell moves up and down with each breath proportionally to the air that is breathed in and out. A pen attached to the bell graphs the movement. Such devices have been used in nursing practice and for nursing research.

Devices such as thermometers and spirometers also exist in electronic form, whereby the displacement is converted to electrical signals. A further example of a displacement phenomenon being converted to an electrical signal is pressure transducers, also used in nursing practice (e.g., to measure arterial pressure, venous pressure, or intracranial pressure) or used in various nursing research studies (e.g., to measure arterial pressure, gastrointestinal pressure, or intracranial pressure) (Table 16-1). A typical pressure transducer has an active element known as a strain gauge. The fluid that applies pressure to the transducer is in contact with a thin flexible diaphragm that is distorted in linear proportion to the amount of pressure applied. This stretches or relieves stretch on various wires within the diaphragm, altering the force applied to the wires. The force applied to the wires causes their length and cross-sectional area to change, changing the resistance of the wire to current flow. When a voltage or current source is applied, the change in resistance is manifested by a change in electrical current for a given voltage or a change in voltage difference for a given current. Such a device also can be used to measure chest or abdominal excursion during breathing.

Electrodes. Sensors that detect electrical events in living tissues are called electrodes. Biopotential electrodes may take the form of skin surface electrodes, needle electrodes, or microelectrodes. Electrodes are conductors that are used to complete a current path between the signal of interest and the signal modifier (DeMarre, 1983). They are usually silver-plated with a silver chloride coating (silver–silver chloride) that provides good current transfer with minimum polarization. Metals such as zinc and nickel are not used because they replace hydrogen upon skin contact, causing ions to gather on the electrodes and blocking signal flow due to polarization. Before electrode application, the skin is prepared to remove oils or dead cells by washing and sometimes by mild abrasion. A conducting gel of potassium chloride is applied to facilitate the movement of ions between the metal of the electrode and the electrolytes of the body. Electrodes commonly are used to measure biopotentials from heart muscle (electrocardiograph), skeletal muscle (electromyograph), eye movements (electrooculograph) and brain (electroencephalograph) both for monitoring in practice or for research (see examples of nursing research in Table 16-1).

Temperature transducers. Thermistors are made of materials that change electrical resistance with temperature. The resistance change is linear within a certain range of temperature. Resistance can be measured by passing an electrical current through the wire and measuring the voltage that develops. Thermistors are made of transition metal oxides (e.g., magnesium, nickel, cobalt, or copper). Electronic thermometers commonly used in clinical practice are thermistors. Temperature is a common variable measured in nursing research (see Table 16-1). Rectal, oral, axillary, skin, bladder, and esophageal thermistors are used to assess body temperature related to fever, hot flashes in women, hypothermia in the elderly, and adaptation to various environments such as operating rooms, delivery rooms, or nurseries. Occasionally in temperature measurement, thermocouples are used in which a voltage develops proportional to temperature at a junction between two dissimilar metals that are in contact with one another, and this is sensed through an electrical circuit.

Flow transducers. In biological flow systems, blood flow has to be measured without impeding it within the vessels. This can be done by using a magnetic flowmeter or an ultrasonic flowmeter. The magnetic flowmeter operates on the principle of voltage induction and requires invasive application. The ultrasonic method uses measurement of sound-wave changes as they are applied to a moving target (blood cells) (see cardiovascular measurement section near the end of this chapter). More recently, blood flow in skin has been measured by nurses using a laser Doppler flowmeter (Huether & Jacobs, 1986). Light from a continuous wave–helium neon source is directed at the skin and moving blood cells. The signal is thereby altered, collected, and directed to a photodiode (see next paragraph).

Light intensity or radiation transducers. A photoelectric cell consists of two electrodes, a cathode and an anode (i.e., a diode) in an evacuated glass tube. Energy or a quantity of light (photons) striking the surface of the cathode (negatively charged pole) transfers energy to electrons contained in the metal of the cathode. Some electrons are emitted from the cathode and attracted to the anode (positively charged pole). This forms a current (a flow of electrons) that is directly proportional to the number of photons striking the cathode. A common application of such a transducer is the photoelectric cell used to signal an automatic door to open when a light beam is interrupted. A photomultiplier tube operates on the same principle—except that as electrons are emitted from the first cathode, they are accelerated to the anode, which releases more electrons that move to another anode. Each diode is held at a more positive voltage to accelerate (impart more energy) the electrons. This means that a smaller initial light source will create a larger anode current. Such a device is used in a scintillation counter to sense energy emitted from radioactive decay.

Radiation is energy propagated through space in the form of waves, which are classified by frequency. Categories include radio frequency, microwave, infrared, visible, ultraviolet, x-rays, gamma rays, and cosmic rays. Radiation also refers to energy such as alpha, beta, and gamma radiation emitted during radioactive decay of compounds. Each form of radiation is detected by a device particular to that frequency (Weiss, 1973). Ultraviolet, visible, and infrared radiation can be detected by electronic tubes whose cathodes are activated specifically by each type of energy. Radioactive decay radiation can be detected directly if it is in the form of gamma radiation, but beta and alpha energy levels must be combined with unique particles called scintillators, which fluoresce (emit light) when joined with alpha or beta rays. If radioactive compounds are mixed with scintillation materials, light pulses are produced that are converted to electrical signals by a photomultiplier tube in a sensing instrument called a scintillation counter. Nursing research that includes the measurement of radiation to detect concentrations of levels of humoral chemicals, particularly hormones, is evident. Radiochemical and radioimmune assays of catecholamines, cortisol, aldosterone, insulin, estrogens, progesterone, the pituitary hormones, endorphins, and others increasingly are being assayed for nursing research (see Table 16-1).

Chemical transducers. Transducers that respond to chemical events are often either electromagnetic or electrochemical. The electromagnetic type is designed to have a chemical sample flow through a cell interposed between a radiation source and a radiation detector. The chemical interacts with a specific radiation frequency and generates a signal proportional to the concentration of the chemical in the sample. Electrochemical transducers use an electrode made of a material that interacts with the specific ion to be detected (e.g., a silver electrode will react with chloride ions and generate an electrical potential related to the chloride concentration). A pH electrode consists of a special thin glass membrane across which a voltage is developed that varies with the pH of the fluid. The voltage difference between the pH and a reference electrode provides a complete circuit for measurement. Electrodes are also available for measuring CO_2 and O_2. A blood gas analyzer, for example, may involve use of these electrodes or consist of a gas absorption chamber. In a gas absorption chamber a volume of gas enters a chamber where volume is measured, and it is exposed to a fluid that absorbs one of the gases (e.g., O_2). As the O_2 is absorbed the volume of gas shrinks proportionally. The difference in amount of gas present before and after the O_2 is absorbed represents the amount of O_2 present (Cromwell, Weibel, & Pfeiffer, 1980). The measurement of pH, Pco_2, Po_2, and chloride concentrations are common in practice and used in research (see Table 16-1).

Signal modification

After being sensed by a transducer, the event of interest passes as a signal into an instrument such as an amplifier for some kind of modifying or processing. Biological signals are frequently low-level signals and must be amplified or built up so an exact analog of the signal can be displayed as output. A signal modulator must faithfully reproduce the signal with a minimum of power dissipated through the system. Often the signals that are sought as amplified analogs of the biological event of interest are accompanied by unwanted energy output called *"noise."* Sources of noise include the biological materials themselves (i.e., cells and organs, material or wires and instrument components, and electrical power radiations that fill our environment). Procedures for shielding wires, cables, and connecting instruments to "ground" are necessary to avoid unnecessary distortion of the amplified signal (Goldstein & Free, 1979).

Output transducers

The results of the measurement process must be displayed in a form that is sensible to human processing. The display may be permanent or temporary, graphic or digital, and discrete or continuous. For example, the output of the sensing and modifying process may be directly written as an ink-lined pattern on a pen recorder or polygraph, imaged on the cathode-ray tube of an oscilloscope, captured in a photograph, transmitted over a loudspeaker, tallied by a digital counter, or sensed as the deflection of a meter needle. It may be stored on magnetic tape or computer discs, although digital printouts or plots are eventually required for information interpretation.

Examples of output transducers

Meters. The magnitude of change in the event of interest may be indicated on a meter by displacement (e.g., a meter on a body weight scale) or transduced into an electrical signal (e.g., an electronic temperature scale). The level of current passing through coils induces a magnetic field in the coils, which are mounted on a pivot with a pointer attached. The meter represents a scale by which to read proportional output. Increasingly, electrical output signals are being sensed as analog information (often voltage

levels) and then converted to digital information for display. Additionally, clinically used monitors display information about blood pressure, arterial pressure, venous pressure, cardiac output, temperature, and so on, as numbers that flash onto the screen and are read like the numbers from a meter.

Oscilloscopes. As an output transducer the oscilloscope visually plots incoming electrical signals against time, depicted as a line or graph being drawn from left to right. The cathode-ray tube contains an electron gun that generates, shapes, and accelerates a fine beam of electrons through a vacuum and against a phosphorescent screen. The collision of electrons with the phosphor produces the pattern of light on the screen. Deflection of the electron beam produces a trace for information display (Goldstein & Free, 1979). Oscilloscopes are also part of many bedside monitoring devices, such as the electrocardiograph, whereby continuous pattern assessment is necessary.

Polygraphs. The polygraph creates an immediate, permanent, and continuous written record of the events of interest. The speed with which the pen can trace the ongoing changes in the amplitude of the electrical output signal is considerably lower than the speed with which the electron gun of an oscilloscope can trace changes. Therefore it is said that the "frequency response" is lower. Polygraphs commonly are used to record electroencephalographic, cardiographic, and electromyographic data, temperature, body movements, galvanic skin response, and other information.

Biochemical measurement

Biochemical function is assayed by procedures that involve binding to—or incorporating a physically detectable molecule into—tissue or cells, measuring the constituents of body fluids, provoking a chemical reaction so that the constituent is detectable through a change in color or optical density, or separating various components in a mixture. Common types of *assays* include radioactive uptake or incorporation, competitive binding assays of which radioimmunoassays are a special type, spectrophotometric, fluorometric, colorimetric, chromatographic, or electrophoretic assays. The following are brief descriptions of these types of assays.

Radiochemical binding studies

Radiochemical binding studies can be used to quantify the amount and/or location of various receptors in cells. For example, ouabain is a drug that binds specifically to the sodium-potassium adenosine triphosphatase enzyme system (Na^+-K^+ ATPase) (an enzyme pump system on the plasma membrane of cells). A tritiated (^3H radioactive isotope) form of the drug can be used to incubate cells or tissue. The drug will bind to receptors on the cell membrane. After washing excess or unbound drug from the tissue, the number of sites on the cells can be estimated under various environmental circumstances and can be assessed by counting the amount of drug bound under the conditions manipulated by the scientist. In a study related to the mechanism of concentration-dilution of urine in the kidney, ouabain binding was used to determine the portions of the kidney tubule having a high density of Na^+-K^+ ATPase and therefore most active in sodium reabsorption (Shaver, 1978).

In *radioincorporation studies* a precursor to some cellular substance is incubated with a biological subsystem (minced tissue, cells) and incorporated into cells as normal metabolism or cell division takes place. For example, thymine, a precursor to the production of deoxyribonucleic acid (DNA) in cells, can be tritiated and added to suspensions of cells or cells in culture (growing outside of the body). The amount of radioactivity incorporated into the cells can be counted and used to indicate cell replication (growth in numbers) or as a check on the viability of the cells in culture and therefore as a check on the validity of their response to manipulation of independent variables. A nursing research study might use such measurement in the following way. Bereaved individuals—perhaps with manifestations of depression—show suppression of immune cell function. A cell culture of immune cells from bereaved (and perhaps depressed) versus nonbereaved (nondepressed) subjects could be used to verify this idea. In a more clinical design, subjects receiving a particular nursing therapy (symptom management or support therapy) could be compared to subjects not receiving systematic nursing therapy, using cell culture of immune cells as one indicator of positive outcomes.

When tissue has a radioactive molecule bound to the cell membrane or incorporated into the cell, a process called "autoradiography" can be used to visualize the location of the radioactive molecules. Thin slices of the tissue are cut in a microtome and placed on slides, and a thin coating of photographic emul-

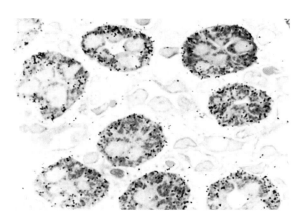

Fig. 16-5. Autoradiograph. Black grains show radioactive molecules of the drug ouabain bound to the cell membranes of kidney distal tubule cells.

sion then is applied over the slides and left to expose in the dark. Energy from the radioactive molecules bound to or incorporated into the tissue reacts with the silver grains of the photographic emulsion that are in close proximity; when developed, the silver grains in the emulsion show as dark spots under the microscope over the portion of the cell having the radioactive molecule. Fig. 16-5 is an example of a radiomicrograph showing ouabain binding to a distal cell of the kidney tubule in rabbits.

Competitive binding assays

Competitive binding assays are used to determine the amounts of individual chemical constituents (often hormones or enzymes) in body fluids and tissues, including blood, urine, saliva, and gland tissue. A competitive binding assay involves the competition of added radioactive molecules (labeled) with unknown amounts of nonradioactive molecules (unlabeled) for tissue binding sites. Four major reagents are involved:

1. The ligand (Li) is the measurand of interest in the assay of a hormone (e.g., cortisol) or chemical. In a radioimmunoassay it is called the antigen.
2. The radioligand (*Li) is a form of the ligand that is labeled with radioisotope.
3. The binder (B) is a compound, usually of high molecular weight, that has a special affinity for the ligand. The ligand and radioligand may exist in the assay in bound form or free form

depending on whether they have combined with the binder. In a radioimmunoassay the binder is the specific antibody for the antigen. In radioreceptor assays the binders fall into three categories:

    a. Tissue receptors (intracellular components or cell membrane components), which are obtained by homogenizing tissues and centrifuging to separate or purify the binding components

    b. Cell membranes derived from cultured or circulating whole cells or tissue preparations allowing accessibility to the cell membrane

    c. Transins, which are plasma proteins

4. The separator has an affinity for either the ligand or the binder. Exposure of the assay reactants to the separator results in dividing a mixture of bound and free ligand and radioligand into that which is bound and that which is free. The separator may be a substance such as dextran-coated charcoal or an antibody to the binder. It also may be a chemical process such as electrophoresis, dialysis, or a combination.

In competitive binding assays (Fig. 16-6) a fixed amount of radioactively labeled ligand (*Li) (hormone) and binder (B) is incubated with samples having an unknown amount of ligand (Li) (hormone). Both labeled and unlabeled ligand compete for the binding sites on the binder. The higher the concentration of unlabeled ligand in the sample, the more

binder that will be complexed with unlabeled ligand. After the time for binding has elapsed, the bound and free forms of the ligand and radioligand are separated. The bound portion then is counted for the amount of radioactivity present. The lower the amount of radioactivity present, the higher the concentration of unlabeled ligand that was present in the original unknown sample. In such experiments a series of tubes containing *known* incremental proportions of labeled and unlabeled mixtures of the ligand are counted, and a standard curve is drawn to show what concentration of ligand is associated with what number of radioactive counts. The concentration for each unknown sample of hormone then is determined by finding the number of counts on the standard curve and reading the concentration (see Fig. 16-6).

In commercially available radioimmunoassay kits an antibody to the measurand may be used to coat the test tubes. Using progesterone as an example, the investigator mixes samples of serum with unknown amounts of progesterone in tubes with a known amount of radioactively labeled progesterone. After allowing the antigen (progesterone) to combine with the antibody that is coating the tubes, the tubes are rinsed and the amount of radioactivity in each tube is counted in a radioactive counter. The greater the amount of unknown progesterone (unlabeled) in the serum samples to compete with the added labeled progesterone, the less radioactivity will be detected in the tube.

The validity of radioimmunoassays is judged in

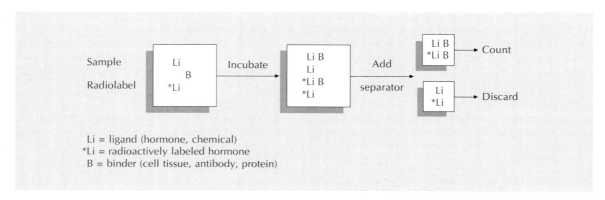

Fig. 16-6. Steps in competitive binding assays.

large measure by the sensitivity and specificity of the assay. The sensitivity refers to the smallest levels of ligand that can be detected accurately by the assay. The specificity refers to the degree to which the antibody is specific for the ligand of interest and does not react with molecules that have a similar chemical structure.

Numerous nursing studies have used or are using radioimmunoassay to determine the effects of normal life transitions, unusual environmental circumstances, and tissue injury or disease pathology on biochemicals (see Table 16-1).

Spectrophotometric methods

Spectrophotometric methods often are used in biochemical measurement. They are based on the property of substances to emit or absorb electromagnetic energy at selected wavelengths. Spectrophotometers are instruments that can be set to detect wavelengths in a small portion of the electromagnetic spectrum. For most applications, wavelengths in the ranges of ultraviolet (200 to 400 nm), visible (400 to 700 nm) and near infrared (700 to 800 nm) are used. In many assays chemical measurands in solution are reacted with agents to form absorption or emission properties, often a color that is detectable to the eye (colorimetric method). The amount of energy absorption that a measurand displays within a certain spectrum band depends on its concentration in the solution.

A source (a hydrogen, deuterium, or tungsten lamp) supplies radiant energy and a monochromator (wavelength selector) allows energy within a limited wavelength band to pass through the chemical sample, which is held in a cuvette (a small holder) in the path of the beam. A detector produces an electrical output that is proportional to the amount of energy it receives after the light has passed through the sample and conveys it to a readout device, often a calibrated meter. Samples of known concentrations are used to generate a standard curve against which samples of unknown concentrations are compared. Such an assay might be used to detect alcohol levels in blood, protein levels in tissues, or an enzyme activity such as acetylcholinesterase (degrades acetylcholine).

Flame photometers are a different type of spectrophotometer. The emission of light by the sample is used in an atomic-emission flame photometer. Atomic-emission instruments operate on the principle that when an atom in an excited state returns to ground state, it emits energy at a characteristic wavelength. Atomic-absorption instruments operate using the principle in reverse. A source of radiant power at the characteristic wavelength of the atom is passed through the flame. As they are raised to an excited state the atoms absorb the energy at their characteristic wavelengths and the amount of absorption is proportional to the concentration of the atoms in the sample. Nursing studies in which the concentration of ions such as sodium and potassium are measured use this assessment (see Table 16-1).

Fluorometric methods

Fluorometric methods can be used on certain chemicals that, when illuminated by light with a short wavelength (ultraviolet range), emit light with a longer wavelength, a phenomenon called fluorescence (Cromwell et al., 1980). They can be used to measure enzymes like monoamine oxidase (degrades norepinephrine) or to measure catecholamines (Heitkemper & Marotta, 1985). Fluorometry has greater sensitivity and specificity than do spectrophotometric methods, partly because only a small number of substances have the property of fluorescence; thus many substances that might interfere with spectrophotometric measures will not interfere with fluorometric methods. Substances that have similar excitation spectrums may have different emission spectrums, improving specificity. However, fluorometry is sensitive to temperature and pH, which must be controlled to have the greatest accuracy (Webster, 1978).

Chromatographic methods

Chromatographic methods involve separating a mixture of chemical components into parts by selective sorption/desorption to or from particular compounds. The components to be separated are distributed between two phases, a fixed phase (liquid or solid) and a mobile phase (liquid or gas). In gas chromatography, inert gas forms the mobile phase, and an absorbent or a liquid distributed over a porous, inert support comprises the fixed phase. In liquid chromatography a low-viscosity liquid (mobile phase) is made to flow through a sorbent bed (fixed phase). The sorbent may be a liquid-coated porous support, a thin-film liquid phase bonded to the sorbent surface, or a compound of particular pore size (Poole & Schuette, 1984).

In adsorption chromatography usually the sample

is added to the top of a glass column packed with some adsorbent material. Various components of the sample adsorb at different levels of the column, and solvents are then percolated through it. A solvent causes adsorbed materials of interest to dissolve and carries them out of the column. The succession and rate at which the materials of interest arrive in the effluent collected at the bottom of the column is assessed. Liquid partition chromatography often involves the use of a dye-sensitive slurry (e.g., silica gel or cellulose) or a layered adsorbed sample, which then is eluted with a solvent (e.g., chloroform).

Gas-liquid chromatography involves injecting a sample with solute contained in solvent into the chromatograph, the temperature of which is set to flash-evaporate the sample and solvent. An inert carrier gas (mobile phase) carries the evaporated sample through the liquid (fixed) phase. The liquid phase is on an inert support or coated with a thick film on the walls of a column. A detector produces an electrical output proportional to the quantity of the solute in the effluent.

Application of chromatography to nursing research might be in the assessment of catecholamines. Epinephrine and norepinephrine are notably responsive to input interpreted by humans as a challenge or threat (stressful). The measurement of elevated catecholamines in severely injured patients, individuals undergoing extensive change, or individuals exposed to stressful environments for purposes of targeting those most in need of health-care intervention (or assessing response of catecholamine levels to various therapeutic interventions) would be appropriate in nursing science.

Electrophoretic methods

Electrophoretic methods are used to measure proteins in body fluids, to separate enzymes into component isoenzymes, and to identify antibodies, as well as for other reasons. Electrophoretic methods consist of initiating the migration of ionized compounds within a medium by applying an electrical field. The mediums may be paper, cellulose acetate, starch gel, acrylamide gel, and sucrose. Separation of the proteins occurs because they are anionic (negatively charged) and migrate to the anode in quantities proportional to their isoelectric position. The strips are developed or stained after electrolyzing, and the concentrations of particular proteins show up as strips or bands of different intensities or den-

sities. Measurement of various serum proteins as indicators of host defense response to injury, illness, nutritional intake, mood status, sleep disturbances, or pain might be incorporated into nursing science.

SPECIFIC BIOLOGICAL MEASUREMENT SITUATIONS

Although the study of human physiological function can be highly particulate to a subcellular level, the phenomena of interest in clinical nursing research are generally those created by the interaction of individuals with their external environments, particularly when the information exchanged with the environment is challenging or threatening and suggests real or potential adversity. The individual is the unit of analysis, and nursing research pursues patterns of responses as they relate to health status. Investigators may study the patterns of responses related to integrated behaviors such as sleeping, eating, or elimination, or they may focus on particular organ subsystems such as the cardiovascular system or reproductive system because a specific pathological condition is present or is a risk. Although clinical nursing research focuses on understanding the whole person, health status still is assessed by observing functional indicators of phenomena that represent parts of the system. The following sections contain descriptions of physiological measurement related to sleep as an example of an integrated behavior measurement and physiological measurement of the cardiovascular system as an example of organ system measurement.

Sleep as an integrated behavior

As a human response to health problems, sleep patterns can be measured both physiologically and by self-report of the subject. Physiologically, measurement of sleep as a behavioral state makes use of the state changes in neuronal and muscular function and is an example of using multiple indicators to describe a phenomenon. Sleep measurement makes use of the natural biopotentials generated by electrical tissues. The electroencephalogram (EEG) is a reflection of the electrical activity of the cortex. By using skin electrodes, this electrical activity can be transduced into electronic signals and recorded. The changes in waveforms that occur with sleep (various forms of synchronized activity as opposed to asynchronous waking activity) can be quantified to indicate various stages of sleep. The electromyogram (EMG) indicates the intensity of tension in skeletal muscle, which also changes in various stages of sleep and helps to identify the particular stage of sleep. The electrooculogram (EOG) senses the activity of muscles that move the eyes and is measured by placing electrodes close to the eyes. It is a major criterion in judging the presence of rapid-eye-movement (REM) sleep.

Surface electrodes are attached to a person's skull and face. The biopotentials are recorded continuously, using a polygraph recorder. The pen-written record is examined in 30-second blocks (epochs), and sleep is scored according to stages by the frequency and amplitude of the electrical signals. Examples of sleep studies recently completed by nurse researchers include sleep and hypnotics in older women (Davis-Sharts, 1986), women and the menstrual cycle (Lee, 1986), and myocardial infarction patients (Erickson, 1987). Research in progress includes sleep and perimenopausal women (Shaver, Giblin, & Woods), sleep and persons with rheumatoid arthritis (Crosby), and sleep and chronic pain (Landis).

The cardiovascular system

The cardiovascular system is responsive to stressors in the external environment and susceptible to stress-related pathological conditions. The function of the cardiovascular system largely depends on cardiac muscle contraction, volume, pressure, and flow within the system. All of these physical phenomena can be assessed through biophysical measurement. Measurement of this system even in humans can include invasive and noninvasive means. Table 16-1 contains several studies incorporating the measurements mentioned as follows.

Electrocardiography. The electrocardiogram (ECG or EKG) is a graphic recording of the time-variant voltages produced as the heart muscle contracts and relaxes through a cardiac cycle (Cromwell et al., 1980). It records the biopotentials of the cardiac muscle, using a number of electrodes. The P, QRS, and T tracings represent the depolarization of the atria and ventricles and their repolarization. To diagnose abnormality, the output is examined for the time intervals between events, polarities, and amplitudes of the waveforms.

Blood pressure. The overall function of the cardiovascular system to promote blood flow to all tissues is dependent on adequate pressure within the system. In routine situations blood pressure usually is measured indirectly, using a sphygmomanometer. It consists of an inflatable cuff that, when inflated to a pressure beyond that in the vessels over which it is placed, will impede blood flow. As the pressure is released so that the cuff only partially occludes the vessels, blood escapes through the opening in the vessel, producing Korotkoff sounds due to turbulence of flow, vortex generation, and arterial wall movements. The sounds can be heard through a stethoscope placed over the artery. Pressure is translated into physical flow that generates a distinctive sound. When carefully done, this auscultatory method is fairly reliable and has an accuracy of about ± 5 mm Hg (Feinberg & Fleming, 1978).

Blood pressure can be measured directly through an invasive procedure. Early measurement involved an external transducer connected to the measuring site by a blood- or saline-filled catheter inserted into a superficial artery or vein. In this system the frequency of response is limited by the natural oscillating frequency of the fluid column, and the measurement is affected by the rigidity of the connecting tubes and any presence of air bubbles. These drawbacks led to the development of miniaturized transducers that are mounted at the tip of the catheter. The signal transmission along the catheter is electrical rather than through fluid.

Blood flow. The majority of blood velocity or flow measurement devices are electromagnetic or ultrasonic. The ultrasonic flowmeter uses principles of sound conductance to measure flow. A Doppler ultrasonic flowmeter sends a beam of ultrahigh-frequency sound into the flowing blood. When a target recedes from a fixed sound source, the frequency of the sound received back is lowered and is referred to as the Doppler effect. A part of the transmitted energy is scattered back and received by a transducer arranged opposite to the source, and a fraction of the transmitted energy reaches the transducer directly with an unchanged frequency. The reflected signal has a different frequency from the first that is directly proportional to the flowing blood. The Doppler frequency can be obtained as the difference between the direct and scattered signal components.

An electromagnetic flowmeter procedure involves

measuring the potential difference generated across a flow channel when a conducting fluid passes through a magnetic field. When a conductor (e.g., blood) moves perpendicular to a magnetic field, a voltage is induced in a direction mutually perpendicular to the direction of the conductor and the direction of the magnetic field. A flowmeter probe consists of a cuff device that can be placed around a blood vessel, a short hollow cylinder that needs cannulation of the vessel, or an intraluminal probe mounted on a catheter tip. Such assessment needs invasive placement.

Blood volume. Plethysmography is a noninvasive procedure used for recording volume variations. A volume-monitoring device, which can be a cuff, a box, a mercury-filled Silastic catheter, or pair of electrodes, is placed around the limb segment being assessed. In arterial plethysmography no other constraint is placed on the limb, and periodic limb volume variation that mirrors the heart contraction is recorded. In venous plethysmography venous return is interrupted temporarily by inflating a cuff to a pressure above normal venous pressure but below diastolic pressure, while the limb distal to the occlusion is monitored for volume change. With outflow blocked but continuous inflow still present, the volume of the limb will increase. The initial rate of volume increase of the limb in this procedure can be used to measure mean arterial flow rate.

SUMMARY

Physiological measurement can be done on several levels, ranging from the function of the whole individual to that of a small molecule within the cell. Biological events tend to be in a low-energy output range and exhibit intraindividual variability, as well as temporal and circumstantial variability. For this reason data are collected on large numbers of subjects to develop norms for comparison. In the process of measurement, biophysical and biochemical events are transduced into a form that can be interpreted and usually quantified by using instruments that act as input transducers, signal modifiers (amplifiers), and output transducers. The events may be externally and noninvasively accessed or internally and invasively accessed.

Factors that influence the acceptability of devices for human monitoring are: (1) any measuring device be preferably noninvasive, (2) the presence of the transducer does not interfere with the phenomenon being measured, (3) any energy imparted by the device is not harmful, and (4) the device reproduces the event in a form that is accurate, precise, specific, and sensitive to very small changes in the event of interest. The measurement of biophysical events usually converts some physical changes into electronic changes, whereas the measurement of biochemical events usually involves the conversion of chemical events to physical events, which may be sensed electronically or in a variety of other ways.

Since all environmental information, including sociocultural information and physical information, gets translated via the biological substrates of the human being, the measurement of physiological phenomena is crucial to our understanding of human function. The behaviors of internal body systems and subsystems and external behaviors performed as individuals interact with their external environments under various conditions need describing. The knowledge must be integrated to define health status and predict the therapeutics that are likely to restore, maintain, and promote health.

REFERENCES

Baun, M. M. (1984). Physiological determinants of a clinically successful method of endotracheal suction. *Western Journal of Nursing Research, 6*(2), 213-225.

Bergveld, P. (1980). *Electromedical instrumentation.* New York: Cambridge University Press.

Coyne, C. (1983). Muscle tension and its relation to symptoms in the premenstruum. *Research in Nursing and Health, 6,* 199-205.

Cromwell, L., Weibel, F. J., & Pfeiffer, E. A. (1980). *Biomedical instrumentation and measurements* (2nd ed.). Englewood Cliffs, NJ: Prentice-Hall.

Davis-Sharts, J. (1986). The effects of a short-acting benzodiazepine triazolam on arousals, body movements and quality of sleep in postmenopausal females. Unpublished doctoral dissertation, University of Arizona, Tucson.

DeMarre, D. A., & Michaels, D. (1983). *Bioelectronic measurements.* Englewood Cliffs, NJ: Prentice-Hall.

Dressler, D. K. (1983). Temperature during O_2 therapy by mask. *Nursing Research, 32*(6), 373-375.

DuBovy, J. (1978). *Introduction to biomedical electronics.* New York: McGraw-Hill.

Erickson, R. (1987). Nighttime sleep and cardiopulmonary function during recovery from myocardial infarction. Unpublished doctoral dissertation, University of Washington, Seattle.

Farr, L., Keene, A., Samson, D., & Michael, A. (1984). Alterations in circadian excretion of urinary variables and physiological indicators of stress following surgery. *Nursing Research, 33*(3), 140-146.

Feinberg, B. N., & Fleming, D. G. (1978). *CRC handbook of engineering in medicine and biology*. Section B instruments and measurements (Vol. 1). West Palm Beach, FL: CRC Press.

Felver, L. (1986). *Circadian rhythms of potassium in hypokalemic rats*. Unpublished doctoral dissertation, University of Washington, Seattle.

Goldstein, N. N., & Free, M. J. (1979). *Foundations of physiological instrumentation*. Springfield, IL: Charles C Thomas.

Goosen, G. B. (1985). *Endorphin levels in burn patients: A descriptive study*. Unpublished doctoral dissertation, University of Arizona, Tucson.

Hathaway, D., & Geden, E. A. (1983). Energy expenditure during leg exercise programs. *Nursing Research, 32*(3), 147-150.

Heitkemper, M., & Marotta, S. F. (1985). Role of diets in modifying gastrointestinal neurotransmitter enzyme activity. *Nursing Research, 34*(1), 19-23.

Huether, S., & Jacobs, M. K. (1986). Determination of normal variation in skin blood flow velocity in healthy adults. *Nursing Research, 35*(3), 162-165.

Kirschhoff, K. T., Rebenson-Piano, M., & Patel, M. K. (1984). Mean arterial pressure readings: Variations with positions and transducer level. *Nursing Research, 33*(6), 343-345.

Lancaster, L. (1986). *Comparison of esophageal temperature to urinary bladder temperature in the trauma victim*. Unpublished master's thesis, University of Washington, Seattle.

Lee, K. (1986). *Sleep patterns, temperature rhythms and health outcomes in healthy women at two phases of the menstrual cycle*. Unpublished doctoral dissertation, University of Washington, Seattle.

Miller, K. (1983). *Serum potassium levels in post surgical patients*. Unpublished doctoral dissertation, University of Arizona, Tucson.

Neff, Janet. (1985). *Incidence of hypothermia in trauma patients*. Unpublished master's thesis, University of Washington, Seattle.

Newport, M. A. (1984). Conserving thermal energy and social integrity in the newborn. *Western Journal of Nursing Research, 6*(2), 175-190.

Osborne, D. (1986). Cardiovascular responses of patients ambulated 32 and 56 hours after coronary artery bypass surgery. *Western Journal of Nursing Research, 6*(3):321-324.

Parsons, L. C., Smith Peard, A. L., & Page, M. C. (1985). Effect of hygiene interventions on cerebrovascular status. *Research in Nursing and Health, 8*(2), 73-81.

Parsons, L. C., & Wilson, M. M. (1984). Cerebrovascular status of severe closed head injured patients following passive position changes. *Nursing Research, 33*(2), 68-75.

Perry, P. (1984). Adrenergic sensitivity in the mesenteric artery of the DOCA hypertensive rat. *Communicating Nursing Research, 17*, 98.

Poole, C., & Schuette, S. (1984). *Contemporary practice of chromatography*. New York: Elsevier.

Randolph, G. L. (1984). Therapeutic and physical touch: Physiological response to stressful stimuli. *Nursing Research, 33*(1), 33-36.

Shaver, J., and Stirling, C. (1978). Ouabain binding to renal tubules of the rabbit. *Journal of Cell Biology, 76*, 278.

Sitzman, J., Kamiya, J., & Johnston, J. (1983). Biofeedback training for reduced respiratory rate in chronic obstructive pulmonary disease: A preliminary study. *Nursing Research, 32*(4), 218-223.

Thomas, H. E. (1974). *Handbook of biomedical instrumentation and measurement*. Reston, VA: Reston Publishing.

Topf, M. (1984). A framework for research on aversive physical aspects of the environment. *Research in Nursing and Health, 7*(1), 35-42.

Webster, J. G. (Ed.). (1978). *Medical instrumentation application and design*. Boston: Houghton Mifflin.

Weiss, M. D. (1973). *Biomedical instrumentation*. Philadelphia: Chilton.

Wells, P., & Geden, E. (1984). Paraplegic body-support pressure on convoluted foam, waterbed and standard mattress. *Research in Nursing and Health, 7*, 127-133.

Woods, S. L., Grose, B. L., & Laurent-Bopp, D. (1982). Effects of backrest position on pulmonary artery pressures in critically ill patients. *Cardiovascular Nursing, 18*(4), 19-24.

17

OBSERVING HUMAN BEHAVIOR

CATHRYN L. BOOTH AND SANDRA K. MITCHELL

Researchers who are interested in studying behavior do not have many options about how to collect data: they can ask people what they do or they can watch them do it. This chapter is about the second choice: approaches to the systematic production, analysis, and interpretation of data that human observers have recorded.

There is no single correct way to conduct observational research, and this chapter is not a "cookbook" with "recipes" for good studies. Instead, it is a "guidebook" to a wide landscape of ways of conducting useful observational research. As with any helpful guidebook, we will try to give readers an idea of the "lay of the land," point out the places of special interest, warn them of potholes in the road, and leave them with a map that will help them find their way by themselves the next time they travel in this area.

WHAT IS OBSERVATIONAL RESEARCH?

An *observational study* is one that asks questions about overt behaviors or events and then answers those questions by having human observers record the behaviors or events over a period of time or a series of occurrences. Please note that the primary definition of an observational study comes from the research question being asked or the hypothesis being tested. Thus studies of attitudes, values, thoughts, and feelings are almost never observational in nature—unless these variables are being compared with or linked to some overt behaviors. We will be discussing only those studies in which a human observer is used to record behavior. There are a vari-

ety of mechanical and electronic ways of recording behaviors that are very useful for a variety of research questions, but they are not the focus of this chapter. Finally, in the kinds of studies we will be discussing, observations are made over a period of time or a series of events. That is, we will not be including studies in which single observations constitute the major data, as they might in a study of voting behavior.

WHY DO OBSERVATIONAL RESEARCH?

The best and most important reason for doing observational research is that a research question or hypothesis requires data that can be produced best through observation. However, beyond this simple rule some kinds of studies are particularly well-suited for an observational approach.

Sometimes researchers are interested in behaviors that individuals are not able to describe through self-report measures of interviews or questionnaires. For example, one might be interested in studying women's facial expressions while they are doing aerobic exercises. These behaviors would be very difficult to self-report and even harder to record. Studies of behaviors like these almost always must be observational.

Researchers also may be interested in groups of individuals who are not able to answer questionnaires or interviews. All animals fall into this category, as do infants and young children, severely ill patients of any age, and people with some kinds of disabilities. Studies that focus on people in any of these categories often use observations to overcome restrictions on measurement and research design.

Finally, researchers often choose to use observational methods when the people being studied would have reason to distort their responses to other kinds of questioning. Office receptionists, if interviewed about their social skills, almost certainly would describe themselves in the most favorable terms possible. They probably would report that they were uniformly polite and helpful to everyone who approached their desks. If the person interviewing the receptionists were a supervisor or were responsible for evaluating their work for some reason, this type of response would be even more likely. Actually observing their behavior under a variety of circumstances probably would give a more accurate and less biased view of the receptionists' social skills.

HISTORICAL INFLUENCES ON OBSERVATIONAL RESEARCH

Because observational research has become much more common and sophisticated over the past decade, some of the historical events and trends that have influenced its development can be overlooked easily. These influences include the child study movement, ethology and ecology, behavioristic psychology, and computer technology.

The child study movement

The child study movement gained momentum during the 1920s and 1930s when several major universities established child study centers and institutes. These centers (most notably those funded by the Laura Spelman Rockerfeller Memorial Fund at Columbia University, the University of California at Berkeley, the University of Minnesota, Yale University, and the University of Iowa) frequently sponsored observational studies of young children attending special preschools and camps. In the early 1930s Mildred Parten (1932) studied the level of social participation among preschool children. She defined six levels of social participation and used these categories to record the behavior of each child she observed frequently over short periods of time. Parten's study was among the first to use systematic observation of behavior in research (Bakeman & Gottman, 1986). Other studies conducted during the early years of the

child study movement also used quite sophisticated ways to collect observational data (see Irwin & Bushnell, 1980, for a history of some of these techniques).

Ethology and ecology

The fields of biology known as ethology and ecology have contributed to the development of observational research by emphasizing the importance of studying organisms in their natural habitats. Moreover, these disciplines also have emphasized the need for complete and detailed recording of the environment, as well as of the animal's behavior. These two aspects—use of the natural setting and interest in describing the environment—have been adopted by those behavioral researchers (for example, Bronfenbrenner, 1979) who are known as "social ecologists." Needless to say, these researchers have used primarily observational methods in their work.

Behavioristic psychology

Although the study of human behavior through observation goes back hundreds of years, behavioral management techniques in practice areas such as counseling, clinical psychology, and education have had an enormous impact on observational research in the last two decades. These clinical techniques, sometimes referred to as behavioral modification, are based on careful recording of specific behaviors and the systematic manipulation of the environmental responses to those behaviors. Changes in the frequency of the target behavior are strong evidence for the occurrence of behavioral change after environmental manipulation. Practitioners and researchers who use behavioral management techniques have contributed to the development of observational research methods by emphasizing the importance of observable behavior. They have pointed out the necessity for careful definitions of behaviors to be recorded and the potential impact of reinforcing and not reinforcing the behavior of interest (Ciminero, 1986).

Computer technology

As the reader will see later in this chapter, one of the characteristics of observational methods is that they yield very large quantities of data that must be managed and analyzed. The increasing availability of computers to do these tasks has enhanced the feasibility of doing observational research. Additionally, modern electronic gadgetry makes it possible to actually collect data in computerized form (by using hand-held microprocessor units, for example), which then can be processed directly by computer (Holm, 1981).

In summary, the child study movement, ethology and ecology, and behavioristic psychology have emphasized the importance of observing behavior and of developing the accurate and detailed records of behavior. These fields of study have developed methods of describing behavior that allow different observers to record activities in a similar manner, and they have developed methods of behavioral recording that can be analyzed for research purposes. Computer technology has made it possible to record and process large quantities of data often obtained from observational methods.

In the remainder of this chapter we will "walk through" the process of planning and conducting a study that uses observational methods. First, we will look at some basic issues that define the kind of study we will conduct. Next, we will construct a coding system, collect data, assess the quality (reliability and validity) of the data, and consider ways of summarizing and analyzing data. Finally, we will reflect on how research studies that use observational methods are reported.

BASIC ISSUES IN OBSERVATIONAL RESEARCH

Clearly, as many different kinds of observational methods could exist as do researchers who choose to make observations! One way to make sense of this variety is to focus on three of the basic issues underlying the research decisions that make one study different from another. The first of these issues is *when* behavioral records will be made; will they be in response to a unit of time or to a unit of behavior? A second issue is *where* observations will be made; which context or setting is best for answering the research question? The third issue is *how* the behavior will be recorded; what role will the observers take in making the behavioral records?

Again, no single way exists to do observational research. Researchers need to design the use of observational methods in ways that make sense for the particular questions being asked or the specific

hypotheses being tested. In the following sections readers may find it helpful to try to evaluate each of the issues for a research problem that interests them.

When to record behavior

When we ask whether an observational system is "event-triggered" or "time-triggered," we are asking what kind of cue or signal the observer uses to know *when* to record a particular behavior. As the names imply, when a specific event is coded as it occurs, an event-triggered system is used, whereas when observations are recorded in response to a specified time period, time-triggered coding is used. The method chosen for data collection depends on the research question and the resources available to the investigator. The following is a more detailed discussion of these factors.

Event-triggered coding. Event-triggered systems require the observer to begin recording behaviors when an event of interest occurs or when an event changes. For example, the observer might be watching children playing on a playground and begin to collect data only when physical aggression is observed, or the observer might continuously collect data about the play activities of the children and simply change codes when aggression is observed.

The researcher can use one of three different schemes for event-triggered coding: frequency only, frequency plus duration, and cross-classified events. A frequency-only coding system is used when the researcher is interested only in whether a behavior occurred, that is, the frequency of occurrence of a behavior or group of behaviors. For example, a researcher who wants to know the number of times an infant smiled during an observation period would use a frequency-only coding system. However, sometimes the length of a behavior is important, and then one uses a frequency-plus-duration coding system. For example, the researcher might want to know the total duration of some behavior or state, such as infant "alertness." In this case the observer would record not only the frequency of alertness but also how long the infant remained alert. A frequency-plus-duration coding system also allows the investigator to determine "time-budget" information, that is, how the observation time is divided into specific mutually exclusive states or behaviors. For example, the investigator can determine the proportion of time that the infant spent in an alert state versus a nonalert state. A time base also would be necessary if the researcher wanted to know how events are coordinated in time. The investigator might want to know what events preceded an alert state in the infant. The final type of event coding, cross-classified events, is used when the researcher is interested in recording a specific sequence of events rather than the general stream of behaviors within a person's repertoire. For example, the investigator interested only in preschoolers' object struggles would not need to record other behaviors but could watch the preschoolers and only begin to record when an object struggle began. The observer might choose to code (1) what happened right before the struggle, (2) what kind of object struggle it was, and (3) how the object struggle was resolved.

Time-triggered coding. In time-triggered observational coding the observer records behaviors at certain predetermined times. For example, the observer might record the occurrence or nonoccurrence of aggressive encounters every 10 seconds on a continuous basis, or the observer might watch the children for 30 seconds and then record the presence or absence of aggressive encounters for 20 seconds. The researcher would take into consideration the expected frequency of the behavior in determining the time interval between observations. For example, the time period for observation would be shorter for behaviors expected to occur frequently than for those that occur only rarely.

The two types of time-triggered coding are called modified frequency and discontinuous probe time sampling. For modified frequency coding the observation period is divided into brief intervals or "epochs," and the observer records whether the behavior occurred during each interval. Note that the observer does not code the actual frequency of the behavior during the time interval but just whether or not the behavior occurred at least once. Discontinuous probe time sampling involves intermittent rather than continuous observation and recording. For example, an observer might watch and record behavior for only 20 seconds of every 1-minute period, or might watch for 30 seconds and record for 10 seconds. This type of recording strategy often is used by the researcher interested in characterizing a group of individuals, rather than being able to distinguish between the behavior of the individual group mem-

bers. For example, the investigator might want to compare children's behaviors in two pediatricians' waiting rooms—one with many toys and books, and one without. The researcher then might sample the behaviors in one room for 30 seconds and then the next room for 30 seconds, etc. In this context the researcher would not be interested in comparing the behaviors of individual children within each waiting room, but in characterizing the differences in behavior across waiting rooms.

In summary, time-triggered coding systems are most useful when (1) behavior is studied that takes place over a substantial period of time, (2) many coding categories exist, and (3) the investigator is not interested in the sequence of behaviors. Event-triggered systems usually provide a less-distorted representation of the behaviors observed and should be used if sequences are important. However, event-triggered systems are frequently more difficult to design and to learn and may be limited in the number of behaviors that can be recorded reliably.

Where to record behavior

The second issue the researcher faces is whether to make observations of naturally occurring events or to contrive a situation or setting. For example, a researcher interested in observing the interaction between a mother and an infant could either conduct a study in the participants' homes (a natural setting) or invite them to a university laboratory (a contrived setting). What differences might those two options make?

One advantage to making the observations in the participants' homes is that their behavior is likely to be most "natural" there. Even though participants may act somewhat differently because they are being watched, a natural setting generally is closer to real life than a contrived setting. Although this is a very important advantage, the naturalistic approach has a number of disadvantages. First, the activities of various participants may be so vastly different that comparing them is nearly impossible. One mother-infant pair might spend most of the time playing together, whereas in another pair the infant may sleep most of the time. Second, the researcher interested in some particular kind of interaction—for example, discipline—may have to make a lengthy observation to be sure that this particular kind of interaction actually takes place (see Kniskern, Robinson, & Mitchell,

1979). Finally, carrying out research in a natural setting tends to be quite time-consuming and expensive.

The advantages and disadvantages of contrived settings are almost the opposite of natural settings. Studies conducted in laboratories may be less generalizable to real life than those conducted in more natural settings. On the other hand, the observations are more likely to be comparable from one participant to the next and are more likely to contain the kinds of interaction or other behaviors that are of interest to the investigator. Finally, most laboratory studies are less time-consuming and less expensive than comparable work in natural settings.

How should observers record behavior?

The researcher also must decide whether to code behavior as it occurs or to record the behavior for coding later. The recent availability of videotaping has many advantages. Once a behavioral sequence is on videotape, it can be coded more than one way. The researcher who decides to consider additional behavior after the study has begun can go back and code it. Videotape can be played back in slow motion so that brief events can be observed in more detail. Videotapes can be archived, so that other researchers can make use of the same material in different ways in the future. And best of all, the researcher who makes a coding mistake or omits something can make corrections later.

Despite all of these advantages, videotaping also has disadvantages. First, making videotapes is expensive. Aside from the initial cost of the equipment, the costs of the tapes, lighting and sound systems, and technicians to operate cameras and recorders are considerable. Coding videotapes can be expensive too; every hour of tape requires at least an hour of coding—and that means another researcher and more electronic equipment. A second disadvantage is that videotape equipment may be very intrusive in the setting being recorded (Kazdin, 1982). Although live observers are also something of an intrusion, the magnitude of equipment needed for high-quality video is clearly a much greater intrusion than is one observer. Third, some aspects of behavior such as facial expressions are not easily caught on tape. Moreover, a camera can look at only part of the scene at any one time. The researcher may not be able to tape a participant who moves or turns. The research-

er interested in social interaction may find that the camera will do a good job for one of the participants and not for the others, for example, if one participant is turned away from the camera.

If the budget is adequate and the researcher has specific plans for repeated use of videotapes, taping can be a big asset to a study. If not, careful "live" coding done by the researcher is probably a better solution.

What function should the observer play?

Traditionally in the context of producing data through observation, observers have had two different functions. At one extreme, the observer is nothing more than a human *detector*—a way of noting whether a particular physical event has or has not occurred. If we ask an observer to record every time a baby moves his or her right arm, we are asking merely for the detection of right arm moving behavior. Taking the position of a behavioral detector, the observer needs to have clear, specific definitions of the behaviors to be observed. Very little judgment is required, except perhaps to decide whether the arm really moved or if the wind was rustling the sheets on the bed. At the other extreme, an observer is an informant, a person who understands the context and meaning of a behavior in a particular setting or situation and reports on it. Thus we might ask an observer to make a rating of how "warm and supportive" a nurse was when interacting with a patient. In this case the observer would still need a careful definition of the category "warm and supportive," but quite a bit of inference on the observer's part also would be necessary. No list of concrete behaviors will define "warm"; rather an entire pattern of behaviors would be scored.

These two different functions make quite different demands on the observer. Observers being trained to detect behaviors must divorce their thinking from their everyday styles. An observer coding smiles, for example, must disregard normal reactions to different kinds of facial expressions and instead apply a set of behavioral criteria to put each expression into a category. The observer might have to learn to break down the components of a smile to give separate codes to eye, cheek, and lip movements, something he or she would almost never do in real life. With careful training, however, most observers can learn to detect behavior effectively.

Observers learning to be informants about behavior have a somewhat more complicated task. Not only must they divorce themselves from their everyday thinking about the behavior they are coding, but they also must adopt a new and specific framework—the one supplied by the framework guiding the research. The framework of the study will direct not only what to watch but how to combine and interpret those events. Many novice researchers are surprised to learn that training informants is often more difficult and time consuming than training other kinds of behavioral observers (Cairns & Green, 1979).

The researcher must never assume that either a detector role or an informant role is necessarily better or more "scientific" or "objective." The quality of a study depends much more on the care with which the questions are asked and the accuracy with which the data are gathered and analyzed than on the specific style of observing.

DEVELOPING CODING SCHEMES FOR OBSERVATIONS

What is the question?

The first step in developing a coding scheme is to ask oneself, "What is the question that the data and their analysis are to answer?" Despite the obvious nature and importance of this step, a surprising number of researchers begin to develop a coding scheme (and even to collect data) without knowing precisely why they are doing it. Knowing why observational data are being collected and what is to be gained by their use is essential; without this awareness the researcher may collect data that are not applicable to the research question (Hawkins, 1982; Rosenblum, 1978). The research question needs to be kept in mind throughout the process of coding-scheme development. Even with a clear question in mind at the beginning, researchers may get off track easily and begin collecting data at a level that is either too detailed or not detailed enough. Another temptation is to try to collect as much data as is physically possible, when half as much will do. To keep clearly focused on the basic research question is therefore crucial.

The researcher's next step in developing a coding scheme is to consult relevant literature in the field for background information and to determine the types of coding systems and behavioral categories used by other researchers. Even if no one else has used observational methods to examine this particular research question, clues are available in the literature about what is important. These clues come from other researchers' empirically based conclusions and their theoretically derived constructs. If previously developed coding schemes exist, parts of them may be useful, or they may be adaptable in some form. In general, other persons' coding schemes are rarely entirely appropriate for new research questions, and their use is limited to those researchers who plan to do an exact replication.

Developing a coding scheme

With a clear notion of the research question the investigator intends to ask and a solid knowledge base in the field of study, the investigator is now ready to develop a preliminary coding scheme.

Field notes. The first step is for the researcher to observe "practice" participants. The researcher should choose a number of participants for whom "real" data will not be collected, but who are as close as possible in their characteristics to the actual participants. Then the investigator must spend a considerable amount of time watching these participants and making extensive field notes. Field notes typically are running descriptions or brief notations about the participants' behavior. At this stage researchers are encouraged not to limit themselves in terms of the behaviors described, because an unexpected behavior may appear that later the researcher will decide is important enough to include in the coding scheme.

In observing practice participants one should try as much as possible to duplicate the setting and techniques one eventually plans to use. For example, if the investigator decides to videotape participants in their home environments, at least some of the practice sessions should involve videotaping and then making field notes from the videotapes. Otherwise the coding scheme could include behavior (such as facial expressions) that is easy to detect "live" but difficult to observe reliably from a videotaped record. While the practice participants are being observed it is useful to keep several important parameters in mind: what level of coding will be most appropriate to the research question (and also feasible for observers to use), what will be the role of time in the observations, and what kind of equipment will be needed.

Levels of coding. The level of coding refers to how "molar" or "molecular" the behavior categories will be. Almost any phenomenon consists of levels. The larger more inclusive levels are referred to as molar concepts, whereas the smaller and more detailed levels are referred to as molecular. For example, consider an infant "smile" behavior. At a very molecular level, such as the one used by Eckman and Friesen (1978), the observer could record all of the specific muscle movements of all parts of the face that together form a "smile." At a less molecular level the observer could record that a particular type of smile occurred, for example, a "full" smile as opposed to a "half" smile. At a more molar level the observer could record that a "smile" occurred, and at an even more molar level that an instance of "positive affect" occurred, with other behaviors subsumed under this category being "laugh" and "chuckle." Another example comes from an observational study of the lifting process and back injury in nurses (Owen, 1985), which involved filming nurses in the process of lifting a 15-pound box from the floor to a table. The molecular coding in this case consisted of precise measurements, such as angles of flexion and distance between the feet, taken from individual frames of the film. A more molar coding scheme might involve viewing the entire sequence of lifting movements and categorizing the method as "straight-back and acutely-flexed-knees," or "kinetic," each of which have several specific defining criteria (Owen, 1985). The point of this is that, once again, the research question must guide the investigator in determining the level of coding, keeping in mind that coding schemes using either extremely molecular codes or extremely molar codes may be very difficult for the observer. Molecular coding schemes tax the observer's ability to be an accurate detector, and extremely molar coding schemes tax the ability of the observer be an astute informant.

Once the investigator has determined whether molar coding or molecular coding will be used, serious consideration should be given to collecting data at a slightly more molecular level than needed for the study. As previously mentioned, observers can sometimes be more reliable with molecular (but not too molecular) coding schemes. Another advantage of collecting data at a more molecular level than is essential to answer the research question is that the researcher can combine the smaller coding categories into larger categories and still have the smaller categories available for data analysis. Additionally, the investigator can combine the smaller categories in different ways, thus allowing analysis at different levels or from different perspectives. For example, suppose a researcher were interested in "positive affect," but not in the individual component behaviors making up the definition of positive affect (smile, laugh, chuckle). By coding the component behaviors (molecular level) the investigator would be able to combine them (molar level) during analysis to get a positive affect score but also would have the frequencies of the specific behaviors. At the end of the study the investigator might realize that laughing and chuckling are really separate in meaning from smiling and might then recombine the behaviors under new headings.

Role of time. Another issue in developing the coding scheme concerns whether or not it is necessary to record the real frequency and real duration of the behaviors of interest or if some time-sampling method is adequate. The answer to this question will depend largely on how precise the time frame should be and whether or not the investigator is interested in accurately capturing *sequences* of behavior. If sequences are of primary importance, then real frequency and, possibly, real duration data should be collected. Otherwise, time-sampling methods may be equally appropriate.

If modified-frequency time sampling techniques are to be used, an epoch length (sampling interval) must be decided upon. In general, the epoch length selected should be shorter than the shortest duration of the observed behaviors but not so short that recording data is impossible. However, an investigator often is interested in behaviors that vary in their average duration. Within the same coding scheme one might be interested in behaviors of very short duration, such as "hiccup," and behaviors of longer duration, such as "sleep." An epoch length must be chosen that can capture both the hiccup and sleep. Previous research may prove helpful in choosing an epoch length. Ideally, the researcher would have sufficient funds and time to carry out a preliminary study to determine the ideal epoch length in terms of the effects on the final distortion of the data. However, often this is not the case.

TABLE 17-1. Real-time frequencies for mother talk and mother touch, and modified frequency distortions for various epoch lengths

	REAL TIME	24-SECOND EPOCHS	12-SECOND EPOCHS	4-SECOND EPOCHS
Mother talk	41	5	10	30
Mother touch	20	4	7	12

Table 17-1 shows an example of the effects of various epoch lengths on the same set of data. In this table the actual instances of "mother talk" and "mother touch" are recorded in the "real-time" column. Notice that a significant amount of data distortion occurs when observations are made for a 24-second epoch; only five and four instances are recorded for mother talk and mother touch, respectively. As the epoch length was shortened, the incidence of mother talk and mother touch behavior more closely approximated the real-time observations. A drawback to the shorter epoch length is the increased training and vigilance required of the observer.

Discontinuous-probe time sampling also requires decisions about how frequently to probe, the length of the probe time, and whether observing and recording should occur simultaneously or if a recording period should follow an observation period. As in modified-frequency time sampling, potential distortions need to be carefully considered.

Another time issue concerns how long to observe each participant in the study. Obviously, one would want to observe long enough to be sure to sample a broad range of behaviors and to be sure that rare but important behaviors would be detected. Practical limitations may also play a role. For example, a study of mother-infant interaction involving 1-month-old infants might, of necessity, be brief because of the limited amount of time that 1-month-old infants are awake and alert. Similarly, a study of hospital patients might be constrained by routine monitoring activities and therapies (unless these behaviors were part of the coding scheme).

Equipment. Consideration of what type of equipment will be needed to collect the data is also important. Recent technological advances have dramatically increased observational researchers' choices among observational data collection methods. A number of portable, hand-held computer systems are currently available that can be used to code "live" or from videotapes.* These computer systems are advantageous for researchers who design complex, real-time coding schemes, although they also can be used for time sampling. Another option, especially when designing a simple coding scheme or one that will use time sampling, is to use paper-and-pencil techniques. A simple battery-operated "beeper" with an ear microphone can be used to let the observer know when one epoch has ended and the next epoch has begun.

An advantage of paper-and-pencil techniques is that they are inexpensive and not intimidating. Furthermore, the worst technological problem that the observer encounters is a dull or broken pencil! A disadvantage of paper-and-pencil techniques is that data that will be computer-analyzed must be transferred from the paper coding forms to a computer data file. Of course, if the database is small, analysis can be done by hand. However, the use of paper and pencil may limit the complexity of the coding scheme.

The final coding scheme

The field notes from the practice participants form the basis for devising the preliminary coding scheme. After the researcher has observed a number of participants, the behaviors of interest should become clearer and clearer. Now is the time to devise a coding form, to define behaviors precisely, to write a coding manual, and to pilot-test the scheme. The first attempts to use a preliminary coding scheme often are frustrating, and the researcher is sent back to the drawing board. Despite the best intentions, antici-

---

*The two most commonly used systems are the Datamyte from Electro General Corporation, 14960 Industrial Rd., Minnetonka, MN 55345, and the OS-3 from Observational Systems, Inc., 15014 N.E. 40th, Suite 201B, Redmond, WA 98052.

pating what an observer actually can and cannot record, or even the amount of coordination that it takes to write and observe at the same time, is difficult. The key is to be flexible and to recognize that many revisions usually are needed before a coding scheme is finalized. Helpful "nuts and bolts" references for designing coding forms and writing coding manuals are, respectively, Hinde (1973) and Herbert and Attridge (1975).

In summary, the process of coding-scheme development is a crucial and often lengthy step whose importance cannot be overrated. As Bakeman and Gottman (1986) have aptly described it, a coding scheme is "the lens with which [the investigator] has chosen to view the world. Now if that lens is thoughtfully constructed and well formed (and aimed in the right direction) a clearer view of the world should emerge. But if not, no amount of technical virtuosity, no mathematical geniuses or statistical saviors can wrest understanding from ill-conceived or wrong-headed coding schemes" (pp. 19-20).

COLLECTING DATA

Choosing observers

Observing, like any other skill, takes lots of practice. However, some people do seem to learn observation skills more easily than others. In recognition of this difference, guidelines for choosing observers need consideration. Although they do not guarantee success, the following characteristics of observers seem important. Yarrow and Waxler (1979) believe that a good observer should be capable of sustained attention and vigilance in the observational situation. An observer who is able to cope with a stimulating environment without confusion usually will find it easier to make the systematic observations required during the research observations. The ability to attend to details is another important characteristic of an observer because the observer will be required to make note of details of behavior. Each observer comes to the research scene with personal biases and theoretical commitments. An observer must be able to recognize those biases and commitments and be able to achieve detachment and distance when observed behavior is in conflict with personal values. Finally, an observer must be analytical and introspective because the research findings will be only as stable and reflective of the behavior as are the observer's records. To this list, we would add that the observer must be highly motivated. Observing behavior over extended periods of time, often in an unvarying context, can become a very tiring activity. The observer who is not motivated to continue with the study will find repeated observations very boring. Second, an observer in a clinical environment must be sensitive to that environment. For example, observers of nurse-patient interaction in the intensive care unit will be able to understand better the context of the behavior if they have had some previous exposure to an intensive care unit and are familiar with the procedures that accompany nurse-patient interactions. Finally, the use of videotape equipment or computers to record observations will require that the observers be comfortable with high-technology equipment.

An interesting technique that one of our colleagues uses (Landesman, 1985) is to interview potential observers about how their houses are organized. We are not sure that we would be selected on this basis because our minds are somewhat more organized than our houses! However, this technique may at least provide some valuable clues about characteristics of the potential observer.

If feasible, more observers should be selected and trained than are actually needed. This advice is especially important if the coding scheme is relatively complex and the training time is lengthy, because the sudden loss of one observer could put the researcher far behind in the research program. Thus having a "backup" observer is important. Some researchers train many more observers than they actually need, and at the end of the training period they select the best observers to collect data in the actual study (Gottman, 1983). This procedure protects the investigator in case initial judgments about an observer are inaccurate. However, employee morale may suffer unless this procedure is made clear from the onset.

Investigator responsibilities toward the observer

To conduct a successful research project involving the use of observational techniques, the investigator must recognize certain responsibilities toward the observers (Reid, 1982). First, the investigator should try to make the observers' job as easy as possible by providing a detailed coding manual. If accurate definitions of the behaviors under study are not provided, then becoming a reliable observer is a much more difficult and frustrating task. Second, it is important to *listen* to what the observers have to say about potential changes that need to be made in the coding scheme or about new codes that need to be added. Since the observers will be collecting the data, they may see something that the researcher did not encounter during the coding scheme–development phase. Thus it may be important for the researcher to incorporate some of their suggestions—or at least to explain why the coding scheme cannot be changed to reflect these suggestions.

A third responsibility of the investigator is either to orient the observers to the specific hypotheses and general background of the project or—if the integrity of the study requires that observers be kept "blind" to the hypotheses—to explain why they cannot be told. A fourth responsibility is to refrain from asking observers to do things that the researcher would not do, such as sending an observer to a home where violent behaviors routinely occur, or setting up an observation schedule that is more demanding than the researcher could handle.

A final, related responsibility is to maintain observer morale, which is important because the considerable time investment in training observers makes them very valuable as long-time employees. We believe that happy observers are good observers and that data quality will suffer when observer morale is low. Several techniques for maintaining morale are (1) to provide incentives for continued good reliability assessments, (2) to make the observation task as scientifically stimulating as possible (by giving the observers relevant articles to read, etc.), and (3) to prepare new observers for the potential frustrations involved in learning a new coding scheme. We have found the last suggestion to be particularly important because good observers often are people who learn new skills quickly and tend to be perfectionists. Being confronted with a new task that is actually quite complex, but which does not seem so on the surface, can be unsettling for many novice observers. Also, we have found it useful to remind observers that coding errors and disagreements among coders will always occur. We expect these errors to occur sometimes because observation is an imperfect process.

Other, less direct methods for maintaining morale are to hire observers for half-time or less because of the exacting demands of observations.

Practical tips for naturalistic observation

One of the issues that always arises in observational research in natural settings is the extent to which the presence of the observer influences or modifies the behaviors of the participants being observed. Although this is one of the drawbacks of naturalistic observation, following some practical tips will minimize the observer's obtrusiveness. First, dark clothing can be helpful to decrease stimuli that would attract attention. Second, movements should be minimized, although some movement may be necessary to keep the participant in view. Third, the observer should stand or sit as far away from the participant as possible, while still being able to get a good view.

The behavior of the observer while in the presence of the participants may also need to vary according to the age or developmental level of the individuals being observed. For example, when observing neonates, the observer would need to be concerned about the neonate's response to him or her only when very close to the baby and when in the baby's direct line of vision. However, older infants present different problems. While observing 10-month-old children at home one of us (CB) found, by trial and error, that the best procedure was to attempt to ignore the infant from the moment the observer entered the house. This plan was explained to the mother before the observation so she would understand the observer's behavior. This ignoring behavior was not easy, but it was mastered with practice. The typical 10-month-old child would look at and approach the observer during the first minutes of observation (this behavior category was actually included in the coding scheme), but when the observer did not respond, the child's approaching behavior gradually diminished. When the baby approached or looked at the observer, the observer continued to collect data but adopted a blank face and looked just past, or to one side of the baby. Also, standing instead of sitting removed the observer from the baby's direct line of view and further minimized the baby's curiosity. This procedure was very successful. With older children the presence in the home of an observer who does not interact or respond affectively seems very bizarre. Thus observers of older children frequently respond to the child's direct questions or else explain that they cannot talk right then and will talk later.

When working with adults, it is important for the observer to clarify that the adults should do whatever they normally do in their natural surroundings and attempt to forget that the observer is there. One often needs to be very specific about the adult not being able to converse with the observer, and participants sometimes need to be reminded of this during the observation. In one study of staff-patient interactions in a psychiatric setting, Niemeier (1983) found that an observer attempting to code "desirable social behavior" between patients was either drawn into the patients' conversation or the conversation was markedly affected by the physical proximity of the observer. Consequently, the coding method had to

be changed so that the observer did not actually need to listen to the content of the conversation and therefore could stand farther away.

Other practical hints for behavioral observation, which are unrelated to obtrusiveness, involve the necessity of establishing equipment integrity before going into the field. This means making sure the observer has enough paper and pencils (how embarrassing to be stuck in the middle of an observation without a good pencil!). If electronic equipment is being used, the observer should check it before the observation period and always bring an extra supply of batteries, tapes, and cords.

Postobservation notes

At the end of an observation, be it "live" or videotaped, several types of systematic notes can be valuable. The first type, *coder resonance*, involves the

---

POSTOBSERVATION REPORT, MODELS OF NEWBORN NURSING SERVICES

1. Are this mother and baby "in step" with each other?
   1. Never
   2. Less than half the time
   3. About half the time
   4. More than half the time
   5. Almost all the time
2. How much did you like this mother?
   1. None
   2. A little
   3. Some
   4. A moderate amount
   5. A great deal
3. How much did you like this baby?
   1. None
   2. A little
   3. Some
   4. A moderate amount
   5. A great deal
4. How difficult was it to observe the behavior of this mother and baby?
   1. Very difficult
   2. Difficult
   3. Average
   4. Easy
   5. Very easy

From Booth, C. L. (1979). Newborn nursing models study (Grant No. NU00719 awarded to K. Barnard). Washington, DC: U.S. Public Health Service.

observer's personal reaction to or evaluation of the participant(s) being observed. The *Coder Resonance, National Institute of Mental Health Study of Child Development and Rearing in Well and Affectively-ill Parents* by Marian Radke-Yarrow, Ph.D. and *Postobservation Report, Models of Newborn Nursing Services* by Cathryn L. Booth, Ph.D. provide examples of these types of forms (see boxes). This information can be a valuable supplement to more objectively collected observational data and can provide a check on

whether the coding scheme is discriminating among individuals to whom the observer has very different reactions.

A second type of postobservation data concerns questioning the participants about their reactions to being observed. For example, in the observation study involving 10-month-old children, we asked mothers the following: "Was this a typical day for your baby?", "What do you think you did differently because I was here?", and "What do you think your

---

CODER RESONANCE, NATIONAL INSTITUTE OF MENTAL HEALTH STUDY OF CHILD DEVELOPMENT AND REARING IN WELL AND AFFECTIVELY-ILL PARENTS

A. Over-all feeling about each participant: (circle)

    Mother — like, ambivalent, neutral, dislike

    Child 1 — like, ambivalent, neutral, dislike

    Child 2 — like, ambivalent, neutral, dislike

B. Characteristic interaction between mother and child:
    _____ Mother is talking *with* child, predominantly
    _____ Mother is talking *at* child, predominantly
    _____ Almost no talking between mother and child

C. What strong feelings are evoked in you: (check 1 to 3 of the following) for each individual and for the interaction:

	Interaction	Mother	Child 1	Child 2
Detached, uninvolved, passive, or bored				
Empathic, prosocial toward				
"High," elated				
Depressed, sad, "down"				
Stirred-up, agitated				
Confused				
Annoyed, angry, aggressive				
Happy, pleasant				
Anxious, uneasy, frightened				
Drained, exhausted, overwhelmed				

From Radke-Yarrow, M. (1982). (Grant No. 79M123). Washington, DC: National Institute of Mental Health.

baby did differently because I was here?" By asking these questions, we were able to attest to our unobtrusiveness in most cases. In fact, most mothers were surprised about the extent to which they were able to forget the observer's presence. Although our presence certainly had some impact on the family, collecting this type of postobservation data (as well as the objective data about the infant's attention to the observer) enabled us to demonstrate that we were able to collect data in a naturalistic setting without gross distortions in the behaviors we observed.

Finally, a third type of postobservation report involves having the observer write a brief paragraph about unusual or disturbing events, environmental variables that may have affected the observation, and clinical notes. These debriefing notes usually are more important to the observer than to the investigator, because they give the observer the chance to record qualitative impressions that the hard data may not be picking up. We have experienced this need as observers—perhaps it relates to a very human tendency to feel that our own perceptions and verbal descriptions are more valid than numerical entries on a coding form, even when we know that other observers might not have the same subjective impressions that we have.

RELIABILITY AND VALIDITY OF OBSERVATIONAL DATA

By now the importance of having reliable and valid measurement instruments for doing high-quality research is probably clear. However, when using observational methods, the researcher will find that the terms "reliability" and "validity" have slightly different meanings than they do when used in relation to a psychological test or a questionnaire.

Reliability

An observational method is considered *reliable* if the scores that it generates are precise, accurate, and consistent. A reliable method is like a good-quality ruler: anyone who has been given appropriate training can use it equally well; it does not stretch or warp while in use (which would distort the measurement process); it gives the same result no matter who is doing the measuring; and if used twice to measure the same object, it will yield the same number. Thus when one uses a reliable ruler—or a reliable observation sys-

tem—the errors of measurement should be small.

How can the researcher tell whether an observational tool is reliable? When we want to check a ruler, we can calibrate it against a standard—a ruler already known to be accurate. However, if we are designing a system of observational recording, probably no standard exists against which we can check ourselves. The best we can do is to compare two or more scores that are made using a particular method and thus determine the extent to which those two assessments are consistent. The several different ways to assess the reliability of observational data are, in fact, different ways to collect and compare two or more scores. (For additional information on these issues, consult Hartmann, 1982; Hartmann & Gardner, 1981; Hollenbeck, 1978; Johnson & Bolstad, 1973; and Mitchell, 1979.)

Interobserver agreement

One of the most basic ways to check the accuracy and precision of a coding system is to determine whether two coders using the same system and observing the same behavior actually make the same record, that is, whether *interobserver agreement* exists. This is usually done by comparing the behavioral records made by the two observers, unit by unit (either time unit or event unit, depending upon which is being used), and noting what percentage of the entries are identical. This number (which is often, and we think confusingly, referred to as "reliability") is an indication of how objective and well defined the coding categories are and how well the observers have been trained.

In most studies observers are required to meet some standard of agreement with an experienced coder (often the researcher) before they begin collecting data. The criterion level sought is usually 85% agreement or more. This may sound like a stringent criterion, but even if an observer were 85% accurate, he or she would still make an error, on the average, every seven codes. If a research question is concerned with a behavior that does not occur very frequently, an even higher standard of agreement may be necessary to ensure that accurate behavioral records are obtained.

Percentages are not the only (or even the best) way of statistically reporting the amount of agreement between observers. Statistical assessments such as Cohen's kappa (Cohen, 1960) and Robinson's *A* (Robinson, 1957) are often more appropriate (see

Hollenbeck, 1978 or Tinsley & Weiss, 1975 for further description of agreement statistics). Whatever way the agreement data are reported, it is important to realize that they really reflect the accuracy of specific observers using a specific system. Such a statistic does not say anything about how well the observers could do with another system or how well the system would work with other observers.

What should a researcher do when observers do not attain an acceptable level of agreement? One possibility is that the coders have not been adequately trained. The investigator can check whether they have memorized definitions, practiced adequately (it may take 10 to 30 practice observations to master even a fairly simple coding system), or have computed their agreement accurately. The other possibility is that the coding system itself needs revision, for example, new or clearer definitions, more or fewer categories, a shorter or longer time unit for sampling. The best way to identify the source of the problem is to look at the practice data and to identify where the disagreements or errors are occurring. Doing this with coders can serve a dual purpose—both improve the system and provide further training for the observers. One final point the investigator should remember is that some behaviors are very difficult to code. If the system and the observers seem to get stuck at some level of agreement, the investigator may need to go back to the beginning and rethink which behaviors are really important to observe, and make changes accordingly.

Statistical reliability

For all of their value, indexes of observer agreement do not give us any information about whether the behavior we are studying is a consistent characteristic of the participant we are observing. We usually choose a behavior to observe because we believe that the behavior reflects some underlying trait or characteristic of the person we are watching. We observe smiling, for example, because we want to study the expression of emotions, or we observe hitting because we are interested in aggression. We are rarely if ever interested in an isolated piece of behavior. Consequently, we need to have some idea whether the behavior we observe is *representative* of the traits or characteristics in which we are interested. This is the issue that statistical reliability addresses.

To determine observer agreement, we compare the records made of one participant by two observers. To determine statistical reliability, we compare the data records made of one participant on two different occasions. We use the general term "occasions" because the two behavioral records might be collected in any one of several ways: (1) on different days, (2) at different hours on the same day, (3) under different environmental conditions, or (4) even during the first and second halves of a longer observation period. When these two records are compared—usually by using a correlation coefficient statistic—we get an index of statistical reliability.

What does a reliability coefficient of this kind really mean? To answer this question, recall that a correlation coefficient reflects the extent to which one set of scores is predictable from another set. If perfect prediction occurs, the correlation is 1.00 or −1.00; if no prediction occurs, the correlation is 0.00. The relatively large correlation (about .60) between height and weight, for example, means that knowing how tall someone is gives you a good deal of information for guessing how heavy that person is. By the same logic, a high correlation between two sets of observations means that the behavior on one occasion is quite predictive of that behavior on the other occasion. In other words, the behavior is quite consistent. A low correlation, on the other hand, means that the behavior is comparatively inconsistent.

The reader should be aware that low reliability coefficients can have different interpretations, depending on how the two occasions for measurement were chosen. If the two occasions were separated in time, for example, some real change may have occurred in the characteristic observed. The baby may have been ill or tired on one day and not on the other. If the two observations were in different situations, the behavior may actually vary systematically from one setting to the other. Consequently, a high reliability coefficient means that a behavior is quite stable, but a low coefficient may have several different meanings, depending on how the data were collected (see Mitchell, 1979, for a more complete discussion of these different meanings).

Although a researcher who finds a low interobserver agreement coefficient can take action to improve the coding system or the work of the observers, one who finds a low statistical reliability coefficient has little action available. The main option is to rethink carefully the behaviors being observed and the two occasions being used for the reliability computation. If the researcher believes that the behavior ought to be consistent over that period of time or circumstances, then he or she will need to consider ways of changing the coding system or study design in hopes of finding such consistency. On the other hand, reliability coefficients do not usually need to look as "large" as agreement percentages; a reliability coefficient of .85 is quite high.

Validity

Whereas reliability concerns accuracy and precision, validity concerns "trueness"—does the measure being used assess the actual trait or characteristic or habit called for by the theory and research questions? Just as several ways exist to establish and discuss reliability, several varieties of validity also exist. (For further details, refer to Cone, 1982; Johnson & Bolstad, 1973).

Face validity. The *face validity* of a measurement is the extent to which it appears to be measuring the right thing. In fact, this is the most common kind of validity claimed for observational systems of collecting data. If one is interested in how often a child hits other children in a classroom, what more valid measure could one have than the number of times a child actually hits other children?

Although that logic sounds persuasive, the fact is that counting something is not necessarily the same as validly measuring it. For example, one could reliably count hits, but if the teacher and other children were really only concerned with *hard* hits, the score obtained might not be a valid measure of the behavior of interest. Moreover, to have a theory that deals only with overt behavior is fairly uncommon; most researchers are interested in classes or types of behavior. Face validity alone cannot answer whether a specific behavior accurately represents the class or type being studied. In short, face validity is not by itself a guarantee of good-quality data, but concerns about face validity should be part of planning every study.

Content validity. A closely related notion is that of *content validity* or the extent to which some general measure is made up of appropriate units or items. For example, suppose that a researcher were interested in recording all of the "noncompliant" behaviors that a child showed in a preschool classroom. The researcher might include disobedience, ignoring the teacher, ignoring other children, and so forth. This measure of noncompliance would have content validity to the extent that the investigator had adequately sampled from all possible kinds of noncompliance. Of course, no way exists of knowing if one really has done that, so researchers sometimes poll other researchers (as experts) to assess whether they have adequately covered the behaviors that ought to be included. In her observational study of staff-patient interactions in a psychiatric facility, Niemeier (1983) used this method to devise a list of appropriate coding categories for "desirable" and "undesirable" patient behaviors. She began with a list of 88 items that exemplified typical behaviors of psychiatric patients. Eight nurses in the psychiatric ward then were asked to rate each behavior on a scale from extremely undesirable (1 point) to extremely desirable (9 points). The mean values of these ratings then were used to select coding categories. Thus much of the preliminary work on developing a coding system is aimed at ensuring the content validity of the system.

Criterion-based validity. The *criterion-based validity* of a measure is assessed by comparing the score on the new measure with an established standard of measurement for that variable. Thus, if you were designing a new test of mental abilities, you could establish its criterion-based validity by correlating scores on the new test with scores on some already existing mental test.

The difficulty for observational measures, of course, is that virtually no criteria exist with which to compare a new measure. Sometimes criterion validity makes no sense at all. What would be the criteria for infant smiling, for example, or for aggressive playground play? Nonetheless, in the few instances where criteria may be available, the investigator should consider this as an index of validity.

Construct validity. *Construct validity* is a way of describing how the scores from a measurement instrument interrelate with other variables. Generally, the theory that guides a research study suggests which characteristics and traits should be related and which should be unrelated. If a new measure shows this pattern of relationships and nonrelationships, it is said to have construct validity. In this sense, nearly every observational measure provides some evidence for the construct validity of its categories. At the same time it is important to realize that failure to find a hypothesized relationship is an important piece of nonvalidating information to which researchers need attend.

Novice researchers sometimes are discouraged by the amount of work that determining the reliability and validity of an observational coding system can require. Although the process can be time-consuming, good-quality data also can be collected in a very straightforward way for many problems, including most of those that beginning researchers are likely to tackle.

DATA REDUCTION AND ANALYSIS

In this section we will discuss various methods of summarizing and reducing (aggregating) observational data at the level of the individual research participant. Compared with other types of assessments, observational data present some unique problems, as well as some unique opportunities. Whereas other measurement methods might yield only one or two scores, observational techniques typically generate hundreds or even thousands of bits of data for each participant. Thus methods of aggregating and summarizing these data at the individual participant level are needed. (For other treatments of this topic, see Bakeman, 1978; Bakeman, Cairns, & Appelbaum, 1979; Gottman, 1978; Kaye, 1982; Notarius, Krokoff, & Markman, 1981; and Sackett & Landsman-Dwyer, 1982.)

Descriptive statistics

One of the simplest methods of summarizing observation data is to use *descriptive statistics*. Rate or frequency is one such statistic that is used to describe how often a behavior occurred. A frequency is calculated by counting how often a particular event occurred. It is easy to count how many times a behavior occurred if it was recorded as real-time data. In the case of the real-time data shown in Table 17-2, the researcher would simply add together the number of times a behavior occurred (e.g., 4 times for behavior *A*) to get the total frequency of that behavior. The total number of seconds during which the behavior occurred would then be added together to get the total duration of that behavior (25 seconds for behavior *A*). When data are time-based, calculating frequency and duration proportions is more useful because observations often differ in their total

TABLE 17-2. **Example of real-time observational data**

BEHAVIOR	DURATION (IN SECONDS)
A	3
D	6
C	18
B	1
C	4
B	8
A	15
D	23
A	4
C	6
D	12
A	3
B	4

length. Consequently, raw frequencies and durations are not comparable across participants. For example, smiling 4 times in 30 minutes for participant *x* would be very different from smiling 4 times in 65 minutes for participant *y*. Thus the relative frequency (also known as the event probability or frequency probability) and the relative duration (also known as the duration probability) are typically calculated instead. The relative frequency of behavior *A* is simply the number of times *A* occurred, divided by the total frequency of all the behaviors (4/13 for behavior *A*, or .31). Similarly, the relative duration of *A* would be the number of seconds *A* occurred, divided by the total number of seconds in the observation (in this case 25/107, or .23).

The average duration of a behavior is another useful statistic when the investigator is interested in how long a particular behavior usually lasts. Average duration is calculated by dividing the total duration of a behavior by the total frequency of that behavior (e.g., 25 seconds/4 behaviors = 6.2 seconds per behavior).

The descriptive statistics we have just described do not convey anything uniquely sequential about the data. Bakeman and Gottman (1986) suggested the use of transitional probabilities to capture the sequential aspect of data. A transitional probability is the probability with which a particular "target" behavior occurs relative to another "given" event that occurred at a different time. Of interest is how often behavior *A,* for example, follows behavior *C.* For example, if we had a sequence of behaviors: *B-B-C-A-A-A-C-B-A-C-B-C,* we would count how many times *C* followed *B* (two times), how many times *A* followed *C* (one time), and so forth. The probability of *B* following *C* or *A* following *B* can be calculated. (See Bakeman & Gottman, 1986, for a detailed description of calculating transitional probabilities.)

Time sampling. When time-sampling methods have been used to collect observational data, descriptive statistics are also very simple to calculate but more difficult to interpret (see the previous discussion of modified-frequency distortions). Thus, instead of calculating the real frequency of a specific behavior, the observer counts the number of intervals during which that behavior occurred (sometimes called the "modified frequency"). Although modified durations also can be calculated, they are much more open to distortion because the researcher has no way of telling if the behavior filled up the entire epoch or just a small portion of it.

Aggregating coding categories

Once the descriptive statistics have been calculated for each participant, the observational researcher is often faced with a dilemma. Coding categories, especially in complex coding schemes, are frequently quite numerous. Some coding schemes incorporate 30 or more specific behaviors. These codes need to be aggregated in some fashion before inferential statistical techniques can be used. For example, in an observational study of falling-asleep behavior of hospitalized children, White, Wear, and Stephenson (1983) compared the behaviors of children who listened to a bedtime story that was tape-recorded by the parent, with the behaviors of children who did not listen to a story. After computing the relative frequencies of 38 different behavior codes for each child (see discussion on descriptive statistics), the researchers might have used a series of 38 *t*-tests to evaluate statistically the difference between the "story" and "no-story" groups on each of the behaviors. However, whenever a large number of statistical tests are calculated for a data set, some results will appear to be significant by chance alone. The phenomenon of finding significance when none really exists often occurs when observational data are used

because of the typical complexity of coding schemes and the larger number of *t*-tests that could be calculated. To avoid the problem of too many statistical tests, some method of data aggregation must be used.

Data can be aggregated conceptually or empirically. Conceptually derived techniques involve aggregation of coding categories based on the researcher's *a priori* ideas about which codes can be grouped together. For example, in the White et al. study (1983) of falling-asleep behaviors, the researchers combined the 38 separate codes into 8 broader categories before analyzing group differences. Thus the behaviors "eye rub," "blinking of eyes," "yawn," and "eyes closed" were combined to form the category "sleepy." Empirically derived techniques, on the other hand, are used to aggregate data when the underlying relationships among the coding categories are not readily apparent to the researcher. *Factor analysis* (see Chapter 27) is the most commonly used empirical data reduction technique.

Factor analysis requires access to a computer-based statistical package such as the Statistical Package for the Social Sciences (SPSS). Although in the case of observational data the purpose of factor analysis would be to provide information about how to aggregate coding categories at the individual participant level, the computational procedures involve all frequencies of all codes for all participants. The output of a factor analysis yields a new set of "components" or factors. Simply put, the factor structure tells us how the specific behavior codes should be grouped together. For example, in a study of nursing home–staff behaviors directed to elderly residents, Kahana and Kiyak (1984) conducted a factor analysis on the frequencies of 10 specific behavioral items such as "general conversation," "criticizes/puts down," and "makes supportive statement or action." The factor analysis yielded three clear factors—negative parenting, treat as equal, and positive parenting. New descriptive statistics then could be calculated on these variables at the individual participant level. Factor analysis is a complex technique that should be studied in depth before it is used.

Sequential analysis

Up to this point we have discussed the frequencies and durations, or relative frequencies and relative durations, of specific behavior codes and combinations of codes. Another type of descriptive technique often used with observational data is called sequential or lag-sequential analysis. Sequential analysis occurs at the level of the individual participant, before using inferential statistics. *Sequential analysis* is used when the investigator has a hypothesis regarding the ways in which specific behavior codes occur in relation to other behavior codes. For example, the researcher might think that two behaviors, "dog bark" and "baby cry," are sequentially related such that baby cry is more likely to follow dog bark than would be expected by chance alone. The basic process of lag-sequential analysis involves comparing conditional probabilities with simple probabilities. In this case we would compare the conditional probability of cry | bark (read "cry given bark") with the simple probability of cry. That is, we must compare the probability that cry follows bark with the simple probability of occurrence of cry. For example, if the simple probability of cry was .25, we would expect cry to follow bark by chance about 25% of the time. If cry followed bark significantly more than 25% of the time, then cry | bark is a contingent behavior pattern, that is, a significantly occurring sequence for that particular participant. We will not attempt to go through the calculations necessary for lag-sequential analysis here, although they involve very simple arithmetic and can be computed with a hand calculator.

The comparison of simple probabilities and conditional probabilities yields a *z*-score, which expresses the contingency of the relationship between two behaviors. Generally speaking, a *z*-score of +1.96 or more indicates that two behaviors are significantly sequentially related. Similarly, a *z*-score of −1.96 or less indicates that the two behaviors are less sequentially related than would be expected by chance alone. For example, "cry" would be unlikely to immediately follow "smile." Inferential statistical techniques then can be used to determine if a significant number of the total participants have the same significantly sequential behavior patterns. For example, if the comparison of the simple and conditional probabilities of "cry" and "cry given bark" yielded a significant *z*-score for 14 out of 18 dog-baby dyads, an inferential technique could be used to inform us about whether this number of participants (14) was statistically significant. This kind of information is useful for determining if a sequential behavior pattern is a generally occurring pattern in a group of participants. *Z*-scores can be treated like any of the other individual-participant descriptive statistics in the sense that inferential techniques can be used to compare, for example, the *z*-scores of two groups of participants to determine if two behaviors are more sequentially related in one group than in another.

Lag-sequential analysis also can be performed on time-based data, to ascertain whether two behaviors are sequentially related in time. As previously mentioned, sequential analyses are rarely appropriate for time-sampled data because the precise order and timing of events is not preserved in the database. For further information on lag-sequential analysis, consult Sackett (1979) or Bakeman and Gottman (1986).

REPORTING OBSERVATIONAL DATA

In this chapter we have introduced the reader to research processes that use observational methods of data production. By now the reader should have a good idea of what observational methods are, what the basic issues are that differentiate one kind of observational approach from another, how to develop a coding scheme, how to collect data, how to evaluate the reliability and validity of the data, and how to analyze the results. One final step remains—reporting the research.

Many of the research questions that are investigated with observational methods simply could not be done otherwise. Our understanding of human social interaction, in particular, has been vastly increased through the use of observation for collecting data. The findings of these studies need to be shared with others in the field in such a way that they can be judged to have internal and external validity. The following list of questions is a helpful guide toward thoughtful appraisal of the quality of studies that use observation. These questions will help the investigator who is reporting a study that used observational methods ensure that sufficient information is included in the written report to allow readers to evaluate the quality of the study, as well as the reliability and validity of the findings.

1. Is observational methodology appropriate for answering the research question raised by this study? The investigator should identify the particular aspect

of the research question that led to the use of observation. It might be the nature of the behavior being studied or the characteristics of the relevant population of participants. Observational methods are complex and require a significant investment of time on the part of the researcher. The investigator should make it clear that observational methods were the optimum choice to answer the research question.

2. What behaviors were recorded and why? The introductory section to the report should provide an overview of the behaviors that were recorded and their relationship to the research question; that is, an obvious match should exist between the way the research problem is stated and the kinds of behaviors included in the methods.

3. In what ways was the time frame used appropriate to the research question? A report of the research should indicate the rationale for choosing a particular time frame. This is an important consideration when a time-sampling method was used. The rationale that the author presents must persuade the reader that an event-sampling method would not have been more appropriate to answer the research question.

4. Under what circumstances were the data collected? The written report of the research study should spell out in some detail why a particular setting or situation was chosen for data collection. Whether the setting is naturalistic or contrived, the choice should be explained. The author should include information about characteristics of the setting that may have contributed to the reported results. Did the data collection setting make demands on the participants that may have altered the findings? Were data collected in a consistent manner from one participant to the other?

5. What apparatus was used for recording the data? The researcher may have used paper and pencil, audio- or videotaping, or electronic data entry equipment. The author should explain how this choice of recording was made and how this choice enhanced the nature or the quality of the data.

6. How were the data used to answer the research question? The researcher must report exactly how the data were handled. Was analysis based on frequency or duration, on patterns or sequences? Were the original coding categories used, or were the data aggregated in some way? Why were these methods of analysis appropriate to the research question?

7. Were the statistical analyses appropriate? The author must provide information about what scores were used for each statistical test. This information must be reported in a way that can be understood clearly.

8. Did the statistical analyses address the major research question? The issue here is whether the study used statistical analyses that matched the statement of the research problem. One common problem in studies using observational methods is that the report will contain a great deal of descriptive detail about the observations (means and standard deviations of 30 or 40 coding categories, for example) and very little information about how the data addressed the original research question. Conversely, the author should avoid reporting so little about the basic data that the reader cannot make good interpretations of the more complex analyses that are reported.

9. Were most of the analyses concerned with differences between groups of participants or with associations among variables for each participant? Although both tests of group differences (t-test or analysis of variance) and measures of association (correlation coefficients or chi-square) are useful, and although they often appear together in research reports, the two kinds of analysis answer quite different questions. If the primary questions of the research are about differences, the investigator should report statistics and summary tables that are about differences. Similarly, if the primary questions are about association, statistical results and tables that reflect that fact should be included. If both kinds of information are important to the study questions, it should be apparent how the various results can be integrated into a "big picture."

10. Did the discussion adequately cover the results that were obtained? The discussion section should summarize the empirical results and explain their significance for the theory or problem that was the origin of the research. Whether the discussion is presented separately or is integrated with the results section does not matter particularly. What does matter is that the discussion include a reasonable interpretation of the study as a whole rather than just restating individual findings in different words or in a different order.

11. Did the discussion include any reference to shortcomings or limitations and/or any suggestions for specific future research to resolve unanswered

questions? A researcher has a responsibility to inform the reader of any aspects of the study that might limit the interpretations that should be made of the data. This does not mean that discussion sections must be apologetic; it does mean that the author should call at least brief attention to shortcomings in the research. Suggestions for further research can come in two different ways. First, most studies raise more questions than they answer, and those new questions are surely subjects for further research. Second, most results can be interpreted in several ways. Choosing among those alternatives frequently requires more study. The discussion section, then, should both summarize what has been found and point to what is yet to be found.

12. Overall, did this study add to our scholarly or clinical knowledge of the participants? This judgment is a summary one, but it is more than just the sum of the answers to the first 11 questions. To answer this question the investigator must make a professional and personal evaluation of how important the question was in the first place and how well, on balance, the researchers have addressed the issues.

In conclusion, the standards for high-quality research that use observational methods are no different from the standards for high-quality research using any other methods. The key is to choose methods that do the best possible job of answering our questions, to use those methods as competently as possible, and to report the study in a complete manner.

SUMMARY

Observational methods are used when researchers ask questions about overt behaviors or events that research participants would have difficulty describing or recording. In this chapter the use of human observers who record behavior was discussed. The child study movement, ethology and ecology, and behavioristic psychology have emphasized the importance of learning about behavior by observing individuals. Computer technology has made manageable the study of complex behaviors.

The recording of behaviors can be event-triggered or time-triggered. In time-triggered coding, behavior is recorded by the clock at predetermined intervals. The occurrence of a particular event triggers coding in an event-triggered coding scheme. Behav-

ior can be recorded in the setting where it naturally occurs or in a contrived setting such as a laboratory. The observer may serve as a detector of behavior, coding whether a particular event has or has not occurred. The observer may also serve as an informant, making a judgment about an entire pattern of behaviors.

The first step in developing a coding scheme for behavioral observations is to select a group of individuals who are similar to those who will be used for the study and to watch their behavior. Field notes are made that will allow the investigator to develop a coding scheme and to define each behavior to be coded.

The investigator must decide whether to record very small (molecular) or very large (molar) levels of behavior. Usually, a coding system that falls between extremely molecular and extremely molar is easiest for observers to learn. Observing individuals as part of the research development process also allows the investigator to decide whether observations should be made continuously or intermittently.

Observers are the human instrument used to collect observational data. They must be chosen with care and trained to carry out the task of observing and recording specific behaviors. The investigator must make every effort to maintain the morale of observers during the long and tedious hours of observing and coding behavior.

As in other types of research, issues of reliability and validity of data are important when observational methods are used. Interobserver agreement and statistical reliability are two ways to ensure that the scores generated from behavioral observations are precise, accurate, and consistent. Validity is concerned with whether the behavioral observations measure the trait or characteristic called for by the theory and research question. Face validity, content validity, criterion validity, and construct validity are typical methods used to establish validity.

Observational methods produce large quantities of data that must be aggregated and summarized. Total frequency, total duration, proportion of frequency, and proportion of duration can be calculated. Observations can be aggregated on the basis of a conceptual scheme or can be empirically aggregated using such techniques as factor analysis. Often, the investigator is interested in the sequence or combination of behaviors. In this case a form of sequential analysis must be used.

Finally, the researcher must report research using observational methods in such a way that readers can understand what was done and why. Guidelines were provided for writing and reviewing a report to ensure that it contains information necessary to understand the study and to evaluate the reliability and validity of the methods used.

REFERENCES

Bakeman, R. (1978). Untangling streams of behavior: Sequential analyses of observation data. In G. P. Sackett (Ed.), *Observing behavior: Vol. II. Data collection and analysis methods* (pp. 63-78). Baltimore: University Park Press.

Bakeman, R., Cairns, R. B., & Appelbaum, M. (1979). Note on describing and analyzing interactional data: Some first steps and common pitfalls. In R. B. Cairns (Ed.), *The analysis of social interaction: Methods, issues, and illustrations* (pp. 227-234). Hillsdale, NJ: Erlbaum.

Bakeman, R., & Gottman, J. M. (1986). *Observing interaction: An introduction to sequential analysis.* Cambridge, England: Cambridge University Press.

Bronfenbrenner, U. (1979). *The ecology of human development: Experiments by nature and design.* Cambridge, MA: Harvard University Press.

Cairns, R. B., & Green, J. A. (1979). How to assess personality and social patterns: Observations or ratings? In R. B. Cairns (Ed.), *The analysis of social interaction: Methods, issues, and illustrations* (pp. 209-226). Hillsdale, NJ: Erlbaum.

Ciminero, A. R. (1986). Behavioral assessment: An overview. In A. R. Ciminero, K. S. Calhoun, & H. E. Adams (Eds.), *Handbook of behavioral assessment* (pp. 3-13). New York: Wiley.

Cohen, J. (1960). A coefficient of agreement for nominal scales. *Educational and Psychological Measurement, 20,* 37-46.

Cone, J. D. (1982). Validity of direct observation assessment procedures. In D. P. Hartmann (Ed.), *Using observers to study behavior* (pp. 67-79). *New directions for methodology of social and behavioral science: No. 14.* San Francisco: Jossey-Bass.

Ekman, P., & Friesen, W. V. (1978). *The facial action coding system.* Palo Alto, CA: Consulting Psychologists Press.

Gottman, J. M. (1978). Nonsequential data analysis techniques in observational research. In G. P. Sackett (Ed.), *Observing behavior: Vol. II. Data collection and analysis methods* (pp. 45-62). Baltimore: University Park Press.

Gottman, J. M. (1983, July 13). Personal communication.

Hartmann, D. P. (1982). Assessing the dependability of observational data. In D. P. Hartmann (Ed.), *Using observers to study behavior* (pp. 51-65). *New directions for methodology of social and behavioral science: No. 14.* San Francisco: Jossey-Bass.

Hartmann, D. P., & Gardner, W. (1981). Considerations in assessing the reliability of observations. In E. E. Filsinger & R. A. Lewis (Eds.), *Assessing marriage: New behavioral approaches* (pp. 184-196). Beverly Hills, CA: Sage.

Hawkins, R. P. (1982). Developing a behavior code. In D. P. Hartmann (Ed.), *Using observers to study behavior* (pp. 21-35). *New directions for methodology of social and behavioral science: No. 14.* San Francisco: Jossey-Bass.

Herbert, J., & Attridge, C. (1975). A guide for developers and users of observation systems and manuals. *American Educational Research Journal, 12,* 1-20.

Hinde, R. A. (1973). On the design of check sheets. *Primates, 14,* 393-406.

Hollenbeck, A. R. (1978). Problems of reliability in observational research. In G. P. Sackett (Ed.), *Observing behavior: Vol. II. Data collection and analysis methods* (pp. 79-98). Baltimore: University Park Press.

Holm, R. A. (1981). Using data logging equipment. In E. E. Filsinger & R. A. Lewis (Eds.), *Assessing marriage: New behavioral approaches* (pp. 171-181). Beverly Hills, CA: Sage.

Irwin, D. M., & Bushnell, M. M. (1980). *Observational strategies for child study.* New York: Holt, Rinehart & Winston.

Johnson, S. M., & Bolstad, O. D. (1973). Methodological issues in naturalistic observation: Some problems and solutions for field research. In L. A. Hamerlynck, L. C. Handy, & E. J. Mash (Eds.), *Behavior change: Methodology, concepts, and practice* (pp. 3-67). Champaign, IL: Research Press.

Kahana, E. F., & Kiyak, H. A. (1984). Attitudes and behavior of staff in facilities for the aged. *Research on Aging, 6,* 395-417.

Kaye, K. (1982). The moral philosophy of microanalysis. In T. M. Field & A. Fogel (Eds.), *Emotion and early interaction* (pp. 237-251). Hillsdale, NJ: Erlbaum.

Kazdin, A. E. (1982). Observer effects: Reactivity of direct observation. In D. P. Hartmann (Ed.), *Using observers to study behavior* (pp. 5-19). *New directions for methodology of social and behavioral science: No. 14.* San Francisco: Jossey-Bass.

Kniskern, J. R., Robinson, E. A., & Mitchell, S. K. (1983). Mother-child interaction in home and laboratory settings. *Child Study Journal, 13,* 23-29.

Landesman, S. (1985, Feb. 7). Personal communication.

Mitchell, S. K. (1979). Interobserver agreement, reliability, and generalizability of data collected in observational studies. *Psychological Bulletin, 86,* 376-390.

Niemeier, D. F. (1983). A behavioral analysis of staff-patient interactions in a psychiatric setting. *Western Journal of Nursing Research, 5,* 269-281.

Notarius, C. I., Krokoff, L. J., & Markman, H. J. (1981). Analysis of observational data. In E. E. Filsinger & R. A. Lewis (Eds.), *Assessing marriage: New behavioral approaches* (pp 197-216). Beverly Hills, CA: Sage.

Owen, B. D. (1985). The lifting process and back injury in hospital personnel. *Western Journal of Nursing Research, 7*, 445-459.

Parten, M. B. (1932). Social participation among preschool children. *Journal of Abnormal and Social Psychology, 27*, 243-269.

Reid, J. B. (1982). Observer training in naturalistic research. In D. P. Hartmann (Ed.), *Using observers to study behavior* (pp. 37-50). *New directions for methodology of social and behavioral science: No. 14.* San Francisco: Jossey-Bass.

Robinson, W. S. (1957). The statistical measurement of agreement. *American Sociological Review, 22*, 17-25.

Rosenblum, L. A. (1978). The creation of a behavioral taxonomy. In G. P. Sackett (Ed.), *Observing behavior: Vol. II. Data collection and analysis methods* (pp. 15-24). Baltimore: University Park Press.

Sackett, G. P. (1979). The lag sequential analysis of contingency and cyclicity in behavioral interaction research. In J. D. Osofsky (Ed.), *Handbook of infant development* (pp. 623-649). New York: Wiley.

Sackett, G. P., & Landesman-Dwyer, S. (1982). Data analysis: Methods and problems. In D. P. Hartmann (Ed.), *Using observers to study behavior* (pp. 81-99). *New directions for methodology of social and behavioral science: No. 14.* San Francisco: Jossey-Bass.

Tinsley, H. E. A., & Weiss, D. J. (1975). Interrater reliability and agreement of subjective judgments. *Journal of Counseling Psychology, 22*, 358-376.

White, M. A., Wear, E., & Stephenson, G. (1983). A computer-compatible method for observing falling asleep behavior of hospitalized children. *Research in Nursing and Health, 6*, 191-198.

Yarrow, M., & Waxler, C. (1979). Observing interaction: A confrontation with methodology. In R. B. Cairns (Ed.), *The analysis of social interaction: Methods, issues, and illustrations* (pp. 37-65). Hillsdale, NJ: Erlbaum.

18

SELECTING AND DESIGNING QUESTIONNAIRES AND INTERVIEW GUIDES

MARCI CATANZARO

Throughout the day we have many encounters with others that take the form of asking questions and getting answers. We meet a friend on the street and ask, "How are you?" or "Did you have a good holiday weekend?" We do not think of these encounters with others as research, yet we are seeking and getting information, often in an unconsciously systematic way. Asking questions of others is our most often-used device for obtaining information. Researchers have two instruments designed to ask such questions: the research interview and the questionnaire. A *research interview* is a face-to-face or telephone encounter with a research participant to obtain specific and systematic information about a given phenomenon. Interviews include special situations such as focus groups, play interviews, role playing, and ethnographic interviews. A *questionnaire* is a paper-and-pencil instrument that a research participant is asked to complete. Questionnaires include techniques that do not require direct interaction between the investigator and the respondent, such as Q-sort and Delphi techniques. Computer technology makes it possible to administer a questionnaire via computer. The respondent's computer terminal displays questions that the respondent answers by keying his or her response into the terminal, possibly at a distance from the originating computer. The actual questions used to achieve the research purpose may be identical on an interview guide and on a question-naire. The method of administration differentiates an interview from a questionnaire.

In this chapter the questions that make up a questionnaire or an interview guide will be referred to as a *schedule*. The chapter begins with a discussion of the uses of interviews and questionnaires and continues with a comparison of these two forms of data generation. The kinds of information appropriate for interviews and questionnaires and the types of schedules and questions are presented. In some cases a schedule may be available that will serve the researcher's purposes; thus sources of existing schedules are suggested, and the effects of altering an existing schedule will be discussed. Finally, the chapter presents strategies for developing and evaluating new schedules. Information about administering questionnaires and interviews, including ensuring the reliability of data, controlling bias, and increasing response rates, follows in Chapter 19.

USES OF INTERVIEWS AND QUESTIONNAIRES

The interview and the questionnaire are useful instruments in nursing research because they allow the investigator to question research participants about facts, ideas, behaviors, preferences, problems, feelings, attitudes, and so forth. Some of this information may not be obtainable any other way. We can observe behavior that is assumed to be motivated by preferences, feelings, or attitudes, but we can understand only a person's perceptions of events and feelings about those events by asking him or her. Interviews and questionnaires may be the main instrument, such as when they are used to identify, measure, or explore the relationship among variables. However, they also may supplement other methods of data generation by allowing the investigator to follow up on unexpected results obtained from other methods or to explore motivations and reasons why persons responded as they did to other instruments. Interviews and questionnaires are the form of data generation most frequently used in nursing research; they are used to generate data for describing phenomena and for testing theories and hypotheses about those phenomena.

Sometimes an interview is used rather than a questionnaire because respondents have not yet learned to write or cannot write because of illness or injury. Lambert (1985) used structured interviews in her study of factors associated with well-being in women who had rheumatoid arthritis because changes in hand joints that result from the disease often make writing difficult. Ritchie, Caty, and Ellerton (1984) used a play interview with preschool-age children to elicit their developmental and hospital-related concerns. Interviews and questionnaires allow the investigator (1) to identify facts and to explore events and their meaning, (2) to explore and test the relationship of variables, and (3) to validate other forms of data collection.

Identifying and exploring events and meanings

Information about age, gender, occupation, income, and other demographic variables used to describe the study sample frequently is gathered through the use of questionnaires. Although this information could be obtained through other sources such as birth certificates, simply asking the respondent is more efficient and may be sufficient for the purposes of the study. Questionnaires also may be used to identify individuals who meet study-inclusion criteria. For example, a questionnaire to determine age and income may be sent to all residents in a particular geographical area. Those respondents to the questionnaire who fall between the ages of 30 and 69 and who have an income over $30,000 per year could be

identified as potential participants in a study of fitness behaviors of middle-aged adults in a middle-income bracket.

Some types of schedules allow the investigator to ask questions about a person's hopes and aspirations and the meaning of certain events; these schedules may provide an opportunity to probe the context and reasons for the answers to the questions. Corbin and Strauss (1985) used interviews with chronically ill persons and their spouses to explore the problems they face when the ill person lives at home. They were able to probe for in-depth information about the many facets of work required to manage the illness along with everyday-life work and the participant's own biographical work.

Respondents may be unable to report their beliefs, feelings, or motivations because they are not consciously aware of them or because they are unable to share intrapersonal matters with others. Sometimes questions require individuals to make inferences or judgments about themselves that they may never have learned to do. The wife of a chronically ill man may be unable to answer questions about how the illness has affected her life because she has never thought about it and thus has not had an opportunity to make inferences about how the disease has affected her behavior.

Exploring and testing relationships

The researcher appropriately uses interviews and questionnaires to identify relationships or to suggest hypotheses for further study. Benoliel (1983) used interviews to explore the factors that influenced identity development in adolescents who had life-threatening disease. She used findings from her early studies to propose hypotheses about the socializing influences on identity development and for developing a theory concerning chronic disease in adolescence.

Validating information

An interview or questionnaire can be used to validate other forms of data collection, to follow up on unexpected results obtained by other methods, and to explore the reasons someone responded in a certain way to other data generating techniques. Tripp-Reimer (1985) used semistructured interviews to augment participant-observation information concerning the practice of *matiasma* (practices associated with the evil eye) in a community of Greek immigrants. She then used interview data to validate what she had observed in the community. Magilvy (1985) used open-ended interview questions and a questionnaire, the Handicap Inventory for the Elderly, to assess the social and emotional aspects of hearing loss and the overall perceived social-hearing handicap in a group of 66 women who were prevocationally deaf or who had experienced a later hearing loss.

CHOOSING BETWEEN INTERVIEWS AND QUESTIONNAIRES

The research interview and the questionnaire are valuable forms of data generation. The decision to ask direct questions of a research respondent will depend on the purpose of the study, the level of knowledge in the field of study, and the variables of interest. When the purpose, the level of knowledge, and the variables direct the investigator to question respondents, the investigator will need to decide whether the questions will be administered as a questionnaire or an interview.

The researcher also must decide how the questionnaire or interview will be administered. Interviews can be administered in face-to-face or voice-to-voice (telephone) situations with individuals or with groups. Questionnaires can be mailed, delivered to the participants in person, or sent to a computer terminal. They can be administered to groups in a classroom or a social or professional meeting, or they can be self-administered in a face-to-face context. When making decisions to use an interview or a questionnaire, the investigator will consider (1) the cost and speed of administration and (2) the likelihood of obtaining useful responses.

Cost and speed of administration

The research interview is costly to use in terms of time and money. Face-to-face interviews are time-consuming for both the participant and the researcher: an open-ended interview can last for hours and may need to be continued at another time, thereby extending the costs associated with interviewer time. Potential participants initially may not realize the extent of the time commitment and withdraw from the study after the interviewer has already spent valuable hours with them. In addition, the interviewer and the respondent must find a convenient time, which may require repeated contacts with the respondent and juggling of schedules. Because of

scheduling conflicts and other demands on his or her time, the researcher may not be able to do all the interviews. When others are needed to help with the interviews, the primary investigator must train them, which adds to the cost of the study. Depending on the structure of the interview, this training may take hours and require that the interviewers understand much of the conceptual framework for the study.

Questionnaires, on the other hand, must be printed and delivered to the respondent. The costs involved will depend on the extent of the questionnaire and the methods of reproduction and delivery used. In general, mailed questionnaires obtain a greater amount of data from a large sample of people in less time. The cost savings gained through use of a mailed questionnaire as opposed to a face-to-face interview can be used to increase the sample size.

The costs of group-administered questionnaires and telephone interviews fall between the costs of face-to-face and mailed data collection. A large quantity of data can be obtained in a short time when a questionnaire is administered to a large group. Administering questionnaires to a group of respondents in one location eliminates the time necessary for postal delivery and return of questionnaires, but it may be balanced by the investigator's time in traveling to the group. When repeated data are needed, mailed or computer-transmitted questionnaires may be most cost-effective.

Telephone interviews are more economical of time because they eliminate the time necessary to travel to the interview site. Interviews can be conducted with groups of people (focus groups), which has the advantage of decreasing interviewer time.

Obtaining useful responses

As noted earlier, the investigator must consider characteristics of participants such as age and the ability to read and write in determining whether participants can be expected to complete a paper-and-pencil questionnaire. The child or adult with a lack of language skills or the inability to read the questions because of visual impairments or language differences cannot be expected to read and respond to questionnaires. Persons who are unable to write because of educational deficiencies or physical limitations also cannot complete questionnaires. In these cases some form of interview will be necessary to obtain data.

The likelihood that the potential study participants will complete the questions on a questionnaire or interview schedule is another important consideration in deciding which data generation method to use. Questions that are administered face-to-face cannot be thrown away or forgotten. Refusing to answer questions is more difficult for many people when facing an interviewer than when being asked to participate by telephone. Completion of a questionnaire on time is more likely if the investigator collects it at a specific time, rather than having the participant mail it. In summary, the more direct contact the potential respondent has with the investigator the more likely it is that timely data will be obtained.

The sensitivity of the information being sought is another consideration when judging the potential usefulness of responses. When the researcher is exploring feelings about and perceptions of situations, the respondent may find it easier to "talk through" those feelings with an interested person than to organize and present those thoughts in a written form. Alternatively, the respondent may be self-conscious about sharing feelings during a face-to-face encounter with the interviewer but may be willing to write those feelings on an anonymous questionnaire or speak them during a telephone interview. Questionnaires that can be completed at the respondent's leisure remove the pressure for an immediate response. The person who is expected to answer a question immediately but who needs time to think about the response may respond with "I don't know" or select any answer from choices offered.

A face-to-face interview provides the investigator with observational data that are not otherwise available. The participant's level of comfort with and understanding of questions can be observed. The length of time required for a participant to formulate an answer may provide important data on the difficulty of the question for that person. The investigator can observe nonverbal responses, such as physically moving closer to or farther away from the interviewer. Information about lifestyle, social class, and educational level is often apparent during face-to-face interviews. However, the interviewer may introduce bias through nonverbal communication or the way in which he or she phrases questions.

The interviewer allows the investigator to explore complex feelings or perceptions with respondents. In the descriptive phase of theory development the investigator may not know enough about the phe-

nomenon under study to structure a paper-and-pencil questionnaire that a respondent can complete. Swanson-Kauffman (1986) was interested in the experience of women who had miscarried. Use of the interview allowed her to explore in depth the feelings that these women experienced as they became aware that they had lost a pregnancy, coped with their loss, and continued to live their lives.

The interview makes it possible for the investigator to clarify or reword questions for the respondent. In her study of the configuration surrounding the evil eye Tripp-Reimer (1985) may have found that fifth-generation Greek immigrants retained *matiasma* practices (practices associated with the evil eye), although they did not recognize the Greek word. Through the use of the interview she would have been able to rephrase her questions so that she could have elicited information about the beliefs and practices surrounding the prevention, diagnosis, and treatment of the evil eye without using the unfamiliar word *matiasma*.

The interview also makes it possible for the investigator to clarify responses that are not fully understood. In response to a question about her first symptoms of multiple sclerosis, a respondent answered, "I had a hot chick pea and bundles of spaghetti in my leg." Such a response written on a questionnaire would have little value to the investigator because its meaning is obscure. During the interview, however, the investigator was able to probe further and learn that the participant had an area about the size of a baseball of intense burning (hot chick pea) on the lateral side of her right leg and that she often felt as if the skin on her leg had insects crawling on it (bundles of spaghetti). The ability to probe, reword, and clarify is counterbalanced by the need for the interviewer to be alert constantly to what the respondent is saying, both verbally and nonverbally.

The interviewer can control the order in which questions are presented. Dai and Catanzaro (1987) were concerned that the responses to questions concerning what paraplegic men actually did to prevent decubitus ulcers would be influenced if they first completed a test of their knowledge about skin care. Use of an interview ensured that the participants completed the questions in the intended order.

In summary, questionnaires and interviews have advantages and disadvantages. The investigator will use information about the purpose of the study, the level of knowledge in the field of study, and the variables of interest to determine which administration of questions will be most appropriate. The cost and speed of administration must be balanced against the probability of obtaining useful responses from the target population. Questionnaires are useful for obtaining a large amount of data in a brief period of time; however, the type of information that can be obtained on a paper-and-pencil instrument may not serve the investigator's needs.

KINDS OF INFORMATION OBTAINED BY INTERVIEWS AND QUESTIONNAIRES

Interviews and questionnaires are useful to obtain information about things that people know. This information may be facts about themselves, other people they know, or events with which they are familiar. These techniques can also elicit information about beliefs, feelings, and attitudes, as well as about the past and present behavior and standards of action used by the respondent or others.

Information about facts

Information about facts can be obtained easily and economically through interviews or questionnaires. Questions about birth date, religious affiliation, income, and occupation are examples of factual data. These data can be verified through documents such as birth certificates, church rosters, and employers' records. Individuals also may be expected to know facts about programs with which they are associated. A dean is expected to know how many students are enrolled in the school of nursing, and a clinic administrator is expected to know the number of patients cared for in a clinic each month. Judging the accuracy of the responses provided requires that the investigator know how the respondent acquired knowledge of the facts reported. Hearsay is less likely to provide accurate facts than direct observation. Memory may also influence the individual's ability to provide accurate facts. A person may have forgotten how many patients were cared for last year. The investigator can verify information by comparing the responses of several respondents. Nurse researchers often elicit facts about an individual's health history and health behaviors, which may be difficult to verify without extended observation of the respondent in situations involving the health behavior of interest.

Information about beliefs, feelings, and attitudes

Questionnaires and interviews can obtain information about beliefs and attitudes that individuals hold. Such questions do not establish what is objectively true but rather what the respondent believes and is willing to share. Nurses may be asked to share how they would respond personally or how others with whom they work are likely to respond to a particular patient situation, such as the birth of a multiply handicapped child. These responses do not, however, indicate how the nurse will actually respond to the given situation. Belief questions may elicit the respondent's knowledge about specific facts or inquire about issues for which no single correct answer exists (see box below).

In response to questions respondents can describe their behavior and the behavior they have observed in others. The box on the right gives examples of questions that elicit information about past, present, and future behavior concerning exercise. When asked to describe the behavior of others, different observers may express different beliefs. A family member, a stranger, or a nurse each may describe differently the behavior of a person with epilepsy during a seizure.

Nurse investigators often are interested in subjective feelings that the patient experiences. Interviews

---

EXAMPLES OF QUESTIONS ABOUT FACTS AND OPINIONS

A. Is this statement true or false? "The incidence of lung cancer in women has risen steadily over the last two decades."
   1. TRUE
   2. FALSE
B. In your opinion is the increased use of tobacco by women responsible for the increased incidence of lung cancer in women?
   1. DEFINITELY YES
   2. PROBABLY YES
   3. MAYBE
   4. PROBABLY NO
   5. DEFINITELY NO

EXAMPLES OF QUESTIONS ABOUT BEHAVIOR

A. Have you, at any time in the past, exercised on a regular basis for at least 20 minutes at least three times a week?
   1. YES
   2. NO
B. Do you exercise on a regular basis for at least 20 minutes at least three times a week?
   1. YES
   2. NO
C. Do you think you will start to exercise on a regular basis for at least 20 minutes at least three times a week at some time in the future?
   1. YES
   2. NO

and questionnaires are the only way of obtaining information about feelings. We cannot see if someone is hungry, nor can we verify hunger when he or she expresses it. We cannot know objectively that a nursing intervention alleviates a woman's perimenstrual pain.

In summary, interviews and questionnaires are used to obtain information about facts, beliefs, feelings, and attitudes of respondents. Questions of fact may be about the respondent or about other familiar people or things. Respondents can be questioned about their own thought processes or about how they believe others feel or believe.

TYPES OF SCHEDULES

Interview or questionnaire schedules may be classified as structured or unstructured. Although this classification often is presented as dichotomous, schedules can vary along a continuum—ranging from the highly structured schedule, where the interviewer and respondent have little flexibility, to totally unstructured conversations with a purpose. Within this classification the investigator must make additional choices about how much information the respondent can provide. These latter decisions determine the types of questions that are asked (open-

ended or fixed-alternative). Structured and unstructured schedules can include both open-ended and fixed-alternative questions; however, fixed-alternative questions are associated more commonly with structured schedules.

Structured schedules

Questions on a structured or standardized schedule are fixed in wording and sequence. Questionnaires always are structured; once the questions are committed to paper, no opportunity for alteration exists. In structured interviews the interviewer is permitted little liberty in asking questions. In extreme cases the interviewer reads the questions to the participant and records the answers. Structured interviews are planned in detail and gather fairly consistent data from one respondent to another. Lincoln and Guba (1985) pointed out that structured interviews are used when the interviewer knows enough about the research problem to formulate appropriate questions.

Structured schedules have several advantages. The information that is generated is relatively easy to process and analyze. When administered as an interview, a structured schedule does not require a high level of skill in the interviewing process. However, a limitation of the structured schedule is that relating the questions to the particular individual and circumstances is not possible. This may make the respondent feel as if the schedule were unnatural and lacked specific relevance to the situation. The respondent may wish to tell the investigator his or her own story and may be annoyed at the fixed sequence of questions, which does not always follow what the respondent has just said.

Unstructured schedules

Face-to-face or voice-to-voice interviews can use questions that are unstructured, open-ended and flexible in their content and sequence. Unstructured schedules are used appropriately when the investigator wants to understand the meaning of the respondent's world, as is the case in most field or ethnographic research. Respondents are encouraged to talk about whatever is relevant to the researcher's interest.

Unstructured schedules may use an interview guide that outlines the topics and issues to be explored before the interview begins but gives no particular order or wording of questions to elicit responses about the topics in advance. The box below contains the first of seven parts of an interview guide developed by Marcella Z. Davis (1970) and used in her study of the transitions to a devalued state that occur in multiple sclerosis.

The interview guide provides a checklist of topics to be covered. Therefore the interviewer must be able to adapt both the wording and the sequence of the questions to the respondent in the context of the interview situation. Use of an outline systematizes data collection to the extent that the same topics are covered with each respondent. The lack of a systematized format for questioning, however, may make it difficult for the interviewer to keep track of the topics covered. Use of a topic outline is particularly difficult for the investigator who is relatively inexperienced in conducting research interviews. When more than one interviewer is participating in a single study, the sequencing and wording of questions can vary considerably and reduce comparability of responses.

The most unstructured of all interviews is conducted much like an informal conversation. Some investigators have referred to this unstructured approach to data generation as the ethnographic or phenomenologic interview (Patton, 1980; Spradley, 1979). The investigator enters the research scene to learn what is going on. Questions emerge from the immediate context, are asked in the natural course of events, and are commonly combined with participant observation. Predetermining a set of questions is not possible because the researcher cannot know beforehand what will occur and what type of questions will be important to ask. The conversational interview increases the salience and relevance of the questions and allows the interviewer full freedom to match the questions to the respondent and the circumstances. The interviewer is allowed to use imagination and ingenuity as he or she tries to develop new hypotheses from the data and test them in the course of the interview (Spradley, 1979).

The data generated by each respondent in an unstructured interview will be different, which makes comparable data unlikely. Questions change over time, and each interview builds on the other, "expanding information that was picked up previously, moving in new directions and seeking elucidation and elaboration from various participants in their own terms" (Patton, 1980, p. 199). The data are not systematic, and their organization and analysis are difficult. A great deal of time is required to sift through responses to find patterns in the data.

Unstructured interviews require a considerable commitment on the part of the respondents and the researcher. Often, more than one interview with each respondent is required to elicit similar information across participants. The interviewer must interact easily with people and be able to think on his or her feet. The essence of the situation must be comprehended and questions formulated quickly and smoothly. There is no time to dawdle over a cup of coffee and ponder the meaning of a word or action in the interview situation.

TYPES OF QUESTIONS

Two basic types of questions can be used for interviews and questionnaires: fixed-alternative questions and open-ended questions (see box on right). A *fixed-alternative question* provides a fixed set of

---

EXAMPLE OF OUTLINE INTERVIEW GUIDE

I. Symptoms
   A. How did you first become aware?
   B. What did you think was happening?
   C. Tell anyone?
      1. Friends, family relatives, etc.
   D. Do anything about symptoms?
      1. See doctor? When?
   E. Age of onset?
   F. Are some symptoms more troublesome than others?
      (Get as specific description as possible)
   G. On medication?
      1. What? Who prescribed?
   H. Treatments?
      1. Psychotherapy, occupational therapy, other?

From Davis, M. Z. (1970). (Doctoral dissertation, University of California, San Francisco, 1970). University Microfilms No. 72-12,768.

responses (example *A*). The respondent must choose from one of the alternative responses provided. An open-ended question does not provide a fixed set of responses but allows the respondent to answer the question in his or her own words (example *B*). An open-ended response category can be included with a fixed-alternative response set (example *C*).

Open-ended questions may be used to generate information that is used as the basis for developing fixed-alternative questions. Lindeman (1975) began her study of priorities in clinical nursing research with open-ended questions that asked panel members to identify burning questions about the practice of nursing. Responses to the open-ended questions were used to generate a list of clinical nursing research topics. Panel members then were asked to use fixed-alternative responses to indicate whether nursing should assume primary research responsibility, how important the topic was for the profession of nursing, and the likelihood that research on the topic would change patient welfare.

Fixed-alternative questions

The fixed-alternative question offers the respondent a choice among two or more alternatives. These choices may be dichotomous such as yes or no, agree or disagree, or they may be scaled to elicit how strongly the respondent agrees or disagrees. Few persons have escaped the telephone survey or mailed questionnaire that inquires about shopping habits or political persuasions. Often the responses requested are of the fixed-alternative type: "Have you pur-chased mayonnaise in the grocery store in the last week?" In nursing research many types of question-naires using fixed-alternative responses are available (see box below). We may ask a patient in pain to select words from the McGill Pain Questionnaire (Melzack, 1975), such as "throbbing" or "stabbing," that best describes the pain. The Health Locus of Control (Wallston, Wallston, & DeVillis, 1978) uses a fixed-alternative type of response in which the respondents must select one of two statements that best describes their belief about the control they have over health-related matters. The Personal Resource Questionnaire (Brandt & Weinert, 1981) uses a

---

EXAMPLES OF FIXED-ALTERNATIVE AND OPEN-ENDED QUESTIONS

A. What is your religious affiliation?
  1. CATHOLIC
  2. PROTESTANT
  3. JEWISH
B. What is your religious affiliation?
C. What is your religious affiliation?
  1. CATHOLIC
  2. PROTESTANT
  3. JEWISH
  4. OTHER (please specify) _____

EXAMPLES OF FIXED-ALTERNATIVE RESPONSES

A. Some of the words on this list may describe the pain you have had in the past week. I would like you to select one word from each category that best describes your pain. You may leave out any category that does not in any way seem to describe your pain.

Flickering	Flashing	Stabbing
Quivering	Shooting	Lancinating
Pulsing	Prickling	Sharp
Throbbing	Boring	Cutting
Beating	Drilling	Lacerating
Jumping		

B. The following statements are about health and illness. Please circle the number before the statement that most clearly describes how you feel.
  1 If I become sick, I have the power to make myself well again.
  2 Health professionals keep me healthy.
C. Please circle the number that most closely describes how much you agree or disagree with each statement.

	Strongly Agree					Strongly Disagree
I have enough contact with the person who makes me feel special.	1 2 3 4 5 6 7					

scale to elicit how strongly the respondent agrees or disagrees with statements about the perceived amount of social support received.

Fixed-alternative questions usually are administered as paper-and-pencil questionnaires. However, the inability of potential respondents to write the required responses because of their age, disability, or lack of facility with English may require that an interview be used. Interview or computer-controlled administration is used when it is critical that questions be answered in a specified order.

The fixed-alternative schedule requires that the investigator construct questions so that all possible alternative responses are included. Not only must responses be inclusive, they also must be phrased so that they are mutually exclusive. These constraints are described earlier in this chapter in the discussion on types of schedules. The fixed-alternative schedule forces the respondent to answer in a way that fits the response categories the investigator provides; they are easy to code and provide a uniformity of measurement with greater reliability of responses across studies. The fixed-alternative format allows many questions to be asked in a short time, which makes this form of data generation appropriate for survey research.

One disadvantage of fixed-alternative questions is that they do not probe beneath the surface of the response. Additionally, some respondents may become irritated when no alternative suitably captures their answer; thus they may fail to complete the questions. Another disadvantage of the fixed-alternative question is that the respondent may feel forced to select one of the alternatives provided rather than expose his or her ignorance about the topic, the true facts, or the opinions that are believed to be socially unacceptable. Investigators who have used fixed-alternative response schedules know that respondents are often unhappy with the responses provided and will either add new responses or make marginal notes that no choice adequately reflected some participants' responses.

Open-ended questions

Open-ended questions are used when the investigator cannot anticipate the ways in which people are likely to respond to a question and when possible responses to a question are too numerous to list. How a group of nurses will respond to the question,

"In your opinion, what is the biggest barrier to preventing young people from smoking?" cannot be predicted. This open-ended question provides an opportunity for the nurses to identify their own beliefs about strategies that could be used to encourage the desired behavior. An investigator who is interested in the number and types of professional journals that are read by a sample of nurses can ask, "What professional journals have you read within the last 30 days?" This open-ended question eliminates the necessity of providing a complete list of all professional journals that have nurses as readers. Such a list would be cumbersome and more difficult to answer than simply to list the journals that are read.

Open-ended items provide a frame of reference for the respondent's answer. Each respondent may be asked the same sequence of questions, which is phrased in essentially the same words. Unlike the fixed-alternative questions, little or no restraint is placed on the way in which the respondent expresses answers. An example of a question that allows an open-ended response would be: "What is this pain like for you?" This question may be part of a structured schedule about the participant's personal experience of pain because each respondent is asked the question in the same way at the same point in the interview. The respondent is not required to select from a list of potential words describing pain, and the question suggests no particular response. The participant may choose to tell the interviewer that the pain is "stabbing" or may explain that the pain represents a lack of control over the situation, which makes him or her feel helpless. Projective techniques such as sentence completion tests are open-ended questions in which the participant is provided with the stem of a sentence and asked to complete the sentence.

Open-ended items are flexible and offer the possibility of exploring the depths of the respondent's answer. After the respondent has described the pain as "stabbing," the schedule can contain questions that seek further clarification about where the pain is felt, how long it lasts, what relieves it, or what effect a nursing intervention has on the pain. The response to open-ended questions may suggest novel possibilities or relationships that the researcher had not considered.

Open-ended questions can take the form of an

outline (see box on p. 306) or can combine an outline with specific probes that may be used if the respondent has difficulty answering the question or does not provide all of the information the investigator seeks. The interview guide shown below (see box) illustrates questions that are asked of persons who are living with a progressive neurological disease. The question in the left column is asked of each respondent, whereas those on the right can be used as necessary to elicit comprehensive information in each area of interest.

Open-ended questions in a structured interview are particularly useful when more than one person is conducting interviews on the same topic and the researcher wants to reduce the variation in responses that may result from differences in the way the interviewers may ask a question. This type of interview schedule allows more flexibility in response than fixed-alternative questions, yet it provides for control over the interview situation and ensures that each respondent is asked for the same information. Responses are easily associated with the questions, which facilitates the organization and analysis of the data.

The investigator who uses open-ended questions encounters several disadvantages as well. Open-ended questions require that the respondent organize and articulate information; this process is demanding and may result in inadequate answers—particularly on a questionnaire when an interviewer is not present to probe and clarify the response. Additionally, open-ended questions encourage free expression, which results in a wide diversity of responses that are difficult to analyze. Poor handwriting on questionnaires can further complicate the task of interpreting and analyzing responses.

In summary, fixed-alternative and open-ended questions can be used for interviews and questionnaires. An open-ended question allows the respondent to answer the question in her or his own words, whereas a fixed-alternative response question provides a selection of answers from which the respondent must choose. Fixed-alternative questions may be difficult to formulate because all possible response options must be identified. This may be difficult if the level of knowledge in the area of study is not highly developed. Responses to fixed-alternative questions are easier to code and more uniform across respondents than responses to open-ended questions. The choice between open-ended questions and

---

EXAMPLE OF INTERVIEW GUIDE WITH PROBE QUESTIONS

Question	*Probe questions*
How has your life changed since you were diagnosed?	Have your symptoms changed?
	Have there been any changes in your marital status (married, divorced, remarried, widowed, separated)? Do you think your disease had anything do to with that?
	Have you always lived here? If not, why did you move?
	Has household composition changed? Birth of children? Children left home? Hired live-in help? Parents came/left?
	Are you still working at the same job? If not, why did things change?
	Has the type or frequency of things you do in the community changed?
	Has your disease made any difference in your social life, e.g., how often you go out or entertain friends at home, the type of leisure activities?

Likert-type scale to elicit how strongly the respondent agrees or disagrees with statements about the perceived amount of social support received.

DEVELOPING NEW SCHEDULES

When a researcher is planning to generate data through the use of an interview or questionnaire, one of the first tasks is to develop a schedule. The schedule is the blueprint that ensures that the different responses that are received represent true differences and do not reflect only the way in which the questions were asked. This procedure involves many steps. Some of the questions that the investigator must ask include the following:

1. What information is needed to fulfill the purpose of the research?
2. What questions will elicit the information needed?
3. How can these questions best be asked?

Purpose of the research

Conceptualizing a schedule requires that the investigator have a thorough grasp of the purpose of the study, the level of knowledge about the phenomenon of study, and the nature of the data needed. Different questions will be needed to provide information about "What is this?" and "What will happen if . . . ?" The study of a poorly understood phenomenon such as the experience of miscarriage (Swanson-Kauffman, 1986) or being infertile (Olshansky, 1985) probably would use an open-ended and possibly unstructured interview guide so that the broadest possible understanding of the phenomenon could be elicited. On the other hand, an experimental study testing the outcome of a nursing intervention for the management of pain may use a structured, fixed-alternative schedule that focuses on the degree and quality of pain the patient experiences before and after the intervention.

An important rule is to gather only the data you need—enough but not too much. Think about how data relate to the purpose of the study. A wealth of information is obtainable about any topic; however, not all interesting data are relevant to the purpose of the study, and all data that are relevant are not necessarily of equal importance. The investigator can list all types or categories of information needed to accomplish the purpose of the study and prioritize this list in terms of importance. Table 18-1 provides

TABLE 18-1. Information needed to describe attitudes of high school students toward smoking

INFORMATION	PRIORITY
Age	Low
Grade in school	Low
Gender	Low
Personal smoking history	Medium
Number of peers who smoke	High
Parents' smoking history	High
Need for peer strokes	High
Importance of role models	High
Knowledge of health hazards of smoking	Medium
School regulations about smoking	Low

an example of the types of information that are needed to describe the attitudes of high school students toward smoking. Prioritizing the information provides a basis for determining where emphasis will be placed when writing questions.

Types of questions needed

When writing a schedule, the first consideration is the type of questions needed to achieve the purposes of the study. Questions that determine a respondent's knowledge of a particular topic will differ from those that assess his or her attitude toward an event. Is the investigator interested in obtaining demographic information, sensory information, knowledge, feelings, or opinions? Age at the onset of a chronic disease may be an important variable in determining how someone copes with the illness. Consider the following list of questions about age:

1. How old were you when you first had symptoms of your disease?
2. What effect do you think your age at onset has had on how well you cope with the effects of your disease?
3. Do you think people who get chronic disease early in life adjust better than people who get the disease later?
4. How did your illness affect what you were able to do with your friends when you were in high school?
5. Were you younger or older than other persons

with your disease when you developed symptoms?

Each of these questions relates to the age that the person was at the onset of a chronic disease. Each question would produce very different information about age and its relationship to the individual's illness. The purpose of the study would determine which of these questions is appropriate.

The time frame covered by the questions is another consideration in developing an interview guide. Is the investigator interested in events of the past, the present, or the future as projected by the respondent? The investigator who is interested in chronic illness may ask such questions as:

1. What was your life like when you first became aware that you had a chronic disease?
2. What is your life like now?
3. What do you think your life will be like next year? 5 years from now?

Phrasing questions

The wording of questions is critically important when structuring a schedule. Questions must be understandable, clear, and unbiased. In most cases respondents will not have the same reading level and degree of sophistication about the topic of study. Therefore it is important to write questions that will be understandable to those respondents who have the least education or sophistication. Short sentences with few modifying phrases are easiest to understand. Technical terminology must be defined when its use is unavoidable. Formulas can be used to calculate the reading difficulty of questions (National Cancer Institute, 1981). Words that can be interpreted in more than one way should be avoided.

Terminology must be clear. Do the participants who are being questioned about the nursing care they received know who the nurses were who cared for them? In some hospital settings similar attire, for example, scrub suits, and lack of identifiers such as name tags make it impossible for the patient to distinguish among nurses, laboratory technicians, and medical students. Patients in this situation may respond to questions about nursing care in terms of care received from everyone in a scrub suit. The educational and cultural background and the age of the respondents may influence the terms they use to describe bodily functions. Teenagers, for instance, may know only the street terms for sexual relationships and be unable to understand questions that use

medical terminology for these relationships.

The investigator must know clearly what information is desired. The question "When do you usually have a bowel movement?" might be answered: "around 8 AM"; "after breakfast"; or "when I eat prunes." The question is short, has no modifying phrases, and, except for "bowel movement"—which may be unfamiliar to the respondent—contains no difficult terms. Yet the unclear intent of the question forces the respondent to imply a meaning for "when" and respond on the basis of that meaning.

The use of a negative word in a question is often confusing. For example, if the respondent were asked either to agree or to disagree with such a statement as "There is no reason for working women to not get married and raise a family," the word "not" may be overlooked and result in a response that is the opposite of the respondent's belief.

Another pitfall in wording questions is the use of "double-barreled" questions or those that contain more than one idea. "What did you think of the nurses and the care they provided during your hospitalization?" is an example of a question that contains two ideas. The respondent may choose to tell the investigator about the personality of the nurses who provided care or may respond to the part of the question about the quality of care provided.

Questions that ask "why" should be used with caution on an interview schedule because they imply that the respondent should know the cause-effect relationships associated with the question. "Why did you like the nursing care provided during your hospitalization?" implies that the person can come up with a logical reason why he or she liked the care. "What did you like about the nursing care you received?" allows the participant to explain the specifics about why he or she liked the care without feeling the need to describe a cause-effect relationship.

The type of information sought will determine how a question is phrased. The investigator who is interested in patients' perceptions of nursing care will elicit different information if patients are asked, "What did you think of the care you received from nurses during your hospitalization?" than if they are asked, "How did you feel about the care you received from nurses during your hospitalization? Would you say that you are (a) very satisfied, (b) somewhat satisfied, (c) not too satisfied, (d) not at all satisfied?" In the latter example the response possibilities are stated clearly and made explicit by the way the question is asked. The former question, however, may not elicit useful information because, although the question does not specify the acceptable responses, the respondent is likely to answer that the care was pretty good or all right. "What things did you like and dislike about the care you received from the nurses during your recent hospitalization?" is an example of an open-ended question that allows the respondent to use his or her own words to describe perceptions about the nursing care received.

The researcher who intends to use open-ended questions must be certain that the questions are structured so that a dichotomous response is not possible. *Dichotomous-response questions* provide a grammatical structure that suggests a "yes" or "no" response to a question. Sometimes the dichotomous structure of the question is obvious; for example, "Were you satisfied with the care you received during your hospitalization?" The structure of the question implies that a "yes" or "no" response is desired. Asking the question, "Is there anything you would like to tell me about your experience with nurses during your hospitalization?" can be interpreted as a dichotomous-response question because the respondent can answer "yes" or "no" without providing any further detail; a dichotomous response is implicit in the way the question is asked. By asking the question "What else would you like to tell me about your experience with nurses during your hospitalization?" allows the respondent to provide information about the nursing care received or to respond that there is nothing else; a dichotomous response is not implied.

Questions also must be phrased in a way that avoids suggesting answers or socially desirable responses. Beginning a question with statements such as "Don't you agree that . . ." makes it difficult for the respondent to disagree. Socially desirable responses may be elicited when the respondent is asked to agree or disagree with the position or attitude of a prestigious or powerful person or group. A nurse may not respond honestly when asked "Do you agree with head nurse that . . . ?"

In summary, the type of information sought will determine how a question is phrased. Questions must be understandable and clear and be written for the respondents who have the least education or sophistication about the topic. When open-ended

responses are desired, the investigator must phrase questions so that a dichotomous response is not possible. Questions should contain only one idea.

Sequencing questions

No fixed rules exist for sequencing questions, although many researchers believe that one should begin with questions that are noncontroversial, that focus on the present, and that require little recall and interpretation. Demographic questions are boring and are better placed after questions that will arouse interest. Questions that require integration of many ideas are easier to answer after the respondent has had an opportunity to think about the topic. The respondents may be more comfortable providing answers to questions that elicit information about their emotional responses after some rapport has been established with the interviewer. Broad questions may be easier to answer before more specific questions.

The interviewer should arrange questions in some natural sequence and group them according to similar content. Asking one question about the onset of symptoms, jumping to questions about current income, and returning to the time of symptom onset makes little sense. Questions about pros and cons of an issue are related and naturally go together. Questions that require the same response ("yes" or "no" versus "agree" or "disagree") should be placed together.

Planning responses

When developing a schedule, the investigator also must consider the type of response he or she expects. In other words, are fixed-alternative questions or open-ended questions appropriate? The extent of information needed and the level of knowledge in the area of study will determine the type of response needed. The investigator may need the exact age of the respondent and thus frame an open-ended question that asks for birth date. On the other hand, if the investigator is interested in placing participants within a specific age-group, a fixed-alternative question that asks respondents to mark the age-group into which they fit will provide the needed information and save the investigator the time of recoding the birth date to establish age ranges. The investigator who wants to know what a patient does to relieve a headache can ask, "What do you do to relieve your headache?" or can provide the person with a list of pain-relieving strategies and ask: "Which of the following pain-relieving strategies do you use when you have a headache?" These examples presume that the investigator knows the possible range of responses. When the research is exploratory in nature, the investigator may not know enough about the topic to frame fixed-alternative questions. The investigator interested in learning about the lifestyles of individuals will not be able to provide fixed-alternative responses to questions.

Fixed-alternative questions require that the investigator carefully consider the responses, as well as the question. The investigator who is developing fixed-alternative questions is referred to textbooks on the topic (Dillman, 1978; Oppenheim, 1966). A few examples here point out the importance of considering the response categories. Responses, for instance, must be inclusive and mutually exclusive. A woman with four children or with no children would have difficulty answering this question:

How many children do you have?
1. 1 to 2
2. 3 to 4
3. 4 or more

Vague categories are also a problem with fixed-alternative questions. Consider these two response sets to this question:

How often have you had a urinary tract infection during the last year?

1. NEVER
2. RARELY
3. OCCASIONALLY
4. OFTEN

1. NOT AT ALL
2. ONCE OR TWICE
3. ABOUT THREE TIMES
4. ABOUT ONCE A MONTH

The investigator needs to know how precise an answer is needed. Is it sufficient to know that the respondent has had a urinary tract infection "occasionally" or is a more precise definition of frequency needed? The categories "rarely," "occasionally," and "often" may be defined differently and not provide the information needed.

EVALUATING NEW SCHEDULES

Newly developed questionnaires or interview guides must be subjected to careful evaluation before, during, and after their use. As soon as the questions are written, the investigator must ask whether the questions are truly related to the research purpose. Comparing the questions to the original outline of types and categories of information needed to fulfill the research purpose will help to answer this question.

Submitting the questions to others for scrutiny is an important early step in evaluating new schedules. Asking a colleague to look at the questions to see whether they are the right type of questions for the data sought is helpful. We often get so accustomed to what we are trying to elicit from participants that we do not notice that questions are not clear or that they are asked in a way that may bias the response. Someone with a fresh perspective on the topic may recognize problems that have not come to the attention of the investigator.

A content expert can evaluate the clarity of the questions and the likelihood that the questions will elicit answers that fulfill the research purpose. The content expert also can assess the inclusiveness of the response set in fixed-alternative questions. A representative of the population that will complete the schedule is also a valuable reviewer of the schedule. That person can help to determine if words are likely to be unfamiliar to the potential respondents, if knowledge and information are requested that the respondent does not have, or if the questions demand personal and delicate material. Review of the questions by someone who represents the population of interest and who is familiar with the culture and customs of others in the group can provide valuable input about whether others will be able to understand and respond to the questions. Review of the questions by someone skilled in measurement can often identify question wording that will threaten the validity of responses or the reliability of the instrument (Waltz, Strickland, & Lenz, 1984).

New schedules must be pretested before they are used to generate data. The pretest is conducted with a sample of individuals who are similar to those for whom the schedule is designed. The pretest will help the investigator determine whether the directions are understandable. A debriefing with those who pretest the schedule can elicit information about their reactions to the questions and format and identify any troublesome portion of the schedule.

The reliability and validity of new schedules are important considerations. Procedures for establishing the reliability of fixed-alternative response schedules are discussed in Chapter 15. Establishing the reliability and validity of unstructured and open-ended response schedules entails considerable time and effort and is therefore often neglected. Reliability of the interview schedule is determined by using the test-retest procedure, where the same schedule is used to interview the same respondent more than once (Waltz, Strickland, and Lenz, 1984). Validity of information obtained through interview is a complex issue that bears on whether the respondent is responding truthfully to questions. Many factors influence the validity of interview data. Since many of these factors—such as the differences in situations and settings and the reactive effects of the interview—occur during the actual interview process, they are discussed in Chapter 19 on administering interviews and questionnaires.

USING EXISTING SCHEDULES

Locating schedules

Developing schedules is a complex process that requires much thought on the part of the investigator. Ensuring that the questions contribute to answering the research question and that the schedule is reliable are time-consuming endeavors. When the investigator knows the exact type of information needed to answer the research question, a review of the literature will indicate whether another investigator has developed a schedule to obtain the needed information. Resource books that contain instruments of use in nursing research are listed at the end of this chapter.

In addition, experienced nurse researchers often know of other investigators who are pursuing similar research questions and who may have as-yet-unpublished schedules. The repeated use of schedules has the advantage of obtaining a larger pool of data and provides the opportunity to compare findings across studies. This is a particular advantage in nursing research because large samples in a single study are often difficult to obtain. The psychometric properties (reliability, validity) of the schedule can be assessed with different samples of participants. Chapter 14 outlines the criteria for selecting an instrument for use in a research study.

Evaluating schedules

After the investigator has identified a questionnaire or interview guide that may be useful in measuring the variable(s) of interest, the next question to be asked is whether the instrument really will meet the investigator's requirements. Is the schedule appropriate for the study population? Can it be administered as intended? Does the schedule indeed answer the question proposed by the research purpose? What are the reliability and validity of the schedule? Many of the resource books listed at the end of this chapter provide information about reliability and validity. Other widely used schedules may have sketchy or inadequate psychometric properties. Some of the resource books evaluate each schedule presented or compare various schedules available to measure the same variable.

Altering schedules

An existing schedule may be nearly what the investigator needs to answer the research question, thus the investigator may decide to use a particular existing schedule with some modification. Structured, fixed-alternative schedules, however, have psychometric properties that are inherent in the way in which the questions are constructed and sequenced. The alteration of items on such a schedule may alter the psychometric properties of the schedule. Even minor modifications, such as changing a word or adding or omitting an item, create a new schedule. Previously reported psychometric properties cannot be assumed to apply to the new instrument. Therefore the investigator must be aware that any alterations made in an existing schedule may change the psychometric properties of that schedule. Reliability and validity of the schedule must be reestablished.

SUMMARY

This chapter has provided an overview of selecting and developing an interview guide or a questionnaire. Interviews and questionnaires are useful to identify and explore events and meanings, to explore and test relationships, and to validate information. Questions can be framed that will elicit facts, beliefs, attitudes, and feelings. The purpose of the study, the level of knowledge in the area of study, and the characteristics of the respondents will determine the type of schedule and questions that are used and the most appropriate means of administering the schedule of questions.

Developing new schedules is a precise art. The

investigator must consider how each question will contribute to accomplishing the purpose of the research. Phrasing and sequencing of questions and responses must be carefully planned. The investigator who has a thorough grasp of the substantive area of study and methods of analysis used to accomplish the purpose of the study will have a good start on developing a useful interview guide or questionnaire. All schedules should be pretested with a representative sample of people who will be included in the study, and the psychometric properties of the schedule should be assessed each time it is used.

REFERENCES

Benoliel, J. Q. (1983). Grounded theory and qualitative data: The socializing influences of life-threatening disease on identity development. In P. J. Wooldridge, M. H. Schmitt, J. K. Skipper, & R. C. Leonard, *Behavioral science and nursing theory* (pp. 141-188). St. Louis: Mosby.

Brandt, P. A., & Weinert, C. (1981). The PRQ—A social support measure. *Nursing Research, 30,* 277-280.

Corbin, J., & Strauss, A. (1985). Managing chronic illness at home: Three lines of work. *Qualitative Sociology, 8*(3), 224-247.

Dai, Y-T., & Catanzaro, M. (1987). Health belief and compliance with skin care. *Rehabilitation Nursing, 12,* 13-21.

Davis, M. Z. (1970). *Transition to a devalued status: The case of multiple sclerosis* (Doctoral dissertation, University of California, San Francisco, 1970. University Microfilms No. 72-12, 768).

Dillman, D. A. (1978). *Mail and telephone surveys: The total design method.* New York: Wiley.

Lambert, V. A. (1985). Study of factors associated with psychological well-being in rheumatoid arthritic women. *Image: The Journal of Nursing Scholarship, 17*(2), 50-53.

Lincoln, Y. S., & Guba, E. (1985). *Naturalistic inquiry.* Beverly Hills, CA: Sage.

Lindeman, C. A. (1975). Delphi survey of priorities in clinical nursing research. *Nursing Research, 29,* 357-361.

Magilvy, J. K. (1985). Experiencing hearing loss in later life: A comparison of deaf and hearing-impaired older women. *Research in Nursing and Health, 8,* 347-353.

Melzack, R. (1975). The McGill pain questionnaire: Major properties and scoring methods. *Pain, 1,* 277-299.

National Cancer Institute. (1981). *Readability testing in cancer communications.* (NIH Publication No. 81-1689). Washington, DC: U.S. Government Printing Office.

Olshansky, E. (1985). *The work of taking on and managing an identity of self as infertile.* (Unpublished doctoral dissertation, University of California, San Francisco).

Oppenheim, A. N. (1966). *Questionnaire design and attitude measurement.* New York: Basic Books.

Patton, M. Q. (1980). *Qualitative evaluation methods.* Beverly Hills, CA: Sage.

Ritchie, J. A., Caty, S., & Ellerton, M. L. (1984). Concerns of acutely ill, chronically ill, and healthy preschool children. *Research in Nursing and Health, 7,* 265-274.

Tripp-Reimer, T. (1985). Combining qualitative and quantitative methodologies. In M. L. Leininger (Ed.). *Qualitative research methods in nursing* (pp. 179-194). Orlando: Grune & Stratton.

Spradley, J. P. (1979). *The ethnographic interview.* New York: Holt, Rinehart & Winston.

Swanson-Kauffman, K. (1986). A combined qualitative methodology for nursing research. *Advances in Nursing Science, 8*(3), 58-69.

Wallston, K., Wallston, B., & DeVillis, R. (1978). Development of the multidimensional health locus of control (MHLC) scales. *Health Education Monograph, 6,* 160-171.

Waltz, C. F., Strickland, O. L., & Lenz, E. R. (1984). *Measurement of nursing research.* Philadelphia: Davis.

19

IMPLEMENTING QUESTIONNAIRES AND INTERVIEWS

MARCI CATANZARO

In the previous chapter we considered the process of developing a schedule of questions to be used for a questionnaire or an interview. The chapter included a discussion of the advantages and disadvantages of questionnaires and interviews, of structured and unstructured schedules, and of open-ended and fixed-alternative response questions. This chapter is about implementing questionnaires and interviews once the investigator has decided how to generate the data. Decisions about the development and implementation of questionnaires and interviews are not made in a linear sequence. The implementation must be considered during the entire development process. The separation of the development and implementation of questionnaires and interviews into two chapters does not imply that they are separate processes.

A number of techniques for administration exist. Questionnaires can be mailed or personally delivered to the potential participant or administered in a group setting. Interviews can be conducted with groups or with individuals in face-to-face settings or by telephone. In this chapter we will discuss each of these methods of implementation. Implementing interviews and questionnaires requires that the investigator (1) ensure response from selected participants, (2) ensure the trustworthiness of data, (3) administer the questionnaire or interview, and (4) record responses of the participants. Decisions about

these steps do not necessarily occur in a linear, step-by-step fashion, but they must be accounted for in planning data collection.

ENSURING RESPONSE FROM PARTICIPANTS

Identifying and sampling respondents for research has been discussed in Chapter 7. However, adequate sampling is not the only consideration in research. No matter how carefully the investigator plans a sampling strategy, the population of interest will be represented inadequately if a large proportion of those sampled for participation do not respond to the questions. Nonresponse on questionnaires is a major factor affecting the validity of study findings. Heberlein and Baumgartner (1978) reported that the return rate for questionnaires ranged from 20% to 80%. Respondents who actually return questionnaires or who agree to be interviewed cannot be assumed to be representative of the intended sample if most of the sample did not respond. Therefore every effort must be made to increase the response rate.

Costs of participation

The tenets of social exchange theory (Blau, 1964) suggest that all activities we perform incur certain costs and that we must maintain a balance between

316

the perceived costs and rewards of doing an activity. Applying social exchange theory to questionnaires and interviews, the respondent must perceive that the personal cost of completing the questions has a reward in terms of goods, services, or experiences that balances the costs incurred. The individual costs of completing a questionnaire or interview include money, time, effort, and power.

The most obvious cost to the participant is in money. Expecting the respondent to provide an envelope and stamp to return a questionnaire involves a small financial cost, but it may have a much larger intangible cost of inconvenience. The participant may not have the right-size envelope or may not know exactly how much postage is required to return the questionnaire. Transportation to the site of an interview and costs of parking may discourage some participants, especially if traffic is heavy and parking is inconvenient. The need to obtain child care while participating in a study is another cost consideration.

Cost also includes the time it will take to complete the study questions. The investigator may tell the respondents the average amount of time required to complete the questionnaire or interview; however, the participant's estimation of the time it will take to complete the questions may be based on appearance. A questionnaire that is crowded on the page, is thick in size, has small print, or has complex response alternatives may be judged too complicated and time-consuming to undertake. Dillman (1978) presented many practical suggestions on format and layout of questionnaires that have been demonstrated to decrease the personal costs of completing questionnaires and thereby to increase response rates. Individually administered questionnaires often can be completed at times and in segments convenient to the respondent. Questionnaires or interviews administered to a group of participants are less flexible because once the time is set it is not easy to make alterations or to interrupt the session.

The availability of time for the respondent to answer is another consideration. Researchers use some population groups more heavily than others. Those with earned doctorates, nursing-faculty members, and those participating in dramatic new treatments are used heavily as research respondents. Woolley (1984) discussed the steadily increasing number of requests to deans and directors of schools of nursing to complete mailed questionnaires. She surveyed a group of deans and directors of baccalaureate and higher degree programs who were attending a national meeting and found that they answered only those questionnaires that they believed to have a sufficiently salient topic to justify the response burden. Woolley suggested that only the least busy deans or directors respond to questionnaires, thereby eliminating the opinions of those who might be most influential. Her respondents admitted that they frequently pass questionnaires on to someone else for completion.

Physical or mental effort required to complete the study is a less tangible cost. Questions that are difficult to understand or that demand complex mental processes on the part of the respondent may require too much effort. The anxiety or discomfort produced by questions of a personal nature may result in the participant abandoning the study or skipping over important questions. The investigator can overcome some of these costs by careful consideration of the way in which questions are worded, ensuring that only necessary information is sought, and by packaging the questions in an attractive way, whether they are part of a mailed questionnaire or are asked in an unstructured manner during a face-to-face interview. Packaging makes it easier for respondents to understand the questions and to decide on the type of desired response.

Blau (1964) also noted that power is an important component of exchange theory. Does the respondent feel powerless or subordinate to the investigator? Consider who has power in the following statements: "If nurses are going to help you, you need to tell us how we can best do that" versus "We are interested in learning what would be helpful to you." In the first instance, the investigators have power, and they are going to do for the respondents that which they may be unable to do for themselves. The respondents need only to say how the investigators can help. In the latter example the respondents have the necessary information, and the investigators would appreciate learning. The respondents have the power to help themselves by sharing their expertise with the investigators.

Referring to the study participants as subjects often sets the tone for feelings of powerlessness. We think of a dictatorial king having subjects under his rule. In common parlance we talk about subjecting metals to stress or of violators of the law being subjected to punishment. Terms such as respondent, participant, or informant establish a collaborative environment in which the participant is seen as contributing to the investigation rather than being subjected to it.

Rewards for participation

The perceived costs of participation in a study must be balanced by the anticipated rewards. What rewards can we offer participants for their completion of a questionnaire or an interview? Thibaut and Kelley (1959) and Blau (1964) believed that the expression of positive regard for another is a reward for many individuals. Several strategies can be used to assure the potential respondents that their participation is important:

1. Make the participants aware that they have been selected carefully to provide information that only they have (e.g., "You are one of a small group of persons who have been selected to help us understand the effects of chronic illness on the daily lives of people").

2. Point out that their responses are critical to the success of the study (e.g., "Your responses are important because you are living with chronic illness and you know how it affects your life").

3. Express verbal appreciation for participation (e.g., "We are most grateful that you are willing to take the time to respond to these questions").

4. Consider the participant a consultant to the study (e.g., "Is there anything else you think we should be asking people to learn how chronic illness affects their lives?").

5. Support the values of the respondents (e.g., "People with chronic illness have different opinions about what is helpful in coping with the illness on a daily basis").

Tangible rewards also can be offered to participants. They can be paid for their participation or offered a sample product or a chance to win a prize. However, the payment of participants ordinarily involves a relatively insignificant amount that is not commensurate with the time and energy contributed to the study. To offer a significant financial reward to potential participants may make someone who needs money participate in the study for the monetary reward offered; in some cases this may be considered a type of coercion to participate. Marketing research often offers participants a sample product as a reward in exchange for completing a questionnaire or interview about the brand they normally use. Nursing intervention studies may offer a product such as incontinence pads or a relaxation tape in exchange for completing questions about how incontinence or stress is managed.

Many Americans have been promised that their names would be entered into a random prize drawing if they returned a questionnaire. This strategy frequently is used to ensure the timely return of the questionnaire, but it also may serve as a reward for participating in a study. An investigator mailing questionnaires to pregnant women might consider offering a month of diaper service to a randomly selected participant who had returned the questionnaire by a specified date.

In summary, people who are asked to respond to a questionnaire or participate in an interview must be able to balance the perceived costs and rewards. The investigator must consider the potential costs versus the rewards available to the participants. For some potential participants the opportunity to share their knowledge, opinions, or expertise with another may be sufficient reward. Others may obtain rewards from the knowledge that they may be able to help others through their participation in the study. More tangible rewards, such as nominal payment for the respondent's time, are also possible. Whatever the reward, participants must perceive a balance between the costs and rewards of participation if the investigator is to have adequate levels of response.

ENSURING TRUSTWORTHINESS OF DATA

Trustworthy data are reliable, valid, and bias free. Reliability, validity, and bias are terms that are used throughout this book in relation to study design, data collection, and data analysis. This section considers threats to reliability and validity of the data obtained from questionnaires and interviews that can occur during the actual administration of the questionnaire or interview.

Reliability and validity

The *reliability* of data is the degree of consistency or dependability with which questions measure the attribute they are designed to measure. Many issues of reliability are managed during the construction of questions and were discussed in Chapter 18. *External reliability,* or whether independent researchers would discover the same phenomena, requires that the methods of data collection be reported precisely and thoroughly. This requirement implies that the researcher have an operating manual in sufficient detail to allow replication of the study. *Internal reliability* refers to the degree to which other researchers code data in the same way as the original investigator. Internal reliability is seldom a major issue with fixed-alternative responses. However, when unstructured interviews are conducted or open-ended questions are asked, the investigator must ensure that the recording of responses is such that all data are preserved in an uncoded and unclassified form either through the use of mechanical recording equipment or the retention of original written responses (LeCompte & Goetz, 1982).

Validity is the degree to which the questions elicit the information that was intended. The truth of responses is a key concern when data are obtained through questionnaires and interviews. The truthfulness of respondents may be altered by their desire to slant the results of the study or to make things seem better or worse than they really are. Hospitalized patients who are questioned about the quality of their care may indicate that the quality is wonderful because they fear reprisal by staff. Conversely, they may respond that their care is awful in an effort to obtain "better" care. Respondents may attempt to please the investigator by responding in the way that they believe the investigator expects. They may also fear that by sharing negative information they will be placed in a devalued position by the investigator. The investigator can increase the validity of responses in such a setting by assuring the informants that the responses will not be shared with care providers and by being alert to response sets that would indicate a tendency to respond extremely positively or negatively to all questions.

Respondents may have difficulty presenting the truth about something in the empirical world because they are unable to verbalize sensitive issues or they attempt to rationalize a fact that they find distasteful. Participants being questioned about their participation in an Alcoholics Anonymous group may find it difficult to discuss their work relationships or may minimize the severity of their drinking problem. The researcher can increase the validity of data obtained in these difficult situations by creating a psychologically comfortable environment for the respondent. When unstructured interviews are used,

the investigator can use active listening and probing to assist the respondent in talking about difficult or distasteful topics. Respondents who are assured of privacy while answering questions and of the confidentiality of their responses have less reason to suspect reprisal than when others are present during the interview or when they believe that the information they share with the investigator will be shared with others.

Bias

Bias, or systematic distortion of responses, can occur in many research situations when a set of personal preferences prevents an impartial judgment. Although bias may occur in many research situations, the unstructured interview provides a significant opportunity for bias to influence the trustworthiness of data. Bias may result from systematic differences from one interviewer to the next or from systematic errors on the part of all interviewers (Kidder, 1981). Davis (1980) reminded us that both the interviewer and the respondent ". . . are social beings with a history of social interaction styles which affects the present encounter between researcher and researched" (p. 215). The views that the participant and the interviewer hold about each other are potential sources of bias. Differing perceptions, judgments, personalities, expectations, and wishes all influence how human beings respond. Bias may be introduced by the appearance and behavior of the interviewer, the way the questions are asked, and the way in which responses are recorded. These sources of bias may be present either in one member of a research team or systematically in all members.

The first step in decreasing bias is to be aware of the possibility of introducing bias at various points during the implementation of interviews and questionnaires. Kidder (1981) suggested that the interviewer dress inconspicuously (i.e., consistent with the norms of the interview environment). Imagine the response of potential respondents at a free healthcare clinic in a low-income area of the city when an interviewer appears in a three-piece business suit and carrying a leather attaché case. Conversely, what quality of data can be expected from a hospital administrator when the interviewer arrives in old jeans and a sweatshirt?

The fewer opportunities that the respondent and investigator have for interpretation, the fewer opportunities occur for introducing bias. Thus the more structured the questions and response alternatives, the greater will be the trustworthiness of the data. Interviewers who conduct unstructured interviews with no predetermined coding system for responses have many opportunities to introduce bias in the way questions are asked, probes are used, and responses are recorded. When more than one person is conducting interviews for a study, each must be trained in the study design and data collection so that possible sources of bias are eliminated.

ADMINISTERING THE QUESTIONNAIRE OR INTERVIEW

The questionnaire or interview can be administered in several ways. Questionnaires can be mailed or personally delivered to potential respondents. The investigator can permit respondents to complete questionnaires alone in the privacy of their home, or the investigator may plan group administration. Computers also can be used to administer a questionnaire. Interviews can be conducted with individuals in a face-to-face setting or by telephone, or the respondents can be interviewed as a group. Each of these methods of administration is discussed in the following section.

Mailing questionnaires

The questionnaire that is mailed or hand-delivered to potential respondents must speak for itself. The investigator will not be present to answer questions, allay anxiety, or clarify items. The appearance of the questionnaire will be the first thing that comes to the respondent's attention. Dillman (1978) made suggestions for increasing response rate that included these points: (1) print the questionnaire as a booklet, (2) do not print questions on the cover pages, (3) photographically reduce the 8¼-inch × 12¼-inch paper, and (4) reproduce the booklet on white or off-white paper. These recommendations result in a questionnaire that is pleasing to the eye and readable to most people. The paper is folded in the middle and stapled to form a booklet that fits in standard Monarch-size or business reply envelope.

The front cover of the questionnaire booklet contains the title of the study, the name and address of the investigator, special directions, and a graphic illustration (Dillman, 1978). The title should be short, easily understandable to the potential respondents, and free of biased wording. An example of a cover used in nursing research is shown in Fig. 19-1.

Getting the questionnaire to the potential respondent is an essential step in obtaining a response. Be certain that the address is correct. Outdated address lists, typing errors, or insufficient postage for return of nonforwardable mail ensure that the questionnaire will never reach its destination.

The information that the potential respondent receives must communicate the message that the benefits of completing the questionnaire outweigh the costs. The cover letter serves as an introduction to the study. Recall some of the ways of increasing participation in research discussed earlier in this chapter. Does the letter make the participants aware that they have been selected carefully to provide information that only they have? Does it point out that their responses are critical to the success of the study? A cover letter that appears mass-produced does little to convey to the potential participants that they have been chosen especially to participate in the study. Computer technology makes it possible to individualize cover letters in a few seconds. Does the cover letter tell the reader why the research topic is important and useful? Is anonymity or confidentiality assured? Is it clear who is to answer the questions and what is to be done with the questionnaire when the answers are completed? Fig. 19-2 shows samples of cover letters.

Postage is a tangible cost of returning a questionnaire. Questionnaires are more likely to be returned when an addressed, stamped envelope is included. This saves the respondent not only the cost of postage but the trouble of finding the correct-size envelope and addressing it to the investigator. Convenience in returning questionnaires that are to be picked up by the investigator is also important. A nurse is more likely to place a completed questionnaire in a box on the nursing unit than to carry it to the nursing office.

An investigator can increase response rates significantly by sending follow-up mailings that remind potential participants to return the questionnaire. Dillman (1978) discussed the timing and content of each follow-up. He suggested that follow-up mailings be done at 1, 3, and 7 weeks after the initial questionnaire was mailed. The first week, a postcard is sent to everyone. This postcard is a thank-you for those who have responded and a reminder to those who have not. A letter and replacement question-

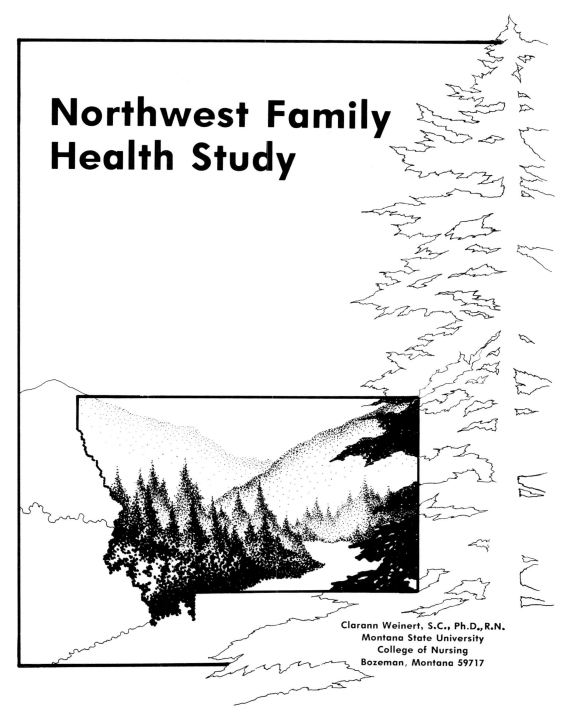

Northwest Family Health Study

Clarann Weinert, S.C., Ph.D., R.N.
Montana State University
College of Nursing
Bozeman, Montana 59717

Fig. 19-1. Cover for mailed questionnaire booklet used for the Northwest Family Health Study conducted by Clarann Weinert.

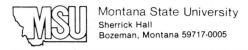

Montana State University
Sherrick Hall
Bozeman, Montana 59717-0005

College of Nursing

NORTHWEST FAMILY HEALTH STUDY
(National Sample)
QUESTIONNAIRE BOOKLET FOR THE SPOUSE WITH M.S.

Thank you for volunteering to participate in our study of families living with M.S. Your time, interest, and information are highly valued. The questions in this booklet are designed to help us better understand those factors which promote "healthy" functioning of families living with a long-term health problem such as multiple sclerosis. Because you are living with M.S. you have valuable insights that can help nurses and other health care professionals provide better care for families. Thank you in advance for participating.

In this booklet you will find the following series of questionnaires: a) Family and Marriage, b) Perceived Stress, c) Religious Beliefs, d) Recent Loss, e) Personal Resource Questionnaire, f) Cost of Support, g) General Health, h) Role Identity, i) Background Information, j) Economic Adequacy, and k) Sickness Impact Profile. Each section has instructions. <u>Please read them carefully</u> before you begin answering the questions. Try not to skip questions and do not spend too much time on any one question.

If you have difficulty with vision or coordination please ask someone (not your spouse) to assist you in answering the questions. **IT IS ESSENTIAL** that you **DO NOT** discuss or compare answers with your spouse until both of you have completed all the questions in the booklet.

Please complete these questionnaires at your convenience. If you get tired or are distracted it is better to quit and return to them at a time that is more conducive for this task. I would like the booklet returned along with your spouse's booklet (<u>WITHIN 10 DAYS</u>) of receiving this packet. Please use the self-addressed pre-stamped envelope which I have provided.

You may be assured of complete confidentiality. Each booklet has an identification number which will allow us to check them off the mailing list when they are returned. Your name will never be placed on the booklet nor identified with the information that you provide. Your participation in this study is, of course, totally voluntary. Returning the completed booklet is considered as your consent to participate. If you decide not to participate please put an "X" in the box at the bottom of this page. If you could share your reasons for not participating that would help me in planning future research.

Thank you for your interest in my research and your thoughtful participation.

Clarann Weinert

Clarann Weinert, S.C., R.N., Ph.D.
Northwest Family Health Study Director

Fig. 19-2. Cover letter enclosed with mailed questionnaire used for the Northwest Family Health Study conducted by Clarann Weinert.

naire are mailed to those who have not responded by the third week. Finally, 7 weeks after the initial mailing, a letter and replacement questionnaire are sent by certified mail.

Group-administered questionnaires

Having a group of people complete a questionnaire at one place may be preferable in some circumstances. The nurse educator who is investigating the cognitive style of nursing students is likely to get a higher completion rate on a questionnaire that is administered to a group of students than on one that is mailed to each student's home. Group administration also has the advantage of the investigator's being present to answer questions about the study or the questionnaire. Additionally, potential respondents cannot put the paper aside until later. Special precautions must be taken to ensure that members of the group do not feel coerced to participate. The investigator can assure anonymity or confidentiality of responses and can make arrangements for group members to return incomplete questionnaires in an unobtrusive manner.

Considerations for group administration of a questionnaire include ensuring that pencils and a comfortable place for writing are available to the respondents. Timing of the group administration is another important consideration. Students who have been in class all day and patients who have just undergone a painful procedure or whose discharge is delayed by participation are not likely to be enthusiastic about completing a questionnaire. Provisions to return the questionnaire must be made for those who decide not to participate, without drawing the attention of others in the group to the fact that these persons are nonrespondents.

Computer-administered questionnaires

Questionnaires can be administered at a computer terminal. This method enables the investigator to control the order in which the questions are presented—an important consideration when the order of presentation may influence subsequent responses. A study of clinical decision making might use a patient-care simulation in which only the patient information that is specifically requested by the respondent is presented. The computer also can be programed to branch questions so that subsequent questions are based on the answer to previous questions. For example, if the respondent indicated that

no children live in the home, the computer can be programed to skip over all questions pertaining to children.

As personal computers continue to become available, more and more people will have the ability to respond to a questionnaire on a computer keyboard or other input device. The availability of compatible computers at many different locations will continue to make this computer administration of questionnaires more feasible. An important advantage of computer administration is that computers can be programed to record and to analyze questionnaire responses; this feature decreases the amount of data-handling required of the investigator.

Face-to-face interviews

Whether an interview is conducted face-to-face or over the telephone, the interviewer needs many skills. Just as the investigator must be aware of his or her philosophical paradigm about the nature of science, the interviewers also must know what they believe about the world. The positivist listens with the idea that the accounts provided by the respondent are subjective and ultimately must be verified by science. The naturalist, on the other hand, believes that common-sense knowledge constitutes the social world and therefore ". . . it must be appreciated and described, not subjected to critical scrutiny as to its validity, nor explained away" (Hammersley & Atkinson, 1983, p. 105). These differences will influence how the interviewer hears what is said and how responses to what the respondent has said are framed. The respondent, too, has a world view. These views of the reality bias the interaction between the interviewer and the respondent.

The manner in which the interviewer presents herself or himself and asks questions will influence the quality of the data obtained. Consider the responses the investigator can expect from the interview (see box on p. 325). Ask yourself:

1. What things in the environment were different? How might that influence the milieu in which the interview takes place?
2. What personal characteristics of the investigator would affect the quality and quantity of the data?
3. What clues indicated that this research was a serious matter?
4. What other influences in this situation would affect the quality and quantity of the data?

Asking questions is only half of the process of conducting an interview. Listening to the content of the verbal responses, the specific words used, and the nonverbal components of the response are critical, particularly in an open-ended interview. Unless fixed-alternative responses are elicited, the interviewer must code what is said into something that makes sense and can be responded to and recorded. In unstructured interviews the interviewer must interpret the meaning instantly so that further questioning can be directed toward understanding the experience of the respondent. The interviewer must know what is expected of respondents. Otherwise knowing what to listen for, being able to stimulate the inarticulate person, or controlling those who respond with irrelevancies or with minutia is impossible. Time is a precious commodity for both the interviewer and the respondent. The interviewer must maintain control of the interview so that the necessary information is obtained and irrelevant information is kept to a minimum.

Exchange theory applies for interviews, as well as questionnaires. The respondents must believe that their effort to answer questions is important and useful. Strategies such as a nod, the expression of verbal appreciation for responses, and body language such as moving closer to the respondent are helpful in communicating the message that what is being said is important enough for the interviewer to listen. The beginning nurse researcher has an advantage over many other social scientists who use interview strategies in research, because communication skills have been an important part of the nurse's education and clinical practice. Techniques such as establishing eye contact, clarifying and checking perceptions, using summary statements, and asking for elaboration and examples serve well in both clinical and research settings.

Many of the nurse's skills in patient interviewing also will be useful in conducting research interviews. However, important differences exist. The nurse-patient interview is directed toward obtaining information that will assist the nurse in caring for the patient. This information will be used immediately to benefit the patient, either through nursing-care planning or patient teaching. The researcher-respondent interview, on the other hand, is intended to obtain information relevant to a research question. Analysis will take place at a later time, and the information obtained will be of no direct benefit to the respondent. Persons who are familiar with nurse-patient interactions in which a sharing of information results in some immediate benefit to the patient expect the same situation to prevail when a nurse is conducting an interview for research purposes. The nurse who is accustomed to providing information to patients and engaging in patient teaching is likely to find the role of a nurse researcher difficult. The nurse investigator who has no contact with the participants outside the research setting will have less difficulty keeping roles separate than one who provides nursing care for the research respondents.

Voice-to-voice interviews

Many of the same communication skills required for face-to-face interviews are required also for voice-to-voice interviews. A major difference is that the telephone does not provide the opportunity to use and to observe nonverbal behavior. Telephone interviews are used for survey research; however, in-depth interviews can also be conducted by telephone.

Bradburn et al. (1981) compared the response rate obtained from personal interview, telephone interview, and self-administered questionnaire. They found that the use of the telephone produced the highest interview completion rate. Completion rates varied among their samples of people who owned library cards, who had registered to vote in Chicago, who were charged with drunken driving, or who had declared bankruptcy recently, but telephone interviews generally were affected least by the respondent's anxiety.

Telephone interviews can be conducted by the investigator from home, with the questions and answers written on notebook paper and analyzed by hand. At the other extreme the interview guide can be computerized (see Appendix A). The interviewer enters the responses to one question, and the next question—based on the previous answer—automatically appears on the cathode-ray tube. Just as in the computer-administered questionnaire, the computer analyzes the data. Thus the telephone interview is perhaps the most flexible method of administering interview schedules, because it allows the investigator to work from home and it offers more flexibility in recording responses.

However, the unexpected telephone call requesting a response to survey questions may result in a

SAMPLE INTERVIEW

Interview A	*Interview B*
(Setting: Hospital room. Door open, possibly roommate in and out; investigator sits on bed; chews gum; dressed casually.	(Setting: Conference room on nursing unit. Door closed, flowers on table; patient and investigator sitting comfortably in chairs; investigator dressed in suit.
Investigator is fidgety, seems to want to get this over with; frequently cuts off interviewee.)	Investigator is relaxed. Keeps interview focused but does not suppress data.)
Hi, Ann. My name's Jean.	Hello, Ms. Brown. My name is Dr. Smith.
I'm doin' some research on what people are afraid of when they are going to the operating room. The nurse told me you were gunna have your gall bladder out in the morning and that you'd answer my questions and do my test.	I am a nurse researcher and am interested in what people think about as they prepare for surgery. I understand that you are going to have surgery in the morning. What kind of surgery will you be having? I would like to ask you some questions and then have you complete a short, written questionnaire. Are you willing to do that?
Some people are afraid they will never wake up after the anesthesia. Do you feel that way?	Is this your first trip to the operating room?
Gall bladder surgery can be painful. What are your concerns about that, for example, are you expecting to have a lot of pain? If so, do you expect the nurses will give you pain medication when you need it?	What are some of the things you have thought about in relation to your planned surgery? What do you think things will be like for you when you awake from the anesthesia? How do you think you will feel? What are some of the things you expect from the nurses after your surgery? How probable do you think it is that you will get those things?
Well, that's all I wanted to know. Is there anything else you want to tell me?	Is there anything else you would like to share with me?
Another thing I want to know is whether people who think others run their lives are afraid of different things than people who think they are in control. You look to me as if you are very much in control of things, especially your health.	This study has two parts. In addition to understanding the concerns you have as you prepare for surgery, I am interested in how these concerns may relate to the control people believe they have over events.
Here's the test. Just use the pencil to answer the questions. Ask if you don't understand something.	I have a 30-item questionnaire that I would like you to complete. It will take about 5 minutes of your time. I will be here if you have any questions.
(Give a stack of loose papers.)	(Give bound booklet and pencil.)

high refusal rate. Dillman (1978) suggested that sending an advance letter to the potential respondent is a reasonable way to avoid refusals or extremely guarded responses. He pointed out, however, that certain groups, particularly ". . . students, ministers, and agency personnel, normally produce such high response rates that a prior letter cannot be expected to influence them" (p. 245). An advance letter for a telephone interview includes the same information as a cover letter for a mailed questionnaire. Additionally, it includes information about when the potential respondent can be expected to receive the telephone call.

Scheduling of telephone interviews will depend on the topic of the investigation, the scope of the interview, and the anticipated time for completion. Anyone who is home between 7 PM and 9 PM on weekday evenings knows that this is a favorite time for telephone interviewers to call. Those who are not home evenings often are called on Saturday afternoon. The investigator who is interested in the health-care utilization patterns of working women would select evening and weekend times to telephone women. If, however, the investigator were interested in the physician's or nurse practitioner's perceptions of working women's utilization of health-care services, telephone calls would be made during normal working hours.

The scope and anticipated time needed for the interview also will determine when calls are made. When extensive interviews are to be done by telephone, making an appointment with the potential respondent is helpful. This may be done through a telephone call or by a return postcard enclosed in the advance letter, asking the potential respondent for the best time to call.

At the beginning of a telephone interview the interviewer introduces himself or herself, briefly states the topic of the interview, and inquires about the availability and willingness of the potential respondent to answer questions at that time. Even when the respondents have preselected the time for the call, confirmation of their ability to participate at this time is appropriate.

Group interviews

Group interviews, also called focus groups, are used commonly in market research. Further information on the mechanics of planning and conducting focus groups can be found in textbooks on market research (Boyd, Westfall, & Stasch, 1981; Smith, 1972; Wells, 1974). Typically, data are collected from a group discussion among four to ten participants who share their thoughts and experiences on a set of topics selected by the investigator. The advantage of a focus group is that the participants have an opportunity to share ideas with other group members; this may trigger additional thoughts or help participants to discuss the topic.

Morgan and Spanish (1984) used the focus group to study what people think about the causes and prevention of heart attacks. Participants between the ages of 35 and 50 who had no history of heart disease were asked to select someone they knew or had heard about who had had a heart attack. This person was to serve as reference point for their subsequent group discussion of "Who has heart attacks and why?" and "What kinds of things prevent heart attacks?" The group discussion was tape-recorded and later transcribed verbatim and coded. Morgan and Spanish noted that they could have obtained information through individual interviews about how people think about the causes and prevention of heart attacks; this method, however, would have required considerably more interview time. In addition to information about the participants' vicarious experience of heart attack, the focus group allowed the investigators to look at what happened when people took differing individual experiences and made collective sense of them.

Special situations

Q-sort and Delphi techniques are used often as scaling techniques. However, they are considered in this chapter as special situations for administering questionnaires. These techniques require a complex set of decisions on the part of the participants in order to respond to the questions.

Q-sort. *Q-sort* is a procedure used to determine respondents' judgment about the degree to which they agree or disagree with a particular idea. Q-sort has been used extensively in nursing to assess the similarity of perceptions about quality of nursing care, behaviors of patients and nurses, and attitudes of nurses about roles and illnesses. Typically, the respondent is presented with a pile of 50 to 100 cards that each contain a word, statement, or message about the object. The respondent is asked to sort the cards into 9 to 11 piles according to a particular dimension, such as approval/disapproval, most like me/least like me, highest priority/lowest priority, or most helpful/least helpful. The investigator specifies the number of cards that can be placed in each pile so that a particular distribution is achieved. For example, a respondent may be given 75 cards that contain statements about nursing actions intended to alleviate pain. The respondent would be asked to sort the cards into nine piles, ranging from most helpful to least helpful. The investigator usually specifies the exact number of cards that may be placed in each category so that all cards are not placed in neutral or extreme categories. Fig. 19-3 illustrates the distribution of cards to produce various distributions. A unimodal distribution is shown in Fig. 19-3, *A*, a rectangular distribution is apparent in *B*, and a U-shaped distribution is shown in *C*. The directions to the respondent for sorting the piles must be clear. For example, the following instructions would yield a unimodal distribution:

"You have been given 75 cards that each contain one nursing action that might be used to relieve your pain. Please sort the cards into nine piles according to the following directions.

"In Pile 1 on the extreme left place the three pain-relieving actions that you feel are the least helpful.

"In Pile 9 on the extreme right, place the three pain-relieving actions that you feel are the most helpful.

A

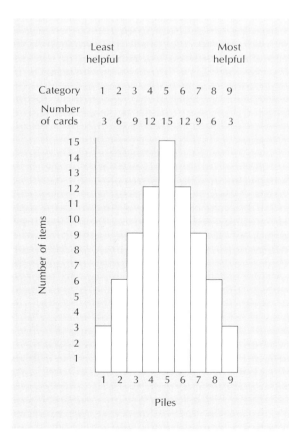

B

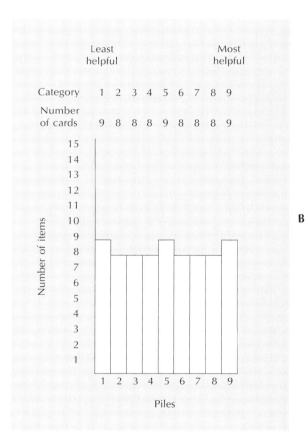

Fig. 19-3. Examples of distribution of Q-sort cards. **A,** Unimodal distribution. **B,** Rectangular distribution. **C,** U-shaped distribution.

Continued.

C

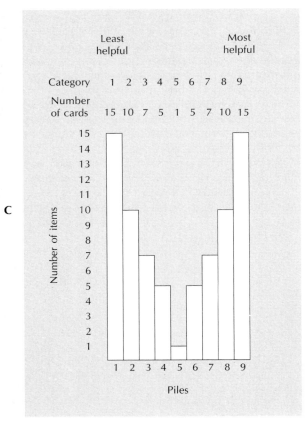

Fig. 19-3, C. For legend see p. 327.

special situation of questionnaire administration that requires considerable ability to follow directions on the part of the participants. The Delphi technique has been used in nursing to assess priorities, to quantify the judgments of experts, and to make long-range forecasts. Typically, a panel of experts are asked to express their viewpoint about the subject of study by responding to a series of questions on more than one occasion. Initially, the experts respond to a questionnaire in much the same way as they would to any questionnaire that elicits a viewpoint. The responses to the questions are analyzed, summarized, and returned to the experts with a second questionnaire. The experts are asked to consider the other participants' responses as they respond to the new questionnaire. This process of analysis-feedback-response, which may involve three or four separate questionnaires, is continued until a consensus is achieved among the expert panel members. Consensus does not imply agreement. The directions to the respondents must clearly communicate the fact that they are members of an expert panel and that the purpose of repeated rounds of questionnaires is to achieve a consensus. Panelists may not agree with the viewpoint expressed by other panel members but can reach a consensus about how items should be ranked or their degree of importance.

RECORDING RESPONSES OF PARTICIPANTS

How will the respondent record the answers to the questions? The answer varies considerably with whether the investigator has chosen to use a fixed-alternative response questionnaire, an open-ended unstructured interview, or something in between. The answer also will depend on the characteristics of the respondents, such as their ability to read and write and their physical proximity to the investigator. In the following section we will survey various ways in which a respondent may record responses to questionnaires and interviews.

Questionnaires

Decreasing the cost of completing a questionnaire requires that the pages be aesthetically pleasing and look easy to do. Dillman (1978) described in step-by-step detail how to formulate the pages of a questionnaire to achieve these ends. Dillman suggested that lower-case letters be used for the questions and

"In Pile 2 place the six next least helpful actions and in Piles 8 and 6 next most helpful actions.

"In Piles 3 and 7 place the nine least and most helpful actions, respectively.

"In Piles 4 and 6 place 12 actions each in terms of their being less or more helpful.

"In Pile 5 place the remaining 15 cards that you believe are of medium usefulness in relieving pain."

The importance of the respondent's understanding and following the directions for sorting cannot be overemphasized. In an effort to ensure that the participants in their study of nursing behaviors in bereavement properly completed the Q-sort, Freihofer and Felton (1976) combined written instructions with a videotape demonstration of how to do the Q-sort.

Delphi technique. The *Delphi technique* is another

upper-case letters be used for the answers. This difference in typeface helps the respondent distinguish between questions and answers. Numbering the responses instead of providing a box or line to check allows the investigator to code the responses more conveniently. Practically speaking, numbers are easier to reproduce than boxes.

Arranging the responses in a vertical column on the page prevents inadvertent omission, something that Dillman noted often occurs when the respondents are required to move back and forth across the page with their answers. Another advantage of the vertical-flow pattern is the psychological effect of enhancing the respondents' feeling of accomplishment as they move rapidly down the page with each answer. The white space on each page that results

from the vertical flow pattern gives the sense that the questions are easy to complete (Dillman, 1978).

Consider the format of the questions shown below (see box). Which format is more visually pleasing and easier to answer? The consistent direction to circle the number eliminates confusion about whether the response line is before or after the response. Although the same questions and responses are used, the questions in part *B* are considerably easier to read and it takes less time to identify all possible response choices. A clear difference exists between the question and the response alternatives. The vertical flow of responses in part *B* decreases the probability that the respondent may inadvertently omit a response when required to look back and forth across the page.

EXAMPLES OF QUESTION AND ANSWER FORMAT

A. What is your sex? ____ Male ____ Female
What is your marital status? ____ Never married ____ Married ____ Divorced
____ Separated ____ Widowed
What was the approximate net family income, from all sources, before taxes, in 1986? Less than $5,000 ____ $5,000 to 9,999 ____ $10,000 to 14,999 ____ $15,000 to 19,999 ____ $20,000 to 24,999 ____ over $25,000 ____ . Please describe your occupation, including title, kind of work, and kind of company or business. If you are not employed, describe your usual occupation.

B. What is your sex? (Circle number)
   1 MALE
   2 FEMALE
   What is your marital status? (Circle number)
   1 NEVER MARRIED
   2 MARRIED
   3 DIVORCED
   4 SEPARATED
   5 WIDOWED
   What was the approximate net family income, from all sources, before taxes, in 1986? (Circle number)
   1 Less than $5,000
   2 $5,000 to 9,999
   3 $10,000 to 14,999
   4 $15,000 to 19,999
   5 $20,000 to 24,999
   6 Over $25,000
Please describe your occupation. (If not employed, describe your usual occupation.)
                    TITLE: _____
          KIND OF WORK YOU DO: _____
KIND OF COMPANY OR BUSINESS: _____

The format of some questions may require that the respondent use a set of identical responses to answer a series of questions. A respondent may be asked to read a series of 25 statements and indicate the level of agreement on a scale that includes: "strongly agree," "agree," "somewhat agree," "neutral," "somewhat disagree," "disagree," and "strongly disagree." An example of questions from the Personal Resource Questionnaire—Part 2 (Brandt & Weinert, 1981) is shown in the box below. One

---

FORMAT FOR CONSISTENT RESPONSE SET QUESTIONS

A. Below are some statements with which some people agree and others disagree. Please read each statement and circle the response most appropriate for you. There is no right or wrong answer.
   There is someone I feel close to who makes me feel secure.
   1 STRONGLY DISAGREE
   2 DISAGREE
   3 SOMEWHAT DISAGREE
   4 NEUTRAL
   5 SOMEWHAT AGREE
   6 AGREE
   7 STRONGLY AGREE
   I belong to a group in which I feel important.
   1 STRONGLY DISAGREE
   2 DISAGREE
   3 SOMEWHAT DISAGREE
   4 NEUTRAL
   5 SOMEWHAT AGREE
   6 AGREE
   7 STRONGLY AGREE
   People let me know that I do well at my work (job, homemaking).
   1 STRONGLY DISAGREE
   2 DISAGREE
   3 SOMEWHAT DISAGREE
   4 NEUTRAL
   5 SOMEWHAT AGREE
   6 AGREE
   7 STRONGLY AGREE
B. Below are some statements with which some people agree and others disagree. Please read each statement and circle the response most appropriate for you. There is no right or wrong answer.

   1 STRONGLY DISAGREE
   2 DISAGREE
   3 SOMEWHAT DISAGREE
   4 NEUTRAL
   5 SOMEWHAT AGREE
   6 AGREE
   7 STRONGLY AGREE

   There is someone I feel close to who makes me feel secure 7 6 5 4 3 2 1
   I belong to a group in which I feel important 7 6 5 4 3 2 1
   People let me know that I do well at my work (job, homemaking)   7 6 5 4 3 2 1

Brandt, P.A., and Weinert, C., The PRQ—A social support measure. ©, 1981, American Journal of Nursing Company. Reprinted with permission from *Nursing Research*, Sept.-Oct., *30*, 277-280.

option would be to place those options after each statement as shown in part *A*. This format would take up considerable space and increase the cost of reproducing the questionnaire; it also would present a formidably long questionnaire. Another response option is to construct a scale that follows each question and to place the key to that scale at the top of each page of statements, as shown in part *B*.

In summary, the format that is used for recording responses to paper-and-pencil questionnaires must decrease the cost to the participant. Making pages aesthetically pleasing and responses easy to mark are two means of accomplishing this end.

Recording interview responses

When fixed-alternative questions are used in voice-to-voice or face-to-face interviews, the interviewer can record the responses directly on the guide by circling the respondent's answer. However, when open-ended questions are used, the investigator must decide whether the interviewer will code the responses or whether the verbatim responses will be captured then and coded at a later time. If the former strategy is used, the interviewers must be trained in the use of the coding scheme and provisions must be made to establish coding reliability. These requirements are similar to those discussed in Chapter 17 on recording observational data. The purpose of the study will help to determine how interview responses are recorded. If the purpose is to count the number of responses that fall into certain categories, coding the responses into those categories will suffice. On the other hand, if the purpose of the study is to understand a complex phenomenon, more precise recording of the respondent's actual answer may be needed.

The debate continues as to whether open-ended interviews should be tape-recorded. If taped, are verbatim transcriptions done? The disadvantages of tape-recording and transcribing interviews are obvious. The respondent may be intimidated by the recording equipment. The recording equipment itself is subject to mechanical failure or may pick up "white noise" from the environment that influences the quality of the recording. To deal with possible problems, the interviewer must be comfortable with the recorder and understand its operation and emergency repair procedures. Strategies for use of tape recorders are listed in the box on p. 332.

When interviews are tape-recorded, the investigator must decide how much of the tapes will be tran-

scribed. Transcribing tapes is costly and time-consuming. At the Minnesota Center for Social Research, Patton (1980) has found that it takes an average of 4 hours to transcribe 1 hour of tape. Verbatim transcripts, however, are enormously useful in data analysis. They are essential for independent analysis of the data and useful for later replication or secondary analysis.

The interviewer can make the task of transcribing easier by attending to the quality of the tape produced. Making a test with each respondent ensures that both the interviewer and the respondent are speaking distinctly and can be heard on the tape. Place the microphone on a stable surface that does not vibrate. A handkerchief under the microphone may improve the tonal quality of the tape. Avoid rustling papers, cups, etc., near the microphone. Check the recording to be certain that a buzz or hum is not created by electrical interference. Correct all distortions of tape quality before proceeding. A loud noise, such as a dog barking or a telephone ringing, will temporarily lower the automatic recording level on the tape recorder. Make a list of proper names and technical terminology for the transcriber.

The interviewer who is busy taking notes during an interaction may miss important information or filter data through preconceived notions and not really hear what the informant is saying. Perhaps a compromise is to tape-record and take some notes during the interviews. The interviewer writes a detailed record of the interview as soon after the event as possible. A complete tape recording of the interaction is available for use to refresh the interviewer's memory concerning details of the situation and for review, when the focus of the study is refined or shifted. Notes will help the interviewer locate salient sections of the tape. Selective transcription of relevant information and quotations illustrating the concepts under study can be done.

Note taking during the interview is an important data-collection technique. Notes help the interviewer to formulate new questions and to check out something that was said earlier. Nonverbal behaviors important in interpreting verbal responses can be noted. Patton (1980) pointed out that note taking can become a kind of nonverbal feedback to the respondent that what is being said is sufficiently important to be written down. Notes become critically important when tape quality is such that verbatim transcription is impossible.

The introduction of small lap or notebook computers has opened another avenue for recording interview data. The interviewer can type notes and verbatim responses during the interview. Experience has demonstrated that respondents are curious initially about the computer, but once the interview is underway, they do not seem to notice it any more than a tape recorder. The expert typist has a consid- erable advantage when using a computer to take notes, because eye contact can be maintained with the respondent. In addition, handwriting does not need to be interpreted. A disadvantage is that the small screen on some notebook computers is inconvenient when trying to refer to something the respondent said.

STRATEGIES FOR TAPE-RECORDING INTERVIEWS

1. A high-quality, dependable tape recorder is essential. One must be available consistently on a moment's notice. Purchasing a recorder for the study may be necessary. Some considerations include the following:
   a. A recorder that operates on both AC and DC current is ideal, because anticipating conditions under which interviews will be conducted is not always possible.
   b. Voice sensitivity and an automatic recording level decrease the possibility of setting the volume too low to hear the playback or so high that feedback makes transcription a challenge. Conversely, the interviewer has no control over the recording level, which is reset each time the volume of input changes. A voice-activated system may result in the loss of the first word with each activation.
   c. A built-in microphone eliminates one more piece of equipment with which to contend. However, a built-in condenser microphone is more sensitive than most external microphones and is likely to pick up background noise in the environment.
2. High-quality tapes intended to record music are not necessary. Cheap tapes, however, have a tendency to malfunction. Very short tapes (C-30) require frequent changing and result in a large accumulation of cassettes, but long tapes (C-120) are thin and fragile and often break or jam when subjected to repeated starting and stopping during transcription. C-60 tapes are recommended. Tapes have a leader that does not record; the tape must be advanced beyond the leader before attempting to record important information.
3. Tapes should be labeled with identifying information, such as the identification number of the participant and the date of the taping. Pressure-sensitive file folder labels can be prepared ahead of time and affixed to the cassettes, not the boxes, at the time of recording. The interviewer should have extra tapes in case the interview lasts longer than expected or a cassette malfunctions.
4. A dependable source of power should be used to operate the tape recorder. Adapters and extension cords should be readily available. If using DC current, the researcher must have a set of batteries that will power the recorder fully for the anticipated duration of the data collection. An investment in rechargeable nickel cadmium batteries is worthwhile.
5. The interviewer should test the recording level with the participant before beginning the interview. Recorders that do not have an automatic recording level need careful adjustment each time they are used.
6. If the tape recorder does not inform the user when the tape has ended, a small timer, such as one designed to remind the user of an expiring parking meter, can be used.
7. The interviewer should take the time to listen to at least segments of the entire tape as soon as possible after recording. Murphy's law is sure to express itself, and recalling lost data is much easier sooner than later.
8. After the tape is transcribed, the interviewer should listen to it while reading the transcription. The typist may be unfamiliar with terminology used or misunderstand or omit words that are important to the study.

SUMMARY

Implementing questionnaires and interviews requires that the investigator attend to many details. This chapter considers the problem of ensuring completion of questions by selected participants. Social exchange theory suggests that the costs and benefits of an activity must be balanced. Costs include both tangible and intangible costs, such as postage or transportation and the inconvenience of purchasing postage or going to an interview site. The investigator must strive to identify and decrease costs and to increase the benefits to the study participants.

Data generated by questionnaires and interviews must be trustworthy; that is, they must be reliable, valid, and unbiased. Strategies for ensuring the trustworthiness of questionnaire and interview data include providing a psychologically safe and comfortable environment for the respondents and identifying and controlling behaviors of interviewers that may bias the responses. Although removing all bias from interview situations is not possible, the investigator must be aware that the appearance and behavior of the interviewer, the way questions are asked, and the way responses are recorded can bias data.

The actual administration of questionnaires can be accomplished by mail, by group administration, or by computer. The questionnaire that is delivered to a potential respondent must speak for itself; the investigator cannot answer questions, allay anxiety, or clarify items. Attention must be given to preparing a paper-and-pencil questionnaire so that it will be visually pleasing and easy to complete. A cover letter is used to explain the importance of the respondent's participation in the study.

Interviews can be conducted in a face-to-face situation with the respondent or over the telephone. Interviews may allow the investigator to probe for depth and breadth of responses and to observe the environment and nonverbal behavior in relation to the verbal responses. Strategies for increasing response rate to telephone interviews include determining the time that potential respondents are likely to be near the telephone, notifying the potential participant of the anticipated telephone call, and making an appointment for the telephone interview. Q-sort and Delphi techniques may be used as scaling techniques; however, in this chapter they are considered as special situations of administering questionnaires.

Strategies are presented for recording responses to questionnaires and interviews. Most commonly, questionnaire responses are written on paper. It must be clear to the respondent whether answers are to be checked, circled, or ranked. Interview responses can be written by the interviewer or can be tape-recorded for later transcription or coding.

REFERENCES

Blau, P. M. (1964). *Exchange and power in social life*. New York: Wiley.

Boyd, H. W., Westfall, R., & Stasch, S. F. (1981). *Marketing research: Text and cases*. Homewood, IL: Richard D. Irwin.

Bradburn, N. M., et al. (1981). *Improving interview method and questionnaire design*. San Francisco: Jossey-Bass.

Brandt, P. A., & Weinert, C. (1981). PRQ—A social support measure. *Nursing Research, 30*, 277-280.

Davis, A. J. (1980). Research as an inactional situation: Objectivity in the interview. *International Journal of Nursing Studies, 17*, 215-220.

Dillman, D. A. (1978). *Mail and telephone surveys: The total design method*. New York: Wiley.

Freihofer, P., & Felton, G. (1976). Nursing behaviors in bereavement: An exploratory study. *Nursing Research, 25*, 332-337.

Hammersley, M., & Atkinson, P. (1983). *Ethnography principles in practice*. London: Travistock.

Heberlein, T., & Baumgarten, R. (1978). Factors affecting response rates to mailed questionnaires: A quantitative analysis of the published research. *American Sociological Review, 43*, 447-462.

Kidder, L. H. (1981). *Selltiz Wrightsman & Cook's Research methods in social relations* (4th ed.). New York: Holt, Reinhart & Winston.

LeCompte, M. D., & Goetz, J. P. (1982). Problems of reliability and validity in ethnographic research. *Review of Educational Research, 52*(1), 31-60.

Morgan, D. L., & Spanish, M. T. (1984). Focus groups: A new tool for qualitative research. *Qualitative Sociology, 7*, 253-270.

Patton, M. Q, (1980). *Qualitative evaluation methods*. Beverly Hills, CA: Sage.

Smith, J. M. (1972). *Interviewing in market and social research*. London: Routledge & Kegan Paul.

Thibaut, J. W., & Kelley, H. H. (1959). *The social psychology of groups*. New York: Wiley.

Wells, W. D. (1974). Group interviewing. In R. Feber (Ed.). *Handbook of marketing research* (pp. 133-146). New York: McGraw-Hill.

Woolley, A. S. (1984). Questioning the mailed questionnaire as a valid instrument for research in nursing education. *Image: The Journal of Nursing Scholarship, 16*, 115-119.

20
USING EXISTING DATA SOURCES: PRIMARY AND SECONDARY ANALYSIS

NANCY FUGATE WOODS

Every literate society records a great deal of information about its members and the important issues of the day. Because health is an important issue in most societies, it is not surprising that a great deal of data exists about human health.

Many sources of data are available about human health and nursing that investigators can use to answer certain research questions. Indeed, a cursory examination reveals a wide range of health-related topics of interest to society. As an example of using available data sources, an investigator concerned about the incidence of chronic illness in the United States could consult a database such as the *Health Interview Survey* to find the proportion of the U.S. population affected by heart disease. Concern with hunger and nutrition in the U.S. could cause an investigator to consult a database such as the *Health and Nutrition Examination Survey* to determine the proportion of women in the United States with iron deficiency. Archives such as those housed at Boston University are useful for investigators concerned with the history of nursing. An investigator concerned about the immunization experiences of children in a health maintenance organization could consult the health records for individuals subscribing to the HMO.

This chapter focuses on using existing data sources for both primary and secondary analysis. *Primary analysis* refers to the initial analysis of data, whether those data were collected orginally to achieve a research purpose or for another purpose. Benoliel (1978), interested in the treatment trajectories of dying patients, studied data abstracted from their hospital records to discern the types of medical and nursing treatments that were given to patients whose diagnosis indicated they were dying. The data in the medical records were recorded for clinical purposes, yet Benoliel abstracted and analyzed them to achieve her own research purposes.

In *secondary analysis* the researcher studies a problem by analyzing data that originally were collected for another study with a different purpose. The data used for secondary analysis may be in several forms, including raw data, statistical databases, or archives. Secondary analysis involves reanalysis of data originally collected and analyzed by another investigator addressing the same question, a different question, or applying different methods of analysis.

In this chapter we will explore existing data sources for nursing research, including personal and public health records, national databases, and databases developed by individual investigators. We will consider the advantages and disadvantages of using existing data for secondary analysis. Finally, we will consider some general guidelines for using personal health records and existing databases.

PURPOSES OF PRIMARY AND SECONDARY ANALYSIS

Investigators may use existing data for primary analysis or secondary analysis. Primary analysis, the initial analysis of data for a specified research purpose, usually involves archives such as personal health records or public health records. Often, the existing data source has not been collected for research purposes, but rather as a record of clinical intervention or surveillance of public health.

Secondary analysis, the analysis of data collected and analyzed for some other research purpose, involves using data in one of several forms, including raw data or a database. As discussed in more detail in Chapter 24, a database is a set of observations for each element in the study population, coded for analytical purposes.

There are several purposes for performing secondary analysis, including:
1. The identification and analysis of significant variables not analyzed in the original study
2. The investigation of relationships or hypotheses not addressed in the original study
3. A change in the unit of analysis from that used for the original study
4. A focus on a subsample not addressed in the original study
5. The use of different analytical strategies in data analysis
6. The application of meta-analysis techniques

Let us consider an application of each of these in the following pages.

Investigators usually collect data that may be used to address multiple purposes. Woods and Hulka (1979) used a database—generated originally by Hulka as part of a study of family needs for primary care—to examine the relationships between women's family and employment roles and illness behavior patterns. The original investigators were concerned with the incidence of health problems and the use of and satisfaction with medical care. Woods and Hulka's later analysis of significant variables not related to the original purpose of the study revealed important influences of family structural variables, but not of employment, on women's response to symptoms.

Investigation of relationships or hypotheses not addressed in the original study is a second application of secondary analysis. Hulka's original interest was predicting use and satisfaction with ambulatory care, whereas Woods's interest was testing a hypothesis related to the complementarity of women's family and employment roles and their subsequent behavior in response to illness.

A change in the unit of analysis is a third application. Although Hulka's original emphasis was on families as a unit of analysis, Woods studied an individual in the family—the woman. The family became the context for women's health rather than the unit of analysis.

A fourth application of secondary analysis is to study a subsample not addressed in the original study. Woods selected only families consisting of a mother, a father, and at least one child, whereas the original study had included single-parent families, families without children, and other types of families.

The use of different analytical strategies is a fifth application of secondary analysis. With the advent of multivariate statistical techniques and expansion of causal modeling strategies, data analyzed by earlier techniques can be studied with more sophisticated methods. Investigators can now apply statistical techniques that permit simultaneous analysis of several independent and dependent variables rather than perform several individual analyses. Advanced statistical techniques are discussed in detail in Chapter 27.

Meta-analysis is a variety of analytical strategies that permit an investigator to summarize mathematically the results of several studies through calculating the size of the effect of the independent variable on the dependent variable (see Chapter 4 for discussion of meta-analysis). Application of meta-analysis to summarize and integrate findings from a body of literature can reveal useful patterns across studies. Meta-analysis can be performed using either raw data from original studies or summary measures to generate effect sizes.

EXISTING DATA SOURCES

Existing data sources that are useful in nursing research include public records, personal records, databases generated by individual investigators, national health databases, and other communications media such as print and film. In the following pages we will consider some of the more common data sources and examples of nursing studies that could be conducted using these sources.

Public records

Every literate society records some statistics about its members. One of the most basic sources of information for planning and programing in many fields, including health, is the United States Census. A census is a periodic count or enumeration of the population. In the United States a census has been taken every 10 years since 1790. Census information is analyzed for the country as a whole and for progressively smaller divisions, including regions, states, counties, municipalities, census tracts, and block groups within census tracts. Two units are created especially for the purposes of the census: Standard Metropolitan Statistical Areas (SMSAs) and census tracts. The SMSA is an area that has at least one city of 50,000 residents and meets other criteria related to social and economic integration of the city and surrounding county or counties, minimum population density, and minimum proportion of the labor force engaged in nonagricultural work. Census tracts are smaller geographical areas within cities that contain 3000 to 6000 persons; they are intended to be relatively homogeneous in ethnic and socioeconomic composition.

Census data provided by individuals are confidential and are only available to agencies or individuals in the form of statistical compilations. Nevertheless, aggregate data from the census can be used in nursing research in several ways. Census data can provide answers to research questions related to indicators of well-being (e.g., income, education) and may be linked to other indicators of health, illness, and mortality. Census data for census tracts can be linked to health variables that reflect the entire census tract, for example, infant death rates or morbidity rates for specific diseases. Investigators also can use census data when defining the sampling frame for a study. For example, census tracts containing a high proportion of individuals who meet certain ethnic and educational criteria could be identified from census data tabulations and subsequently used as a sampling frame for a study.

Other data sources related to health include vital statistics—the data collected from ongoing recording or registration of all "vital events": births, adoptions, deaths and fetal deaths, marriages, divorces, legal separations, and annulments. The vital Statistics Registration System in the United States centralizes information filed through local governments. Information then is processed through city and county health departments for allocating services, planning programs, measuring the effectiveness of services, and conducting research. The state registrar or bureau of vital statistics compiles statistics for the state for use in planning, evaluating, and administering state and local health activities and conducting research. In addition, the state transmits information to the National Center for Health Statistics (of the United States Public Health Service), which publishes vital statistics for the nation, conducts research based on vital statistics, and controls the quality of the information collection system.

Death certificates include information about the deceased person's characteristics such as age, sex, race, and usual occupation and about conditions that led to the death. The diagnostic terms on the death certificate follow an internationally accepted classification, the International Statistical Classification of Diseases, Injuries, and Causes of Death (ICD), revised every 10 years. Certificates of Live Birth include both public and private information. Public information identifies the child and its parents. The confidential section of the birth certificate includes data about the race and education of the parents, previous pregnancies, amount of prenatal care, birth weight, complication of pregnancy and delivery, and congenital abnormalities.

Morbidity data for the population also are compiled and include information about reportable diseases. Diseases considered "reportable" vary from state to state, but certain diseases are reportable in all states; some are governed by International Quarantine agreements. In some states communicable diseases constitute the majority of reportable diseases, whereas in others occupationally linked disease and cancer are reportable. States use various reporting procedures, but most report to local and state health departments, to the Centers for Disease Control, and in some instances to the World Health Organization. Some states have disease registries—for example, for cancer—in which all cases of cancer are recorded. These databases are accessible to nurse investigators and may serve as the basis for sampling for population-based studies or as a data source.

Schultz and Kerr (1986) explored the relationships of community factors, interorganizational relationships, organizational factors, and health system outcomes in communities that were identified as medically underserved and well served. As an indicator of health system outcomes, they included data about death rates for heart disease, cancer, stroke, and arteriosclerosis from death rates reported by the respective counties. Small, rural underserved communities with older populations had fewer diagnostic screening tests. Moreover, these communities had the highest death rates.

Personal health records

Many sources of data about personal health exist. Medical and nursing records are the most commonly used records for research. Personal health records can be a source of data that can be abstracted for analysis, as well as a source for identification of a sample. Nursing records, particularly those employing nursing diagnoses and chronicles of the outcomes of nursing therapeutics, offer a great deal of promise for future research applications. In addition to medical and nursing records, documents such as referrals to other agencies, discharge summaries, and incident reports can be rich sources of nursing data.

Benoliel (1978) used hospital records to describe and compare types of dying, including duration of dying, time of death, place of dying, cause of dying, and personal-social characteristics of the person; to describe the relationship between types of dying and location and time of the death; and to describe the shape of the trajectory of dying.

One challenge for the future is linking vital statistics and health records so that they might provide a chronicle of individual or family health status over the years. Although many technical and ethical challenges are associated with record linkage, the knowledge gained about patterns of health over the life span makes the idea important for nursing.

Investigator-generated databases

Many individual investigators willingly provide access to databases they have generated. Literature searches of published works help to identify their work. In some instances unpublished works that are abstracted or cited in publications point to a database that appears to meet the purposes envisioned for secondary analysis. The investigator who is anticipating use of the database must contact the individual investigator to determine the adequacy of the database to meet the goals of the secondary analysis, to obtain permission to use the data, and to obtain the raw data and documentation regarding it. Raw data, such as questionnaires or interview transcriptions, may not be shared in some instances because of conditions imposed by agreement with the original participants.

National databases

To provide for a more comprehensive picture of the health of the population than is possible with vital statistics, the federal government sponsors large scale sample surveys. The most extensive and well known of these is the National Health Survey, which has been conducted for decades. Established by an act of Congress in 1956 and conducted by the National Center for Health Statistics, the *National Health Survey* includes several components that are directed toward the description of the health status and needs of the U.S. population. The *Health Interview Survey, Health Examination Survey, Health and Nutrition Examination Survey, Health Records Survey, National Family Growth Survey,* and the *National Ambulatory Medical Survey* are all components of the *National Health Survey.*

The *Health Interview Survey* (HIS) is based on interviews conducted with about 800 households sampled from throughout the country. Weekly samples are combined to reflect the health status of the U.S. population for the month and the year. Questions included in the survey address whether anyone in the family experienced an illness and sought medical care. The *Health Examination Survey* (HES) augments the information from the HIS with physical examinations and laboratory tests. The *Health and Nutrition Examination Survey* augments the HIS and the HES with specific items related to the nutritional status of the population.

The *Health Records Survey* involves collection of information from medical and residential institutions providing health care. Nursing homes and hospitals serve as the source of data for this survey, which is designed to describe health services, the characteristics of the population being served, and the types of diagnoses and treatment they experience. The *National Family Growth Survey* is a household survey of patterns of fertility and family planning practices. The *National Ambulatory Medical Care Survey*

TABLE 20–1. Data sources by subject classification

| | SUBJECT CLASSIFICATION | | | | |
DATA SOURCE	NURSING PERSONNEL	NURSING EDUCATION	HEALTH-CARE DELIVERY SYSTEM	CLIENT POPULATION	DATA TAPES AVAILABLE
Directory of Nurses with Doctoral Degrees	x				x
Health Interview Survey				x	x
Hospitals, Annual Survey of			x		x
Index of Help-Wanted Ads for Nursing	x				x
National Ambulatory Medical Care Survey			x	x	
National Health and Nutrition Examination Survey				x	
National Hospital Discharge Survey			x	x	
National Nursing Home Survey	x		x	x	
National Sample Survey of Licensed Practical/Vocational Nurses	x				
National Sample Survey of Registered Nurses	x				
Nurse-Faculty Census		x			
Schools of Nursing, Annual Survey of		x		x	
Special Surveys of School of Nursing— Minority Students					
Yearly Review			x		

Modified from Interagency Conference on Nursing Statistics. (1984). Unpublished manuscript.

includes a sample of physicians' practices from which reports about the types of problems patients seen in office visits experience. In 1985 a National Nursing Home Survey will be launched, the first since 1977 and the first ever to seek follow-up interviews with patients' next of kin. The survey involves 1200 nursing homes in the United States and asks detailed questions about staffing, services, expenses, and recruiting of nurses, as well as questions about the patients' families and reasons for admission to the nursing home. These databases are described in detail in *Inventory of U.S. Health Care Data Bases, 1976-1983.*

In addition to databases that describe the health of the population, databases are published about nursing and nurses, based on various samples of nurses. These include the *National Sample Survey of Registered Nurses,* conducted by the Bureau of Health Professions, Health Resources and Services, United States Public Health Service.

The National League for Nursing conducts several surveys regarding nurses and nursing-education programs. The *Nurse Faculty Census,* updated biennially, contains a census of nurse faculty in schools of nursing by level of preparation. The *Annual Survey of Schools of Nursing* contains data regarding admissions, graduations, enrollments in RN, baccalaureate, masters, doctoral, and LPN programs. A *Special Survey of Schools of Nursing—Minority Students* also is conducted every 3 years by the National League for Nursing. The *Yearly Review,* also sponsored by the National League of Nursing, is a study of policies, practices, and trends in community health nursing throughout the country.

The American Nurses' Association Center for Research conducts a survey of nurses with doctoral degrees that was updated most recently in 1983 with updating planned again for 1987 (Table 20-1). ANA also conducts a *Help Wanted Ad* survey for nursing positions, advertised in 22 newspapers spanning the country—a database useful for estimating RN supply and demand.

The *Annual Survey of Hospitals,* conducted by the American Hospital Association, contains current and trend information on hospital facilities and utilization, and financial and personnel data. These databases are described in greater detail in *Interagency Conference on Nursing Statistics* (ICONS), 1984.

Media

Other sources of data include media such as print and film productions. Newscasts, editorials, television shows, advertisements, films, and novels all can provide rich databases for studies that document historical trends or current viewpoints about nursing and health. Each month, from 1978 to 1981, Kalisch, Kalisch, and Belcher (1985) analyzed newspaper articles about nursing. They subsequently constructed a model to show the effects of key nursing issues on the image of nursing. Newspapers that showed nurses in clinical settings and articles that showed nurses as playing a major role were the most important factors in projecting positive nursing images.

ADVANTAGES AND DISADVANTAGES OF USING EXISTING DATA

Many rich existing sources of data are available. With imagination, investigators frequently can find existing data sources that address their research questions. Nevertheless, the investigator must consider some important advantages and disadvantages associated with the use of existing data sources.

Existing data are attractive to investigators because the data exist. Although this statement may seem self-evident, it implies several advantages to the investigator who is contemplating the use of existing data for primary or secondary analysis. The investigator who wishes to study changes in birthing practices over a 10-year period in which the home-birth movement became influential in a community would have access to 10 years of hospital and clinic records for retrospective review. The data are already recorded and need not be generated from new observations. In the case of secondary analysis the time and money involved in collecting the data have already been spent; the initial effort already has been made. Obvious economic advantages accrue from ordering a computer tape that contains the data versus conducting interviews and coding and entering the data before beginning the analyses. The initial investigator has borne the costs of time, personnel salaries, personnel training, and supervision.

Additionally, existing data often allow the tracking of trends over time. For example, an investigator using data from the *Health Interview Survey* can trace patterns of health status for women over 2 decades. An investigator tracing the development of the concept of caring in the nursing literature has 100 or more years of archival material to review. Collecting longitudinal data could be prohibitively expensive and perhaps consume most of one's research career.

Using existing databases, especially national databases, allows investigators to study a larger sample size and a broader geographical area than is possible when the investigator must depend on his or her funding for the study. The investigator can use secondary data for testing ideas before designing a study. Using secondary data for learning database management and analytical techniques is helpful. The investigator can refine the research hypotheses and learn from the inadequacies of the secondary database to plan a study.

Using existing databases also carries many disadvantages. For example, using personal health records as a data source has many limitations. Benoliel (1978) found great variability among records kept by three hospitals due to idiosyncratic methods of record keeping. Moreover, she encountered records that were totally or partially missing; gross omissions of information from the record; haphazard methods of recording; microfilmed records suffering from poor quality of film, poor photography, or omissions of sections of the chart; illegible handwriting; sparse information; and excessive redundant information (Benoliel, 1978, p. 39). Another problem Benoliel encountered was the changing patterns of medical diagnosis. Because the diagnostic categories used over a 5-year period changed, it was difficult to compare causes of death and associated diagnoses for the two cohorts of patients she studied. Another problem was the inconsistency in data collection, transcription, and coding of some variables from the health record by the data collectors.

Investigators studying nursing information in personal health records might anticipate finding omissions of descriptions of nursing care and the application of many different taxonomies of nursing diagnoses. Nevertheless, these problems do not occur in all agencies, and many nursing records are exemplary in their completeness and utility for research purposes.

When using existing statistical databases, the investigator also is faced with many challenges. First, the definition of terms the investigator proposes may be inconsistent with the technical definitions employed by the investigators who conceived of the database. For example, the *Health Interview Survey* asks about morbidity experiences in the family over the last 2 weeks. The investigator who is interested in studying family health may find that morbidity experiences do not completely reflect her definition of health.

Adequacy of methods is another concern for investigators using existing databases. The investigator must accept the database as it exists, with no recourse to redesigning the study. In some instances the disparity between the preferred and actual study methods is so great that the investigator may reject the use of the existing database in favor of personal data collection efforts.

Quality of the database cannot be assumed. Missing data, lost data, and coding and data entry errors are sometimes the unfortunate legacy of the original study. The secondary analyst must cope with them. Ideally, the secondary analyst can contact the original investigator to determine whether the errors or omissions can be rectified. Often the researcher using the databases was not part of the original study team, and the original investigator may not be accessible to the secondary analyst. In some instances the unknowns may make the use of the data too risky. Unforeseen problems may increase the time, monetary cost, and personnel needs beyond the estimated budget. Glitches in file structure, junk in the database, and other surprises are not uncommon, but they are not insurmountable with good documentation and access to the person who created the original database. With the advantages and disadvantages of using existing data sources in mind, let us consider some guidelines for their use.

GUIDELINES FOR USING EXISTING DATA

Regardless of the type of data being used, the investigator must become intimately familiar with the data. Indeed, becoming aware of existing data sources is perhaps the major challenge in exploiting them for research purposes. Creativity and ingenuity may lead investigators to identify sources of data that others in the discipline could not imagine. The work of the Kalisches (1985) on films that depict nursing is exemplary in this regard.

A major consideration for secondary analysis is the match or mismatch between the framework of the initial investigator and the investigator proposing secondary analysis. Intellectual flexibility in the framing of the research question, the construction of indicators of the concepts to be studied, selection of cases, and data analysis procedures are essential to using existing data. The investigator who wishes to study the illness experiences of families might be willing to begin with an existing database if the nature of illness experiences contained in the database were symptomatic episodes but not instances of a major catastrophic illness. He or she may be able to justify learning about family morbidity patterns under conditions of less acute illness as a prelude to understanding responses to critical illness.

An investigator cannot impose indicators on the database that are not present in the data. Alternatively, the investigator can create new indicators from the data to reflect the construct of interest. For example, although measuring women's attitudes toward women's roles (traditional or modern) may not be possible, education may be used as an indicator of the construct "sex-role orientation" because earlier studies have shown that education correlates highly with sex-role attitudes.

Selection of the sample and data analysis procedures are not likely to be exactly as the investigator intended. Consideration of the disparity between the actual and desired sample may lead to rejecting the use of the existing database or to reconsidering the generalizability of the findings. Often, using an existing database provides the investigator with a larger sample than would be possible to obtain with only the investigator's own support.

The nature of the sampling and measurement may constrain analyses. For example, use of a specific sampling strategy such as stratification implies the necessity of a stratified analysis. Nevertheless, many of these challenges need not preclude the use of existing databases.

Validity of the existing data is an important issue for investigators who use either primary or secondary analysis. Validity of archival data has been discussed in Chapter 15. Benoliel (1978) found validity of hospital records troublesome because of the inconsistencies among individual practitioners in the use of nomenclature about patients' conditions and medical diagnoses. As discussed earlier, omissions in records or missing records also contributed to her concerns about validity of the data sources. To enhance validity in the abstraction and coding of data from hospital records, Benoliel used several procedures. She developed extensive lists of alternate words subsumed under each of the established coding categories that subsequently were applied to the records. An abstracting form used in the study of dying in teaching hospitals is shown on pp. 342-345. The coding information used to complete the form is included in Table 20-2. Note the specification of the alternate words that would indicate each category. Benoliel (1978) also developed specific directions for using clearly identified sections of the hospital record as the data sources for coding complex variables. Finally, she reviewed all coded instruments and jointly reviewed all the completed instruments with the data collectors.

Validity of the data also is of concern to the investigator who is using statistical databases. Not only do questions arise about internal validity, for example, those pertaining to adequacy of fit between the indicators and the construct, but also concerns arise about the external validity of the study—the extent to which the study findings are informative about the population of interest. These questions must be weighed carefully before commitment to the use of an existing database is made.

Recommendations for investigators contemplating using existing data sources

Investigators contemplating using existing data sources such as personal health records will find performing a small pilot study useful before committing large amounts of time and money to a study. The pilot study will contribute understanding of the degree to which the research purpose can be achieved, given the existing data source. If the data simply are not recorded in the personal health record, or are recorded so inconsistently or haphazardly that their validity is dubious, the data source cannot support the proposed study.

Access to records is another important issue. When many records are missing in whole or in part, the investigator will need to weigh whether the representation of the phenomenon being studied is adequate. An investigator interested in studying changing patterns of nursing diagnoses will be frustrated in that aim if the nursing recordings are consistently missing from the hospital record. Finally, investigators will discover the need for careful abstracting and coding rules, such as those employed by Benoliel, before initiating the study.

Recommendations for investigators contemplating secondary analysis of databases

Some recommendations designed to assist the investigator contemplating secondary analysis include the following:

1. Obtain the best possible documentation regarding the raw data, variable transformations, directionality of scales, and any other modifications made on the original database.

2. Be certain to a have a complete code book before considering secondary analysis.

3. Supplement the documentation with access to

Text continued on p. 347.

MAIN POPULATION CODING FORM

Patient Identification Number:			

Age Class:	(1) Premature (2) Newborn (3) Stillborn	(4) Infant (5) Preschool Child (6) School Child	(7) Adolescent (8) Adult	

Age: (in years) (Year of birth)	

Sex: (0) Not Indicated (1) Female (2) Male	

Race/ Ethnicity:	(0) Not indicated (1) Caucasian (2) Negro	(3) Oriental (4) Spanish surname	(5) American Indian (6) Eskimo	

Marital Status:	(0) Not indicated (1) Single	(2) Married (3) Separated	(4) Divorced (5) Widowed	

Religion	(0) Not indicated (1) Protestant	(2) Catholic (3) Jewish	(4) No preference (5) Other	

Birthplace:	(0) Not indicated (1) Metropolitan (2) (3) USA, except	(4) Outside USA (5) (6) (7) (8) No city given	

Residence City:				

Residence State:	

Type of Residence:	(0) Not indicated (1) Own home or apt. (2) Family member's home (3) Nursing home	(4) Other hospital (5) Cust. unit, Hosp. 1 (6) Other institution (7) Other_____	

Employment Patient:	(0) Not indicated (1) Employed	(2) Unemployed (3) Retired (4) Housewife	

Occupation Patient:	

Employment Spouse:	(0) Not indicated (1) Employed	(2) Unemployed (3) Retired (4) Housewife	

Occupation Spouse:	

Payment Class:	(0) Not indicated (1) Self (2) Insurance	(3) Medicare (4) Medicaid (5) Welfare	(6) Veterans (7) Other_____ Room Rate_____	

Relationship of Person to Notify:	(0) Not indicated (1) Spouse (2) Parent (3) Child (4) Sibling	(5) Other relative (6) Friend (7) Legal guardian (8) No one	

In Hospital During Previous Year:	(0) NI	(1) Yes	(2) No

Hospital Identification Number:	(1)	(2)	(3)

University of Washington
7/74 Comparative Nursing
Care Systems

MAIN POPULATION CODING FORM, Care–Cure Project

1/4 MM

Type of Physician:	(0) Not indicated (1) House Staff (2) Private MD	(3) Cancer Team (4) Attending/Academic	Primary Alternate	
Specialty of Physician:			Primary Alternate	
Date of Admission (Month/Day/Year):				
Time of Admission:				
Admission Ward:				
Reason of Admission:				
Clinical Service:				
Date of Death (Month/Day/Year):				
Time of Death:				
Number of Hospital Days:				
Coroner's Case:	(0) Not indicated	(1) Yes	(2) No	
Autopsy:	(0) Not indicated	(1) Yes	(2) No	
Terminal Event:	(0) Not indicated (1) Found dead (2) CP Cessation (3) CP Arrest/Resus. (4) CP Arrest/ No Resus. (5) CP Arrest during treatment	(6) CP Failure on machine with resuscitation (7) CP Failure on machine without resuscitation (8) Surgical Death		
Place of Death:				
Persons Present at Death Site:	(0) Not indicated (1) No one (2) Staff only	(3) Family only (4) Family and Staff (5) Other		
Type of Chart:	(1) Unfilmed (2) Roll film	(3) Microfiche		
State of Chart:	(1) Complete (2) Purged	(3) Sections Missing _____		
Coding Team:	(1) JB (2) VF	(3) PO (4) DM	(5) LD	
Date of Coding:				

University of Washington
7/74 Comparative Nursing
Care Systems

MAIN POPULATION CODING FORM, Care–Cure Project

1/4 MM

Continued.

Patient Identification Number: | | | |

Address (if Seattle, Everett, Tacoma):

Admitting Diagnosis:

_____

_____

Immediate Cause of Death:

_____

_____

Underlying Cause of Death:

_____

_____

Recent Other Conditions: (1) Present   (0) Absent

☐ (1) Sepsis/infection
☐ (2) Renal Failure
☐ (3) Major Post-operative
   Complications, this
   hospitalization
☐ (4) GI Obstruction
   Perforation, Infection
☐ (5) Acute Respiratory Disorder

☐ (6) CV Critical State
☐ (7) Poison Ingestion
☐ (8) Injury
☐ (9) Post-op Complications
   (Post Rx), prior to
   hospitalization

Chronic Other Conditions: (1) Present   (0) Absent

☐ (1) Malignancy
☐ (2) Diabetes Mellitus
☐ (3) Chronic CNS Disorder
☐ (4) Chronic CV Disorder
☐ (5) Chronic Respiratory Disease

☐ (6) Chronic Renal Disorder
☐ (7) Chronic GI Disorder
☐ (8) Liver Disease
☐ (9) Alcoholism
☐ (10) Drug Dependence

Death Certificate Information:

Cause of Death:_____

Due to_____

Due to_____

University of Washington
7/74 Comparative Nursing
Care Systems

MAIN POPULATION CODING FORM, Care–Cure Project

1/4 MM

Condition on Admission:
(0) Not indicated
(1) Terminal
(2) Grim prognosis

(3) Critical
(4) Serious
(5) Noncritical

Consciousness of Admission:
(0) Not indicated
(1) Unconscious
(2) Deep stupor
(3) Stuporous

(4) Confused
(5) Dull alert
(6) Alert but aphasic
(7) Alert

Treatment Effort on Admission:
(0) Not indicated
(1) Comfort orientation
(2) Recovery orientation
(3) Heavy recovery

(4) Life support
    maintenance
(5) Active CPR

Condition on Day of Death:
(0) Not indicated
(1) Terminal
(2) Grim prognosis

(3) Critical
(4) Serious
(5) Noncritical

Improving—code 1 level up from day before
No improvement–no change—code same as day before

Consciousness on Day of Death:
(0) Not indicated
(1) Unconscious
(2) Deep stupor
(3) Stuporous

(4) Confused
(5) Dull alert
(6) Alert but aphasic
(7) Alert

Treatment Effort on Day of Death:
(0) Not indicated
(1) Comfort orientation
(2) Recovery orientation
(3) Heavy recovery

(4) Life support
    maintenance
(5) Active CPR

Therapy Misadventure, This Hospitalization:
(0) No record of misadv.
(1) Surgical misadv.
(2) Suspected surg. misadv.
(3) Therapy misadv.
(4) Suspected tx. misadv.
(5) Dx. proced. misadv.
(6) Other misadv.

(7) Suspected other
    misadv.
(8) Suspected dx.
    proced. misadv.
(9) Suicide in
    hospital
(10) Multiple misadvs.

Specify briefly:

GRAND TOTAL WORK EFFORT SCORE

TABLE 20–2. Coding information

VARIABLE NAME	CODE CATEGORIES	INSTRUCTIONS
CONSCIOUSNESS ON ADMISSION		Recorded M.D. statements of patient's level of consciousness (awareness); sources: history, progress notes, admitting and discharge notes
	(0) Not indicated	Includes stillbirth
	(1) Unconscious	Unresponsive, unresponsive and flaccid, totally unresponsive, unresponsive to all stimuli, deepening coma terminally, coma
	(2) Deep stupor	Little response, obtunded, responds to stimulation only; responds to deep pain, unresponsive except to pain, largely unresponsive, unresponsive to commands
	(3) Stuporous	Semiresponsive, semicomatose, very somnolent, responds occasionally with nod, minimal response to physical and verbal stimuli, increasingly obtunded
	(4) Confused	Confused, disoriented, difficulty maintaining contact, confused and agitated, intermittent confusion, conscious but not reliable, not oriented, incoherent, senile, delirious, hallucinating
	(5) Dull alert	Mildly obtunded, responsive, can respond to simple commands, less responsive, responsive but not alert, lethargic, increasingly lethargic, slightly more responsive
	(6) Alert by aphasic	Unable to speak but can comprehend
	(7) Alert	Implied alert, alert, answers questions relevantly, responds intelligently, awake and oriented, awake and responsive, mental status good, oriented to place and time, good historian
TREATMENT EFFORT ON ADMISSION		Represents M.D. orientation toward treatment as reflected in the medications/treatments given; select the highest level of code category which includes one or more treatments/medications received by the patient on that day
	(0) Not indicated	No information available
	(1) Comfort orientation	Receiving one or more comfort drugs only, items 01-05 on work effort tally sheet; if only potassium added to IVs, use this code
	(2) Recovery orientation	Receiving one or more recovery drugs/treatments, items 06-31 on work effort tally sheet
	(3) Heavy recovery orientation	Receiving one or more heavy recovery drugs/treatments, items 32-40 on work effort tally sheet
	(4) Life support orientation	Receiving one or more life support maintenance drugs/treatments, items 41-51 on work effort tally sheet
	(5) Active CPR	Any type of cardiopulmonary resuscitation. Resuscitation includes mechanical and chemical methods; oxygen alone does not count

Modified from Benoliel, J. (1978). Unpublished manuscript.

someone who knows the database intimately.

4. Screen the data by means of frequency distributions and displays, for example, to become familiar with each variable.

5. Reproduce tables and correlations that were published by the initial investigators as a check on your data manipulation and the database itself.

6. Become a student of the data. Study the frequencies, correlation matrixes, and other simple analyses before embarking on multivariate analyses.

7. Finally, do not assume the original investigator performed a perfect analysis. There is no reason to be shocked by errors in the database unless you replicate the error.

SUMMARY

Existing data sources for nursing research include public records, personal health records, investigator-generated databases associated with earlier studies, national databases, and mass media. These data sources can be used for primary analysis or secondary analysis. Primary analysis refers to the initial analysis of data for a specified research purpose. Secondary analysis is the study of problems through analysis of data that were originally collected for another study with a different purpose from the secondary analysis.

There are many advantages to using existing data. Because the data are available, the investigator does not spend the time and money in collecting the data. Moreover, existing data enable the investigator to trace patterns over time. Databases such as the large national databases offer the advantage of a large sample size and broad geographical area. Disadvantages of using existing data include missing data, omission of needed data, idiosyncratic methods of recording, poor quality of documents, inconsistency in definitions between the investigator's proposed study and the existing data, and adequacy of the methods used to collect the initial data. Familiarity with the data is essential before the investigator can make an informed decision to use the data. To make a sound decision about performing secondary analysis with an existing database, the investigator needs to consider the match between the framework of the initial investigator and that of the investigator proposing secondary analysis, the adequacy of indicators in the database, sampling and possible data analysis procedures, and validity of the data.

REFERENCES

Benoliel, J. (1978). *A care-cure problem: Dying in teaching hospitals.* Final Report to the Division of Nursing, Bureau of Health Manpower, Health Resources Administration, Department of Health, Education and Welfare. Unpublished manuscript.

Boruck, R. (1978). *Secondary analysis.* San Francisco: Jossey-Bass.

Glaser, B. (1963). Retreading research materials: The use of secondary analysis by the independent researcher. *American Behavioral Scientist, 6,* 11-14.

Hyman, H. (1971). *Secondary analysis of sample surveys: principles, procedures, and potentialities.* New York: Wiley.

Interagency Conference on Nursing Statistics (1984). *Nursing related data sources.* Unpublished manuscript.

Kalisch, B., Kalisch, P., & Belcher, B. (1985). Forecasting for nursing policy: A news-based image approach. *Nursing Research, 34,* 44-49.

Lobo, M. (1986). Secondary analysis as a strategy for nursing research. In P. Chinn (Ed.), *Research methodology: Issues and implementation* (pp. 195-220). Rockville, MD: Aspen.

McArt, E., & McDougal, L. (1985). Secondary data analysis: A new approach to nursing research. *Image, 18*(2), 54-47.

Miller, J. (1982). Secondary analysis and science education research. *Journal of Research in Science Teaching, 19,* 719-725.

Mumma, C., & Benoliel, J. (1984-85). Care, cure, and hospital dying trajectories. *Omega, 15*(3), 275-288.

Schultz, P., & Kerr, B. (1986). Comparative case study as a strategy for nursing research. *Methodological Issues in Nursing.*

United States Department of Health and Human Services. (1984). *Inventory of U. S. health care data bases, 1976-1983.* Washington, DC: U. S. Department of Health and Human Services, Health Resources and Services Administration.

Woods, N., and Hulka, B. (1979). Symptom reports and illness behavior among employed women and homemakers. *Journal of Community Health, 1979*(5), 36-45.

21

USING HISTORICAL SOURCES

OLGA MARANJIAN CHURCH

Nursing by definition is a humanist discipline; nurses deal with all levels of the human condition. Yet we often lose sight of this unifying truth. In our desire to be as "scientific" as possible, we forget to connect in human terms the *here* and *now* with the *there* and *then*. Historical inquiry provides the methodology for researchers to examine this essential connectedness that one generation has with the next.

This chapter introduces some of the basic concepts and approaches in historical methodology as a means for interpreting the past, as well as ongoing developments in nursing. The basic premise that a historical awareness is a prerequisite to a professional mentality is founded on the belief that through a collective sense of history, a profession creates and recreates ideas and possibilities that ultimately contribute to the development of its discipline.

History as a kind of research or special form of inquiry uses a particular methodology to answer questions about the past. This methodological approach is referred to as "historiography."

According to Kerlinger (1986):

Historical research is the critical investigation of events, developments, and experiences of the past, the careful weighing of evidence of the validity of sources of information on the past, and the interpretation of the weighed evidence. The historical investigator, like other investigators, then, collects data, evaluates the data for validity, and interprets the data. Actually, the historical method, or *historiography,* differs from other scholarly activity only in its subject matter, the past, and the peculiarly difficult interpretive task imposed by the elusive nature of the subject matter. (p. 620)

The potential of historiography in nursing research remains limitless. Our history holds so much as yet undiscovered data, and we in nursing are at such a primitive stage of our excavations, that *we don't even know what we don't know.* Collingwood (1956) states that ". . . all science begins from the knowledge of our own ignorance: not our ignorance of everything but our ignorance of some definite thing" (p. 9). He also maintains that history as a special form of thought or inquiry generally belongs to what we call the sciences: "Science is finding things out and in that sense history is science. More specifically, history is the science that attempts to answer questions about human actions done in the past via interpretations of evidence left behind" (p. 9). Quite clearly for those of us involved in the pursuit of truth through historiography, the elusive nature of the quest holds a certain fascination that is difficult to describe.

Yet if history, as a science, is defined as a search for "truth," one must at all times be aware of the many facets of "the truth" and the multiplicity of witnesses to and interpretations of "the truth." As such, the historian must be satisfied with the tentative nature of the research findings and accept the age-old dictum that "the past is real but the truth is relevant."

However, by means of a critical examination of the available evidence, the reconstructed past becomes knowable through the skill and efforts of the historiographer. The historiographer may choose from many diverse options in studying nursing's past. But whether the focus is on social history, intellectual history, political, organizational, or institutional history, biography, or oral history, the research process remains essentially the same: (1) defining the problem; (2) stating the objectives; (3) collecting the data; (4) evaluating the data; and (5) reporting the findings. Thus the fundamentals of historical research do not differ from those of all research as described in the initial chapters of this text.

In addition, historiography contains elements of art (i.e., contemplation, imagination, and creative interpretation), science (i.e, the discovery of facts), and philosophy (i.e., approaching the subject under consideration by way of an individual frame of reference).

The knowable truth then—the available data that can be collected and processed as objectively, accurately, and systematically as is humanly possible—requires some measure of interpretation. Further, the evaluation and synthesis of evidence should result in defensible conclusions. The process includes asking what happened (the search for facts), as well as why—thus the interpretive task. In addition, historians attempt to satisfy what is commonly referred to as the "so what" factor: the issues of implication and relevance. The concept of relevance directly relates to the social utility of history.

History, according to Charles Beard (Morison, 1985, p. 94) is a combination of fate, contingency, and character, all unstable forces. So why should we try to rely on it? Or for that matter, why use it? Can it be utilized? In response to such questions it is well to remember the functions that history serves

to preserve and perpetuate the social tradition; to harmonize, as well as ignorance and prejudice permit, the actual and the remembered series of events; to enlarge and enrich the . . . present common to us all, to the end that society . . . may judge of what it is doing in the light of what it has done and what it hopes to do. (Winks, 1968, p. 17)

Of the many models used by historians/historiographers in their approach to data, most can be classified into one of two fundamental approaches: the empirical and the structural. The empiricist chooses to have the facts speak for themselves, and the structuralist prefers to use data to explain and interpret the larger issues under examination.

Thus history can be viewed as an interpretive science; that is, it has understanding rather than control as its fundamental concern. Whereas the goal of the empirical approach of inquiry is to control the phenomenon under study, the goal of the structural approach is always open to interpretation, that is, subject to arguments and reinterpretation. As such, we rewrite our history even as we live it.

INITIATING THE INVESTIGATION

In historiography, as in any research effort, the most decisive step is to define the problem: What is the subject of the investigation? One may begin with a contemporary issue and trace it backward (searching for the roots), or one many identify a particular event (or individual) from the past and demonstrate, through data newly discovered or recovered, the impact and evolution of the event (or individual's work) on the present. In either case the intent is to connect the here and now with there and then—or the reverse, the there and then with here and now. The importance of the connection cannot be overstated. One is striving to show the relevance of historical circumstances, which in turn serves to satisfy the "so what" factor. Without this step one's effort may be reduced to "trivial pursuit."

The subject under study may be an individual, as in biographical studies, or an issue, such as collective bargaining within nursing. Whatever the subject the historical perspective brings with it certain expectations that must be met if the subject is to be presented in an in-depth and balanced fashion.

STATING THE OBJECTIVE OF THE RESEARCH

Having identified the issue, event, or individual to be studied, one must state the objectives of the research as specifically as possible. The researcher may make a simple statement, develop a working hypothesis, or pose specific questions that will guide the investigation. In any event the objectives of the research are directly related to the questions that will be asked. Some general questions that guide the research at this stage are:

1. Is the historical approach the most appropriate for this investigation?
2. Is the question researchable? Are data available? What/where are the resources?

3. Is this investigation feasible? The length of time, energy, and financial resources are considerations to deal with here.

Once the decision has been made to go forward, the researcher must develop and focus specific questions to guide the investigation. The more specific one is in the beginning, the more manageable the investigation is likely to be. One way to focus on the topic is to use "time frames" that define the period of time under investigation. For example, the study of psychiatric nursing from 1882 though 1946 clearly limits the time scope of the study.

However, when defining time frames, the researcher must state explicitly a rationale for the choice of both the beginning and end points. In the case of the example provided here, the rationale for choosing 1882 is that it was the year of the official opening of the first formal training program for psychiatric nursing. The rationale for choosing 1946, the year of the passage of the National Mental Health Act, is that it is recognized as an important milestone in the history of psychiatric care, which in turn is viewed as significant to the chosen subject. The arbitrary choice of dates is not only meaningless; it may be counterproductive in the ongoing efforts toward depth, scope, and specificity.

Obviously one must have some background information before developing specific questions. This can be acquired only through the extensive initial general literature review required of all serious researchers in any given area of study. Without an adequate general knowledge base, specifying a time frame or developing comprehensive questions would be very difficult if not impossible.

In general, then, knowing what to study and in what time frame comes from familiarity established through an extensive review of the literature about the topic of concern, as well as through experiences that might provide ideas for questions and time-frame possibilities. Milestones in nursing specifically and important events in history in general, such as wartime, political turning points, and periods of social reform, all hold implications for the study. For nursing does not exist in a vacuum today, nor did it in the past. The truism that nursing is a response to social needs holds here, and as such the *context* out of which nursing issues emerge is as important as the issues themselves.

The questions that give direction and focus to the research can be viewed as part of the working hypothesis and are obviously developed through the researcher's own interests and concerns. As stated earlier, the historiographer's philosophy determines to some extent the approach to be used. Therefore it is vital for individual researchers to be aware of their personal frames of reference. The concern here is the possibility of the unconscious introduction of personal bias. As Winks (1968) has aptly stated, "Self knowledge therefore takes pre-eminence among the historian's tools" (p. 17). The problem of personal bias is a reality in any form of human endeavor, but awareness of its impact is a first step toward minimizing and neutralizing its effects.

The steps of the research process discussed thus far, identifying the subject and developing the questions, are vulnerable to personal bias as are the steps that follow. The next stage of the research involves the collection of data.

COLLECTING DATA

A certain amount of selectivity in collecting data is supported by the individual researcher's personal view of the subject. In addition, why one set of data was sought and another not pursued has as much to do with availability and convenience as with the persistence required to continue the search. Knowing oneself in terms of strengths and weaknesses benefits the researcher's efforts toward objectivity.

Collecting the data also implies sorting the materials (documents, letters, artifacts) that provide the historical evidence for the research into two main categories: primary source data and secondary source data. Data considered to be primary sources are those events that the author/observer directly witnessed. Secondary sources are those data that the author/observer did not directly witness but instead reported from the observations of others. The priority for the historiographer is collecting primary sources whenever possible, since first-hand evidence is considered more credible.

PERFORMING CRITICAL ANALYSIS

Once the data have been evaluated and sorted into primary and secondary sources, they must then be subjected to a form of critical analysis that tests the historical evidence. Similar to tests for determining reliability and validity, the rigorous tests involved in this critical analysis are intended to discover truth and meaning.

The first test, often referred to as a lower form of criticism, is the test of *external criticism*. The question asked of the data is: Is the document/artifact/information authentic? For example, is the letter reported to have been written by Florence Nightingale really the genuine article? Once the authenticity is determined, then the researcher may proceed to the second or higher form of criticism, referred to as *internal criticism*, which deals with establishing the true meaning of the content. Historical source materials must pass both tests if they are to be used with confidence.

In addition, when evaluating data, historians distinguish facts from possibility or probability. According to Christy (1972), "Proper methodology requires two corroborating primary sources: that is, two primary sources must agree with each other that this is what actually did happen. If they agree, then you can say that indeed this is a fact."

Probability is established if only one primary corroborating source exists. Establishing that the individual was there does not necessarily mean that a reported occurrence is a fact. Only the probability that it did occur exists. The cautious historian, or the historiographer, concludes that probably the event occurred.

"Often when only secondary sources are available but repeated evidence appears from a variety of secondary sources that suggest the data to be accurate, the researcher states that the event was a *possibility*." (Christy, 1972)

With few or no primary sources to add weight to the validity of an occurrence, the wise historiographer carefully states the findings in terms of possibilities and probabilities.

AVOIDING COMMON ERRORS AND CONCERNS

Some common errors to avoid if one is to engage in a scholarly effort in historiography have been alluded to but bear repetition.

First, the subject should not be so broad as to be meaningless. One must abandon the notion that any investigation will reveal everything the researcher wants to know. Instead, the investigation must focus on a manageable aspect of the subject. Second, using too many secondary sources strains the credibility of the work, as well as the worker. It also limits the generalizability and utility of the findings.

Another issue, that of personal bias, can be a problem if the investigator is unaware of the bias. Since all researchers are personally involved in their work, bias is a reality—one that should be acknowledged and dealt with by balancing the evidence and presenting the findings as objectively as possible.

Another pitfall to avoid is offering as history merely the recitation or chronology of names, dates, and places without integration or synthesis. Given the structuralist perspective, the facts do not speak for themselves, for in selecting which facts to present the historian also is offering a particular view of particular facts. Offering "just the facts" is really a misguided notion of objectivity.

SUMMARY

The goal of the historiographer/historian then is to find the available facts and to produce as unbiased a report as possible in an integrated and interesting manner. The significance of the account relies on the extent to which it provides a demonstration of the relationship between past and present—their connectedness—that in turn supports its relevance.

Thus it is vital that the historian develop and maintain an attitude of healthy skepticism, which will assist in challenging the evidence at hand. In addition, Barzun (1985) pointed to many problems or fallacies in historiography. Overexpansion—that is, generalizing beyond the facts, the failure to think of the negative instance, and the use of careless language—all contribute to misapprehensions, misstatements, and misguided accounts of fiction as history.

As in any investigation, the basic questions remain who, what, how, where, when, to what extent, and, last, why? Generally, *how* takes precedence over *why*. The historical interpretation must remain tentative. In human history, multiple causation of events is always likely. More important, as scientific interpretations change with each new discovery, so do historical interpretations. For in the final analysis the promise of discovery—to find the knowable truth and to shape new knowledge from old truths—reveals history's ultimate relevance.

Historical research provides an alternative view of the world as it was and as it is, and it shapes the vision of what it could be. It can provide a keen sense of appreciation of who and what went before, as well as a sense of awareness of nursing's continuing journey through time. The scholarly inquiry into nursing's history can provide insight into the evolution of nursing as a profession and into determining the historical imperatives of the nurse's role in the present delivery of health care.

As a viable area of research, nursing's heritage is available, knowable, and usable. At a time when we must be accountable for our actions, we should be no less accountable for our historical knowledge. Such accountability implies an awareness of the parameters of the past, as well as a mature acknowledgment of ownership. That is, by knowing something a person owns it, it becomes his or hers, and he or she cannot "un-know" it. So it is with history. The self-knowledge that comes with such ownership can be powerful. In turn, historical knowledge serves to engage and empower the imagination. As we link up with events and individuals who paved the way for us to follow, we experience precious moments of recognition and reassurance, and for all those willing to examine the past, history offers the hope of an enlightened vision of the future.

REFERENCES

Barzun, J., & Graff, H. F. (1985). *The modern researcher* (pp. 145-161). Chicago: Harcourt Brace Jovanovich.

Christy, T. E. (1972, March). *Problem forum on historical research: Characteristics of historical research and problems of the historian*. Paper presented at the American Nurses' Association Eighth Nursing Research Conference, Albuquerque, NM.

Collingwood, R. G. (1956). *The idea of history* (p. 9). New York: Oxford University Press.

Kerlinger, F. N. (1986). *Foundations of behavioral research*. Chicago: Holt, Rinehart & Winston.

Matjeski, M. (1986). Historical research: the methods. In P. Minhall and C. Oiler (Eds.), *Nursing research: A qualitative approach* (pp. 173-192). Norwalk, CT: Appleton-Century-Crofts.

Morison, E. E. (1985). Knowledge beyond numbers. *American Heritage, 36*(6), 94.

Winks, R. W. (1968). *The historian as detective: Essays on evidence* (p. 17). New York: Harper & Row.

RESOURCES

Selected Listing of Sources and Resources for Historical Investigators in Nursing

Important and Well-Documented Information

Dzuback, M. A. (1981). Nursing historiography: 1960-1980: An annotated bibliography. In E. C. Lageman (Ed.), *Nursing history: New perspectives, new possibilities* (pp. 181-120). New York: Teachers College Press.

James, J. W. (1984). Writing and rewriting nursing history: A review essay. *Bulletin of the History of Medicine, 58*(4), 568-584.

Palmer, I. S. (1986). Nursing's heritage. *Annual Review of Nursing Research, 4*, 237-257.

Other Recent Sources

Chinn, P. L. (Ed.) (1985, January). Nursing history. *Advances in Nursing Sciences, 7*, (2).

Downs, F. S. (Ed.) (1987, January). Nursing history issue, *Nursing Research.*

Recent Guides/Bibliographies

Bullough, B., et al. (1981). *Nursing: A historical bibliography*. New York: Garland.

A survey of manuscript sources for the history of nursing and nursing education in the Rockerfeller Archives Center. (1981). Pocantico Hills, NY: Rockerfeller Archives Center.

Archives/Libraries

American Journal of Nursing, Sophia F. Palmer Memorial Library, New York, NY.

M. Elizabeth Carnegie Nursing Archives at the Hampton University School of Nursing, Hampton, VA.

Mary Adelaide Nutting Historical Nursing Collection at Teachers College, Columbia University, New York, NY (Collection also available on microfiche).

Nursing Archives, Mugar Memorial Library, Boston University, Boston, MA.

Regional Research/Resource Center

Midwest Nursing History Research Center, University of Illinois at Chicago, College of Nursing, Chicago, IL (Attention Olga Moranjian Church, PhD., FAAN).

Nursing History Center, University of Pennsylvania, Philadelphia, PA (Attention Joan M. Lynaugh PhD., FAAN).

Nursing History Center, University of Texas at Austin, Austin, TX (Attention Eleanor Crowder, Ed.D).

Organizations

American Association for the History of Nursing, P.O. Box 90803 Washington, DC 20090-0803

The Society for Nursing History, Box 150, Nursing Education Department, Teachers College, Columbia University, New York, NY 10027

22

PLANNING STATISTICAL ANALYSIS

NANCY EWALD JACKSON

Nurse researchers have good reason to feel at ease about the role of statistics in their work. The historical connection between the practice of nursing and the science of statistics is an intimate one that honors both disciplines. In the middle of the nineteenth century when the science of statistics was so new that no British university professorships existed in the field, Florence Nightingale recognized the potential power of statistical evidence and developed creative new ways of presenting it (Grier & Grier, 1978; Kopf, 1916/1978). Nightingale's contributions to applied statistics were memoralized in a 1916 issue of the *Journal of the American Statistical Association*. The article concludes with a tribute to her perception of the purpose of statistics: "her control over laborious detail . . . her scrupulous care in testing the statistical foundations of her premises . . . [and] her careful regard for the competent counsel which she so often consulted. In all these respects, Miss Nightingale exhibited the prime qualities of one thoroughly versed in the art of preparing and reflectively analysing social data" (Kopf, 1916/1978, pp. 101-102).

The effectiveness with which Nightingale used statistics to bring about social change probably is well known to readers of this volume, but her substantial contributions to the practice of statistics itself are not so familiar. Statistics of the nineteenth century was concerned with the development of techniques for quantitative description that we now take for granted, such as the frequency histogram. Nightingale, who was exceptionally well educated in mathematics, invented a graphic technique for representing frequency data, called the "coxcomb," based on polar coordinates. When information is graphed in polar coordinates, meaning is carried by the radial distance of a point from the central pole of the graph and by degrees of arc around the pole. One of Nightingale's coxcomb charts, reproduced in Fig. 22-1, provides a dramatic summary of changes in hospital mortality rates at Scutari and Julali hospitals from the fall of 1854 through the fall of 1855. The chart shows monthly rates in comparison with one another and with the much lower mortality rate at military hospitals in or near London during the same period.

Nightingale used a variety of tabular and graphic techniques to present comparisons between observed and expected frequencies, and the statistician Karl Pearson credited her with foreseeing the line of reasoning that he later developed into the chi square test (Grier & Grier, 1978). Even more basic to the development of applied statistics was Nightingale's proposal of improved, uniform methods for computing mortality rates (Grier & Grier, 1978). She was a fellow of the Royal Society of Statistics and an honorary member of the American Statistical Association.

Nightingale's career provides an excellent example of how nursing research and nursing practice can benefit from the nurse researcher's mastery of statistics. However, both the nature of the questions nurse researchers seek to answer and the nature of the sta-

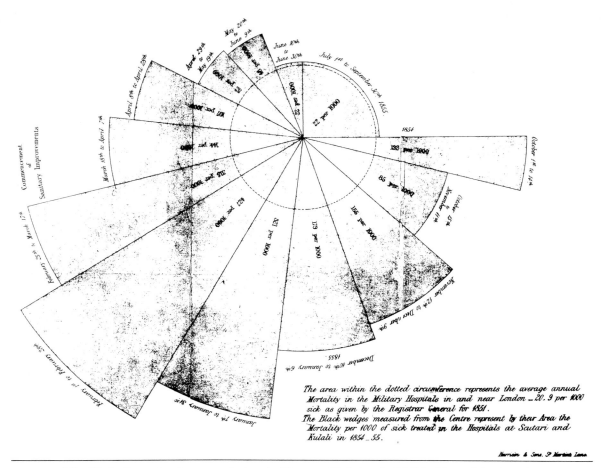

Fig. 22-1. Example of a coxcomb chart by Florence Nightingale (1858). (From Grier & Grier, 1978, *Research in Nursing and Health, 1,* 103-109.)

tistical techniques that can be used to address those questions have become much more complex since Nightingale's day. Today, investigators easily may become so involved in specifics that they lose the perspective and control that distinguished Nightingale's use of statistics.

The purpose of this chapter is to promote the effective use of statistics by introducing readers to some key features of the nature of statistical knowledge and to strategies that characterize skilled statistical problem solvers such as Nightingale. In current educational and psychological jargon this could be called a chapter about "metastatistics." Researchers

in cognitive psychology (e.g., Bransford & Stein, 1984) have found that effectiveness in solving complex new problems is related to the extent to which problem solvers have a general, high-order understanding of what they are doing and why they are doing it, but such an understanding is not likely to come from taking an introductory class in statistics or any other science (Altman, 1981; Schoenfeld, 1983). This chapter is intended for readers who have had at least one course in statistics. Readers without any prior exposure to statistics may find the chapter hard to comprehend, but getting even a partial understanding of the material should provide a helpful context for future learning. In other words, readers can use this chapter both as a guide to reflecting on the statistics they have studied previously and as an outline to organize the statistics they will study in the future.

DOMAINS OF STATISTICAL KNOWLEDGE

Statistics is a scientific discipline with roots in mathematics and with diverse applications in the social, behavioral, and natural sciences. It involves the understanding and use of quantitative information about real-world phenomena. Within statistics itself work varies from basic theory development to refinement of practical applications. Those of us who are consumers of statistical knowledge must remember that this knowledge is complex, theory based, constantly growing, and not absolute.

The domain of applied statistics can be partitioned in many different ways, but one distinction of particular importance to most users is that between descriptive and inferential statistics. We need to be aware of the nature of each of these aspects of statistics and of the ways in which they work together.

Descriptive statistics

In Nightingale's day, statistics was essentially descriptive. *Descriptive statistics* provide precise, standard ways to summarize, understand, and communicate complex information. Nightingale's charts and tables illustrate her mastery of descriptive statistics such as frequency distributions, rates, and proportions. She used these statistics to clarify what was happening in the military hospitals and to make arguments so precise that they could not be dismissed (Grier & Grier, 1978). The techniques of descriptive statistics are just as important today, but beginning researchers sometimes overlook their importance, perhaps because the most common ones are so simple to understand that they receive relatively little attention in introductory courses. However, descriptive statistics must not be neglected. These are the "facts" on which an analysis is based; they are a summary of the key characteristics of the sample being studied.

The *sample,* or *subgroup, mean* may be the most familiar of descriptive statistics. In the first weeks of an introductory course, we learn that the *mean* is one of several statistics that can be used to define the

average of a set of scores, the other being the *median* and the *mode*. We are taught that the mean is simple to compute as the sum of all the scores divided by the number of scores and that it has several desirable properties that contribute to its widespread use. We also are taught that the mean is not a good indicator of the average of a set of scores when the distribution of scores is severely asymmetrical, or skewed. A common example used to illustrate this point is the distribution of incomes in a group such as the population of the United States. There are many poor people in the United States but very few who are extraordinarily wealthy. In statistical terms the distribution of income has a strong positive skew. In everyday language a positively skewed distribution is one with a hump of greatest frequencies toward the low end of the scale and relatively few cases strung out in a wag tail toward the upper end (Chapter 25). Because the mean is pulled toward the tail of a skewed distribution, describing the income of people in the United States by giving the population mean would create an inappropriately rosy picture of the resources available to most people. The median, or middle value, is a better average to use for describing income because it is not unduly influenced by the wealthy few.

Most of the principles of descriptive statistics are as simple as the one just described, but researchers often neglect them. For example, the mean is used so commonly in nursing and related literatures that one may easily forget to ask oneself whether it is the most appropriate descriptor for a particular set of data. Nursing research often is concerned with skewed distributions in which most of the scores are within a range that indicates acceptable functioning, but in which a few cases exist that are doing very poorly. Nonetheless, many researchers do not remember to consider the median as an alternative average score to report for their data. Without careful attention to such basics, the researchers cannot fulfill the purposes of descriptive statistics or build a sound foundation for moving beyond description of the current sample of inferences about the population it represents.

Inferential statistics

Providing probabilistic guidelines for inferences beyond the present set of data is the purpose of the second kind of statistics (Hays, 1981). Inferential tests such as the *t* test for evaluating the difference between two means and the chi square test of independence are what most researchers think of when they think of statistics. The teaching of these tests and of the theory of probability that underlies their application absorbs much of the time in introductory statistics courses. Inferential statistical methods are harder to understand than descriptive statistics, but students sense their importance because they are the immediate source of those magical *p* values that determine whether or not test results are significant (Jacobsen, 1981).

The importance of inferential statistics should not be denigrated. Inferential statistics enable us to go beyond the immediate description of the results of individual research studies in ways that provide the best possible bases for clinical practice or further research. These twentieth-century advances have provided precise and systematic ways to generalize from the findings of individual studies with limited samples. The two kinds of statistics complement one another, but the descriptive ones are the most basic. When the researcher reports that the mean diastolic blood pressures of groups receiving two different kinds of treatment are significantly different from one another at the $p < .05$ level, the reader also needs to know the mean level and variability (standard deviation) for each set of pressures. These descriptive statistics are components of the *t* test formula used in deriving the inferential test of significance, but they also have value in their own right. Without the descriptive statistics, a reader has no way of knowing such important facts as whether the mean blood pressure of one or both groups was within healthy limits or the extent to which the pressures of patients within each group differed from one another.

SOME COMPLEXITIES OF APPLIED STATISTICS

The practice of statistics is a craft as well as a science. As in any other craft, those who know the rules well break them occasionally. Within statistics there is a large body of research on the effects of violating the assumptions of tests such as the analysis of variance or the chi square test of independence (e.g., Glass, Peckham, & Sanders, 1972). These studies often show that under some conditions certain violations are highly unlikely to have any effect on the interpre-

tation of a statistical result. Breaking statistical rules through ignorance can be disastrous, but there is nothing improper about informed violations that serve a useful purpose. Beginning users of statistics tend to think that because statistics involves numbers it is absolute, and they tend to be distressed at the prospect of doing anything inconsistent with the rules presented in an introductory text. However, the expert statistician is much like the expert nurse (Benner, 1984) in having a knowledge that is deep and rich enough to provide a basis for appropriately flexible decision making.

Several different correct ways may exist to define a question in applied statistics; each of these questions will have a different answer. Awareness of the possibility of alternative conceptualizations of statistical problems is especially important for nurse researchers. The nursing discipline draws on basic knowledge from many different sciences, and nurse researchers need to communicate their findings to diverse audiences. My early years in nursing research were enriched by discovery of the different ways in which statisticians oriented toward epidemiology, laboratory sciences, and sociology approach problems. For example, both psychologists and sociologists are likely to use statistics in the context of a rich set of prior theoretical predictions about the nature of their data. Statistical tests often are corollary to nonstatistical reasoning. Biostatisticians working on epidemiological problems typically operate in a very different way. Relatively little theory exists in epidemiology that is not in itself statistical, so statistics is central to answering epidemiological questions. This means that biostatisticians are much less likely than psychological or sociological statisticians to want to use nonstatistical considerations to structure or reduce the data or to allow any operation that might bias the interpretation of tests of statistical significance.

Statisticians and researchers trained in different substantive disciplines also may vary in the extent to which they emphasize the importance of random sampling as the basis for the use of inferential statistics, in the degree to which they are concerned about the level of measurement represented by the numbers being analyzed (Chapter 14), and in the balance they seek between the error of falsely claiming a significant effect and the error of failing to detect an effect that actually exists (Chapter 26). To use statistics as wisely as Nightingale is said to have done, today's nurse researchers need to have their own research objectives clearly in mind and to learn enough about statistical alternatives to make informed choices among them.

HOW TO ACT LIKE AN EXPERT STATISTICAL PROBLEM SOLVER

The small amount of research that has been done on the characteristics of skilled statistical problem solvers (Allwood, 1984) and the kinds of instruction that help students become effective applied statisticians (Taney, 1985) suggest that expertise in statistics is much like expertise in other, more thoroughly studied, domains. Studies comparing methods by which experts and novices solve problems in physics, mathematics, medical diagnoses, and other fields have shown that experts have several key advantages (Chi & Glaser, 1985; Larkin. McDermott, Simon, & Simon, 1980). Consideration of these advantages suggests several strategies that novice statistical problem solvers can use to improve their own effectiveness.

Perhaps the most essential characteristics of expert problem solvers are that they have a richly interconnected, logically organized understanding of the knowledge in their area and that they are able to use this knowledge to maintain purposeful control of the problem-solving process. Experts "know where they are going" when they begin to solve problems, and every step is a meaningful part of the whole process (Larkin et al., 1980). A beginning researcher may not have an expert statistician's understanding, but anyone can share in part of the expert's advantage simply by remembering that statistics is supposed to make sense and that statistical information should help the researcher understand and communicate the results of a study. Can one imagine Nightingale badgering Parliament with numbers that had no meaning for her? She knew what each of her statistics meant and why it was important. Even though the novice researcher may not be able to reach Nightingale's level of mastery, active and dogged pursuit of understanding inevitably will result in better statistical problem solving and a better research project.

An expert can handle many routine aspects of a problem almost automatically. Because executing familiar component processes need not command much of the researcher's attention, the expert can more easily direct attention to other activities such as monitoring whether the results of calculations are reasonable. The surest route to working automatically—that is, without the need for conscious attention—is practice, but the novice can also use a variety of strategies to avoid wasting limited time and attention. The first strategy is the most useful, although it may be the hardest to put into practice. Relax! Attention devoted to worrying about the possibility of failure or whether one might appear ignorant to others is better spent on the problem itself. Another enormous help is for the researcher to take notes and make outlines or charts of everything needing consideration while solving a statistical problem. As each part of the problem is tackled, the researcher can keep a complete record of what has been done. When something is written down, it can be cleared out of the researcher's head until it is needed. Although this advice may seem superfluous for experienced scholars, many of the nursing students who seek statistical consultation need to be prodded to take notes. Without such a written record, they would be unlikely to remember enough of a lengthy discusssion to complete their analyses.

Another characteristic of the expert compared to the novice is that the expert is much better able to represent a problem mentally in a way that facilitates its solution—to recognize the key elements of a situation and to use an organized representation of these elements to guide problem solving. Problems in statistics can be represented in several different ways. Sometimes a verbal statement of the problem will be sufficient, but graphic or algebraic representations are likely to be more precise and helpful. Algebraic representation of statistical problems may not be a comfortable strategy for the beginner, but anyone can diagram a research design or graph a set of results. A student researcher often begins the process of data analysis by drawing figures summarizing the data for individual cases or groups. These figures help both student and teacher to understand the nature of the student's statistical problems.

Another key feature of expert knowledge is that the expert can spot trouble quickly and reliably. In statistics trouble can occur early in the conceptualization and design of a study. A novice often proposes research questions and designs that will lead to serious statistical difficulties. The most sensible thing a novice researcher can do is seek expert statistical help before, rather than after, a study design is fixed. The benefits of "preventive statistics" are comparable to those of preventive health care (Jackson, 1982; 1983).

Although novice statisticians may fail to detect some actual and potential problems in a statistical analysis, beginners should trust any feelings they do have that something doesn't fit or isn't working correctly. When nursing graduate students have such feelings, they are almost certain to have discovered a real problem. When one notices that the research question doesn't seem to match any of the statistical procedures learned in an introductory course or the computed significance level does not seem consistent with what is known about the data, one can be proud of oneself because detecting such problems is the first step toward the development of expertise (Allwood, 1984).

PLANNING DATA ANALYSIS

Introductory textbooks sometimes present the development of a research project as a linear process, beginning with a literature review and conceptualization of the research questions or hypotheses and ending with analysis and interpretation of the data. This is a dangerous oversimplification. A good research design develops through back-and-forth or circular interplay among issues related to the scope and nature of the research questions; the choice of an overall approach and design structure; the specification of measures, hypotheses, and analytical techniques; and consideration of specific sample characteristics. In any quantitative research project, the plan for statistical analysis is an essential link between conceptualization and fulfillment of a study's purpose. When studies fail, they often do so because no way exists to analyze the available data to address the researcher's questions or hypotheses.

The sequence of activities involved in development of an analysis plan is depicted in Fig. 22-2. Note the events at any stage of the process can lead to reconsideration of earlier stages. For example, one may want to do a study comparing job satisfaction between male and female pediatric nurse practitioners (PNPs). The investigator identifies a measure that is expected to yield a broad distribution of job satisfaction scores and then states the hypothesis that male and female PNPs will differ significantly in their mean scores on this measure. A t test for independent means might be proposed as the statistical test of the null hypothesis that gender differences in job satisfaction do not exist. The researcher hopes to be able to reject this null hypothesis by obtaining a statistically significant difference in mean satisfaction scores for the male and female samples.

After specifying the analysis, the researcher's next step is to consider whether the available sample of PNPs will include enough men to provide a good chance of rejecting the null hypothesis, if it is indeed false. What if only five or six men are likely to be in the sample? No matter how many female PNPs are available, such a small group of males is not likely to yield t test results that will permit rejection of the null hypothesis. Techniques are available for estimating how good—or bad—are the odds of rejecting a false null hypothesis. The process is called *statistical power analysis*. However, to use these techniques the investigator must know something about the characteristics of the measure to be used and be able to specify the form of the analysis (Cohen, 1977). If the power estimation techniques reveal that the study is unworkable as planned originally, the investigator can reconsider decisions made at earlier stages of the planning process.

Perhaps the study of gender differences in PNP job satisfaction could be salvaged with a revised sampling plan in which the small population of men would be sampled more intensively than the large population of women, but a more radical revision of the design might be a better choice. If only a few male PNPs are available, more interesting and useful data might be generated by intensive examination of each man's feelings about his job. Such a study might rely on open-ended questions that would yield responses that could be content analyzed using qualitative techniques such as those discussed in Chapter 28. In terms of Fig. 22-2 consideration of the gender distribution of the available sample might lead the investigator to reconsider how to measure job satisfaction and even how to define the overall purpose and design of the study. Perhaps, exploring aspects of attitudes of male PNPs toward their jobs would be more productive than contrasting male and female attitudes on a single measure. This example illustrates just one of many ways in which the process of working out an analysis plan can change the whole thrust of a study, enabling the investigator to make

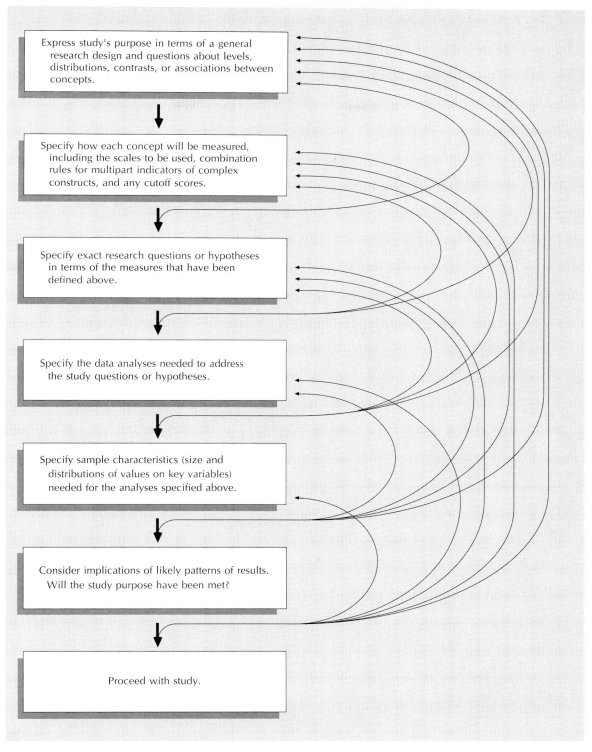

Fig. 22-2. Steps in developing a data analysis plan. At any step the researcher may have to return to a previous step.

sound design choices while change is still possible. In a simple yet extreme case such as the one just described, limitations imposed by the characteristics of the sample might become obvious during initial discussions of the study's feasibility. However, working through an analysis plan is likely to reveal problems that did not become apparent during preliminary explorations.

COMPONENTS OF AN ANALYSIS

The analysis phase of research is itself a complex process that includes a number of points at which important choices are made. The test of significance (*t* test) proposed for the hypothetical study of gender differences in job satisfaction would actually be only one part of the data analysis. Much of the work in data analysis consists of preparing the raw data and inspecting their characteristics to make sure that the planned descriptive and inferential statistics will indeed be appropriate for this data set. After planned tests of significance have been done, further post hoc analyses may be needed to explore aspects of the data that would qualify interpretation of the planned analyses or suggest new ideas for subsequent research.

Data analysis includes the instrument development and evaluation activities described in Chapter 14. The full sequence of activities, from initial checking of the data set for errors to planned and post hoc analyses, is described in subsequent chapters. While reading about these specific activities, the nurse researcher should keep trying to picture how they all fit together.

The data analysis process can be illustrated in terms of other complex, creative activities, such as Chinese wok cooking. Much of the hard work in cooking a Chinese dish is in the initial preparation of the ingredients. Vegetables have to be cleaned and their bad spots cut out. Each ingredient is chopped or sliced into the form that will be needed for the final dish. Some combinations of ingredients may be blended into a sauce in which their diverse flavors are reduced to a smooth combination. Typically, one works first with individual ingredients, then with combinations of small subsets of ingredients. Just before serving, everything is stirred together in the wok. At this point, tasting the dish may suggest the need for some changes in seasoning that were not part of the original recipe.

In data analysis, as in cooking, the researcher starts by cleaning up each kind of score or measure—transforming, blending, and reducing as needed. When each measure of indicator has been considered fully in itself *(univariate analysis)*, pairs of variables may be considered in conjunction with one another (bivariate analysis). If the research questions are complex and involve multiple measures, a grand stirring-together in multivariate analysis may be required. Finally, inspection of the results as planned may reveal the need for some unanticipated, post hoc analyses. Whether cooking chicken with walnuts or analyzing a complex data set, the researcher knows that the quality of the final product depends on the thoroughness with which each step of the preparation has been executed.

Living up to the example of Florence Nightingale as statistician is no easier than living up to her example as bedside nurse, administrator, or political activist. Nonetheless, even beginning nurse researchers can be more effective statistical problem solvers if they adopt Nightingale's commitment to understanding the purpose of statistics, to maintaining vigilant control over every detail of a statistical analysis, and to using consultation wisely. The investigator must be aware that data analysis is integral to the design of a study and that analysis consists of a series of informed choices, not just of applying a test of significance to a set of scores.

SUMMARY

Planning data analysis requires that the investigator consider the domains of descriptive and inferential statistics. Descriptive statistics summarize information about a sample, whereas inferential statistics allow the investigator to make conclusions that extend beyond the sample studied to the population of interest.

When planning data analysis, the researcher must recognize that many correct ways exist to analyze data. The investigator begins by considering the study's purposes as they relate to research design and the questions the study attempts to answer regarding levels, distributions, contrasts, or associations between concepts. Specification of how each concept was measured and the precise research questions or hypotheses precede specification of the necessary data analysis. Sample characteristics such as size and distribution of the values of the key variables need to be specified before selecting the analytical strategy. Finally, implications of the most likely patterns of results need to be considered before the analysis of the data can begin.

References

Allwood, C. M. (1984). Error detection processes in statistical problem solving. *Cognitive Science, 8*, 413-437.

Altman, D. G. (1981). Statistics and ethics in medical research. VIII. Improving the quality of statistics in medical journals. *British Medical Journal, 282*, 44-47.

Benner, P. (1984). *From novice to expert: Power and excellence in nursing practice.* Palo Alto: Addison-Wesley.

Bransford, J. D., & Stein, B. L. (1984). *The ideal problem solver.* New York: Prentice-Hall.

Chi, M. T. H., & Glaser, R. (1985). Problem-solving ability. In R. J. Sternberg (Ed.). *Human abilities: An information processing approach.* (pp. 227-250). New York: W. H. Freeman.

Cohen, J. (1977). *Statistical power analysis for the behavioral sciences* (rev. ed.). New York: Academic Press.

Glass, G. P., Peckham, P. D., & Sanders, J. R. (1972). Consequences of failure to meet assumptions underlying the fixed-effects analyses of variance and covariance. *Review of Educational Research, 42*, 237-288.

Grier, B., & Grier, M. (1978). Contributions of the passionate statistician. *Research in Nursing and Health, 1*, 103-109.

Hays, W. L. (1981). *Statistics* (3rd ed.). New York: CBS College Publishing.

Jackson, N. E. (1982). Choosing and using a statistical consultant. *Nursing Research, 31*, 248-250.

Jackson, N. E. (1983). The statistically simple study: A guide for thesis advisers. *Journal of Nursing Education, 22*, 351-354.

Jacobsen, B. (1981). Know thy data. *Nursing Research, 30*, 254-255.

Kopf, E. W. (1978). Florence Nightingale as statistician. *Research in Nursing and Health, 1*, 93-102. (Reprinted from the *Journal of the American Statistical Association, 1916, 15.* 388-404)

Larkin, J. H., McDermott, J., Simon, D. P., & Simon, H. A. (1980). Models of competence in solving physics problems. *Cognitive Science, 4*, 317-345.

Schoenfeld, A. H. (1983, April). *Theoretical and pragmatic issues in the design of mathematics "problem solving" instruction.* Paper presented at the annual convention of the American Educational Research Association, Montreal, Canada.

Taney, S. (1985). Statistics: A course students love to hate. *American Psychological Association Monitor, 16* (7), 27.

23

USING COMPUTERS TO ANALYZE NURSING RESEARCH DATA

NANCY FUGATE WOODS

The use of computers in nursing research has increased dramatically over the last 20 years as nursing research has become more sophisticated. Most recently published nursing research studies include multiple variables or several measurements of a small number of variables, as well as complex analyses of data. The primary contribution of computers to nursing research is their ability to process large amounts of data with a great deal of accuracy and speed. If the data for many of these complex studies were analyzed with a hand calculator, the essential analyses would be considerably slower if not impossible because of the complexity of the calculations. In this chapter we will consider the contributions and limits of computers in nursing research, the components of a computer system, modes of communicating with computers, and the programs commonly used in nursing studies. We will conclude with a discussion of the applications of computers in nursing research.

CAPABILITIES AND LIMITATIONS OF COMPUTERS IN NURSING

Computers can perform many functions that support research, as well as other endeavors. The earliest computers performed simple counting operations and became popular because of the speed with which they could operate. The speed with which computers can perform mathematical and logical operations remains one of their greatest contributions to

research today. Because of their speed, computers can produce answers that would be useless if the time for hand calculations were required. For example, a rocket would crash before its trajectory could be corrected on the basis of calculations performed with a hand calculator. Computers also can perform simulations that help project consequences of human actions, such as the effect on hospital costs of increasing nursing salaries or the effects on delivery of services produced by changing current educational patterns of health-care personnel. Furthermore, computers can store large amounts of information, as well as retrieve, organize, manage, and present large data banks. The *Index Medicus* information is stored, retrieved, organized, and managed through computers. Computers also can be used to gather data from experiments and to monitor those data. Monitoring of cardiac output in intensive care units is accomplished by means of computer calculations. In some instances vital signs can be monitored by computers, and medication dosage can be adjusted on the basis of complex calculations. Computers also can be programed to display intelligence by learning to perform tasks, improving their success rates as their experience increases. Finally, in many health sciences settings clinicians use computers to assist with diagnosis by identifying patterns among data such as symptoms and laboratory findings.

Computers now contribute to nursing research in many ways. Their main contribution lies in their ability to perform complex analyses of data with accuracy, speed, and flexibility. Computers are able to perform accurate calculations. In contrast to humans, who make calculation errors and who get tired, computers are unflagging in accuracy that does not deteriorate with their use. In a few seconds, computers can perform calculations that would require several weeks of work for a human.

Computers also are very flexible. An investigator can use the same computer to analyze research data by using a statistical program, to write a final report by using a word-processing program, and to balance the budget for a project by using an accounting program. In addition to these contributions, computers can provide permanent storage for subsequent analysis and shared use of data. A computer's memory has the capacity to store billions of bits of information. In addition, data can be stored in media that are readily accessible to the computer user.

Computers are not without their limitations. Indeed, computers only do precisely what humans tell them to do, even when the human commands are wrong. When instructed to execute a program that has no command to end, some computers may continue to execute the program forever. Fortunately, procedures are available to stop that kind of error.

Computer use also requires spending an initial time investment to learn to use the system. Investigators cannot escape the necessity of learning the features of each computer system they use and of learning some basic information about using computers in general. When investigators use computers to analyze their data, they also must invest a significant amount of time in coding and entering data. The investigator must provide detailed instructions (often referred to as programs) for the computer to use in analyzing the data. In addition, when investigators rely solely on the computer to analyze the data, they easily lose the "feeling" for the data that they gain when they perform hand statistical calculations. Also, the accessibility of the many analyses provided by computers is both a major contribution and a limitation. Although investigators have a myriad of analyses available to them, they may have a poor understanding of them and apply them inappropriately. They may be tempted to short-circuit rigorous thinking about hypothetical relationships and appropriate tests of hypotheses and to employ a shotgun approach in which they examine every possible relationship simply because they can do so. If faced with the prospect of hand calculations of statistical analyses, investigators would be considerably more selective in the analyses they apply to their data. A final limitation of using computers for data analysis is cost. Usually, the investigator or the investigator's employer pays for "computer time," the amount of time the various components of the computer actually were used for the project. In addition, there is a human cost, as well as monetary, in preparing the data for computer analysis and transfering them to a medium acceptable to a computer.

COMPONENTS OF COMPUTER SYSTEMS

The three types of computers, mainframe computers, microcomputers, and minicomputers, differ in speed, cost, capacity to store information, and the number of users who can simultaneously share their use (Figs. 23-1 through 23-3). Mainframe computers are large, high-speed, expensive computers that typically are leased or purchased by large organizations for many people to use simultaneously. Microcomputers, also known as personal computers, are the small desktop computers typically used by one user or only a few. The minicomputer is an intermediate-size computer, capable of more rapid functioning than a microcomputer and intermediate in expense. Several investigators can share minicomputers.

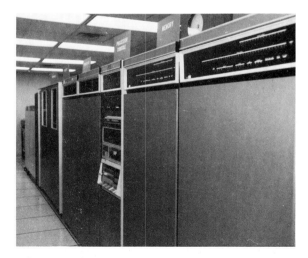

Fig. 23-1. Mainframe computer.

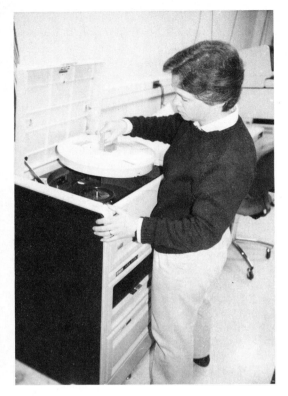

Fig. 23-2. Minicomputer.

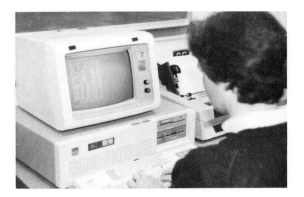

Fig. 23-3. Microcomputer, also called a personal computer.

Each computer system is somewhat different, but several components are common to each system. Each component of a computer system can be classified as hardware or software. *Computer hardware* is the electronic equipment that processes, controls, and stores data. *Computer software* is the group of instructions and procedures required to operate the computer.

Computer hardware

Most computer operations depend on one rather basic mechanism. Computers perform highly complex logical and mathematical maneuvers by means of changes in on-off states, and the basic element of a digital computer works much like the on-off switch of a lamp. One on-off switch is called a "bit." There are eight bits in a byte, and a byte may represent one character of information. A character may be a letter, a number, or a symbol such as + or −. Each character derives from the pattern of on-off configurations of the bits in a byte.

In its most basic form a computer is composed of an input device, central processing unit, and an output device. Input and output devices are sometimes referred to as "peripherals" (Fig. 23-4).

Input devices. The *input device* allows a human to interface with the machine by transforming data into a form the computer can process. The input device enables the investigator to provide commands and information about how the computer should function. Commonly used input devices include the keyboard of a terminal into which commands and data are typed; a card reader, which reads information from punched cards; and optical scanners, which recognize marks such as those used on computer-scored answer sheets for examinations. Other input devices include wands, which recognize characters such as those printed on items in the grocery store; magnetic ink–character readers, which can read numbers from items like checks; and light pens, which allow the investigator to enter data by indicating choices on the screen of a cathode-ray tube (CRT). In the future the options for input devices will include voice input, to allow the investigator to talk into a device that will transform sound waves to electronic signals. Currently, the most commonly used input devices in nursing research are terminal keyboards and card readers.

Investigators who enter their data on a terminal keyboard recognize its similarity to a common type-

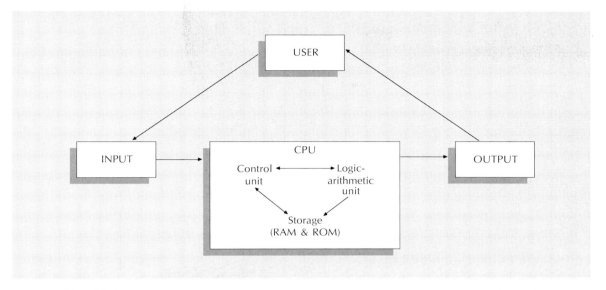

Fig. 23-4. Relationship of computer components. Input devices, central processing unit (CPU), output devices, and their relationship to the user.

writer keyboard. A computer keyboard has several additional keys that allow the investigator to perform special functions. The data or commands that are entered on the keyboard usually also appear on the CRT. (The program also may send messages back to the investigator on the same screen.) Investigators can use keyboards to enter data on *input media* such as magnetic tape, disks, or diskettes (sometimes referred to as floppy disks).

Magnetic tape can store an immense amount of data in relatively little space. The tape itself looks similar to the tape commonly used in a reel-to-reel tape recorder. More than 6000 bits of information can be stored on 1 inch of its magnetized surface. Although it can store a great deal of information, magnetic tape must be treated with care. Extremes of temperature and rough handling can damage it and ruin the data from an entire study.

Another commonly used input medium is a magnetic disk, which resembles a phonograph record in appearance. They are grouped together in a disk pack. Data are stored as magnetized spots on the disk surface. The major advantage of using disks for storage of data is that they allow users to go directly to the data they want to use. With a magnetic tape users must read through all the data on the tape before

getting to the data they are interested in analyzing. The ability to access data directly increases efficiency. Many disk packs can store millions of characters of data. However, disk packs may cost a few hundred dollars, in contrast to $10 to $15 for tape. Diskettes, sometimes called floppy disks, also are coded magnetically and are used commonly in personal computers. Each disk can hold up to half a million characters. Floppy disks cost a few dollars apiece and often can hold as much as 300 pages of typewritten material.

Card readers "read" data from computer cards by transforming the codes (punched holes) on the cards into electrical impulses that the computer can interpret. A computer card consists of 80 columns of potential codes, which may stand for letters or numbers. A keypunch machine is used to punch holes in the card that correspond to the data or commands the investigator wishes to enter. The keypunch machine has a keyboard like a typewriter, and the investigator types the characters on the keyboard that correspond to the data or commands. After punching a batch of cards, the investigator can use a machine called a "verifier" to determine if the codes were punched accurately. The investigator simply types in the same codes again; if an error is encountered, a light on the verifier signals the mistake. The errors can be corrected after they are verified with the original data.

Use of a keyboard for entering data or commands is advantageous in several respects. Entering data through a terminal usually is faster than entering it through a card reader. In addition, the tapes or disks can be erased and new data can be entered, whereas computer cards cannot be reused.

Central processing unit. The *central processing unit* (CPU) controls and coordinates all activities of the computer. It runs programs requested by the user, moves program instructions and data in and out of the central memory, and monitors the machine's activities. It is composed of thousands of electronic components, in particular, silicone chips that contain integrated circuits. The CPU can be thought of as the computer's brain. To function, the computer needs a control unit to coordinate its activities, an arithmetical logic unit that performs arithmetical or logical processing of data, and storage registers for storing short-term memory or the intermediate results of calculations.

The *memory* stores program instructions and data while the program is actually executing. It is connected directly to the control unit and the arithmetic-logic unit of the CPU. The two kinds of memory are (1) permanent, read only memory (ROM) and (2) changeable, random access memory (RAM). ROM is permanent, nonerasable memory built into the computer by the manufacturer to command its internal operations. RAM temporarily stores data and instructions for data processing while a program is being executed. The CPU can perform complex calculations, rearrange data, read input, write input and output, store a great deal of information, and transfer that information to another medium.

Output devices. *Output devices* transmit information from the computer's CPU to the investigator. Many of the input devices we have discussed already can serve as output devices. The user can output information to a CRT screen, a tape, a disk, or a diskette or have it punched into cards. A commonly used output device is a printer. The printer can output lines of information very rapidly. Some line printers can print over 1000 lines of information per minute. Character printers print character by character across the page. Several new types of printers are available that do not require impact with the page,

including laser printers, electrothermal printers, electrostatic printers, xerographic printers, and ink jet printers. Another commonly used computer output device is the graphics plotter, which displays graphs and charts in multiple colors and patterns. Other new devices produce voice output, photographs, and microfiche. The most common users of the line printer, the plotter, and the CRT are people who want to use the information from a research project immediately. Output to punched cards, tape, or disk is used frequently for storage of information or when transfering the data to another investigator.

Software

Software is a special set of instructions *(program)* written for a computer. The person who writes programs is a *programer*. The computer's ability to perform complex arithmetical and logical operations depend on the programer's capability. Communication with computers is carried out in special languages. Machine language is the extremely complex code that the particular type of computer understands. *Programing languages* are reasonably easy to learn and use compared to machine language; they allow the programer to construct a simpler set of commands than would be the case with machine language. Programs can be written in programing language and then translated into machine language by a program called a *compiler*.

Of the many programing languages, the most common are FORTRAN, PL/1, PASCAL, PILOT, and BASIC. FORTRAN and PL/1 are used commonly in the sciences; BASIC is one of the simplest programing languages for beginners to learn.

In addition to programing languages that allow investigators to create their own programs, several program packages (collections) for statistical procedures are available. Software packages commonly used in nursing research for statistical analysis procedures include Statistical Package for Social Sciences (SPSS-X), Statistical Analysis System (SAS), and Biomedical Statistical Software Package (BMDP). These packages contain multiple statistical analysis procedures. Many statistical packages are available for personal computers (see box above, right and Appendix A). In addition, a number of packages are available to assist with qualitative analyses (see Appendix A).

Some software is in the public domain and can be

Selected Statistical
Procedures Available with
SPSS-X, SAS, and BMDP
Statistical Packages

Descriptive statistics
Measures of central tendency
Plots
Histograms
Bar charts
Cross-tabulations

Inferential statistics
Chi square
Pearson's *r*
Nonparametric correlations
t tests
Analysis of variance (ANOVA)
Analysis of covariance (ANCOVA)
Partial correlation
Multiple regression
Discriminant analysis
Factor analysis
Loglinear regression
Time series analysis
Canonical correlation

---

accessed and copied free of charge. Other software packages range in price from a few dollars to several hundred dollars. Ethical and legal issues surrounding the use of software face each investigator who uses programs or packages protected by copyright.

COMMUNICATING WITH A COMPUTER

Several modes are available for communicating with a computer. The most common is the *batch processing mode*. In this mode the investigator submits a program or a group of programs in a single batch, and the programs are executed simultaneously. When using this mode, a delay occurs between submitting the program and getting the results; this lag is referred to as turnaround time. Turnaround time may range from a few minutes to hours, depending on how busy the system is and what the investigator's priority is when using the system. Batch pro-

cessing can be used with almost any input device.

Interactive mode refers to the ability of the investigator to interact with the computer program at various intervals. When operating in interactive mode, the computer receives commands from the investigator and executes them immediately, providing feedback to the investigator on a CRT screen or a printer. *Time-sharing* is a processing mode that is possible on larger computers and is similar to the interactive mode. Time-sharing permits parts of several different programs to be executed at the same time by different users.

APPLICATIONS OF COMPUTERS IN NURSING RESEARCH

To appreciate the applications of computers in nursing research, consider the following study being conducted by two investigators, only one of whom uses a computer. Both investigators are conducting a telephone survey of elderly residents and their families in a county that is served by community health nurses. The investigator's goal is to determine the kinds of services needed by families who have an elderly resident living in the home. The first investigator creates a complete enumeration list of the families in the county and randomly samples households from the enumeration list, choosing every third family. He or she then telephones each of the randomly selected households to interview the elderly person and a family member about their needs, recording the information on an interview guide during each interview. After the interviews are completed, the investigator transfers the data to a coding sheet and tabulates the frequencies of responses to the questions. Using a hand calculator, the investigator then computes the percentage of the elderly population needing various types of assistance, measures of central tendency for the variables, and some correlations between age and types of needs. He or she types a report and mails copies to the supervisor and colleagues. The second investigator uses computer-generated random digits to access a sample through random-digit dialing. The data from the telephone interviews are placed directly into a computer file during the interview, using a copy of the interview displayed on the screen of a CRT. With a data management program, the investigator edits the database and, using selected statistical programs from a program package, analyzes the data with multivariate statistics, as well as univariate and bivariate statistics. The investigator uses a word-processing package to write a report on the computer and includes summary tables generated by the statistical analysis program. The report is transmitted to the supervisor and to colleagues in other parts of the country via a computer network.

As seen in the comparison of these investigators' approaches, the applications of computers in nursing research are nearly endless. Investigators frequently use computers to generate literature citations when they begin a literature review by conducting a Medline or other computerized search. Researchers use computers to manage databases by means of programs that edit and rearrange data. Computers also offer the investigator the opportunity to conduct many complex statistical analyses, as well as to store their data and results. Computers can be "networked" (connected by communications linkups) with other computers, thus extending access to databases, varied programs, and computer capabilities. Finally, when they are part of a network, computers can offer investigators a vehicle for exchanging messages, often referred to as "electronic mail."

Application of computers in data analysis requires some special characteristics on the part of the investigator. First, the realization that using a computer is partly an art and partly a science creates a mindset that facilitates comfort with the process. Although some aspects of using a computer are strictly mechanical, other aspects can be regarded as creative art forms. Using a computer requires adjustment similar to traveling in another country. Understanding a new language and customs is similar to understanding the new jargon and rules that are necessary for interacting with a computer. Both can be stressful experiences for the person who is learning. Often the rules seem arbitrary and even unreasonable. Patience and willingness to experiment with new procedures and programs can make using a computer fun and challenging.

SUMMARY

The use of computers in nursing research has increased dramatically, paralleling the increased sophistication of statistical analyses in nursing studies. Computers are capable of performing rapid calculations that enable investigators to perform in a few seconds analyses that would require weeks of human work. Computers are flexible and are able to perform functions such as storing large amounts of data, word processing, and financial accounting. Nevertheless, computers only are capable of doing precisely what humans tell them to do. Computers differ in size, speed, cost, and capacity to store information. Listed in decreasing order of size, three types of computers are mainframe, minicomputers, and microcomputers. A computer consists of input devices, a central processing unit, and output devices. Computer systems include hardware and software. Hardware is the electronic equipment that processes, controls, and stores data. Software is the instructions and procedures required to operate a computer. There are several modes for communicating with a computer: the batch processing mode, the interactive mode, and the time-sharing mode. Computers have multiple applications in nursing research. Patience and willingness to understand new languages and rules for computers can make using computers fun and challenging.

REFERENCES

Dixon, W. (1975). *Biomedical computer programs*. Berkeley, CA: University of California Press.

Nie, N., Hall, C., Jenkins, J., Steinbrenner, K., & Bert, D. (1979). *Statistical package for the social sciences*. New York: McGraw-Hill.

Nie, N., Hall, C., Jenkins, J., Steinbrenner, K., & Bert, D. (1983). *SPSSX user's guide*, New York: McGraw-Hill.

Norusis, M. (1982). *SPSS Introductory guide*. New York: McGraw-Hill.

Norusis, M. (1985). Advanced statistics guide. New York: McGraw-Hill.

SAS Institute. (1979). *SAS user's guide, 1979 Edition*. Cary, N. C.: SAS Institute.

Sweeney, M., & Olivieri, P. (1981). *An introduction to nursing research: Research, measurement, and computers in nursing*. Philadelphia: Lippincott.

24

PREPARING DATA FOR ANALYSIS

NANCY FUGATE WOODS

After data are collected from the study participants the investigator can begin a series of important processes to prepare the data for analysis. Before data are collected, the investigator develops a general analysis plan and answers questions such as:

1. In what form will I record the data? Will I record them as handwritten responses to questions? Will the data be options on precoded items? Will the data be marks on a visual analog scale? Will the data be recordings from a strip chart recorder?

2. Will I be using a computer program to analyze the data? Will I be using a calculator? Will I be analyzing the data with such methods as content analysis? Will I be using a combination of these methods? Will I perform quantitative or qualitative analyses?

With the answers to these questions an investigator can proceed through the essential processes of preparing the data for analysis.

The six essential processes for preparing data for quantitative or qualitative analysis are: editing for legibility and completeness, coding data, transferring data to a computer file or to another analysis system, editing the data file, reducing or modifying the data, and editing the modifications (Fig. 24-1). Although some of these processes may seem tedious and boring, the careful performance of each is essential to the accuracy of the data. Let us consider each of these processes in greater detail.

EDITING THE DATA

Once the data collection records are complete the investigator edits each questionnaire, interview guide, or recording to be certain that the information is legible and usable. When data are not recorded in legible handwriting they can be unintelligible and worthless. One can take several precautions against this, but there are few remedies after it has occurred. Careful and complete editing immediately after the data are collected is the best precaution. Within a short period of time after an interview or questionnaire is completed, the recorder can usually recall what the unintelligible scribble means. Interviewers can be trained to edit their interviews immediately after completing them. When study participants are accessible to the investigator after the data have been collected, and when the investigator can screen the data immediately, the participants can be asked to interpret their writing. Physiological recordings can be monitored for legibility and completeness at the time they are made.

In addition to editing for legibility the investigator also edits data collection records for completeness. Identifying each data collection record is extremely important; labeling each piece of paper with the participant's identification number is an example of a simple but essential process that ensures that the investigator can attribute the data to the correct participant. An investigator must often make a decision about whether to omit a record from the

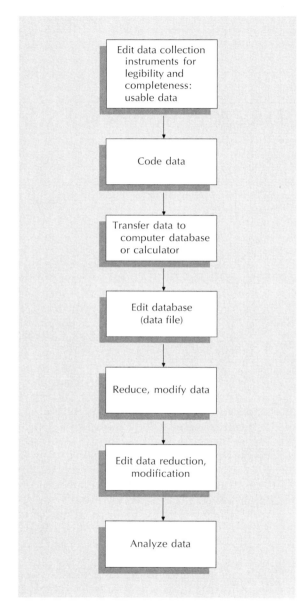

Fig. 24-1. Process for preparing data for analysis.

study. For example, if a participant skipped several sections of a questionnaire or ended the interview prematurely, the investigator may determine that the data from that individual are so incomplete as to be unusable. In some cases the investigator will disregard all the data obtained from that individual and in others will simply regard a portion of the data as incomplete. Decision rules to guide such judgments help the investigator maintain consistency across all cases. Careful documentation of these decision rules is important to ensure consistency and to assist the investigator in the interpretation of some of the study's results. For example, when a large number of participants do not provide complete data for the same portion of the study, the results may be strangely skewed and difficult to interpret. This systematic omission of a section of a questionnaire or interview requires careful attention to avoid making spurious interpretations of findings that represent only the subset of participants who completed the section of the instrument in question.

A third level of editing incorporates a final check on eligibility criteria for the study. Despite the investigator's earlier caution in stipulating and adhering to inclusion and exclusion criteria, individuals who do not meet the study's sample selection criteria may have been included in the study. A final check on these criteria, such as making certain that all the participants were in the correct age range, can be performed in the early editing. Identifying data that are inappropriate to include in the final analyses before they have been coded and incorporated as part of the final database saves time and money and reduces the likelihood that the investigator will need to repeat an entire series of analyses to correct this error later.

CODING

After carefully editing the original data (sometimes referred to as "raw" data) the investigator is ready to begin coding. Coding is the process by which the original data are transformed into symbols compatible with computer-assisted analysis or other types of analysis. Coding decisions establish how many values a variable can take in an analysis.

Most computer programs for statistical analysis require that all data be coded as numbers (numerical) rather than as letters (alphabetical). Coding for computer analysis frequently involves transforming phrases or words to numbers. The following paragraphs will discuss coding procedures for computer-assisted statistical analyses of the data. Special coding procedures for qualitative analyses are discussed in Chapter 28.

Coding procedures for various types of variables

Most research projects include several different types of variables. It is not unusual for a nursing research project to include variables that are inherently quantitative as well as qualitative. A person's age, height, weight, income, and years of education can be obtained as quantitative variables and incorporated directly into the database without being transformed from the form in which they are reported to a new code.

In some instances investigators ask participants to indicate information in one of several categories. These variables are termed "nominal" or "categorical variables." For example, an investigator might ask the participants to choose which ethnic group best describes them. Some may report black American, some Japanese American, some Hispanic, and some Irish American, to name a few. When data are reported in this way, the variable must be coded as some number before it can be entered in a computer file. For example, black American could be coded as *1*, Japanese American as *2*, and so forth. Variables from questionnaires and interviews often can be precoded, that is, the responses to questions can be anticipated and assigned a numerical code before the instrument is administered. For example, the person's rating of health could be coded in this way:

Compared to the health of other people your own age, how would you rate your health?

Poor	1
Fair	2
Good	3
Excellent	4

The person who answered "fair" would be given a code of *2* for that response, the person who answered "good" would be given a *3*, and so on. In some instances the numerical codes used have some implic-

it value. Here, *4* reflects better health than *3*. Other coding schemes, such as in the example below, have no implicit numerical value; rather the codes correspond to the alphabetized list of responses.

Almost everybody in the United States has ancestors who originally came from somewhere else. As far as you know from what countries or parts of the world did your ancestors come?

Africa	01
Asia	02
Australia	03
Europe	04
North America	05
South America	06

When participants have the option of indicating multiple responses, the investigator can treat each response as a separate variable, for example:

Has a nurse practitioner or physician ever told you that you have any of these problems?

	Yes	No
Endometriosis	1	0
Fibroids	1	0
An abnormal Pap smear	1	0

When there are several responses to the same general question, each response would be treated as a separate dichotomous variable and coded *0* for "no" and *1* for "yes."

Investigators often incorporate open-ended questions in their studies because the types of answers cannot be anticipated. Sometimes the investigator does not want to impose a frame of reference on the participant but instead emphasizes the participant's individual perception of the phenomenon. A question such as "What does being healthy mean to you?" can elicit a wide variety of responses. Depending on the purposes of the study the investigator can create a very simple or very extensive category schema to accommodate responses. Scanning the responses might reveal that people think being healthy is associated with feeling good, being able to function, or not having any symptoms. The investigator could categorize the responses as:

Feeling good	01
Able to function	02
Absence of symptoms	03

The coding categories must be exhaustive, that is, they must account for every possible response to the item. In addition, the categories must be mutually exclusive, meaning that a statement can be coded in one and only one category. Thus a statement coded as reflecting feeling good could not also be classified as able to function. Alternatively, the investigator could create an elaborate taxonomy to describe each dimension of being healthy and several subdimensions of the construct. Several aspects of feeling good could be elaborated. More elaborate coding schemes for qualitative data are discussed in Chapter 28. Regardless of the extensiveness of the coding scheme the qualitative statements can be reduced to numerical codes for purposes of statistical analysis.

One can code data in many ways. In general, including as much detail as possible in the data file is preferable. When data are reported as continuous variables the investigator need not code them but can enter them directly into the data file. Later in the analysis, if it is necessary to transform a quantitative variable to categories, a new coding scheme can be incorporated into the computer program to group responses into categories. For example, age can be readily transformed from the exact ages reported by participants to categories that are relevant to the researcher's purpose. These relevant categories can be determined after the age distribution is known. A person who is 26 could be classified into a category of 20 to 30 years of age through the use of a short computer command. When data are entered into the data file in categories, however, retrieving the original value is impossible. The investigator would not be able to determine the precise ages of the individuals who are in the 20 to 30 category when their ages are coded as a categorical variable rather than ratio variables.

Coding conventions

A few widely used coding conventions facilitate using computer programs for data analysis. Coding missing data is important so that it is possible to distinguish them from zeros or blanks in the data. When a participant skips an item or refuses to answer a question in an interview or when the observer misses an observation, it is important for the investigator to recognize that the datum is missing. Often the number 9 or multiple 9s (99 or 999 for multicolumn variables) are used to indicate a missing val-

ue. Some investigators choose to code missing values as blanks in the data. This is not an incorrect convention, but some computer programs do not distinguish between blanks and zeros unless given a specific command to do so. (The SPSS-X program reads blanks for missing values.) The use of blanks for missing data may result in spurious values for some variables because some computer programs may read the blanks as zeros, thus giving an artificially low value for the variable. A similar problem may occur with other missing value indicators if the investigator does not designate the missing values correctly within the analysis program.

Sometimes an item is not applicable to the participant. For example, in an interview only pregnant women who are partnered are asked a series of questions about the amount of support they anticipate receiving from their partners. The responses of women who are not partnered are not missing; rather they are not applicable. A commonly used coding convention for nonapplicable responses is 8 or multiple 8s. Some investigators use other coding conventions. For example, in some instances it may be important to distinguish those individuals who did not know an answer to an item from those who refused to answer the item. Some other digit that is not already used to code the responses to the item can be used to indicate the individual did not know the answer.

There is no "correct" method for coding missing or nonapplicable values. However, it is imperative that an investigator use a consistent method for coding missing values or nonapplicable values for all data for a study in order to increase the likelihood of accurate coding for all values.

Developing a code book

It would be impossible for most investigators to remember all the rules that guided the coding and all the conventions used in coding their data. For this reason an investigator develops a code book before the data are coded, usually before data collection is initiated. A *code book* is a directory of the kinds of data the investigator anticipates or collects. A code book usually includes the following items: a list of all variables in the study, a shorthand name for each variable, code numbers for the possible values of each variable, a summary of the possible values for each variable, the location (columns) in which the values

TABLE 24-1. **Code book for "Problems After Mastectomy"**

VARIABLE (VARIABLE NAME)	CODE		VALUES	COLUMNS	FORMAT
DEMOGRAPHIC VARIABLES					
ID number (ID)	Code as is (CAI)		01 to 43	1-2	F2.0
Age (AGE)	CAI		21 to 70	3-4	F2.0
Race (RACE)	Black = 1		1 to 5	5	F1.0
	Native American = 2				
	Mexican American = 3				
	Asian American = 4				
	White = 5				
Income (INCOME)	<2000 = 1		1 to 7	6	F1.0
	2000-3999 = 2				
	4000-6999 = 3				
	7000-9999 = 4				
	10,000-14,999 = 5				
	15,000-24,999 = 6				
	≥25,000 = 7				
Education (EDUC)	Elementary school = 1		1 to 6	7	F1.0
	Junior high school = 2				
	High school graduate = 3				
	Some college or technical				
	school = 4				
	College graduate = 5				
	Masters/doctorate = 6				
TYPE OF MASTECTOMY SURGERY					
Type of surgery (SURGERY)	Lumpectomy = 1		1 to 5	8	F1.0
	Partial mastectomy = 3				
	Simple mastectomy = 3				
	Modified radical = 4				
	Radical = 5				
POSTOPERATIVE SYMPTOMS RELATED TO SURGERY					
Swelling in arm (SWELL)	Yes = 1	No = 0	0 to 1	9	F1.0
Weakness in arm (WEAK)	Yes = 1	No = 0	0 to 1	10	F1.0
Stiffness in arm (STIFF)	Yes = 1	No = 0	0 to 1	11	F1.0
Trouble moving arm (TROUBLE)	Yes = 1	No = 0	0 to 1	12	F1.0
Numbness in arm (NUMB)	Yes = 1	No = 0	0 to 1	13	F1.0
PROBLEMS IN DAILY LIVING					
Can't do light housework (HOUSE)	Yes = 1	No = 0	0 to 1	14	F1.0
Can't do laundry (LAUNDRY)	Yes = 1	No = 0	0 to 1	15	F1.0
Can't entertain (ENTER)	Yes = 1	No = 0	0 to 1	16	F1.0
Can't visit friends (VISIT)	Yes = 1	No = 0	0 to 1	17	F1.0
Can't do heavy cleaning (CLEAN)	Yes = 1	No = 0	0 to 1	18	F1.0
Can't drive car (DRIVE)	Yes = 1	No = 0	0 to 1	19	F1.0
Can't prepare meals (MEALS)	Yes = 1	No = 0	0 to 1	20	F1.0
Can't care for children (CHILD)	Yes = 1	No = 0	0 to 1	21	F1.0
Can't do shopping (SHOP)	Yes = 1	No = 0	0 to 1	22	F1.0
Can't play sports (SPORTS)	Yes = 1	No = 0	0 to 1	23	F1.0

Conventions: 8 = not applicable, 9 = missing value.

appear, and the format of the digits and decimal point placement for each variable. The code book for a study entitled "Problems After Mastectomy" is shown in Table 24-1. The purpose of the study was to identify the types of problems women experienced several years after mastectomy for breast cancer.

In the left column is the name of each variable in the study, beginning with the participant identification number and the abbreviation of the variable name, in this instance ID. The next variable is age, and the last variable in the code book is "can't play sports," abbreviated "sports".

When constructing a code book it is important to remember that each distinct variable must have a different variable name. For example, if we had called each of the problems in daily living "problems" instead of "house," "laundry," and so forth, we would not be able to distinguish one variable from another. As an alternate example, if we had three blood pressure measurements for each person in a study, we could call them BP1, BP2, and BP3, but we could not call each of them BP. Another important consideration is that the definition of the variable must remain constant for each case. For example, BP1 would always be the first, BP2 the second, and BP3 the third blood pressure measurement.

The next column includes the coding instructions and the code numbers to be given to the possible values for the variable. Notice that the instructions for the ID number are to code it as is, meaning as it is reported on the questionnaire. Specific instructions are given for coding race, where black will be coded *1*, native American, *2*, and so forth.

The next column contains information about the possible values for the variables. This column is useful when the investigator is screening values that have been entered into a computer file. Note that the values for ID number can range from 01 to 43, age from 21 to 70, and race from 1 to 5. A value of 44 for ID number would be incorrect, as would a value of 6 for race.

Each case can have only one value per variable. When a questionnaire item has several answers it may be translated into several variables. For example, an item that has multiple responses, such as the question about postoperative symptoms, can be coded so that each possible answer is a separate variable. That is why the answers to this item have been treated as the separate variables "swell," "weak," "stiff," "trouble," and "numb."

The column labeled "columns" denotes where the variable resides in the computer file. Before the location of variables can be discussed in greater detail, it is important to understand the concept of data matrix. The *data matrix* is usually arranged so that data from each case (usually individuals in the study) appear in one or more rows, with the values for the variables occupying designated columns. ID number is in columns 1 and 2, and age is in columns 3 and 4.

The far-right column (Table 24-1) contains information about the format of the variable. A format statement tells the computer program how the data are organized into columns. For the most commonly used statistical packages, two types of format can be used: freefield or fixed. In freefield format the variables are always in the same order but are not necessarily in the same column for each person. The code values for each variable are separated by either commas or blank spaces. Fixed format is used more commonly and is the format shown in the sample code book. Each row of data contains information about only one participant, and a given variable always appears in the same column(s) for all participants. A column is the space occupied by a single character, either a number, letter, decimal point, symbol, or blank space. To match each variable with the actual data values, one needs to tell the computer program exactly which columns contain that information. For example, the first variable in the sample code book is the participant's ID number (ID). Since there were 43 women in the study some will have two-digit ID numbers; columns 1 and 2 were assigned for this variable. The first woman has ID number 01. The leading 0 may be left out, but the 1 must be right-justified, that is, it must appear in the right-most column for that variable. The investigator specifies that two columns (the field width) have been set aside with the format statement F2. The F2 means that information for the ID variable takes up two columns. The next variable, "age," also needs two columns and has the format F2. However, the third variable, "race," has only a one digit code, so its format is F1.

All the individual format specifications are combined into a statement called the input format statement in some programs. The statement must account for each variable's format in the same order in which the variables appear. When several adjacent variables have the same format, the number of repetitions can

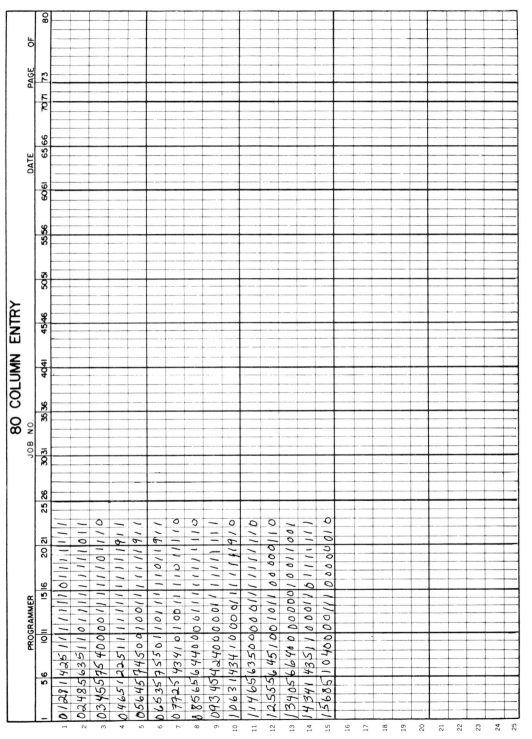

Fig. 24-2. Data for 15 women for variables described in code book (Table 24-1).

be indicated in front of the common format specification. For instance, if 10 variables have F2 formats all can be represented by writing 10F2. If those 10 variables were followed by three variables with an F1 format, the entire group of 13 variables would be represented by the format statement (10F2,3F1). Other information may be communicated to a statistical program in the input format statement. An X indicates a column that should be left blank. A Tn (where n is some number) tells the cursor to go to that column number and start reading data at that point. Data values for the first 15 participants (of the total of 43) in the postmastectomy problems study are shown on the sample sheet of data in Fig. 24-2. Each person has one row of data, with 23 columns of information in each row.

The investigator can use many options in developing a plan for coding and entering the data. Generally, the same participant's data are given in rows, and the individual variables are represented in columns. In the database (data matrix) for the postmastectomy problems study, data for each woman are given in a single row. When the data for a single individual extend beyond the number of columns desired in a single row, the next row is identified with the ID number of that participant, and the data are continued on the next row. The variables in the study are given in the columns, with the same columns used for each variable for each woman. Sometimes entering the data is easier when spaces are left between variables. This variation can be done at the investigator's discretion. The code book reflects the structure of the database as the investigator has defined it and as data are represented in computer files. A computer file can be thought of as a collection of information; a data file contains the data matrix described earlier.

Coding the data

Coding may be a very simple, straightforward, and quickly accomplished aspect of a research study or a very complicated and time-consuming one. Data that are precoded on questionnaires require no coding before they are added to a computer file. A precoded questionnaire such as the one shown in the box below may include precoded answers and an indication of the column on the instrument. In this example there are column numbers in the far-right margins under the heading "edge coding." The column numbers correspond to the column in the database where that datum will be entered. These data can be entered directly into a computer file by typing

---

EXAMPLE OF PRECODED QUESTIONNAIRE WITH EDGE CODING

After breast surgery, women sometimes notice swelling, redness, or warmth in their arms. Some women have trouble moving their arms or notice other changes.

INTERVIEWER: CIRCLE CORRECT RESPONSES.

	b. "Do you *now* have:"		Edge coding
a. Swelling of your (surgical) arm(s)	Yes 1	No 2	9
b. Weakness in your arm(s)	Yes 1	No 2	10
c. Redness in your arm(s)	Yes 1	No 2	11
d. A feeling of stiffness in your arm(s)	Yes 1	No 2	12
e. A feeling of warmth in your arm(s)	Yes 1	No 2	13
f. Trouble moving your arm(s)	Yes 1	No 2	14
g. Problems with your incision healing	Yes 1	No 2	15
h. A feeling of numbness in your arm(s)	Yes 1	No 2	16

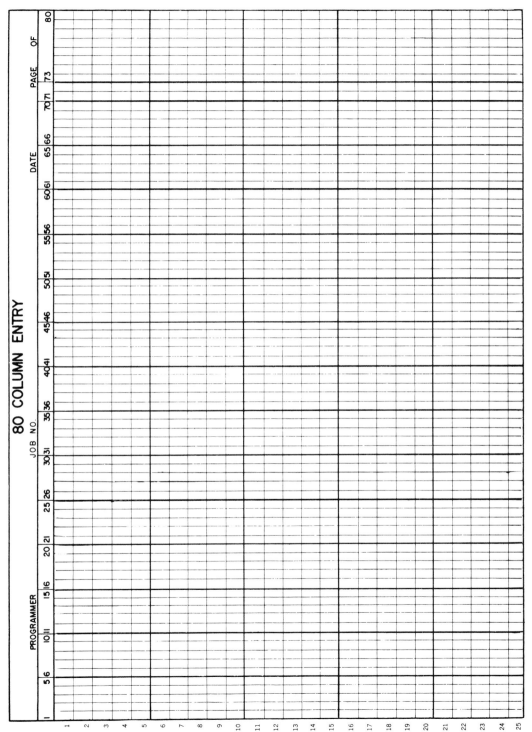

Fig. 24-3. Coding paper for 80 columns of data.

the code number corresponding to the response in the column indicated by the edge coding.

It is not always possible to anticipate responses and thus to precode instruments. In these instances the investigator must develop a coding scheme after the data are collected. The investigator may code the data directly on the questionnaire or transfer the data from the questionnaire to a coding sheet such as that shown in Fig. 24-3. This paper, often referred to as Fortran paper or coding paper, contains 80 columns per row. Each column corresponds to one column on a computer card or to a field on a computer disk or tape. Coding directly on a questionnaire is faster than coding from a questionnaire to a code sheet. Moreover, coding directly on the questionnaire reduces the chance of error that occurs when information is recopied. On the other hand, some would argue that the use of a coding sheet generally speeds data entry and decreases the likelihood of entering data in the wrong field when they are entered into a computer file.

Training coders

When more than one individual are coding the data, it is important to train them to implement the coding rules contained in the code book. This is especially important when the data are not precoded. Ideally coders practice coding and subsequently receive feedback about the accuracy of their coding. Reliability checks of the coding should yield a 90% or better agreement between the coders. In addition, it is important to reassess reliability throughout the coding process to enhance accuracy and agreement among the coders and to avoid *drift,* the tendency to code differently as the coding process continues. Documentation of the coding decision rules is extremely important for consistency of coding, especially when many coders are working with the same data.

TRANSFERRING DATA TO A COMPUTER FILE

Once data are coded they are transferred to a medium that is compatible with computer analysis. Data may be transferred to computer cards, disks, or magnetic tapes with the original data records or code sheets serving as the source. Each participant's record generally begins with an identification num-

ber that is unique to that participant. Following the identification number are the data. When the data exceed the limits of the field (usually 80 columns), they are continued on a second card.

The transfer of data from code sheets or the original instruments to a computer file can be achieved by using one of the types of input devices discussed in Chapter 23, that is, a key-punch machine to punch cards, a terminal to create a record on magnetic tape or a computer disk, or an optical scanner that directly transfers the data from a coding sheet designed to be completed with a no. 2 lead pencil and to be used with an optical scanner.

Regardless of the mechanism used to create a computer database, a careful check of the accuracy of the data is essential. A computer file on magnetic tape or a disk can be checked for errors by proofreading a hard copy printout or a video display of the file with reference to the original data or the coding sheet. Another option is entering the data twice into separate files and using a computer program to match or compare the two files. The program will print a listing of differences between the two files.

EDITING A DATABASE

Once the file has been created the investigator edits the database for data entry errors, coding errors, and reporting errors. Data entry errors are those mistakes in the file attributable to typographical errors. Coding errors result from inappropriate application of the coding rules. Reporting errors occur when the participant in the study reports information inconsistently; for example, the participant indicates in one part of the questionnaire that she has never been hospitalized but refers to a hospitalization in response to another part of the questionnaire. These types of errors can be detected in several ways. A first check can be done by printing out the content of the database (Fig. 24-4). This step allows one to check the completeness of the data. The investigator can look for missing cases by checking the identification numbers of all the cases against a listing of the eligible identification numbers. Printing a frequency distribution of 10 numbers allows the investigator to discover duplicate entry of cases. The investigator also can look for a pattern in the database. For example, if the first line of data entered for each participant

ID Number	Age	Race	Income	Education	Surgery	Swell	Weak	Stiff	Trouble	Numb	House	Laundry	Enter	Visit	Clean	Drive	Meals	Child	Shop	Sports
01	25	1	4	2	5	1	1	1	1	1	1	1	0	1	1	1	1	1	1	1
02	40	5	6	3	5	1	1	0	1	1	1	1	1	1	1	1	1	0	1	1
03	45	5	7	5	4	0	0	0	0	1	1	1	1	1	0	1	1	1	1	0
04	65	1	2	2	5	1	1	1	1	1	1	1	1	1	1	1	1	0	1	1
05	64	5	7	4	5	0	0	1	0	0	1	1	1	1	1	1	1	0	1	1
06	53	5	7	5	5	0	1	1	0	1	1	1	1	1	0	1	1	0	1	1
07	72	5	4	2	4	1	0	1	0	0	1	1	1	1	0	1	0	1	0	
08	56	5	6	4	4	0	0	0	0	1	1	1	1	1	1	1	1	1	1	0
09	34	5	4	2	4	0	0	0	0	0	1	1	1	1	1	1	1	1	1	1
10	63	1	4	3	4	1	0	0	0	0	1	1	1	1	1	1	0	1	0	
11	46	5	6	3	5	0	0	0	0	0	1	1	1	1	1	1	1	1	0	
12	55	5	6	4	5	1	0	0	1	0	1	1	0	0	0	0	0	1	1	0
13	62	5	6	6	4	0	0	0	0	0	0	1	0	0	1	1	0	0	1	
14	34	1	4	3	5	1	1	0	0	0	1	1	0	1	1	1	1	1	1	
15	68	5	1	2	4	0	0	0	0	1	1	1	0	0	0	0	1	0	1	0
16	50	5	7	3	3	0	0	0	0	0	1	1	1	1	1	1	1	1	1	
17	48	5	6	3	4	0	0	1	0	0	1	1	1	1	1	1	1	1	0	
18	48	5	5	4	5	0	0	0	0	0	1	1	1	1	1	1	1	1	1	
19	62	5	2	3	5	0	1	0	0	1	1	1	1	1	1	1	1	1	0	
20	42	5	6	3	4	0	1	1	1	0	0	0	0	1	1	0	0	0		
21	67	5	3	3	4	0	0	0	0	1	1	1	0	1	1	1	1	1	0	
22	59	5	7	3	4	0	0	0	0	0	1	1	1	0	0	1	1	0	1	0
23	59	5	5	4	4	0	0	0	0	0	1	1	1	1	1	1	1	1	0	
24	50	5	7	3	4	1	0	0	0	1	1	1	1	1	1	1	1	1	0	
25	54	5	5	2	4	0	0	0	0	1	1	0	1	1	0	1	1	1	0	
26	(75)	1	8	2	3	0	0	0	0	1	1	1	1	0	1	1	1	0		
27	61	5	0	3	4	0	0	0	0	1	1	1	1	0	1	1	1	0		
28	62	5	2	2	3	1	0	0	0	1	1	1	1	1	1	1	0	1	0	
29	59	1	1	1	5	0	1	1	1	1	1	1	1	1	0	1	0	1	0	
30	65	5	2	3	3	0	0	0	0	0	1	1	0	1	1	0	1	0	1	1
31	57	5	3	4	4	0	0	0	0	0	1	1	1	1	0	1	1	1	0	
32	64	1	(8)	1	5	0	0	0	0	0	1	1	0	1	1	0	1	0	1	0
33	49	5	0	3	3	0	0	0	0	0	1	1	1	1	1	1	0	1	0	
34	61	5	4	2	5	0	0	0	0	0	1	1	1	0	1	1	1	0		
35	80	1	2	3	4	1	0	1	0	0	1	1	0	1	0	0	1	0	1	0
36	47	5	5	2	5	0	1	0	0	1	1	1	1	1	1	1	1	1	1	
37	(7)3	5	7	3	3	0	0	0	0	0	1	1	1	1	1	1	0	1	1	
38	43	5	(8)	3	4	1	0	0	0	1	1	1	1	1	1	1	1	1	1	
39	54	5	3	1	5	1	0	0	0	0	1	1	1	1	1	1	0	1	0	
40	64	5	7	4	3	0	0	0	0	0	1	1	1	1	1	1	1	1	1	
41	41	5	5	3	5	1	1	1	0	1	1	1	1	1	1	1	1	1	1	
42	44	5	6	5	4	1	0	0	0	0	1	1	1	1	1	1	1	1	1	
43	61	5	7	4	4	1	1	0	0	1	0	1	1	0	1	1	0	1	0	

Fig. 24-4. Computer printout of the data after being entered for the mastectomy study described in the code book. This database consists of 43 cases with 23 columns of data per case. Circled values are wild codes.

should contain data in 80 columns and the second line should contain data in 40 columns, the investigator could see a pattern of 80 and 40 columns in alternating rows throughout the database. A series of 80/40/80/80/40 would suggest that a line is missing. In addition, duplicate records would be indicated by identifying too many records with the same identification number and with exactly the same data included in all the columns of both records. Next, the investigator can obtain a frequency distribution for all the variables in the database. The frequencies can be checked against the code book to determine if there are any wild codes in the database. Wild codes refer to values that are not included in the code for the variable in question. For example, if there were two values for gender, 1 and 2, the value 3 or 20 would be considered a wild code. It is also possible to write simple computer programs to screen for wild codes. A third type of problem exists when there are logical inconsistencies among the responses to questions. For example, a record might indicate that a woman reported that she had never used oral contraceptives but later reported the brand of contraceptive she had used. In this instance it would be important to check the coding against the original data. Logical inconsistencies can be identified by cross-classifying the two variables, in this case, oral contraceptive use and contraceptive brand. Women who deny using oral contraceptives logically would not name a brand. Once these errors are identified they are corrected, and the file is checked again for accuracy.

DATA REDUCTION AND MODIFICATION

Another aspect of preparation of data for analysis includes data reduction and modification. Data reduction refers to the translation of information from several variables to a smaller number of variables to simplify problems of analysis, storage, and dissemination to other scholars (Selltiz et al., 1976). Data reduction involves processes by which data are summarized or put into smaller units. The process of data reduction encompasses scaling (discussed in Chapter 14), as well as some coding procedures. *Scaling* involves the assignment of a numerical score to an attribute; this score is a combination of several measurements. For example, instead of enumerating 50 different types of stressful events, an investigator might choose to summarize the total number of stressful events, allowing a single score to represent the construct.

Data modification refers to procedures that transform the original data to another form but do not necessarily reduce the data to smaller units. Suppose an investigator originally used two scales to measure well-being. One of the scales is scored so that high scores indicate well-being, and the other is scored so that low scores indicate well-being. The investigator might wish to compare the relationship between the two scores. The investigator can score two scales in the same direction by recoding the scores on the second scale so that the high scores on both instruments reflect well-being. When data are reduced or modified, checking their accuracy is important for precise interpretation.

EDITING . . . AGAIN

A frequency distribution of the reduced or modified data can be helpful to the investigator in several ways. Review of the frequencies can aid in the identification of wild codes produced by some arithmetic error or logical error in data reduction or modification. For example, the bounds of each scale can be compared with the theoretical minimum and maximum scores. A scale with seven items that are scored from 1 to 7 should have a theoretical total minimum score of 7 and a theoretical total maximum score of 49. As with coding rules, rules for data reduction and modification need to be carefully documented for future reference. When errors are found in the data reduction or data modification results, the investigator must rethink the mathematical and logical processes used to create the reduction or modification.

EXAMPLE OF A COMPUTER PROGRAM FOR DATA ANALYSIS

Once the investigator has completed the data preparation processes just outlined, it is time to begin analysis. SPSS is one of several packages used in nursing research and has had a dominant influence in nursing and social sciences owing to its comprehensiveness and excellent documentation. For this reason the SPSS-X package (one version of SPSS) will be used to illustrate a computer program for data analysis. Basic SPSS-X programs contain three types of commands: file definition commands, variable transformation commands, and statistical procedure commands.

File definition

Computer files may be of several types. Raw data files have been discussed thus far; this kind of file contains the data matrix. Command files contain a list of commands used to transmit information regarding the data file, transformations of the data, and statistical procedures to the program.

The several commands for file definition pertain to data contained in raw data files. FILE HANDLE is a command that references the data file on SPSS-X commands. The file handle can contain up to eight alphanumeric characters, beginning with an alphabetical character or the symbols $, #, or @. In the example in the box on the right the file handle assigned to our data file is QUALITY. The file specifications that appear after the file handle refer to specifications required by the particular computer system being used.

DATA LIST is a command that points SPSS-X to a data file and indicates the format of the file, the number of records in the file, and the format of the data and defines the variables. In this particular example the DATA LIST command specifies that the file handle is QUALITY, that the format of the file is fixed, and that there is one record per case. Following the slash is the number *1*, indicating that the variables that follow are located on record number *1*. The variables follow in the order of their appearance in the file and are the same variables that were included in our code book (Table 24-1). Following the variable name is the column or columns in which the values for that variable appear in the file. When the variables contain values to the right of the decimal place, the number of places to the right of the decimal place are indicated in parentheses after the column specification (e.g., "HEIGHT 6-8 (1)" would indicate that height is recorded in three columns with one integer to the right of the decimal place).

VARIABLE LABELS associates a label or name with the variable specified in the command. The VARIABLE LABELS command is usually used when the investigator wishes to assign a more complex name to the variable than is contained in the DATA LIST command. VALUE LABELS associ-

FILE HANDLE	QUALITY/specifications
DATA LIST	FILE = QUALITY, FIXED, RECORDS = 1 / 1 ID 1-2 AGE 3-4 RACE 5 INCOME 6 EDUC 7 SURGERY 8 SWELL 9 WEAK 10 STIFF 11 TROUBLE 12 NUMB 13 HOUSE 14 LAUNDRY 15 ENTER 16 VISIT 17 CLEAN 18 DRIVE 19 MEALS 20 CHILD 21 SHOP 22 SPORTS 23
VARIABLE LABELS	EDUC EDUCATION / SURGERY TYPE OF SURGERY
VALUE LABELS	RACE (1) BLACK (2) NATIVE AMERICAN (3) MEXICAN AMERICAN (4) ASIAN AMERICAN (5) WHITE
MISSING VALUES	ID, AGE (99) / RACE TO SPORTS (9)
COMPUTE	PROBLEMS = HOUSE + LAUNDRY + ENTER + VISIT + CLEAN + DRIVE + MEALS + CHILD + SHOP + SPORTS
MISSING VALUES	PROBLEMS 99
SELECT IF	AGE LE 60
RECODE	EDUC (1,2,3 = 1) (4,5,6 = 2)
IF	SURGERY GE 4 RADICAL = 1
FREQUENCIES	VARIABLES = ALL / STATISTICS = MAXIMUM MINIMUM MODE MEDIAN MEAN STDDEV

The program commands describe a file named QUALITY contained on one record beginning with a variable called ID and ending with SPORTS
Each of the first two variables occupies two columns, and each of the remaining 19 variables occupies one column. The VARIABLE LABELS command assigns "education" to EDUC and "type of surgery" to SURGERY. VALUE LABELS assigns "black" to the value 1 for the variable of race, "Native American" to the value 2, and so on. The MISSING VALUES command indicates the value 99 for missing values for ID and AGE and a value of 9 for all the other variables. The COMPUTE statement adds HOUSE through SPORTS, for the total number of problems. The SELECT IF command selects only women who are 60 years of age or younger. The RECODE command assigns the value 1 to women with a high school education or less and a 2 to women with more than a high school education. The IF statement creates the new variable RADICAL, which takes the value 1 if a woman had a modified radical or radical mastectomy. The MISSING VALUES command assigns a value of 99 to the computed variable PROBLEMS if one or more of the variables comprising problems has a missing value. The procedure command FREQUENCIES requests a frequency distribution and the statistics specified for all the variables in the file.

ates a label with each value of the variable specified. The VALUE LABELS command is usually used when the investigator wishes to assign a more complex statement to the values for the variable than the number coded in the data file. MISSING VALUES informs the SPSS program which values for a given variable are to be considered missing. Each of these commands defines one or more aspects of the data file.

Another type of command is the variable transformation command. Variable transformation commands change the value of the variable as it is coded in the data file. The COMPUTE command creates new variables or new values for existing variables by means of combining existing variables via one or more arithmetical operators or special functions. The arithmetical operators include addition, division, subtraction, multiplication, and exponentiation. Special functions include logarithms, square roots, cosines, and so forth. The SELECT IF command selects for processing only those cases that meet the criteria specified. The SELECT IF command is used when the investigator wishes to perform the analyses on a special subset of the cases. The RECODE command is used to change variable values to group values when transforming a continuous variable to a categorical variable or when reverse-scoring items for a scale. The IF command can be used to create new variables. When the logical expression is true for the case, a new variable is created based on specifications in the IF command. The investigator can use the MISSING VALUES command to assign a missing value for variables that have been computed with a COMPUTE or IF command, or the SPSS-X system will generate a missing value for the new variable.

The third kind of command is a procedural command. The procedural commands implement the statistical procedures contained in the SPSS package. Usually they follow the form: procedure command, OPTIONS command, STATISTICS command, or subcommands. The Procedure command specifies the procedure to be implemented, the OPTIONS command specifies the optional features to be used with the procedure, and the STATISTICS command specifies the particular statistical analyses to be carried out. Some SPSS-X procedures have subcommands instead of the options and statistics specifications. In the example in the box on p. 383, the procedure FREQUENCIES will generate a frequency table as well as the minimum, maximum, mode, median, mean, and standard deviation for each variable. Notice that not all statistics are meaningful for each variable (e.g., the mean for race is meaningless but would be generated by the program without regard to the type of variable).

Although our example used the SPSS-X package there are many other statistical packages that perform similar functions (see Appendix A). Many of the packages have unique advantages and disadvantages that can be considered with help from a computer consultant or statistical consultant in one's educational organization and computer facility.

Many computer centers offer consultation as well as instruction on application of available packages.

SUMMARY

There are six essential processes for preparing data for analysis: editing for legibility and completeness, coding the data, transferring data to a computer file or to another analysis system, editing the data file, reducing or modifying the data, and editing the modifications. Once data have been transferred to a computer system, the investigator creates a computer program for analyzing the data. Using one of the computer packages available, the investigator must define the characteristics of the data file, transformations of any of the variables, and the statistical procedures to be applied to the data.

REFERENCES

Babbie, E. (1973). Survey research methods. Belmont, CA: Wadsworth.

Barhute, D., & Bacon, L. (1985). Approaches to cleaning data sets: A technical comment. *Nursing Research, 34,* 62-64.

Jacobsen, B. (1981). Know thy data. *Nursing Research, 30,* 254-255.

McElmurry, B., & Newcomb, B. (1981). Clarification of the database concept. *Nursing Research, 30,* 155.

Nie, N., Hull, C., Jenkins, J., Steinbrenner, K., & Best, D. (1983). *SPSS user's guide.* New York: McGraw-Hill.

Selltiz, C., Wrightsman, L, & Cook, S. (1976). *Research methods in social relations.* New York: Holt, Rinehart, & Winston.

Sonquist, J. A., & Dunkelberg, W. C. (1977). *Survey and opinion research: Processing and analyses.* Englewood Cliffs, NJ: Prentice Hall.

25

USING DESCRIPTIVE STATISTICS

NANCY FUGATE WOODS

Once the data have been collected, coded, and entered into a computer file or tabulated with a calculator for analysis, the temptation to immediately see the results of the most complex statistical tests that are contemplated may be overwhelming. Nevertheless data analysis requires a state of mind that tempers urgency with skepticism and openness. Investigators need to employ more than complex statistical tests for data analysis. Indeed, data analysis takes place in the mind of the investigator, not in the central processing unit of a computer or the circuitry of a calculator. To be open to unanticipated findings, as well as errors, investigators need to look for them. Likewise, researchers need to be skeptical of measures that summarize several data points or many variables, particularly those from complex statistical procedures. The summary measures can often camouflage errors and mask unanticipated but informative findings. Investigators would be wise to assume that the greater their knowledge of their data, the better information they can provide to the consumers of their research. Maintaining openness and skepticism throughout the analysis of data is particularly important when using computers to perform statistical tests because it is more difficult to become familiar with the data when calculations are done by computer than it is when calculations are done by hand. Concern about the importance of openness and skepticism in data analysis has precipitated development of an approach to data analysis called *exploratory data analysis*. Exploratory data analysis emphasizes familiarity with data as a means of understanding what they convey. Exploration is contrasted with

confirmation and description with hypothesis testing. The techniques of exploratory data analysis help the investigator study unusual and unanticipated aspects of data rather than only the usual and anticipated. For example, exploratory data analysis techniques include ways of emphasizing extreme values of a variable, not just the average values.

This chapter will explore several techniques that are useful to investigators during the initial phases of data analysis, techniques that support openness and skepticism and that promote careful understanding of the data. These techniques also promote careful description of the phenomena of nursing research and include those commonly termed "descriptive statistics" and techniques used in exploratory data analysis. Descriptive statistics summarize in precise, standard ways the characteristics of observations from a sample.

This chapter emphasizes description of data through the use of frequency distributions and several characteristics of distributions: shape, location, and spread. In addition, the chapter contains discussion of measures of central tendency and dispersion. The chapter addresses the use of contingency tables and correlations to describe associations between variables.

FREQUENCY DISTRIBUTION

In the earliest stages of data analysis the investigator needs an overall picture of the data. A set of data to which descriptive statistics would be applied consists of numbers that represent some phenomenon. Con-

TABLE 25-1. Frequency distribution for problems

NUMBERS OF PROBLEMS	ABSOLUTE FREQUENCY	PERCENTAGE
2	1	3.0
4	3	9.1
6	2	6.1
7	2	6.1
8	8	24.2
9	9	27.3
10	8	24.2
TOTAL	33	100.0

TABLE 25-2. Tally for data in Table 25-1

VALUE	TALLY	COUNT
2	I	1
4	III	3
6	II	2
7	II	2
8	IIII III	8
9	IIII IIII	9
10	IIII III	8

sideration of the possible number of problems women experience 5 years after mastectomy would be overwhelming and confusing if the investigator simply examined each woman's data. The values might look like this:

2 8 8 7 6 4 4 6 7 9 9 9 9 9 10 10 4 8 8 8 8 10 10 10 10 9 8 8 10 9 10 9 9

Imposing some order on this meaningless sequence of numbers is clearly necessary if the investigator is to make meaning of the data.

A *frequency distribution* allows the investigator to apprehend several features of a set of data. In constructing a frequency distribution the values of a particular variable are arranged from lowest to highest, and the frequency with which each value appeared in the study sample is counted. Often the percentage of the total sample that had a particular value for the variable is given also. Let us consider the example of scores obtained from the study of women's experiences 5 years after mastectomy mentioned in Chapter 24. The left column in Table 25-1 contains the possible numbers of problems women could have at the time of the interview. The middle column contains the number of women who reported having that number of problems. The right column contains the percentage of the total sample who had that particular number of problems. Although the frequency distribution constitutes a definite improvement over the scrambled enumeration of data given earlier, the investigator can learn more about the distribution of the data through examining the distribution's shape, location, and spread.

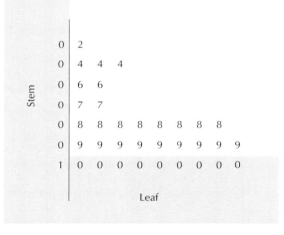

Fig. 25-1. Stem-and-leaf diagram for data in Table 25-1.

Shape

The investigator can learn many features of a distribution by simply looking at a frequency distribution. First, the investigator can apprehend the shape of the distribution and its similarity or dissimilarity to other distributions, including the normal distribution, discussed in detail later in this chapter. Usually the best way to apprehend the shape of a distribution is by using visual techniques that involve displaying data in a graphic form.

The frequency distribution in Table 25-1 can be displayed with a simple tally, a stem-and-leaf diagram, a histogram, or a frequency polygon. A simple tally for the data given in Table 25-1 appears in Table 25-2. The number of times each value appears in the distribution is tallied and then counted. This approach allows the investigator a quick overall impression of the shape of the distribution. Areas of the most frequent scores can be identified by the number of marks in the tally column. One disadvantage of this approach is that when some values are skipped or when there are many possible values and each occurs no more than once or twice, the shape of the distribution is difficult to see.

Another quick technique that allows the investigator to see the shape of the distribution is the stem-and-leaf display. A stem-and-leaf diagram for the data in Table 25-1 is given in Fig. 25-1. In constructing the *stem-and-leaf display* the stem (column to the left of the vertical line) reflects the highest digit in the distribution of scores, and the leaves (rows to the right of the vertical line) reflect the individual digits. For a score of *9* in our distribution the stem would be *0* and the leaf *9*. For a score of *10* the stem would be *1* and the leaf *0*.

One could also use a frequency polygon, as in Fig. 25-2, to graph the data given in Table 25-1. To construct a *frequency polygon* one plots the number of times a given value appeared in the data (the frequency) on the vertical axis, and the value of the variable (or score) on the horizontal axis. The points are then connected with a straight line. A variation on a frequency polygon is a histogram, shown in Fig. 25-3. To construct a *histogram* the investigator draws bars at the point where the frequency and value intersect.

Some distributions do not lend themselves to application of these simple displays of shape. In some instances there are too many scores in a distribution to allow the investigator to apprehend the distribution's shape. For example, some instruments could yield as many as several hundred possible values. When this is the case the investigator can group values into categories, such as 0 to 50, 51 to 100, 101 to 150, and so forth. The class or category then replaces the value of the variable in the display of the distribution.

Another case that does not lend itself to easily apprehending shape of a distribution is the distribu-

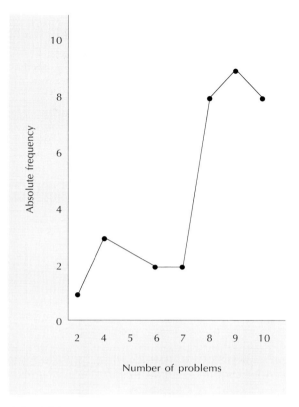

Fig. 25-2. Frequency polygon for data in Table 25-1.

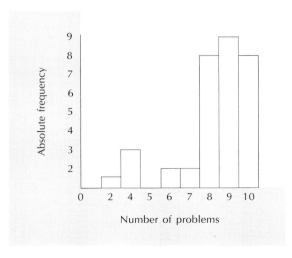

Fig. 25-3. Frequency histogram for data in Table 25-1.

tion for nominal (or categorical) data. The same techniques used for ordinal, interval, and ratio data could be used to illustrate the distribution of a variable such as gender or race, but because no inherent numerical value can be attached to the values for these variables, the order or sequence in which the values are presented has no inherent meaning.

Distributions assume many possible shapes. A distribution can be described as symmetrical or asymmetrical. A *symmetrical distribution* consists of two halves that are mirror images of one another, whereas an asymmetrical distribution consists of two halves that do not resemble one another. Fig. 25-4 gives examples of symmetrical and asymmetrical distributions. When a distribution is asymmetrical it is usually described as a *skewed distribution*. When the longer tail of a distribution points to the right (and the higher values of the variable), the distribution is *positively skewed*. When the longer tail points to the left (and the lower values of the variable), the distribution is *negatively skewed*. In Fig. 25-2 the frequency distribution of problems women experienced after mastectomy is negatively skewed, with the tail pointing to the left. This means that only a few women reported each of the values, indicating a low number of problems after mastectomy.

Distributions can also be described in terms of the number of peaks in the values, or in terms of *modality*, as shown in Fig. 25-5. The mode is the most frequently reported value in a frequency distribution. A *unimodal distribution* has only one peak, but a *bimodal distribution* has two and a *multimodal distribution* has several peaks. The data in Fig. 25-2 are unimodal, with the mode being 9. Nine women reported nine problems, whereas fewer women reported other values.

Distributions also can be described as platykurtotic or leptokurtotic. A *platykurtotic distribution* is flat at the peak, and a *leptokurtotic distribution* is very peaked. The frequency distribution in Fig. 25-2 could be described as leptokurtotic because of the clustering of values at 8, 9, and 10. The *normal curve* (discussed in greater detail later in this chapter) refers to a special kind of distribution that is bell-shaped, symmetrical, unimodal, and not too peaked (Fig. 25-6).

It is extremely important for investigators to recognize the shape of the distribution of variables as a basis for selecting appropriate statistical tests. Most

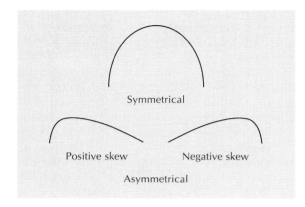

Fig. 25-4. Shapes of distributions—symmetrical versus asymmetrical.

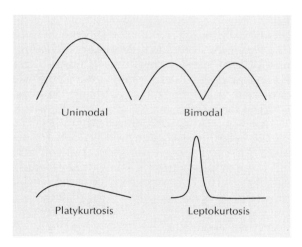

Fig. 25-5. Shapes of distributions. Shapes appear unimodal or bimodal and may be platykurtotic or leptokurtotic.

of the inferential statistical procedures discussed in Chapter 26 are based on the assumption that the variables are normally distributed. Departures from the assumption of normality imply that one should use alternative statistical tests that are not predicated on meeting the assumption of normality.

Location: Central tendency

In addition to apprehending the shape of a distribution, the investigator can ascertain the *location of the*

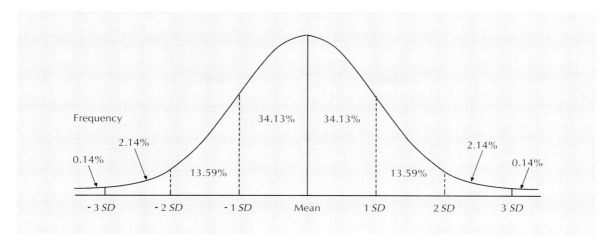

Fig. 25-6. Normal distribution. Notice that the distribution is bell-shaped, symmetrical, unimodal, and not peaked.

distribution (that is, the point at which a distribution is anchored) from displays of the distribution. The location of a distribution is usually summarized as a measure of central tendency. *Measures of central tendency* describe the center of the distribution or the most typical values in the distribution.

The three most common ways of summarizing central tendency in a distribution are the mode, the median, and the mean. The *mode* is the most frequently occurring value in a distribution. One can identify the mode by simply looking at a frequency distribution. In our earlier example the modal number of problems women experienced was 9. Because distributions can have more than one mode, it is not always the best way to summarize central tendency. The mode is the most appropriate summary for nominal variables such as gender or race because it does not require algebraic manipulation of the values that have no mathematical meaning.

The *median* is the value that marks the midpoint of the distribution. Half of the values fall above and half below the median. In our example the median number of problems women experienced was 8.5. The median gives the middle value of the distribution but does not take into account the actual values of the scores above or below it. For this reason the median can be a good estimate of central tendency: it is not greatly affected by extreme scores in the distribution. For example, adding the value 50 to the fre-

quency distribution in Table 25-1 would not alter the median of the distribution in a dramatic way; it would only shift the median from 8.5 to 9. On the other hand, the median does not take into account the actual values of the extreme scores, so it could underestimate the highest or lowest scores in a distribution. By looking only at the median an investigator could miss the extreme value of 50 in the example.

A third way to measure central tendency is use of the *mean,* the arithmetical average of all the scores. The mean is usually represented by the symbol $\overline{X}$ or M, and its computational formula is:

$$\overline{X} = \frac{\sum\limits_{i=1}^{N} X_i}{N}$$

where $\overline{X}$ = mean, X_i = individual scores (X_1 to X_N), N = total number of cases, and Σ = sum. The formula is read as follows: The mean is the sum (Σ) of all observed values of X (X_i) divided by the total number of observations (N). In other words, the sum of all the observations is divided by the total number of observations.

The mean is the most commonly used measure of central tendency, and most tests of statistical significance are based on the mean. Nevertheless, in some cases the information provided by the mean is inappropriate or needs to be supplemented by other information. The mean is intended for interval or ratio level data. Nominal data are summarized by the mode. Calculation of a median or mean for these data is meaningless because the numbers indicating the values of nominal variables have no mathematical meaning. Because ordinal-level data can be ranked and because the intervals between the ranks cannot be assumed to be equal, ordinal-level data are most appropriately summarized by the median, which gives the midpoint of the range of the values in the distribution and does not require algebraic manipulation of the ranks. Because interval-and ratio-level data have the property of equal intervals between values, it is appropriate to add, subtract, multiply, and divide them. Thus the mean is an appropriate measure of central tendency for interval- and ratio-level data.

Unlike the median, the mean is affected by the value of each score in the distribution, no matter how unusual that score might be. For this reason the mean for a skewed distribution may not coincide with the mode or the median. When a distribution is markedly skewed it is wise to consider the median as well as the mean.

Spread: Variability

The investigator can also apprehend the *spread of a distribution*, that is, the variability or dispersion of values in the distribution, width of distribution, and the distance between values. The variability of a distribution can be described in three ways: the range, the interquartile range, and the standard deviation.

The range is the simplest and most crude measure of variability. The *range* is computed by subtracting the lowest score from the highest score in the distribution. The range for the data in Table 25-1 is 8. The lowest score (2) is subtracted from the highest score (10). Although it is easy to compute, the range is sensitive to extreme scores. For example, if the value 20 were added to the distribution in Table 25-1, the range would jump from 8 to 18.

The *interquartile range,* another measure of variability, is the range of scores that encompasses the middle 50% of the scores, leaving 25% above and 25% below it. To identify the interquartile range the investigator simply orders the scores and divides the array of scores into quarters. Q_1 represents the category in and below which one quarter of the scores

fall, and Q_3 represents the category in and below which three quarters of the scores fall.

$$\text{Interquartile range} = Q_3 - Q_1$$

where Q_1 = category into and below which 25% of scores fall and Q_3 = category into and above which 25% of scores fall. The interquartile range in our example is 8 to 9. The presence of extreme values in a distribution does not greatly alter the interquartile range, because no mathematical operations incorporating each value in the frequency distribution are performed on the data. The interquartile range is an appropriate estimation of variability for ordinal data because it does not involve mathematical operations that can only be performed on data meeting the requirement of equal intervals.

The variance and the standard deviation are the most commonly used measures to summarize the variability of a distribution for interval- and ratio-level data. The *variance* is computed by finding the mathematical difference (deviation) of each individual score from the mean, squaring each of these differences, summing all of the differences, and dividing the sum by the number of scores in the distribution. The *standard deviation* is the square root of the variance. The formula for computing the variance is as follows:

$$S^2 = \sum_{i=1}^{N} \frac{(X_i - \overline{X})^2}{N - 1}$$

where S^2 = variance, X_i = individual scores (X_1 to X_N), $\overline{X}$ = mean, and N = total number of cases. The denominator of $N - 1$ is used for calculating the sample variance, whereas N is used for calculating the variance for an entire finite population.

The standard deviation is a useful statistic for summarizing the average deviation about the mean of a distribution, that is, for discerning the degree to which individual scores differ from one another. Indeed, the standard deviation is an index of the average deviation in the scores included in a frequency distribution. In addition, the standard deviation is useful when interpreting the scores of an individual within a distribution. A score of 25 in a distribution with mean 12 and standard deviation 5 is approximately 2.5 SD above the mean, considerably higher than the average score for the distribution. A score of

TABLE 25-3. Relationship between level of measurement and descriptive statistics

LEVEL OF MEASUREMENT	CENTRAL TENDENCY	VARIABILITY
Nominal	Mode	Range
Ordinal	Median	Range
		Interquartile range
Interval/ratio	Mean	Range
		Interquartile range
		Standard deviation
		Variance

10 is below the mean but within 0.5 SD of the mean.

The meaning of a standard deviation becomes clearer if one considers its relationship to the normal distribution. The *normal distribution* (also called *normal curve* or Gaussian curve) is a symmetrical, unimodal curve with mean 0 (see Fig. 25-6). Half of the observations lie above the mean and half below. The mean, median, and mode of this distribution are the same. The standard deviation is located at the point on the curve at which the curve starts growing faster horizontally than it grows vertically, the point of inflection of the curve. When the distribution resembles the normal curve, we know what proportion of cases fell within specified standard deviations about the mean. We know that 99.7% of observations will fall within 3 SD of the mean, 95% of cases within 2 SD of the mean, and 68% within 1 SD of the mean. This information is useful in interpreting how extreme or typical a given score might be.

Appropriate application of descriptive statistics to reflect central tendency and variability depends on the level of measurement for the variable being summarized. The statistics used to reflect central tendency and variability for each level of measurement are indicated in Table 25-3. It is best to use the statistic appropriate for the level of measurement, although in some instances an investigator may select a statistic appropriate for a lower level of measurement. Despite the fact that a variable is measured at an interval level, an investigator may use the median and semiquartile range appropriately to describe a skewed distribution. Note that one can use statistics appropriate for both nominal- and ordinal-level variables to summarize interval- and ratio-level variables, but it is inappropriate to use the statistics for central tendency and variability that are appropriate for interval- and ratio-level variables to describe nominal and ordinal variables.

DESCRIBING RELATIONSHIPS BETWEEN VARIABLES

In addition to describing characteristics of a distribution for a single variable, investigators usually are concerned with the relationships between variables in a study. Many nursing research studies address questions such as:

1. What is the relationship between social support and depression in young adult women?
2. What is the association between reports of anxiety and electromyographic levels during labor?
3. What is the association between use of kith-and-kin support and family cohesion when a diagnosis of cancer is made for a family member?

Contingency tables and correlation coefficients are the most commonly used means of summarizing relationships between variables.

Contingency tables

A *contingency table* is a two-dimensional frequency distribution in which the frequencies of two variables are cross-tabulated. Contingency tables are most commonly used to describe relationships between two nominal or categorical variables. One variable is given in the rows of the table and the other in the columns. Each cell of the table contains frequencies for the joint distribution of the two variables. In Table 25-4, cell A contains the frequency of cases that had low scores on both variable 1 and variable 2. Cell B contains the frequency of cases that had

TABLE 25-4. Sample contingency table

		VARIABLE 2	
		Low	High
VARIABLE 1	Low	A	B
	High	C	D

TABLE 25-5. CMI-MR scores by the complement of women's roles (Woods, 1985)

ROLES		CMI-MR SCORES			ROW TOTAL
	n	<10 (%)	*n*	>10 (%)	
Employed only	31	79%	8	21%	39
Parent only	21	66%	11	34%	32
Employed and parent	44	67%	22	33%	66
TOTAL	96		41		137

low scores on variable 1 and high scores on variable 2. Cell C contains the frequency of cases that had high scores on variable 1 and low scores on variable 2. Cell D contains the frequency of cases that had high scores on both variable 1 and variable 2.

Woods (1985) used contingency tables to assess the relationship between young adult married women's roles as parent and employee and their mental health. She found that the percentage of women with Cornell Medical Index–mental health (CMI-MR) scores above 10 (an indicator of poor mental health) was greater among women who had children than among women without children. Table 25-5 contains information about the women's roles in the rows and their CMI scores in the columns. As seen in the row totals, 39 women were employed, 32 were parents only, and 66 were employed and were parents. The table indicates that 21% of the women who were employed had CMI-MR scores greater than 10, whereas 34% of those who were parents and 33% of those who were parents and were also employed had CMI-MR scores greater than 10. The higher percentage of women with high CMI scores were found in the two groups of women who had children.

The data in contingency tables can be used to describe the association of two variables. Use of the contingency table is appropriate to analyze nominal variables and also to analyze the association between ordinal-level variables with a few values. In some instances contingency table analysis is extended to interval- and ratio-level variables that are recoded as categorical variables, as was done with the CMI scores in the example in Table 25-5. Contingency table analysis is also used in conjunction with statistical tests of association such as the chi square test and others discussed in Chapter 26.

Correlation

Correlation is used most commonly to describe the relationship between two variables that are of ordinal-, interval-, or ratio-level measurement. A correlation coefficient informs us of the extent to which two variables are related to one another. In the example relating parenting and symptoms of poor mental health, parenting and poor mental health were treated as categorical variables, and contingency table analysis was used. The same relationship could be examined by treating each of the variables as ordinal- or interval-level variables and by calculating a correlation coefficient to indicate the strength of the relationship between the two variables. Computation of a correlation coefficient will be discussed in Chapter 26.

In addition to calculating a correlation coefficient graphic plotting of the relationship between two variables reveals information about the direction, strength, and shape of a relationship. The correlation between number of children and CMI-MR raw score values produced the plot seen in Fig. 25-7. Number of children is graphed on the X (horizontal) axis, and CMI-MR scores are graphed on the Y (vertical) axis. The relationship could be described as weakly positive, indicating that women who had children reported more symptoms of poor mental health than did women without children.

When exploring the relationship between two ordinal, interval, or ratio variables, the investigator can first employ a scatterplot or scattergram such as that seen in Fig. 25-6. Each point on the diagram represents the position of one individual on both X and Y axes. The X (horizontal) and Y (vertical) axes represent the two variables being related. Usually the independent or predictor variable is plotted on the horizontal axis and the dependent or outcome vari-

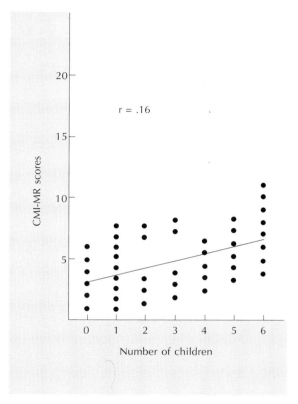

Fig. 25-7. Relationship between CMI-MR scores and number of children.

able on the vertical axis. From the scattergram the investigator can determine the direction, shape, and the magnitude of the relationship.

The direction of the relationship refers to whether it is positive or negative. A positive correlation exists when high values on one variable are associated with high values on the second variable. A negative correlation exists when high values of one variable are associated with low values on another variable. The relationship in Fig. 25-7 is positive. As the number of children increases from *0* to *1*, the CMI-MR scores increase also.

Investigators can usually assess the strength of the relationship by looking at how closely the points in a scattergram cluster around the diagonal slope of the plot. When the points are clustered closely about the diagonal line, the relationship is strong. When they are scattered far apart, the relationship is weak or

nonexistent. A perfect relationship exists when it is possible to predict the value of one variable from the value of another.

The strength of a relationship is expressed by an index called a "correlation coefficient." The magnitude of the correlation coefficient describes the number of units of change in the Y variable given an increase of 1 unit in the dependent variable. A correlation coefficient of 1 implies that for each increase of 1 unit in the X variable, an increase of 1 unit will occur in the Y variable. A correlation coefficient of 0 implies that for each increase of 1 unit in the X variable, an increase of 0 units will occur in the Y variable. The greater the absolute value of the correlation coefficient, the stronger the relationship between the two variables. Correlation coefficients range in magnitude from -1.00 to $+1.00$, where the negative correlations range from 0.0 to -1.00 and positive correlations range from 0.0 to $+1.00$. The value of a perfect positive correlation is $+1.00$ and the value of a perfect negative correlation is -1.00 (Fig. 25-8). When two variables are positively correlated they are also said to be directly related. When they are negatively correlated they are described as inversely related.

Perfect correlations are rarely seen in research with humans. The magnitude of a correlation depends to some extent on the nature of the variables being studied and the precision with which they are measured. When investigators are measuring physiological variables with a high degree of precision, a correlation of 0.8 may seem low. When psychosocial variables are measured, however, a correlation of 0.8 would be quite high.

The shape of a relationship refers to its contour when it is plotted. Visual representation of a relationship, such as in a scattergram, is a typical way of studying the shape of a relationship. The plot allows the investigator to see clustering of points as well as *outliers*, points that are remote from other values on the graph. It is also possible to see many types of relationships. In linear relationships, when X changes, Y changes at the same rate throughout the entire distribution. A *monotonic relationship* is one in which an increase in X is associated with an increase or a decrease in Y throughout the entire range of X (Fig. 25-9). A *nonmonotonic relationship* changes directions so that an increase in X may be associated with an increase in Y over part of the distribution but

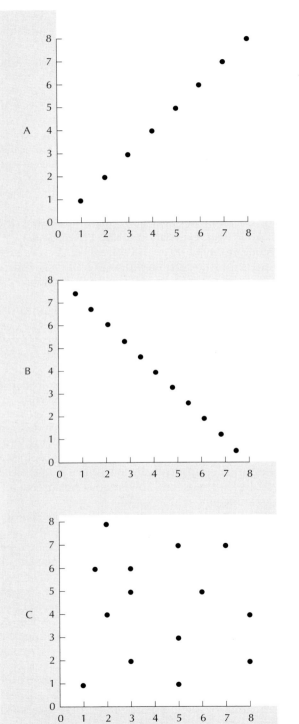

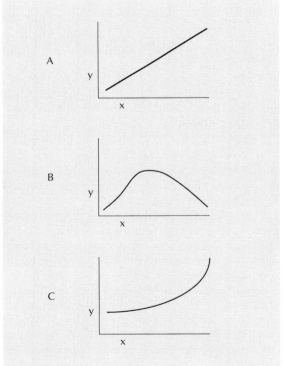

Fig. 25-8. Examples of various correlations. **A,** Perfect positive correlation (high correlation). **B,** Perfect negative correlation (high correlation). **C,** A scattergram of unrelated variables (low correlation).

Fig. 25-9. Graphing relationships reveals their pattern. **A,** Linear, monotonic relationship. **B,** Nonmonotonic relationship. **C,** Nonlinear, nonmonotonic relationship.

with a decrease in Y over other parts of the distribution. In a linear monotonic relationship the rates at which X and Y change are similar, producing a straight line. In a nonlinear monotonic relationship the rate at which Y increases or decreases along with X changes. The shape of relationships can be assessed only through inspection of graphic displays of relationships between two variables. An investigator who relies on a correlation coefficient alone to summarize the relationship between two variables may discover that when the relationship is graphed, the variables are related in a U-shaped fashion despite the fact that the correlation coefficient was moderately large. Moreover, an investigator could discover that despite a small correlation coefficient, a strong linear relationship exists between two variables but only in a portion of the distribution. There are many ways of estimating correlation coefficients, and these are discussed in Chapter 26.

SUMMARY

Descriptive statistics summarize in precise, standard ways the characteristics of observations from a sample. Frequency distributions specify the frequency with which certain values occur in a sample. From a frequency distribution an investigator can determine the shape, location (central tendency), and spread (variability) of a variable. Descriptive statistics can also characterize the relationships between two or more variables. Contingency tables and correlation coefficients can be used to characterize the relationship between variables. Correlation coefficients provide information about the direction, strength, and shape of relationships.

REFERENCES

Blalock, H. (1978). *Social statistics*. New York: McGraw-Hill.

Bruning, J., & Kintz, B. (1977). *Computational handbook of statistics*. Glenview, IL: Scott, Foresman.

Chambers, J., Cleveland, W., Kleiner, B., & Tukey, P. (1983). *Graphical methods for data analysis*. Boston: Duxbury.

Conover, W. (1971). *Practical nonparametric statistics*. New York: Wiley.

Daniel, W. (1978). *Applied nonparametric statistics*. Boston: Houghton-Mifflin.

Edwards, A. (1954). *Statistical methods for the behavioral sciences*. New York: Rinehart and Co.

Elzey, F. (1974). *A first reader in statistics*. Monterey, CA: Brooks/Cole.

Ferketich, S., & Verran, J. (1986). Exploratory data analysis: Introduction. *Western Journal of Nursing Research, 8*, 464-466.

Hartwig, F., & Dearing, B. (1979). *Exploratory data analysis*. Beverly Hills, CA: Sage.

Huck, S., Cormier, W., & Bounds, W. (1974). *Reading statistics and research*. New York: Harper & Row.

Jackson, N. (1982). Choosing and using a statistical consultant. *Nursing Research, 31*, 248-250.

Siegel, S. (1956). *Nonparametric statistics for the behavioral sciences*. New York: McGraw-Hill.

Tukey, J. (1977). *Exploratory data analysis*. Menlo Park, CA: Addison-Wesley.

Verran, J., & Ferketich, S. (1987). Exploratory data analysis: Examining single distributions. *Western Journal of Nursing Research, 9*, 142-149.

Verran, J., & Ferketich, S. (in press). Exploratory data analysis: Comparisons of groups and variables. *Western Journal of Nursing Research.*

Waltz, C., & Bausell, R. (1981). *Nursing research: Design, statistics and computer analysis*. Philadelphia: F. A. Davis.

Willemson, E. (1974). *Understanding statistical reasoning*. San Francisco: W. H. Freeman.

Williams, F. (1979). *Reasoning with statistics*. New York: Holt, Rinehart, & Winston.

Woods, N. (1985). Employment, family roles, and mental ill health in young married women. *Nursing Research, 34*, 4-10.

26

USING INFERENTIAL STATISTICS FOR ESTIMATION AND HYPOTHESIS TESTING

NANCY FUGATE WOODS

The preceding chapter considered the use of descriptive statistics to summarize the values of certain variables within a study. In addition to careful description of the data, investigators usually are concerned about generalizing to the population from which they drew the sample. For example, data about the outcomes of two different community health nursing approaches for high-risk, low-income pregnant women may be extremely enlightening to the community health nurses working in the particular center in which the study was conducted. They may be concerned with the specific population of that neighborhood and the effectiveness of the nursing approaches in reducing the incidence of low birth weight infants, decreasing the incidence of child abuse, and enhancing mother-infant relationships within families in the neighborhood. Although these concerns are specific to the neighborhood involved in the new nursing intervention program, nurses in a large number of health centers around the country are also likely to share them. By designing a study to ensure that the population involved was representative of the population of consumers served by the health center and by using inferential statistics, the investigator is able to generalize to the larger underlying population served by the health center but not included in the study. With an awareness of the specific characteristics of the population, nurses in other health centers serving similar populations might also be able to apply the results of the study in their own communities. To make an inference from the individuals who participated in a study to the larger underlying and unstudied population, the investigator uses *inferential statistics*.

This chapter includes a discussion of inferential statistics for purposes of estimating population parameters and testing hypotheses. Following a discussion of inference from a sample to a population is a discussion of estimation. Use of inferential statistics, including tests of differences and association, to test hypotheses concludes this chapter.

INFERRING FROM A SAMPLE TO A POPULATION

Before proceeding further in a discussion of inferential statistics, two terms need clarification. *Statistic* refers to a characteristic of a sample, such as the arithmetical mean, the variance, or the standard deviation. A *parameter* is a characteristic of a population. *Statistical inference* is the process of estimating parameters from statistics by generalizing from the sample to the population (Fig. 26-1).

Sampling distribution and error

One important assumption when using inferential statistics is that the sample was obtained from the underlying population by means of random sam-

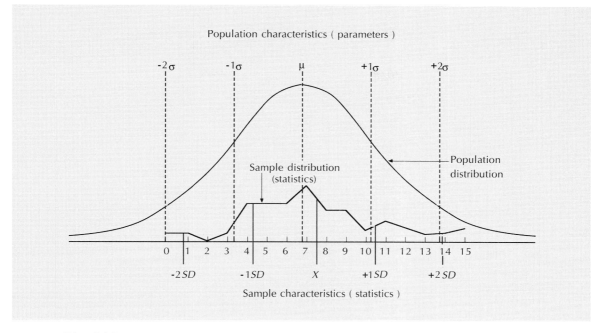

Fig. 26-1. Comparison of sample and population distributions. Population parameters are estimated by sample statistics. Population parameters include the mean designated by μ and the standard deviation designated by σ. Sample statistics include the mean designated by M or $\overline{X}$ and the standard deviation designated by s or SD.

pling procedures. As discussed in Chapter 7 use of random sampling procedures is the optimal way to ensure that the sample is indeed representative of the underlying population. Despite the use of these procedures, however, if samples were repeatedly drawn at random from the population, each sample would yield slightly different values. Let us consider a study of height and weight among 4-year-old children in one community. From 10,000 children 100 different random samples of 100 children could be selected, with the names of the children being replaced each time a representative sample was drawn. In each of the samples there would likely be slightly different values for average weight and height. The fluctuation from one sample to another is termed *sampling error*. If a large number of random samples were drawn from the population, with the units used for each sample being replaced each time, the distribution of the sample means could be plotted. The plot would illustrate the *sampling distribution* for the pop-

ulation. This distribution would approximate the normal distribution curve seen in Fig. 26-2.

The sampling distribution, which is a theoretical distribution rather than one actually obtained in practice, is basic to the inferential statistical procedures discussed in this chapter. From the distribution of sample means the *population mean* could also be calculated; this is an average of the sample means. In addition, how much the sample means deviated around the population mean could be calculated. The standard deviation of a distribution of sample means from the population means is called the *standard error of the mean*. Sampling error is an estimate of how statistics may be expected to deviate from parameters when sampling randomly from a population. The smaller the standard error, the more precise the estimates of the parameter. Because taking a large number of samples from the underlying population is impractical, statisticians have derived a formula that enables investigators to estimate standard error.

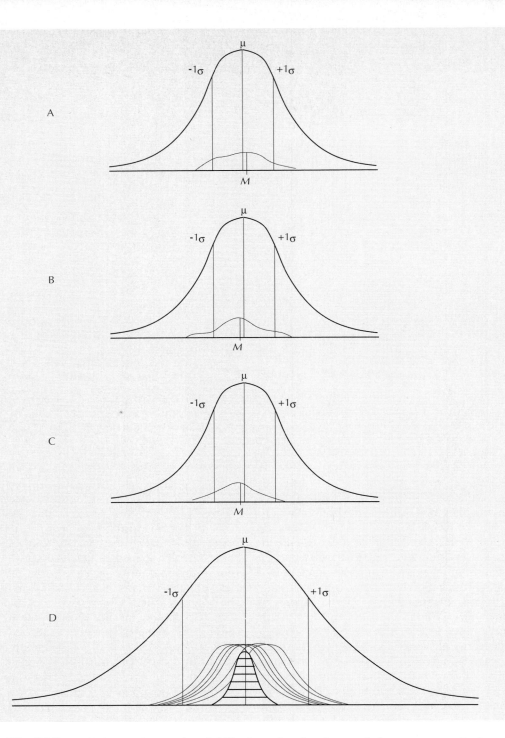

Fig. 26-2. Multiple samples vary in reliability for estimating the population parameters. In **A** the sample mean *(M)* is higher than the population mean *(μ)*, whereas in samples **B** and **C** the sample mean is lower. **D** shows how when many samples are averaged together, the sampling mean approaches the population mean, thereby reducing sampling error. From *Reasoning with statistics,* 2nd ed., by Frederick Williams. ©, 1979, 1968, by Holt, Reinhart, & Winston. Reprinted with permission from Holt, Reinhart, & Winston, Inc.

The standard error of the mean is estimated by the formula:

$$SEM = \frac{s}{\sqrt{n}}$$

where s = the standard deviation of the sample, n = the sample size, and SEM = the standard error of the mean.

Considering the formula for estimating the standard error of the population mean illustrates the relationship between sample size and precision of estimates. Consequently, one way of minimizing the size of the standard error of the mean is by increasing the sample size; that is, the likelihood of drawing a sample that is very unusual with respect to the population decreases as the number of units in the sample increases. Likewise, when the standard deviation of a parameter (s) is small, the sample size required for a precise estimate is small.

With the normal distribution curve as a reference point, the probability with which different sampling means would occur could be determined. From the diagram of the normal distribution given in Fig. 25-6, it is known that 34% of the scores for the distribution will be within 1 SD above the mean and 68% within 1 SD above and below the mean. *Standard scores,* sometimes called *z scores,* can be calculated to determine exactly how far away from the mean any given score (x) lies. With the following formula the z score for a given value could be calculated and then referred to a table to determine what percentage of the distribution would lie below and above the corresponding score:

$$Z = \frac{(X - \overline{X})}{SD}$$

where Z = standard score, X = an individual score, $\overline{X}$ = mean score, and SD = standard deviation. The use of a z score can indicate to an investigator the probability of getting a certain value. For example, a z score greater than 2 would be unusual, since only 2% of scores lie 2 SD above the mean.

ESTIMATING PARAMETERS

Estimating parameters and testing hypotheses constitute two major types of inferential statistical techniques.

Point estimation allows the investigator to use information from a random sample to determine a single numerical value that would be a good indicator of the value of an underlying parameter. In determining the average raw score on the Denver Developmental Screening Test for a population of 2-year-old children, there is a problem of point estimation. The investigator desires an estimate that is as close as possible to the parameter, in this case, the average score.

Although point estimates are informative about a population value such as the mean or median, having some information about the accuracy of the estimate is also important. *Interval estimation* allows investigators to calculate, with a certain degree of confidence, a range of values within which the population value lies. Appropriate point and interval estimates for variables according to their level of measurement are given in Fig. 26-3. *Confidence intervals,* a type of interval estimate, are a measure of the variability associated with the estimate. *Confidence limits* are two boundary points between which one has a specified level of confidence that the population parameter lies. Short confidence intervals indicate little variability about the point estimate for the population. Long confidence intervals indicate great variability about the point estimate. A 95% confidence interval indicates with 95% probability the two values within which the population parameter lies, whereas a 99% confidence interval indicates with 99% probability the two values within which the population parameter lies. The point estimate (such as the mean) is usually followed by the confidence interval:

Mean ± Confidence interval *or*
Lower confidence limit < Mean < Upper confidence limit

The confidence interval for a distribution of height for a population of 5-year-old children would be given as 43 ± 2 inches or as 41 < 43 < 45 inches.

The computational formula for confidence intervals is:

$$CI = \overline{X} \pm (SND\ SEM)$$

where CI = confidence interval, $\overline{X}$ = mean score, SND = standard normal deviate, and SEM = standard error of the mean. To calculate a confidence interval one only needs to know the mean and standard error associated with the representative sample. Suppose that the mean is 43 and the standard error is 1.02. In order to calculate a 95% confidence interval the investigator would refer to the normal distribu-

ESTIMATES	NOMINAL	ORDINAL	INTERVAL
Point estimator			
Measures of central tendency	Mode	Median	Mean or median
Measures of variability (dispersion)	Most and least frequently occurring categories	Range	Standard deviation—variance (semiquartile range)
Interval estimator		Confidence intervals for the median	Confidence interval for the mean

Fig. 26-3. Appropriate estimates for variables according to their levels of measurement.

tion table and note that 95% of the scores lie within 1.96 SD of the mean. The value of the standard normal deviate in this case is 1.96. The confidence interval is obtained by multiplying 1.96 by the standard error, in this case 1.02. Next, the upper confidence limit is obtained by adding the confidence interval to the mean $(43 + 2)$; the lower confidence limit is obtained by subtracting the confidence interval from the mean $(43 - 2)$. These values indicate the range within which the population mean can be estimated to lie with 95% certainty.

TESTING HYPOTHESES

In earlier discussions of inferential statistics the focus was on how statistical concepts underlie reasoning from the data to descriptions of what the data are believed to represent. The focus has been on estimating a value for an entire population based on data from a sample drawn from that population. In hypothesis testing the concern is with making a decision about statements being tested by conducting a study. Hypothesis testing concerns making correct decisions about research findings. Let us consider an example of this type of decision making. Geden and associates (1985) found that nulliparous women who were taught individual elements of Lamaze preparation for childbirth (breathing, relaxation, and instruction) and combinations of these elements

demonstrated different pain ratings, systolic and diastolic blood pressure levels, electromyographic levels, and heart rate. Were the differences between the groups treated attributable to the different treatments? Were the differences due simply to chance or to fluctuation in the population means? To make an informed decision regarding which of these treatments might be most effective with women in labor, investigators and clinicians need to sort out answers to questions like these. The discussion that follows will review the processes involved in sorting out the answers to these and related questions.

The logic of statistical hypothesis testing is concerned with sorting out results attributable to chance from those representing the probable effects of a treatment or the characteristic of an outcome or dependent variable. Statistical hypothesis testing is based on a process of disproof or rejection. Because the statistical procedures used in hypothesis testing are based on rules of negative inference, they require the investigator to formulate two hypotheses: the null hypothesis and the alternative hypothesis, or the research hypothesis. The research hypothesis reflects the investigator's reasoning about the differences she or he expects to find. For example, Geden and associates (1985) anticipated finding that some elements of Lamaze had more effect than others on women's pain levels, muscle tension, and vital signs. The *null hypothesis* asserts that no difference or no relationship

TABLE 26-1. Investigator's decisions regarding the null hypothesis based on sample data

	Null hypothesis true	Null hypothesis false
Do not reject	Not rejecting the null hypothesis when it is in fact true: correct decision	Not rejecting the null hypothesis when it is in fact false: type II error (β)
Reject	Rejecting the null hypothesis when it is in fact true: type I error (α)	Rejecting the null hypothesis when it is in fact false: correct decision ($1-\beta$)

exists between the variables. In this case all the groups in Geden's study would have similar outcomes.

Statistical procedures for hypothesis testing are based on rules of negative inference. This means that proving that the research hypothesis is correct is not possible; instead, the investigator can only prove that the null hypothesis is incorrect. The decision to accept or reject the null hypothesis is based on a consideration of the likelihood that the observed differences or associations are due to chance.

A chance exists that even when closely following the rules for hypothesis testing, the investigator may make the wrong decision regarding rejection or acceptance of the null hypothesis. Because the data used for hypothesis testing were obtained from a sample of the underlying population, the results obtained from the sample could be different from those for the entire population. Two types of error can occur when testing hypotheses. As seen in Table 26-1, *type I error* occurs when the null hypothesis is true for the population, but the investigator rejects the null hypothesis in favor of the research hypothesis. *Type II error* occurs when the null hypothesis is false for the population, but the investigator accepts the null hypothesis. If in the study of preparation for women in labor (Geden et al., 1985) no differences existed in the outcomes (such as pain level) of any of the treatments, the null hypothesis would have been true for the sample data. If no differences truly existed in the effects of the treatments, and the researchers accepted the null hypothesis, they would have made a correct decision. Had the researchers concluded that differences did exist, they would have made a type I error by rejecting the null hypothesis when it was true. If the researchers found differences between the treatment groups and differences indeed existed between the groups, they might have concluded that the null hypothesis was false. This would have been a correct decision. Had they concluded that the null hypothesis was true when differences actually existed in the treatment groups, they would have made a type II error (see Table 26-1).

Level of significance

Unfortunately investigators do not really know whether they are in error in accepting or rejecting the null hypothesis because knowing the real conditions of the total population is impossible. Nevertheless, the investigator can control the likelihood of committing errors in decision making.

The investigator's choice of a *level of significance*, also referred to as the *alpha level* or *p value*, can control the risk of a type I error. The alpha level is the probability of making a type I error. The investigator commonly chooses to use an alpha level such as 0.05 or 0.01 when testing hypotheses. With an alpha of 0.05 the investigator accepts the risk of making a type I error in 5 of every 100 samples selected from the underlying population. With an alpha level of 0.01 the investigator reduces the likelihood of making a type I error to 1 of 100 samples. An alpha level of 0.05 is common in most social science or behavioral research. When life-threatening consequences are associated with the decision or when the decision has an important impact on health or human welfare, a stricter (smaller) alpha level is more appropriate. Because the consequences of a type I error (e.g., believing an alternative treatment is better than the standard when it is not) are more dangerous than those associated with a type II error (failing to detect small differences), investigators are usually more willing to make a type II error. The investigator chooses the magnitude of error that is acceptable, and the size of the alpha in turn determines the likelihood of rejecting the null hypothesis. When investigators state that the results of a study were *statistically significant*, they are referring to the fact that their results were unlikely to be attributable to chance and at a level of probability (alpha) that they specified for the statistical test.

The investigator also can control the probability of making a type II error. The probability of making a type II error is referred to as beta (β), the failure to reject a null hypothesis when it is in fact false. The probability of making a correct decision to reject the null hypothesis when the null hypothesis is false is referred to as the power of the test and is represented as 1-β. The investigator can increase the power of the test and decrease the chance of type II errors by increasing the sample size. The relationships between power (1-β), alpha, and beta are illustrated in Fig. 26-4.

Investigators need to weigh the consequences of type I versus type II errors for each study. In one instance, missing an important relationship or difference (type II error) may be more important than accepting evidence for relationships that are not reliable (type I error). Contemporary nursing studies

typically test multiple hypotheses. For this reason the investigator faces a complicated task in choosing alpha and beta levels for the study.

As the alpha level becomes smaller the probability of a type I error decreases, and as the beta level becomes smaller the probability of a type II error decreases. Unfortunately, the investigator cannot minimize the probability of both type I and type II errors with a fixed sample size (Fig. 26-5 and Table 26-2). As seen in Fig. 26-5, as the significance level is

TABLE 26-2. **Probabilities for a fixed sample size**

ALPHA	BETA	1-β
0.1	0.3231	0.6769
0.01	0.6593	0.3407
0.001	0.9095	0.0905

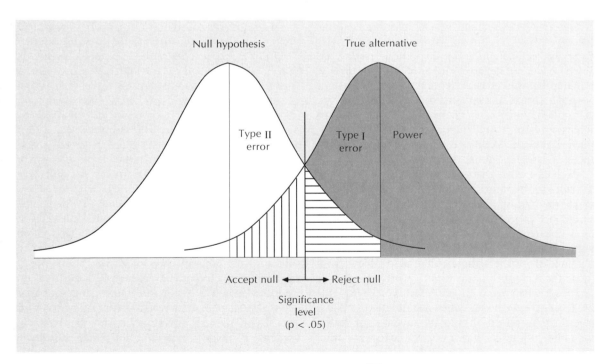

Fig. 26-4. Comparison of type I (α) and type II (β) errors. ▤, The probability of a type I error when the null hypothesis is true but has been rejected; ▥, the area in which the alternative hypothesis is true but the null hypothesis has been accepted.

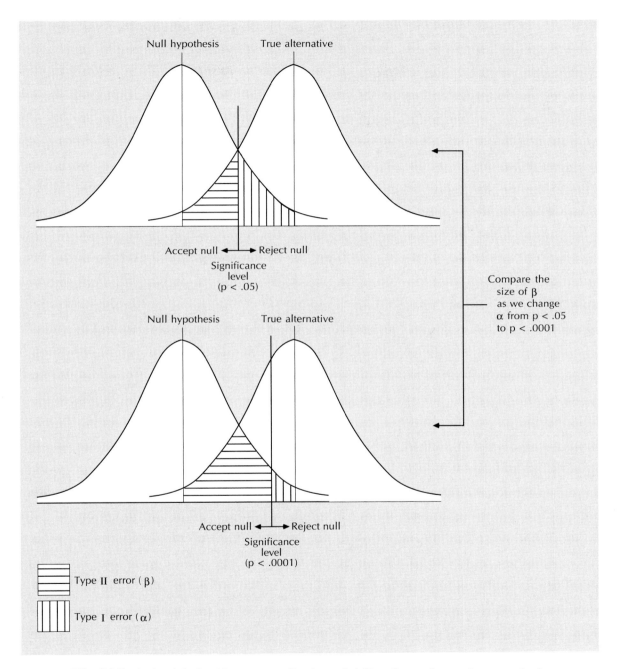

Null hypothesis   True alternative

Accept null ◄——► Reject null
Significance
level
(p < .05)

Compare the
size of β
as we change
α from p < .05
to p < .0001

Null hypothesis   True alternative

Accept null ◄——► Reject null
Significance
level
(p < .0001)

Type II error (β)

Type I error (α)

Fig. 26-5. As the alpha level becomes smaller the probability of a type I error decreases. As the beta level becomes smaller the probability of a type II error decreases. As alpha increases beta decreases.

adjusted from 0.05 to 0.0001, the probability of a type I error decreases, but the probability of a type II error increases. Table 26-2 illustrates the effects of adjusting alpha on beta for a fixed sample size.

The process of statistical hypothesis testing

The following pages will reveal some of the many types of statistical tests that nursing researchers most commonly use. Regardless of whether investigators are testing a hypothesis of difference between groups or a hypothesis of association between two variables, they use some general approaches in testing hypotheses.

Step 1: Checking that the assumptions associated with the statistical test can be met. The first step involved in hypothesis testing is checking whether the assumptions concerning the distribution of the variables being measured can be met with the collected data. The two classes of statistical tests are parametric and nonparametric.

Parametric tests of significance require that the variables being tested are distributed normally in the population, that is, their frequency distributions would resemble the normal curve. Parametric tests involve estimating at least one parameter from a sample for the population. The assumption that the variable is normally distributed in the population can have serious consequences on the accuracy of the test of the hypothesis.

Nonparametric tests are not based on the estimation of a parameter for the underlying population. They do not require normal distribution of the variables. Indeed, nonparametric statistics are also called distribution-free statistics. A simple scattergram should reveal whether the variable is normally distributed.

Step 2: Specifying the null and alternative hypotheses. The next step in testing a hypothesis is to specify the null hypothesis and the alternative hypothesis. The investigator has specified the research hypothesis to be tested in building the plan for the study. At this point the investigator translates the research hypothesis into a statistical hypothesis. The hypothesis that women who had relaxation training would have significantly less pain in labor than those who had instruction about the stages of labor or instruction about breathing techniques could be translated into the following statistical hypotheses:

Null hypothesis: $M_R = M_I, M_B$
Alternative hypothesis: $M_R < M_B, M_I$

where M_R = mean for the relaxation group, M_B = mean for the breathing instruction group, and M_I = mean for the labor instruction group. Translated, the statistical expression of the null hypothesis suggests that the mean pain level for women in all three groups would be the same. The alternative hypothesis suggests that the women in the relaxation group would have less pain than the women in the group who received instructions in the stages of labor or in the group who received instruction in breathing.

Step 3: Specifying the test statistics. In the next step in testing a hypothesis the researcher specifies the test statistic to be used and its distribution under the null hypothesis. Each statistical test is associated with an underlying theoretical distribution that indicates probable and improbable values for the test statistic. This theoretical distribution of values is the basis for finding the point at which the magnitude of the test statistic (as computed on the data from the study) exceeds the values that are likely to occur owing to chance. The theoretical distributions for test statistics are given in most basic statistics texts. Most statistical tests are designed so that the larger the test statistic, the less likely the finding will be due to chance. The test statistic is selected with several criteria in mind: the distribution of the variables studied, the nature of the research question(s), the design used in the study, and the level of measurement used in measuring the variables.

Step 4: Specifying the significance (alpha) level. The next step is to specify the significance (alpha) level. As discussed earlier, the alpha level controls the likelihood of type I error. The smaller the alpha level (or *p* value), the less likely that the null hypothesis will be rejected inappropriately. In other words, compared to an alpha level of 0.05 an alpha level of 0.01 further reduces the likelihood of accepting a finding that was due to chance. When the results of a study have important implications for life and well-being, the investigator selects a stringent alpha level to protect against the likelihood of inappropriately rejecting the null hypothesis.

Step 5: Forming the decision rule. The next step in testing a hypothesis is forming the decision rule for rejecting and not rejecting the null hypothesis. In this step the researcher specifies acceptance and rejection regions for the test. To identify the acceptance and rejection regions for the test, the researcher computes the degrees of freedom, which reflect the size of the samples and the number of samples being tested. The concept of degrees of freedom is used in most tests of statistical significance; the appropriate method for calculating degrees of freedom is specified for each statistical test. *Degrees of freedom* refers to the number of sample values left to vary. For example, if the investigator knows the mean for a distribution, the degrees of freedom would be $n - 1$, as all but one value are free to vary. The investigator uses the information about the degrees of freedom as well as the alpha level to locate the critical value on a table of values for the particular statistical test, such as an *F*, *t*, or chi square table. When the computed test statistic exceeds the critical value, the null hypothesis is rejected.

Step 6: Computing the value of the test statistic. Once the critical value is identified, the investigator computes the value of the test statistic from the data. The calculations of a *t*, *F* or x^2 value for a given sample exemplifies this step.

Step 7: Drawing conclusions about the rejection of the null hypothesis. The final step in hypothesis testing involves drawing conclusions regarding the rejection or the non-rejection of the null hypothesis. When the value of the test statistic exceeds the critical value, the null hypothesis is rejected in favor of the alternative hypothesis.

An example of hypothesis testing is given in the box below.

Example of Hypothesis Testing by Step

Suppose an investigator is studying the difference between men's levels of depression before and after coronary artery bypass grafting. Depression is measured with a scale with scores ranging from 0 to 100. The investigator makes two sets of measurements, one before and one after the operation. The mean score for the premeasures is 52 (SD = 11), and the postmeasure mean is 50 (SD = 10).

Step 1: Check that assumptions associated with statistical tests can be met
The investigator can assume that the distribution of depression in the underlying population is normal and can inspect the distribution of depression scores in the sample by looking at the frequency distribution or a plot of the scores.

Step 2: Specify the null hypothesis and alternative hypothesis
The null hypothesis for the study is that no difference exists between the mean depression scores for men before and after surgery. From the research literature the investigator may propose the hypothesis that depression scores after surgery will be significantly greater than scores before surgery.

Step 3: Specify the test statistic
The appropriate test statistic for this study is a paired *t* test (described in latter part of chapter).

Step 4: Specify the alpha level
The investigator selects an alpha level, in this instance 0.05.

Step 5: Specify the decision rule
The critical value of *t* for which the null hypothesis would be rejected can be checked in a table of the *t* distribution. For the sample size of 100 there are $n - 1$ degrees of freedom, or df = 99. The critical point for a df of 99 and an alpha of 0.05 is $t = 1.660$. Therefore the null hypothesis will be rejected if $t > 1.660$.

Step 6: Compute the test statistic
Calculation of *t* indicates that $t = 1.3$.

Step 7: Draw conclusions about rejection of the null hypothesis
Because *t* is smaller than the critical point, the null hypothesis is not rejected. Therefore the depression scores before and after surgery were not significantly different.

TESTING HYPOTHESIZED DIFFERENCES

Investigators are commonly concerned about testing whether the differences observed between two or more groups or the differences between measures obtained on the same individuals on two or more occasions are statistically significant. When investigators design an experiment to assess the effects of a treatment, such as the effects of a health promotion program on an outcome such as blood pressure, they are interested in determining whether the effect of the program on the outcome was attributable to the program or whether the outcome was simply due to chance. Comparing the outcome for the group or groups that received the health promotion intervention with the outcome for those who received no intervention can be accomplished using tests of difference. In addition, investigators may want to determine whether the changes that occurred in individuals in the treatment group between the premeasure and the postmeasure were statistically significant. In both of these situations tests of difference can be helpful in deciding whether the differences were statistically significant or whether they are of a magnitude that they can be attributed to chance.

Several statistical tests allow investigators to assess group differences. The most commonly used tests that can be applied when assumptions of a normal distribution can be met are the *t* test and analysis of variance. In addition, several nonparametric tests may be applied when distributions do not meet the assumption of normality. Each of these will be discussed, and their use will be illustrated with examples from contemporary nursing research. The computation of the test statistics will not be presented in detail here because such information is readily available in statistical textbooks. Instead, the appropriate application of these tests is emphasized, and references to appropriate statistical texts are included.

The *t* test

Investigators commonly use *t* tests to assess differences between group means. The two types are the *t* test for independent samples and the *t* test for dependent (also referred to as related, paired, or matched) samples. Investigators use the *t* test for independent samples to compare the means obtained from two different samples, such as experimental and control groups or the differences between samples of people who are living with a chronic illness versus those

who are not. They use the *t* test for dependent samples or to compare two measures obtained from the same individuals, for example, the premeasures and postmeasures on the same group of people who were given relaxation training.

The following considerations will help the investigator determine whether the *t* test is appropriate, which form to use, and whether the hypothesis is directional or nondirectional:

1. The *t* test is designed to compare two sets of scores when the dependent variable is measured on an interval or ratio scale.
2. The data should conform with the distribution assumptions for the *t* test; that is, the frequency distribution of the scores should resemble the normal distribution.
3. To use a *t* test for independent samples the means for the two groups should be from two different sets of individuals, not the same individuals.
4. When the scores are from two occasions of measurement on the same individuals and in other cases, for example, the observations are from members of a couple, the investigator should use the paired *t* test.
5. In addition, the investigator should consider whether the hypothesis is directional or nondirectional. When the research hypothesis predicts that one group will have a greater or lesser value for the dependent variable (i.e., the hypothesis is directional), then a one-tailed statistical test can be used. A one-tailed test is sensitive to differences in only one direction. When the researcher does not predict the direction of difference, then a nondirectional test or a two-tailed test is used. When a one-tailed test is used a smaller difference between the means will be statistically significant than would be true if a two-tailed test were used (Fig. 26-6).

t **Tests for independent samples.** When the research question concerns group differences the *t* test for independent samples is an appropriate test.

The following example illustrates the use of a *t* test for two independent samples. Shannahan and Cottrell (1985) compared the effects on mothers of delivering their infants in a birth chair versus the effects of delivering on a traditional delivery table on duration of second-stage labor, fetal outcome, and maternal blood loss. These investigators used a *t* test for independent samples to compare the hemoglobin

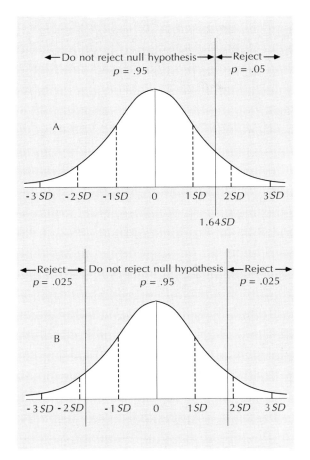

Fig. 26-6. One-tailed (**A**) versus two-tailed (**B**) tests. Notice that with a one-tailed test (directional hypothesis) the critical value for the test statistic is different from the critical values for a two-tailed (nondirectional) test.

TABLE 26-3. Admission and postdelivery hemoglobin and hematocrit values

GROUP	HEMOGLOBIN (grams)	HEMATOCRIT
ADMISSION		
Delivery table	12.8	37.7%
Birth chair	13.3	39.5%
	($t = -2.27$,	($t = -2/37$,
	df = 58,	df = 58,
	$p = 0.27$)	$p = 0.022$)
POSTDELIVERY		
Delivery table	12.1	36.0%
Birth chair	11.3	33.7%
	($t = -2.27$,	($t = 2.37$,
	df = 58,	df = 58,
	$p = 0.027$)	$p = 0.022$)

Data from Shannahan, M., and Cottrell, B. (1985). *Nursing Research*, 34, 89-92.

The *t* test statistic for independent samples tests the null hypothesis that no significant differences exist between sample means:

$$H_0: M_A = M_B$$

$$H_A: M_A \neq M_B$$

where M = mean values, A = group 1, and B = group 2. Computation of the *t* test for independent samples involves subtracting the mean of one group from the mean of another and then dividing the mean difference by a value that reflects the variability of the two groups. The computational formula for the *t* test for independent samples follows:

$$t = \frac{\overline{X}_A - \overline{X}_B}{\sqrt{\frac{\Sigma X_A^2 + \Sigma X_B^2}{n_A + n_B - 2}\left(\frac{1}{n_A} + \frac{1}{n_B}\right)}}$$

where $\overline{X}_A$ = mean for group A, $\overline{X}_B$ = mean for group B, ΣX_A^2 = sum of the group A deviation scores squared, ΣX_B^2 = sum of the group B deviation scores squared, n_A = number in group A, and n_B = number in group B. The calculated value for *t* is compared to the theoretical distribution for the *t* statistic. The alpha level and the degrees of freedom determine the critical value of *t* to be used in deciding whether or not to reject the null hypothesis. The

and hematocrit values for the two samples of women. They found that, although the women who delivered their babies in the birth chair had significantly higher hemoglobin and hematocrit values before delivery, they had significantly lower hematocrit values after delivery. The means for hemoglobin and hematocrit and the *t* test results are given in Table 26-3. Because the investigators predicted, before they collected the data, the greater blood loss for the women in the birth chair, they appropriately used a one-tailed test.

degrees of freedom associated with the t test for independent samples is computed by

$$df = n_A + n_B - 2$$

We can apply this information to the Shannahan and Cottrell (1985) example. In the study 30 women delivered in the birth chair (BC) group and 30 women delivered on the delivery table (DT) group; therefore df = 58. Comparing the hemoglobin values obtained after delivery for the DT and the BC groups, Shannahan and Cottrell found that women in the BC group had lower hemoglobin levels (11.3) than those in the DT group (12.1). The calculated value of the t statistic was 2.27. Using an alpha 0.05 and df = 58 and consulting a table for the distribution of the t statistic, we find that a value of t larger than 2 is sufficient to reject the null hypothesis. The investigators appropriately conclude that the differences in hemoglobin levels with the use of the birth chair and the delivery table are significant, with the greater blood loss occurring with the use of the birth chair.

Using the t test for independent samples requires the investigator to inspect the variances of the two samples. When the variances of the samples are sim-

ilar the investigator can assume homogeneity of variances and uses the formula given above. When the variances of the two samples are not homogeneous, the investigator must use a different denominator than that given. (For a description of alternate formulas refer to Blalock [1982] and Bruning & Kintz [1977].)

t Tests for paired samples. In some studies the investigator is concerned with assessing the difference between measures made on two occasions on the same individuals. In other instances the measures made on two individuals such as members of a couple may be considered as related or matched measures. The t test for paired or matched samples is appropriate for these situations, and the t test for independent samples is inappropriate.

In a study of parental network structure and perceived support after the birth of a first child, Cronenwett (1985) investigated the differences in men's and women's network size, density, contact with preschool children, coworker contact, friend contact, emotional support, and informational support from antepartum to 8 months postpartum. Her findings are given in Table 26-4.

Men's networks decreased significantly in size,

TABLE 26-4. Changes in social network structure after birth of a first child

NETWORK CHARACTERISTICS	PARENTAL GENDER	n	FREQUENCY OR PERCENT		PAIRED t	p
			ANTE PARTUM	8 MONTHS POST PARTUM		
Size	M	31	9.1	7.4	4.32	0.0002
	F	38	8.5	7.9	1.37	NS
Density (%)	M	31	27.1	39.3	−2.42	0.02
	F	31	28.2	35.7	−1.41	NS
Preschool children (%)	M	31	17.2	32.4	−4.29	0.0002
	F	38	17.6	36.1	−7.08	<0.00001
Coworker contact (frequency)	M	31	4.3	3.4	1.09	NS
	F	38	2.6	0.9	3.13	0.003
Friend contact (frequency)	M	31	1.9	1.7	0.26	NS
	F	38	2.4	3.8	−2.06	0.047
Emotional support (%)	M	31	74.9	85.8	−2.17	0.038
	F	38	91.2	89.3	0.73	NS
Informational support (%)	M	31	53.4	62.3	−1.50	NS
	F	38	50.5	68.9	−3.75	0.0006

From Cronenwett, L. (1985). Reprinted with permission from *Nursing Research, 34,* 347-353. ©, 1985, American Journal of Nursing Company.

and density of overlap of the men's network with the women's network increased. Moreover, men perceived that they were receiving emotional support from a higher percent of their network post partum than they had ante partum. Both the men's and women's networks had an increase in the number of members with preschool children. Women experienced a significant decrease in contact with coworkers but an increase in contact with friends. In addition, women's postpartum networks included a higher percentage of members providing informational support. The hypotheses tested with the paired *t* test were:

$$H_0: M_A = M_B$$

$$H_A: M_A \neq M_B$$

where M = the mean, A = antepartum measure, B = postpartum measure, and H_0 = null hypothesis. The *t* statistic for paired measures is computed with the following formula:

$$t = \frac{\overline{D}_{a\text{-}b}}{\sqrt{\dfrac{\Sigma d^2}{n(n = 1)}}}$$

where $\overline{D}_{a\text{-}b}$ = the mean differences between the paired scores, d = the deviation scores for the difference measure, Σd^2 = sum of the squared deviation scores, and *n* = number of pairs. The *t* distribution is used to identify critical values of *t*, but when a paired *t* test is used the degrees of freedom reflect the number of pairs rather than the number of individuals and are calculated as

$$df = n - 1$$

where *n* is the number of pairs.

Other tests of difference

Median test. When investigators find that their data do not meet the assumptions for using the *t* test (as, for example, when the size of the groups is small, the distribution is not normal, or measures are not of at least interval level), they may find several alternative tests appropriate. The median test allows comparison of the medians from two independent groups and is based on the calculation of the deviations from the median instead of from the mean. The *median test* assesses the null hypothesis that the two groups being compared come from populations having different medians. To test the hypothesis of no

difference between medians, a median is obtained for both groups combined. Next, the individual scores in both groups are divided into those above and those below the median for the combined group. If the medians of both groups were the same, we would expect to see an equal number of observations above and below the median in the combined group. The *p* value associated with the median test indicates the probability that whatever discrepancies are observed between the two groups could have occurred under the null hypothesis.

Mann Whitney U test. The *Mann Whitney U test* tests the hypothesis that the two independent groups come from populations having different distributions rather than merely different medians. The scores for both groups are ranked together, and each is labeled as coming from one of the two groups. Next, U is calculated. U is merely the total number of times that scores for group 1 preceded the scores for group 2. The *p* value associated with the Mann Whitney U test indicates the probability that a value of U of this size or smaller could occur under the null hypothesis.

Sign test. When the data are paired but do not meet the assumptions for the paired *t* test, the sign test may be used. The *sign test* involves assigning a plus or a minus sign to the differences between a pair of scores. For example, an investigator comparing preexercise and postexercise depression scores of people with arthritis would assign a + to the higher scores of people each pre-post pair of scores. The number of plus pairs is then calculated and compared to the total number of pairs. The *p* value associated with the sign test is the likelihood that the proportion of positive results would have occurred under the null hypothesis. The *Wilcoxon signed rank test* is a similar test but involves calculating the arithmetical difference between paired scores and then ranking the differences.

In general, use of nonparametric tests of difference involves minimal assumptions about the underlying distributions of the variables being tested. These tests are relatively easy to compute by hand. On the other hand, they tend to be less sensitive, partly because they disregard the scale of measurement, and some involve assignment of ranks or a nominal value to the numerical score. Finally, these tests are not designed for estimating a parameter for the underlying population as is the case with the *t* test.

Analysis of variance

Analysis of variance (ANOVA) is an inferential statistical test used to test the significance of differences between the means of two or more groups. (Investigators could use a *t* test or ANOVA for two groups and obtain exactly the same *p* value with either test.) The statistic computed as part of the ANOVA procedure is the *F* ratio, which is tested against a table of the theoretical distribution of *F*.

ANOVA helps the investigator ascertain the sources of differences in scores obtained from individuals within two or more groups. ANOVA decomposes the total variance in the dependent variable into two components: the variability resulting from one or more independent variables and the variance from all other sources such as individual differences, measurement error, and so on.

All the many different varieties of ANOVA employ the *F* ratio. The *F ratio* is obtained by contrasting variation between groups with variation within groups. When the difference between groups is large relative to the difference within groups, the difference in scores is likely to be due to the effect of the group (such as a treatment group effect) rather than to random fluctuation. The variability between groups is reflected in a calculation of the sum of squares between groups, abbreviated SS_b. SS_b is the sum of squared deviations of individual group means from the overall mean for all the data. SS_b reflects variability attributable to the groups rather than to individual differences. The variability resulting from individual differences and measurement error is reflected in the sum of squares within groups, SS_w. SS_w is the sum of squared deviations of individual scores from their own group means.

The mean square between groups (MS_b) is calculated by

$$\frac{SS_b}{df_b}$$

where $df_b = k - 1$ and k is the number of groups. The mean square within groups (MS_w) is calculated by

$$\frac{SS_w}{df_w}$$

where $df_w = (n_1 - 1) + (n_2 - 1) + \ldots (nk - 1)$. The *F* ratio is then obtained by dividing MS_b by MS_w:

$$F = \frac{MS_b}{MS_w}$$

The *F* statistic is compared with the tabled values of the theoretical *F* distribution by use of the specified *p* value and the df_b and df_w to locate the critical value.

Single-factor analysis of variance. As an example of a single-factor ANOVA let us turn to the analysis of data from a study of patient self-disclosure among individuals with hypertension, diabetes, and no known chronic illnesses. Dawson (1985) hypothesized that hypertensive patients would attribute less importance to self-disclosure to clinicians than would diabetics or non-chronically ill patients. In Dawson's design the factor (independent variable) was the type of disease the patient had. The factor had four levels: hypertensive patients, diabetics, individuals without chronic illness who had male health-care providers (control 1), and individuals without chronic illness who had female health-care providers (control 2). Table 26-5 gives means and standard deviations for the importance of disclosure related to responses to health care. Dawson found a significant difference between the groups in their ratings of the importance of self-disclosure. Using a one-way ANOVA Dawson found that the *F* statistic was 3.26 with 3 and 214 degrees of freedom. The associated *p* value was 0.02. These findings indicate that the difference between the patient groups was statistically significant, but they do not tell us which groups differed. Contrasting the groups with another statistical

TABLE 26-5. Average scores for importance of self-disclosure regarding responses to health care*

	n	M	SD
Hypertensive patients	54	43.56	4.58
Diabetics	47	39.36	10.01
Control 1	65	42.03	6.06
Control 2	50	42.10	5.97
Total sample	216	41.85	6.92

Data from Dawson, C. (1985). *Research in Nursing and Health, 8,* 191-198.

*F = 3.26; df = 3, 214; *p* < .002.

test (a test for the hypothesized contrasts, which will be discussed in greater detail in a later section of this chapter), Dawson found that the hypertensive patients attributed greater importance to disclosing responses to health-care clinicians than did the diabetics.

As we have seen with Dawson's use of a single-factor ANOVA, ANOVA indicates whether or not a significant difference exists between the groups but does not tell us which groups differ. Determining which groups' scores differ significantly requires the use of additional tests, referred to as a priori contrasts, post hoc contrasts, or multiple comparison tests, to determine exactly where the differences lie. Dawson used a *t* test to test her a priori hypothesis that the hypertensive patients would attribute less importance to the responses to health care by clinicians than would diabetics. She found that, contrary to her expectations, the hypertensive patients attributed greater importance to responses to health care by clinicians than did the diabetics.

Although simply using a *t* test to test for differences between every pair of groups might seem logical, when multiple tests of significance are used with the same data, the likelihood exists that some significant results will be due simply to chance. To guard against this, some statisticians recommend using a correction formula, termed the Bonferroni correction, to alter the *p* value associated with the tests:

$$\frac{p}{n}$$

where *p* = the alpha level and *n* = the number of tests. This formula gives a *p* value corrected for the number of tests.

Several post hoc tests or multiple comparison tests can be used to detect where significant differences lie. Their advantage is that they adjust the level of significance to decrease the influence of chance that occurs with more than one comparison. Liberal tests, such as Fisher's exact test, detect small mean differences, whereas conservative tests (for example, the Scheffé and Tukey tests) work when the means are far apart. For a more detailed discussion of post hoc comparisons see Holm and Christman (1985), Hays (1981), and Blalock (1982). Table 26-6 lists some of the more commonly used post hoc comparison tests in order of decreasing power, with the Fisher least significant difference test being the most

TABLE 26-6. Commonly used post hoc comparison tests

TEST	COMPARISON
Fisher least significant difference	All pairwise comparisons tested
Duncan	All pairwise comparisons of ordered means tested
Newman-Keuls	Comparisons or ordered means tested
Tukey honestly significant difference	All pairwise comparisons tested
Dunnett	All means compared with control mean
Scheffé	All pairwise comparisons and complex comparisons tested

From Holm, K, & Christman, N. (1985). *Research in Nursing and Health, 8,* 207-210.

powerful and Scheffé's test being the most conservative.

Multiple-factor analysis of variance. In the example in Table 26-5 ANOVA was applied to the influence of a single factor on an outcome variable. The focus was the influence of patient group on ratings of the importance of self-disclosure to a clinician about the responses to treatment. Because this problem dealt with the effects of a single factor, it was termed a one-way ANOVA, or single-factor ANOVA. Investigators are commonly concerned with more than one factor and their individual and joint effects on a dependent variable. This kind of problem requires the use of a more complex statistical procedure termed *multifactor analysis of variance.* Multifactor ANOVA helps researchers determine the influence of two or more factors on a dependent variable.

An example in which multifactor ANOVA was used to examine the effects of several factors is the study by Winslow, Lane, and Gaffney (1985), who were concerned with the physiological responses before, during, and after three types of baths among individuals who were recovering from myocardial infarction. They designed an experiment in which 18 male and female patients who had experienced

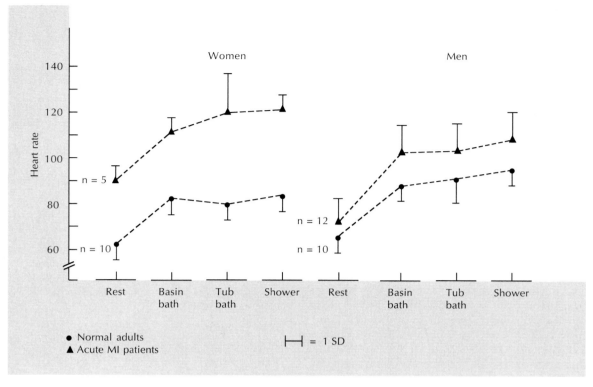

Fig. 26-7. Mean heart rate during rest and mean peak heart rate during basin bath, tub bath, and shower in normal adults and acute myocardial infarction patients.

TABLE 26-7. Analyses of variance for heart rate (beats per minute) during rest and peak heart rate during basin bath, tub bath, and shower

SOURCE	SS*	df	F	p
Group	8129.20	1	22.04	0.0001
Sex	0.51	1	0.00	0.9704
Group by sex	3729.16	1	10.11	0.0030
Error: Subject within group by sex	13277.62	36		
Type	18638.10	3	106.20	0.0001
Group by type	187.17	3	1.07	0.3677
Sex by type	144.74	3	0.82	0.4859
Group by sex by type	306.69	3	1.75	0.1606
Error	5791.76	99		

From Winslow, E., Lane, L., and Gaffney, F. (1985). Reprinted with permission from *Nursing Research, 34,* 164-169.
©, 1985, American Journal of Nursing Company.
*SS = sum of squares.

infarction 5 to 17 days previously had their vital signs measured after they had rested for 10 minutes and after they took one type of bath (basin bath, tub bath, or shower) on each of the next 3 days. A comparison group of 22 individuals who had not had a myocardial infarction participated in the same experiences. The order in which the patients and controls took the three types of baths was randomized. Pulse rates were measured at two points: midway through the bath and when the bath was completed.

The investigators used a three-way ANOVA (group × sex × activity type) with repeated measures over one factor (activity type). There were two levels of the group factor (controls and patients), two levels of the sex factor (male and female), and four levels of the activity type factor (rest, basin bath, tub bath, and shower).

The ANOVA data given in Fig. 26-7 and Table 26-7 show the statistically significant effects of the group (cardiac vs. noncardiac), a significant group by sex interaction, and significant effects of rest and type of bath (basin, tub, or shower). Fig. 26-7 shows the heart rates for the patients were higher than those for the controls, but the heart rates for women with cardiac disease were higher than those for men with cardiac disease. The figure also shows that the type of bath was associated with different levels of heart rate.

This example illustrates two kinds of effects that can be studied with multifactor ANOVA: main effects and interaction effects. Main effects refer to the effects of a single factor, for example, the effects of being in the patient group or in the control group. Interaction effects refer to the joint effects of two factors, in particular to whether the effect of one factor is consistent over all levels of another individual factor. In the study of bathing the investigators found a significant interaction effect for group by

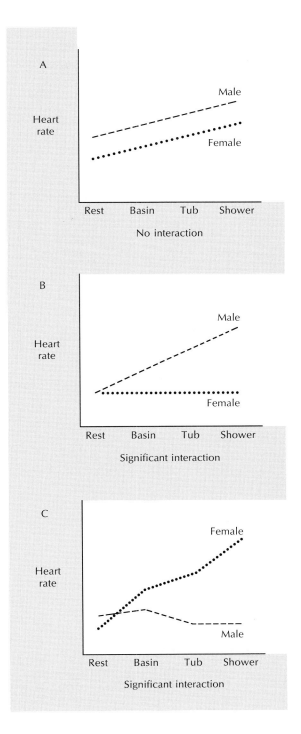

Fig. 26-8. Hypothetical examples of interaction effects. **A,** No interaction: heart rate increases from rest to basin bath, tub bath, and shower both for men and women. Type of bath has the same effect for both men and women. **B** and **C,** Significant interactions: heart rate changes at a different rate for men and women across bathing conditions.

sex. This means that the effects of group (patient or control) on heart rate differed across levels of sex (male or female). In other words, the influence on heart rate of having had a myocardial infarction was different for males than for females. Some other hypothetical examples of interactions are graphed in Fig. 26-8.

Interaction effects may suppress or enhance individual effects on the dependent variables. In cases of disordinal interactions, effects are fully crossed, meaning that the lines drawn across levels of both factors cross (see Fig. 26-8). In cases of ordinal interactions, the rank order of one factor remains the same across treatments, but the effect is different across groups. Because of floor and ceiling effects associated with the measures used in a study, interactions are difficult to interpret. That is, it is difficult to know whether the interaction is a function of lack of sensitivity of measurement rather than a true joint effect. Interactions that are fully crossed most likely are true interactions (Neale & Liebert, 1986).

With multifactor ANOVA the investigator tests multiple hypotheses: hypotheses related to each of the main effects and to the interaction effects. Winslow, Lane, and Gaffney tested for each of the main effects (group, sex, and type) and for all possible interactions (group by sex, group by type, sex by type, and group by sex by type).

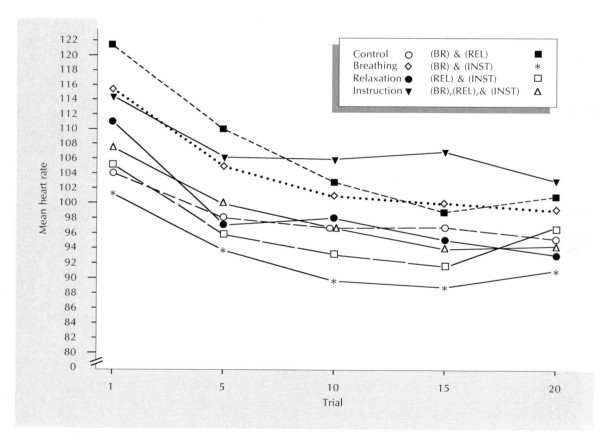

Fig. 26-9. Mean heart rate per stimulus exposure across trials (N = 80). Note that heart rate tends to decrease across trials for almost every group. Analysis of variance for repeated measures revealed a significant effect of trials. (From Geden, E. et al. [1985]. *Research in Nursing and Health, 8,* 155-166.)

Repeated measures. Occasionally investigators are concerned about the effects of a series of measures made on individuals in a study. In the study by Geden et al. (1985) of the effects of several components of the Lamaze method for preparing women for labor, a series of 20 measures of pain, heart rate, and frontalis electromyography were made. To determine whether these values changed over time, the investigators used repeated-measures ANOVA. This form of ANOVA tests for a significant effect of the number of trials. A significant effect indicates that significant variability exists across trials. As with other types of ANOVA a priori (planned) as well as post hoc comparisons can be done to determine at which points in the trials the significant differences occur. As seen in Fig. 26-9 heart rate tends to decrease across trials regardless of the treatment group of the participants.

Nonparametric tests. In addition to parametric tests some nonparametric tests can be used to analyze the effects of multiple factors. The *Kruskal Wallis test* is performed with ordinal data and is based on the assignment of ranks to the scores for the various groups. The *Friedman test* can be used when several measures are obtained from a single sample or when the investigator has studied paired groups. For more information about these tests consult Siegel (1956), Hays (1981), Daniel (1978), or Connover (1971).

Table 26-8 summarizes appropriate tests of hypotheses of difference according to sampling and level of measurement of the dependent variable. Note that a variety of parametric and nonparametric tests exist to achieve the purposes of testing for difference.

TESTING ASSOCIATIONS

An investigator may be concerned with the extent to which one variable is associated with another variable. For example, evidence from many nursing studies indicates that the level of social support is associated with the experience of illness and complications of pregnancy. Many studies link the exposure to stressful life events to illness. The two most common ways of assessing association between two variables is by using the chi square test and correlation coefficients.

The chi square test

The chi square statistic is used to test hypotheses about the association between variables that can be (or are) divided into categories (nominal or categorical variables). The variables being tested are crossed in a contingency table. Then the chi square statistic is used to test the hypothesis that the observed frequencies (given in the contingency table) are not different from the frequencies to be expected if no asso-

TABLE 26-8. Appropriate tests of hypotheses of difference according to sampling and level of measurement of dependent variable

SAMPLE	PURPOSE	NOMINAL	ORDINAL	INTERVAL
Paired observations from one sample	Test differences in proportions	McNemar's test	Wilcoxin signed rank test	
	Test differences in ranks		Friedman test	
	Test differences in means			Paired *t* test
Two independent samples	Test differences in medians		Median test	
	Test differences in means			*t* Test ANOVA
	Test differences in ranks of scores		Mann Whitney U test, Kruskal Wallis test	
	Test differences in proportions	Chi square test		

TABLE 26-9. The relationship between parents' reports of impact on family life and outside help

	PARENTS' REPORTS		
	NEUTRAL	NEGATIVE	TOTAL
OUTSIDE HELP			
No*	18	7	25
Yes**	16	21	37

From Knafl, K. (1985). *Western Journal of Nursing Research, 7*, 151-167. Copyright © 1985. Reprinted by permission of Sage Publications, Inc.
*Includes cases from "alone" category.
**Combines cases from "some help" and "delegation" categories.
$p < 0.05$ by chi square test.

ciation existed between the variables. The chi square test assesses whether the two variables are independent of one another.

Let us consider an example. Knafl (1985) studied how families manage a hospitalization of a child. One of the relationships she explored was the association between parents' reports of having outside help to manage the hospitalization and their judgments of the impact on the family. She found that proportionately more of the families who received outside help were likely to view the hospitalization as negative and disruptive of the family than were parents who managed the hospitalization alone. The data in Table 26-9 produced a satistically significant ($p<0.05$) chi square statistic.

The chi square statistic is computed by comparing two sets of frequencies: those that were observed and those that would be expected under conditions of no association. Expected frequencies are calculated so that

$$f_E = \frac{f_R\, f_C}{N}$$

where f_E = expected frequency for a cell in the table, f_R = observed frequency for the row, f_C = observed frequency for the column, and N = the total number of participants in the study. The chi square statistic is computed from the formula:

$$\chi^2 = \frac{\Sigma(f_o - f_E)^2}{f_E}$$

where f_o = observed frequency for a cell and f_E = expected frequency for a cell. The chi square statistic is compared to a table of values with df = $(R - 1)$ $(C - 1)$, where R = number of rows and C = number of columns in the contingency table.

Appropriate use of the chi square statistic depends on meeting several requirements. All observations should be independent. Therefore the data from a pretest and a posttest given to the same subjects cannot be analyzed by means of the chi square test of independence. In this case McNemar's (1969) test for matched samples would be appropriate. Given that the observations are independent the expected frequency in any cell cannot be 0. In addition, expected frequencies of less than 1 can never occur in more than 20% of the cells.

Correlation coefficients

Chapter 25 discussed the use of the Pearson correlation coefficient as a descriptive measure and interpretation of its direction and strength. Used inferentially, the Pearson correlation coefficient also can be used to test hypotheses concerning relationships in the population when variables are assumed to be of at least interval level of measurement. The usual hypothesis is:

$$H_o: \rho = 0$$

where ρ = the population parameter rho and H_o = null hypothesis.

Uphold and Sussman (1985) were concerned about the relationships between the roles women enacted and their experiences of menopausal symptoms. The investigators used a Pearson product-moment correlation coefficient (also called Pearson's r) to assess the strength and direction of the relationships between variables related to women's roles and the number and severity of menopausal symptoms. As seen in Table 26-10 only marital adjustment was related significantly and negatively to the number and severity of menopausal symptoms. This means that women who had the best marital adjustment had the fewest and least severe symptoms. Pearson's r is calculated by the computational formula

$$r_{xy} = \frac{\Sigma_{xy}}{nS_xS_y}$$

where y = deviation scores for y, x = deviation scores for x, xy = the products of the deviation scores, S_x = the standard deviation of x, S_y = the

TABLE 26-10. Relationship between women's roles and menopausal symptoms—Pearson's *r* (*N* = 185)

	NUMBER OF SYMPTOMS	SEVERITY OF SYMPTOMS
Work hours	0.03	0.03
Marital adjustment	−0.29*	−0.37*
Maternal obligation	0.08	0.11
Number of children	0.04	0.02

Data from Uphold, C., & Sussman, E. (1985). *Research in Nursing and Health, 8,* 73-82.
*$p < 0.05$.

TABLE 26-11. Example of ranking system for which Spearman's rho may be computed

PARTICIPANT	EDUCATION	HEALTH RATING
1	6 (8)	100 (9.5)
2	4 (5.5)	90 (8)
3	1 (1)	10 (2)
4	5 (6)	70 (7)
5	2 (2.5)	30 (4.5)
6	6 (8)	10 (2)
7	3 (4)	30 (4.5)
8	2 (2.5)	10 (2)
9	6 (8)	100 (9.5)
10	4 (5.5)	40 (6)

standard deviation of y, and *n* = the number of participants in the study. The value for Pearson's *r* is then compared to a table of the theoretical distribution of *r* with df = n − 2.

Because Pearson's *r* is a parametric statistic, when the assumptions of normality cannot be met or when one or more of the variables is ordinal, then Spearman's rho, Kendall's tau, or gamma is a more appropriate correlation coefficient.

Spearman's rho, Kendall's tau, and gamma are each computed from rankings rather than the raw data value for each variable. *Spearman's rho* is computed by ranking individuals' scores on each variable. Consider a study of education and health in which individuals were given a measure of educational

attainment and then given a health rating based on a physical examination and a questionnaire. Suppose the ratings for the two variables for 10 participants are those given in Table 26-11. Each participant would be assigned a rank for each variable as seen in the numbers in parentheses. Where two or more individuals were tied for a rank, the rank would be computed by assigning the median of the ranks they would have received if they had not been tied. The difference in ranks for each pair is then computed, and the sum of the squared differences is calculated. The formula for rho is:

$$\rho = 1 - \frac{6\Sigma D^2}{n(n^2 - 1)}$$

where 6 = a constant always used in the formula, D = difference between ranks for each pair, D^2 = squared difference between ranks, ΣD^2 = sum of squared differences between ranks, and *n* = number of pairs.

Kendall's tau and *gamma* both use information regarding the ordering of categories of variables by comparing every possible pair of cases. The easiest way to understand the computation of both is to consider a contingency table for two variables (Table 26-12). Suppose variable 1 is education and variable 2 is health. Each pair of cases is checked to determine (1) if its relative ordering on the first variable is the same (concordant) as its relative ordering on the second variable or (2) if the ordering is reversed (discordant). Suppose person 1 has low education and poor health, whereas person 2 has high education and excellent health. The rating for this pair (persons 1 and 2) would be concordant; both are low or high on both variables. Suppose person 1 has low education and poor health, whereas person 3 has low education and excellent health. The rating for this pair (persons 1 and 3) would be discordant. The first step in computing both gamma and tau involves computing the number of concordant (P) pairs and the number of discordant (Q) pairs. If P > Q then the statistic will be positive, indicating that a relationship exists between the two variables. The computational formula for gamma is quite simple:

$$\gamma = \frac{P - Q}{P + Q}$$

Gamma takes a positive value when concordant pairs predominate and a negative value when discordant pairs predominate.

TABLE 26-12. Contingency table for two variables (education and health)

		HEALTH		
		POOR	FAIR	EXCELLENT
EDUCATION	Low			
	High			

TABLE 26-13. Tests of association according to level of measurement

LEVEL OF MEASUREMENT—VARIABLE 1	LEVEL OF MEASUREMENT—VARIABLE 2		
	NOMINAL	ORDINAL	INTERVAL
Nominal	Chi square	Kendall's tau	Kendall's tau Pearson's r if nominal variable takes values of 0, 1
Ordinal	Kendall's tau	Spearman's rho Kendall's tau Gamma	Spearman's rho Kendall's tau Gamma
Interval	Kendall's tau Pearson's r if nominal variable takes values of 0, 1	Spearman's rho Kendall's tau Gamma	Pearson's r

Kendall's tau takes ties into account and has a more complex computational formula; tau b is more appropriate with tables in which the number of rows equals the number of columns, whereas tau c is more appropriate with asymmetrical tables. The computational formula for tau b is

$$\tau_b = \frac{P - Q}{[\frac{1}{2}(N^2 - \Sigma T_1^2)\frac{1}{2}(N^2 - \Sigma T_2^2)]^{1/2}}$$

where P = number of concordant pairs, Q = number of discordant pairs, N = number of pairs, T_1 = number of ties in row variables, and T_2 = number of ties in column variables.

There are many options for testing hypotheses of association. Appropriate tests of association according to level of measurement are given in Table 26-13.

SUMMARY

Inferential statistics enable investigators to make inferences from a sample to a larger population. Inferences may involve estimating a population parameter from a sample or testing hypotheses. Hypothesis testing involves seven steps: deciding whether to use parametric or nonparametric tests; specifying the null and alternative hypotheses; specifying the test statistic; specifying the significance (alpha) level; forming the decision rule regarding whether or not to reject the null hypothesis; computing the value of the test statistic; and drawing conclusions about the results. Hypothesis testing can be applied to test differences between groups or across occasions or to test associations between two or more variables. There are many statistics available for testing hypotheses of difference: t test for independent samples, *t* test for paired samples, median test, Mann Whitney U test, the sign test, and several variations of ANOVA (see Table 26-8). Likewise, there are many statistical tests available for testing associations: the chi square test and correlation coefficients, including Pearson's *r*, Kendall's tau, and Spearman's rho (see Table 26-13).

REFERENCES

Blalock, H. (1982). *Social statistics*. New York: McGraw-Hill.

Bruning, J., & Kintz, B. (1977). *Computational handbook of statistics*. Glenview, IL: Scott, Foresman.

Burckhardt, C. S. (1982). The measurement of change in nursing research: Statistical considerations. *Nursing Research, 31*(1), 63-65.

Burkhardt, C. S., Goodwin, L. D., & Prescott, P. A. (1982). The measurement of change in nursing research: Statistical considerations. *Nursing Research, 31*, 53-55.

Cohen, J. (1977). *Statistical power analysis for the behavioral sciences*. New York: Academic Press.

Conover, W. (1971). *Practical nonparametric statistics*. New York: Wiley.

Cronenwett, L. (1985). Parental network structure and perceived support after birth of first child. *Nursing Research, 34*, 347-353.

Cronbach, L. J., & Furby, L. (1970). How we should measure "change"—or should we? *Psychological Bulletin, 74*, 68-80.

Daniel, W. (1978). *Applied nonparametric statistics*. Boston: Houghton-Mifflin.

Dawson, C. (1985). Hypertension, perceived clinician empathy, and patient self disclosure. *Research in Nursing and Health, 8*, 191-198.

Edwards, A. (1976). *An introduction to linear regression and correlation*. San Francisco: W. H. Freeman.

Egger, M. J. (1983). Testing for experimental effects in the pretest-posttest design. *Methodology Corner, 5*, 306-312.

Everitt, B. (1977). *The analysis of contingency tables*. New York: Wiley.

Feldman, M. J. (1983). Evaluating change using noninterval data. *Nursing Research, 33*(3), 182-184.

Geden, E., Beck, N., Brouder, G., Glaister, J., & Pohlman, S. (1985). Self-report and psychophysiological effects of lamaze preparation: An analogue of labor pain. *Research in Nursing and Health, 8*, 155-166.

Hartwig, F., & Dearing, B. (1979). *Exploratory data analysis*. Beverly Hills, CA: Sage.

Hays, W. (1981). *Statistics for the social sciences*. New York: Holt, Rinehart, & Winston.

Henkel, R. (1976). *Tests of significance*. Beverly Hills, CA: Sage.

Holm, K., & Christman, N. (1985). Post hoc tests following analysis of variance. *Research in Nursing and Health, 8*, 207-210.

Huck, S., Cormier, W., & Bounds, W. (1974). *Reading statistics and research*. New York: Harper & Row.

Huck, S. W., & McLean, R. A. (1975). Using a repeated measures ANOVA to analyze the data from a pretest-posttest design: A potentially confusing task. *Psychological Bulletin, 82*, 511-518.

Kerlinger, F. N. (1986). *Foundations of behavioral research* (pp. 230-250). New York: Holt, Rinehart & Winston.

Knafl, K. (1985). How families manage a pediatric hospitalization. *Western Journal of Nursing Research, 7*, 151-167.

Kviz, F., & Knafl, K. (1980). *Statistics for nurses: An introductory text*. Boston: Little, Brown, & Co.

Loftus, G. R. (1978). On interpretation of interactions. *Memory and Cognition, 6*(3), 312-319.

McNemar, Q. (1969). *Psychological statistics*. New York: Wiley.

Neale, J., & Liebert, R. (1986). *Science and behavior: An introduction to methods of research*. Englewood Cliffs, NJ: Prentice-Hall.

Pedhazur, E. J. (1982). *Multiple regression in behavioral research*. New York: Holt, Rinehart & Winston.

Shannahan, M., & Cottrell, B. (1985). Effect of the birth chair on second stage labor duration, fetal outcome, and maternal blood loss. *Nursing Research, 34*, 89-92.

Siegel, S. (1956). *Nonparametric statistics for the behavioral sciences*. New York: McGraw-Hill.

Uphold, C., & Sussman, E. (1985). Child-rearing, marital, recreational and work role integration and climacteric symptoms in midlife women. *Research in Nursing and Health, 8*, 73-82.

Waltz, C., & Bausell, R. (1981). *Nursing research: Design, statistics and computer analysis*. Philadelphia: F. A. Davis.

Weiner, E. E., & Weiner, D. L. (1983). Understanding the use of basic statistics in nursing research. *American Journal of Nursing, 83*(5), 770-774.

Willemson, E. (1974). *Understanding statistical reasoning*. San Francisco: W. H. Freeman.

Williams, F. (1979). *Reasoning with statistics*. New York: Holt, Rinehart, & Winston.

Winer, B. (1971). *Statistical principles in experimental design*. New York: McGraw-Hill.

Winslow, E., Lane, L., & Gaffney, F. (1985). Oxygen uptake and cardiovascular responses in control adults and acute myocardial infarction patients during bathing. *Nursing Research, 34*, 164-169.

27

USING ADVANCED STATISTICAL PROCEDURES

NANCY FUGATE WOODS

Nurses study complex phenomena. As we have seen, our understanding of how individuals and families experience health-related phenomena, the interrelationship between human health and the environment, and the influence of nursing therapies on human health requires consideration of multiple dimensions of the concepts being studied and conceptual frameworks that address multiple concepts. Because of the complexity of the phenomena being studied, nurses' use of sophisticated statistical techniques has increased. These techniques allow investigators to consider multiple concepts or multiple dimensions of concepts simultaneously. *Multivariate statistical procedures* are designed to help the investigator consider multiple variables concurrently. In the pages that follow, we will consider several options available to investigators and illustrate their applications. For more specific information about individual techniques and their computations, the reader should consult one of the multivariate statistics texts cited in the references.

The advanced statistical techniques discussed in this chapter can be grouped according to their purposes. The purposes of advanced statistical techniques include testing the relationship between multiple independent variables and a single dependent variable, testing the relationship between multiple independent and multiple dependent variables, grouping variables or individuals, examining the relationship between several repeated measures of the same variable, and testing complex causal models.

TESTING THE RELATIONSHIP BETWEEN MULTIPLE INDEPENDENT VARIABLES AND A SINGLE DEPENDENT VARIABLE

Several techniques can be used to test the relationship between multiple independent variables and a single dependent variable: multiple regression analysis, analysis of covariance, and discriminant analysis. Each has special applications. Multiple regression analysis tests the relationship between multiple independent variables that may be nominal or interval level and an interval level dependent variable. Analysis of covariance tests the relationship between two or more independent variables, one of which is an interval level covariate, and an interval level dependent variable. Discriminant analysis tests the relationship between two or more independent variables and a single nominal level dependent variable. Generally the sample size required for the procedures is at least 15 participants per variable or a total sample size of at least 50 more than the number of variables. (See Cohen [1977] for further information on estimating sample size for multivariate procedures.)

Multiple regression analysis

Multiple regression analysis is a multivariate statistical method used to understand the relationship between multiple independent variables and one dependent variable. The purpose of multiple regression analysis is to describe the extent, direction, and strength of the relationship between several independent variables and a single dependent variable. The dependent variable is normally distributed and continuous (usually interval or ratio level of measurement), and the independent variables may be continuous or categorical, or a combination of these.

Multiple regression analysis is an extension of simple linear regression. In simple regression one variable (X) predicts a second variable (Y). A simple regression equation takes the form:

$$Y' = a + b\ X$$

where

Y′ is the predicted value of variable Y, the dependent variable

a is the intercept, a constant—the point on the X axis where Y intercepts it

b is the regression coefficient, a measure of slope

X is an independent variable

Regression analysis solves for both *a* and *b*. Linear regression fits a straight line to the data such that deviations (Y′ − Y) from the line are minimized, where Y represents the observed value of Y and Y′ represents the predicted value of Y. A regression equation is a type of linear combination. The combination of the products of the constants and observed (measured) values produces a line.

Suppose a nurse wished to predict the birth weight of an infant from extrauterine measurements made at the beginning of labor. Using measurements of abdominal girth of the mother and the infant's birth weight, the investigator could calculate a regression equation such that

Birth weight (grams) = a + b (abdominal girth)

The task would be to predict the birth weight for a new infant by using the equation derived from earlier data. By knowing the mother's abdominal girth, nurses could predict the birth weight of the infant. To solve the equation, the investigator needs to solve the equation for a and b where the formula used to solve the equation is

$$b = \frac{\varepsilon xy}{\varepsilon x^2} \qquad\qquad a = \overline{Y} - b\overline{X}$$

where

b = regression coefficient
a = intercept constant
$\overline{Y}$ = mean of variable Y
$\overline{X}$ = mean of variable X
x = deviation scores from $\overline{X}$ ($X_i - \overline{X}$)
y = deviation scores from $\overline{Y}$ ($Y' - \overline{Y}$)

Regression analysis solves for a and b in a way that minimizes errors of prediction where the errors of prediction are defined as the difference between Y′ and Y or

$$Y' - Y$$

minimizes the errors of sums of squares of prediction and is referred to as a "least-squares solution." The error term (Y′ − Y) is referred to as a "residual."

Fig. 27-1 contains a plot of hypothetical data based on work by Engstrom and Chen (1984) where birth weight was predicted from several variables. Using the variable "abdominal girth" as a predictor of birth weight, note that the regression equation would approximate

Birth weight (grams = −.46 + (27.49 × abdominal girth in centimeters)

The general form for multiple regression analysis is an extension of simple linear regression. The multiple regression equation is

$$Y = a + b_1X_1 + b_2X_2 + \ldots + b_KX_K + \varepsilon$$

where

Y = the dependent variable
a = an intercept (constant)
$b_1 \ldots b_K$ = regression coefficients
X_1 = independent variable 1
X_2 = independent variable 2
X_K = independent variable k
k = the number of independent variables in the equation
ε = an error term

A complex series of equations is solved in which the independent variables are analyzed as a group to determine their relative influence on the dependent variable.

Let us consider an example of the application of multiple regression in a nursing study. Laborde and Powers (1985) used multiple regression analysis to explore the relationship between health perception, health locus of control, and illness-related factors to life satisfaction for individuals with osteoarthritis. To test the hypothesis that health-related variables influenced the arthritic person's perception of present life satisfaction, the investigators used hierarchical multiple regression analysis. They included each independent variable in the model in sequence so that the first variable was analyzed alone with the dependent variable, the second variable was added to the equation that already included the first variable, and the third variable was added to the equation that already included the first and second variables, and so on.

The order of the variables in hierarchical regression can be determined theoretically or according to size of the correlation between each of the independent variables with the dependent variable. Based on the principle of logical causal priority (Cohen & Cohen, 1983), Laborde and Powers (1985) entered health perception first because of strong evidence for the salient effect of that variable on life satisfaction. Health locus of control, being related to perception of health, was also entered early. The researchers entered illness-related variables on the basis of logical progression from duration of illness to joint involvement to pain.

In the multiple regression analysis table in Table 27-1, we see the result of the series of regression equations. First, health perception was included as an independent variable. Next, health locus of control was added as a second independent variable and then illness duration, number of diseased joints, and finally pain.

Multiple correlation coefficient

Now let us consider the information given in the columns of the table. R refers to the *multiple correlation coefficient*, which represents the correlation between the independent variables and the dependent variable. Notice that R is a simple correlation for the first variable but a multiple partial correlation coefficient for the second equation, in which both health perception and health locus of control are included. A multiple partial correlation coefficient represents the correlation between X_{k+1} and Y given the correlation between X_K and Y.

R has several important characteristics. First, R is no smaller than the largest correlation coefficient between any independent variable and the depen-

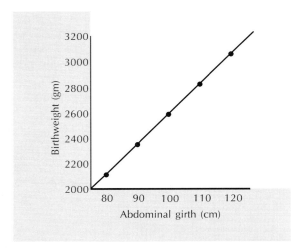

Fig. 27-1. Example of regression equation showing birth weight as a function of a constant $(-.46) + (27.49 \times \text{abdominal girth})$. (Data from Engstrom, J., & Chen, E., [1984]. *Research in Nursing & Health, 7,* 314-323.

TABLE 27-1. Hierarchical regression of present life satisfaction on health-related variables for 160 osteoarthritics

LEVEL/VARIABLE	R	R²	BETA*	df	F
I. Health perception	.49	.24	.43	1,158	40.99†
II. Health locus of control	.54	.29	−.17	2,157	6.49‡
III. Illness duration	.54	.29	.03	3,156	0.21
IV. Number of diseased joints	.55	.30	−.08	4,155	1.33
V. Pain	.57	.32	−.15	5,154	4.43‡

From Laborde, J., & Powers, M. (1985). Reprinted with permission from *Research in Nursing and Health, 8,* 187. ©, 1985, American Journal of Nursing Company.
*Standardized partial regression coefficients (Beta weights) control for other independent variables at the same or lower levels, but not for independent variables at higher levels (as indicated by Roman numerals).
†p < .01.
‡p < .0001.

dent variable. When the independent variables are highly correlated with one another, the change in R with the addition of each independent variable is smaller than when the independent variables are not highly correlated with one another. When the correlations among the independent variables are high, each successive variable included in the equation does not contribute much new information to account for the variance in Y because of the redundancy among the independent variables. Another noticeable feature in Table 27-1 is that each successive independent variable usually contributes a smaller increment to R. This occurs because of redundancy among the independent variables.

R^2 represents the proportion of the variance in the dependent variable accounted for by the independent variables included in the equation. R^2 is sometimes referred to as the *coefficient of determination*. Fig. 27-2 shows how each successive variable included in the regression equation contributes to explaining the variance in the dependent variable.

Beta weights

Beta weights are the weights that would need to be applied to the independent variables in the regression equation to predict the value of the dependent variable. To predict life satisfaction for the persons in the sample studied by Laborde and Powers (1985), an investigator would multiply the beta weight for that particular independent variable by the individual's value for the corresponding independent variable. The beta values given in this example are standardized regression coefficients, meaning that all the variables have been transformed to standard scores with a mean of 0 and a standard deviation of 1. The use of standardized beta values allows the investigator to compare the relative contribution of each of the independent variables within the same equation for the same sample. For example, the beta associated with health perception is approximately three times as large as the beta associated with health locus of control.

Beta weights also are directional. The results in Table 27-1 imply that health perception (defined as perceived level of health) has a positive influence on life satisfaction, whereas health locus of control (defined as the belief that health is controlled by fate)

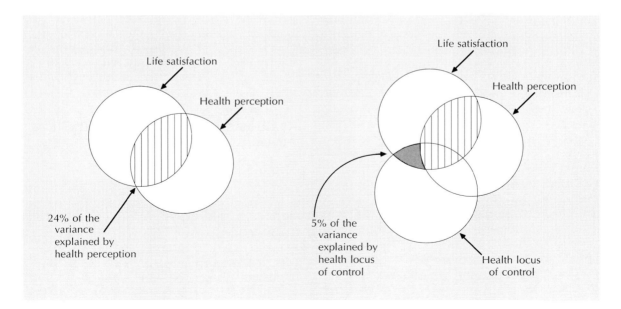

Fig. 27-2. Successive variables entered in the regression equation explain more of the variance in life satisfaction

has a negative influence on life satisfaction. Because beta weights fluctuate from sample to sample, the results pertaining to the size of the beta weights of the regression equation are applicable only to the sample from which they are generated.

F = statistic

Multiple regression analyses can test many hypotheses, but all involve the use of the F-statistic. In the case of multiple regression, the relationship

$$F = \frac{SS \text{ due to regression/df regression}}{SS \text{ due to residuals/df residuals}}$$

is tested, where SS denotes the sums of squares and df the degrees of freedom. The variance explained by the independent variables is contrasted to the variance due to individual differences or chance (called the residual variance), much as is the case with the use of the F-statistic in analysis of variance. The degrees of freedom (df) in Table 27-1 reflect the number of independent variables in the equation (df regression) and $(N - k - 1)$ where N is the total number of participants in the study and k is the number of independent variables in the equation. In the example in Table 27-1 notice that the Fs for the first and second equations are statistically significant, but the F associated with the addition to the equation of the third variable, illness duration, is not statistically significant. This implies that illness duration does not significantly improve the amount of variance that is already explained by health perception and health locus of control. In addition to testing whether each independent variable contributes significantly to explaining the variance in the dependent variable, that is, whether X_{k+1} improves the ability to predict Y over X_K, multiple regression analysis can also be used to test the significance of the full model, that is, whether R^2 for the full model including all independent variables is statistically significant.

Order of variables

The investigator can control the order in which variables are included in multiple regression equations. When there is theoretical justification for entering the variables into the equation in a certain order, the investigator can use a procedure called *hierarchical multiple regression analysis*. This procedure was used to generate the data in Table 27-1. Investigators can use a similar procedure to enter groups of variables, instead of one variable at a time. An alternative is to enter the independent variable that is correlated most highly with the dependent variable first, followed by the one with the next highest correlation with the dependent variable until all the independent variables have been included in the regression equation. This procedure is referred to as *forward stepwise multiple regression analysis*. A procedure called *backward elimination* also may be used in which all predictors are entered first and then variables are deleted one at a time, each time assessing whether the decrease in R^2 is statistically significant.

Analysis of covariance

Analysis of covariance (ANCOVA) is related to both multiple regression and analysis of variance. The purpose of ANCOVA is to describe the relationship between a continuous dependent variable and one or more categorical variables while controlling for the effect of one or more continuous independent variables. ANCOVA is used often in nursing research to control for the initial value of a variable that is being manipulated experimentally. Another application of ANCOVA is to control for one or more values that are not manipulated experimentally but are associated with the dependent variable.

Chang and her associates (1985) used ANCOVA to investigate the influence of selected components of nurse practitioners' care on the likelihood of elderly women adhering to health-care regimens. They examined the influence of several variables, including the women's personal characteristics (such as their preexisting satisfaction with health care) and the

TABLE 27-2. Analysis of covariance of care by intent to adhere (N=268)

SOURCE	df	MS	F	SIG
Covariates	5	4.52	6.22	.001
Psychosocial care	1	1.95	2.69	NS
Technical quality	1	.36	.50	NS
Patient participation	1	.16	.22	NS
Residual	232	.73		

From Chang, B., Uman, G., Linn, L., Ware, J. & Kane, R. (1985). Reprinted with permission from *Nursing Research, 34*, 27-31. ©, 1985, American Journal of Nursing Company.

TABLE 27-3. **Rotated standardized function coefficients**

PLANS AND VALUES	FUNCTION 1	FUNCTION 2
1. Intention to leave present job	−.63	−.45
2. Intention to get a degree outside nursing	.50	.09
3. Plan to work only in home	−.38	−.08
4. Plan to get degree in nursing	.55	.75
5. Value for friendly coworkers	.01	−.67
6. Value for nursing as a career	.23	−.53

From Taylor, M., & Covaleski, M. (1985). *Nursing Research, 34,* 240.

influence of videotaped visits of patients to nurse practitioners (demonstrating high and low levels of several components of care, including technical quality, psychosocial elements, and patient participation components) on women's intentions to adhere to a treatment regimen. The investigators were concerned because the covariates (in this case the personal characteristics) were related to the dependent variable. They used ANCOVA to control for the influence of the personal characteristics when examining the influence of the components of nurse practitioner care on intention to adhere to a regimen. They found that the covariates of marital status (widowed vs. nonwidowed), religion (Jewish vs. non-Jewish), preexisting satisfaction with health care, importance of a physical examination, and social network all contributed significantly to the women's intent to adhere to treatment. As seen in Table 27-2, the independent variables, that is, psychosocial care, technical quality, and patient participation, did not have significant effects on the intent to adhere to a treatment regimen after the effects of the covariates were controlled.

Discriminant analysis

Discriminant analysis is related to multiple regression analysis. Like multiple regression analysis, discriminant analysis allows investigators to examine the effects of multiple independent variables on a dependent variable. The dependent variable in discriminant analysis is a categorical or nominal variable. The purpose of discriminant analysis is to determine how one or more independent variables can be used to discriminate among different categories of a nominal dependent variable. The different categories of the dependent variable are referred to as "groups." Discriminant analysis develops a type of regression equation called a *discriminant function.* The function includes the variables that best discriminate between two groups and is derived by maximizing the ratio of the between-groups variance to within-groups variance.

Taylor and Covaleski (1985) used discriminant analysis to identify a group of factors that best predicted nurses' internal job transfer and turnover (Table 27-3). In the first analysis, (Table 27-3, "Function 1" column), they compared nurses who left their jobs with those who stayed. They found that the group of factors that best separated the nurses who left from those who stayed included their intentions to leave their present job, their intentions to get degrees outside nursing, and their plans to work only in the home. In a second analysis (Table 27-3, "Function 2" column), they compared nurses who transferred to other work areas with those nurses who left their jobs. They found that another set of factors, that is, plans to get degrees in nursing, value for friendly coworkers, and value for nursing as a career, differentiated those nurses who transferred to other areas from those who left their jobs.

The information presented in Table 27-3 includes the standardized discriminant function coefficients that are analogous to multiple regression coefficients. The first three items listed under function 1 separated the nurses who left their positions from those who stayed. The last three items in function 2 separated the nurses who transferred from those who left.

SETS OF VARIABLES EXAMINED IN KANG'S STUDY OF PATTERNS OF INTERDEPENDENCY BETWEEN TWO SETS OF VARIABLES RELATED TO PARENTAL COMPETENCE

Independent set of variables

Parental Awareness
  Interview (PAI)
Knowledge of Infant
  Development Interview (KIDI)

Total reflective solutions
  (problem-solving solutions)
Total restrictive solutions
  (problem-solving solutions)
Total supportive solutions
  (problem-solving solutions)

Dependent set of variables

Home Observation for Measurement
  of the Environment (HOME)
Total Parent Nursing Child
  Assessment Teaching Scale (NCATS)
Total Child Nursing Assessment
  Teaching Scale (NCATS)

Modified from Kang, R. (1985). Unpublished doctoral dissertation, University of Washington, Seattle.

TESTING THE INFLUENCE OF MULTIPLE INDEPENDENT VARIABLES ON MULTIPLE DEPENDENT VARIABLES

Two procedures commonly used to test the influence of multiple independent variables on multiple dependent variables are canonical correlation and multivariate analysis of variance. *Canonical correlation* relates multiple interval level independent and multiple interval level dependent variables, whereas *multivariate analysis of variance* (MANOVA) relates multiple nominal level independent variables to multiple interval level dependent variables.

Canonical correlation

Canonical correlation is a statistical procedure designed to analyze the relationship between two or more independent and two or more dependent variables. Canonical correlation produces two linear combinations, one consisting of the independent variables and another consisting of the dependent variables. The relationship between the two linear combinations is expressed by the canonical correlation coefficient, R_C. R_C^2 indicates the proportion of variance explained in the dependent variable function.

Kang (1985) used canonical correlation to define patterns of interdependency between two sets of variables related to parental competence. The purpose of Kang's study was to explore the relationship among components of a model of parental competence, including parental cognitive structure, parental cognitive process, and parental behavior. Parental awareness about the nature of children and the parenting role was assessed through the Parental Awareness Interview (PAI) and the Knowledge of Infant Development Interview (KIDI). Solutions for child rearing problems included reflective, restrictive, and supportive solutions developed by parents in response to a hypothetical problem. The home environment and the way parents taught tasks to their infants were assessed by observation. The two sets of variables examined using canonical correlation are listed in the box above. The canonical correlation between the variables was .675, <.001.

The canonical correlation coefficients (see box on p. 427) indicate that the PAI and KIDI contributed almost equally to the variance of the canonical variate of the first set, which reflects parental awareness. The HOME contributed most of the variance of the canonical variates of the second set, which reflects parental behavior. The relationship between the independent and dependent set was thus largely dependent on the influence of the PAI and the KIDI

Coefficients of Canonical Correlation for Variables Related to Parental Competence

Variates of the first set	
PAI	.524
KIDI	.632
Total reflective solutions	.073
Total restrictive solutions	.013
Total supportive solutions	.127
Variates of the second set	
HOME	.811
Total parent NCATS	.273
Total child NCATS	.042

From Kang, R. (1985). Unpublished doctoral dissertation, University of Washington, Seattle.

on the HOME, that is, parental awareness and knowledge of infant development influenced the home environment. Parental problem-solving skills did not appear related to the quality of the home environment or the way parents taught tasks to their infants.

Multivariate analysis of variance

MANOVA extends procedures for analysis of variance to cases with more than one dependent variable. MANOVA allows the investigator to take into account the variation in more than one independent and more than one dependent variable simultaneously. The advantage of MANOVA over the use of two or more separate ANOVAs is that MANOVA considers the intercorrelations of the dependent variables in computing the test statistics, whereas separate ANOVAs ignore the interrelationships among the dependent variables. MANOVA can be used as the first step in complex data analysis to protect against attributing chance results to the dependent variable, such as occurs when multiple statistical tests for each dependent variable are used.

Johnson, Christman, and Stitt (1985) used MANOVA to evaluate the effects of interventions that provided different means of exerting personal control over the postoperative experiences of black and white women having hysterectomies. The investigators used MANOVA to analyze the effects of several variables on measures made during and after hospitalization: race (black or white), the type of information provided to patients (concrete sensory information), instruction in a coping technique (cognitive coping, behavioral coping, or usual care), and discharge information (experimental care or usual care). In addition to these independent variables, several covariates were included in the analysis, such as physician ratings, complication scores, preoperative anxiety, confusion, and anger scores. The dependent variables included pain and discomfort during hospitalization, mood state, physical activity, and resumption of normal activities. In this very complex example the application of MANOVA allows the investigator to analyze multiple independent and multiple dependent variables simultaneously.

Johnson and her colleagues (1985) used MANOVA to evaluate multiple indicators of recovery during hospitalization: anxiety, confusion, and vigor scores, physical recovery index, pain sensation scores, number of times of ambulation, number of doses of parenteral narcotics, and length of postoperative hospitalization. Four scores produced significant multivariate effects: covariates (F 40, 626.12 = 6.46, *p*. 001), coping technique (F 16, 286 = 1.59, $p < .07$), race (F 8, 143 = 3.52, $p < .001$) and race × coping interaction (F 16, 286 = 1.58, $p < .07$). Covariates explained a large amount of the variance in recovery. Univariate analysis revealed that the effect of the interaction of race and coping techniques was the result of their effects on anxiety and confusion scores (Table 27-4). No significant differences occurred in the effects of coping for blacks. For whites, behavioral coping techniques decreased anxiety (Dunnett's *t* 3, 150 *df* = 3.45, $p < .001$), while both cognitive coping (Dunnett's *t* 3, 150 *df* = 2.74, $p < .025$) and behavioral coping techniques (Dunnett's *t* 3, 150 *df* = 2.75, $p < .025$) decreased confusion. In this example MANOVA was useful for analyzing complex relationships. In conjunction with MANOVA, univariate post hoc analyses using Dunnett's *t* or another post hoc comparison are essential to determine exactly where differences exist (see Chapter 26 for discussion of post hoc tests).

TABLE 27-4. Mean mood scores 3 days after hysterectomy*

RACE	COPING TECHNIQUE					
	COGNITIVE		BEHAVIORAL		NONE	
	ANXIETY	CONFUSION	ANXIETY	CONFUSION	ANXIETY	CONFUSION
White	6.13	3.09	2.72	3.10	9.64	6.56
	($n = 12$)		($n = 13$)		($n = 22$)	
Black	5.26	4.01	7.97	4.82	7.01	4.91
	($n = 36$)		($n = 34$)		($n = 50$)	

From Johnson, J., Christman, N., & Stitt, C. (1985). *Research in Nursing and Health, 8,* 131-146.
*Means have been adjusted for covariates; higher scores indicate increased presence of the mood. Coping Technique × Race for anxiety, $F (2, 150) = 5.15, p < .01$; for confusion, $F (2, 150) = 3.06, p < .05$.

GROUPING VARIABLES AND GROUPING INDIVIDUALS

Advanced statistical techniques are also useful for grouping a large number of variables into a smaller number of variables. Factor analysis is used commonly for this purpose. In addition, grouping individuals according to their profiles on certain variables is another useful advanced statistical procedure. Cluster analysis is commonly used for this purpose.

Factor analysis

Factor analysis is a multivariable statistical procedure designed to identify one or more new composite variables called "factors." Factor analysis commonly is used to reduce a large set of variables to a smaller number of summary measures. For example, an investigator could use factor analysis to reduce a scale with many items to a few subscale scores. The statistical procedure involved in factor analysis is analogous to multiple regression analysis in that a linear combination of variables is identified. Exploratory factor analysis does not test hypotheses, but it does help the investigator to identify a set of variables that group together. The underlying dimension that the variables have in common is called a "factor." A *factor* is a linear combination of variables that contains the scores of N persons on k measures. A factor can be defined as

$$F = b_1X_1 + b_2X_2 + b_3X_3 + \ldots b_kX_k$$

where X_1 to X_k are the original variables (such as items on a scale) and b_1 to b_k are weights. The use of

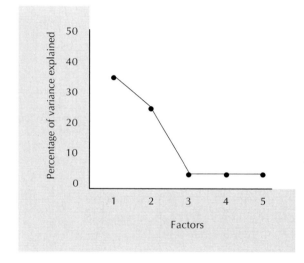

Fig. 27-3. Scree test. When a sharp drop-off occurs in the percent of variance explained, factors following the drop-off are usually omitted. In this graph factors *3, 4,* and *5* would contribute very little to the explained variance.

factors allows the investigator to group a large set of items so that a factor score can be computed.

Factor analysis involves two phases: factor extraction and factor rotation. *Factor extraction* consists of intercorrelating variables to identify clusters of highly correlated variables. The result of this step is an unrotated factor matrix. *Principal components analysis* is a procedure frequently used to extract the factors.

TABLE 27-5. **Factor loadings and eigenvalues using principal factor analysis and varimax orthogonal rotation for two factors of the scales of the questionnaire, "what being the parent of a new baby is like" (N-49)**

ITEM	FACTOR 1	FACTOR 2
11—Baby is on parent's mind	.11091	.56873
12—Changes for parent/family	−.13693	.56161
13—Difficulty in leaving baby	−.07837	.60990
14—Satisfaction in being a parent	.62502	−.01019
15—Sense of being in tune with baby	.73933	.01126
16—Parent's knowledge of baby	.64877	−.15062
17—Parent's meeting of self-expectations	.80904	−.02896
Eigenvalue	2.56	1.64
Percent of the total variance explained	36.6	23.5
Cumulative percent	36.6	60.1

From Pridham, K., & Chang, A. (1985). *Research in Nursing and Health, 8*, 25.

With the principal components method, weights for the first factor are defined so that their average squared weight is maximum; a maximum amount of variance is extracted by the first factor. The second factor is formed so that the maximum amount of variance is extracted from the variance remaining after the first factor has been extracted.

Several criteria are used to determine when no more factors should be extracted. These include the eigenvalue, percentage of explained variance, and discontinuity. An *eigenvalue* represents a value equal to the sum of the squared weights for each factor. When eigenvalues associated with each factor are less than one, the amount of weight assigned to that factor reflects little variance explained by that factor. When the factor explains less than 5% of the variance, it is often eliminated. The *principle of discontinuity*, or scree test, requires graphing the percentage of variance explained by each or the eigenvalue factor associated with each factor. When a sharp drop-off occurs in the percentage of variance explained, the factors following the drop-off are usually omitted (Fig. 27-3). Usually a combination of these criteria guides the decision regarding the number of factors to retain.

Factor rotation is the second phase of factor analysis. Because the factor matrix obtained from the principal components analysis is often difficult to interpret, investigators use a procedure called "factor rotation" to distinctly associate groups of items with factors. *Orthogonal rotation* keeps the factors at right angles to one another, or independent, so that the factors are uncorrelated with one another. *Oblique rotations* allow the rotated axes to depart from a 90-degree angle. The oblique rotation produces correlated factors. The oblique rotation approach is defensible, particularly when the concepts being factored are correlated with one another. The rotated factor matrix is the basis for most of the researcher's decisions about factor structure.

Let us consider a common application of factor analysis, the identification of underlying dimensions in an instrument. Pridham and Chang (1985) used factor analysis to determine the grouping of items on an instrument they developed to measure "what being the parent of a new baby is like." The seven items of the scale are grouped into two underlying factors: factor *1* includes three items dealing with the centrality of the infant, and factor *2* includes four items dealing with success in care of the infant. Table 27-5 contains the results of the factor analysis of the Pridham and Chang scale.

The *factor loadings* reported in Table 27-5 represent the weights of each item on that particular factor. Computation of *factor scores* involves using the factor loadings as coefficients and multiplying them by the participants' scores on each item. Below the factor loadings are three different pieces of information: the eigenvalue for the factor, the percentage of the total variance explained by the factor, and the cumulative percentage of variance explained by the factor. The eigenvalue represents the sum of the squared weights for the factor. The percentage of the total variance explained by the factor refers to the variance in the total item pool accounted for by that factor. The cumulative percentage of variance is the total variance accounted for by the addition of factors; in this example the total variance in the item pool explained by the factors jumps from 36.6% to 60.1% when the second factor is added.

Cluster analysis

Cluster analysis, a procedure used to classify people or things, pertains to a variety of procedures that can be used to create classifications. These procedures are used most commonly to group people according to profiles of their values on several variables. Both variables and people can be clustered. The purpose of using cluster analysis is to group highly similar entities. Clustering methods are multivariate statistical procedures that begin with a set of data containing information about a sample of entities. Cluster analysis yields a reorganization of these entities into relatively homogeneous groups. Most applications of cluster analysis are directed toward one of the following goals: to develop a typology or classification, to investigate useful conceptual schemes for grouping entities, to generate hypotheses by exploring groupings of data, or to test hypotheses (e.g., test for the presence of data verifying types of entities that have been defined through other procedures) (Aldenderfer & Blashfield, 1984).

Cluster analysis methods are relatively simple mathematical procedures that do not involve tests of statistical significance. Indeed, few rules or assumptions are necessary with the use of cluster analysis. Simple inspection of the results confirms the clusters.

Because cluster analysis has evolved from several different disciplines, various approaches exist, each with its own disciplinary biases. Clustering methods begin with the calculation of a matrix of similarities or distances between entities. These methods are discussed in detail in Aldenderfer and Blashfield (1984), Everitt (1980), and Lorr (1983). Applica-

tion of different clustering methods to the same data can yield different solutions. The structures produced by one cluster analysis approach should be cross-validated by applying another clustering approach to the same data or by replicating the structures with another dataset.

To create a typology of perimenstrual symptoms, Woods, Lentz, Mitchell, Lee, and Taylor (1987) used the average distances method of cluster analysis to group women. The researchers grouped 313 women according to scores that reflected several symptom groups occurring during the premenstruum and menstruum. They identified nine different symptom groups as shown in Table 27-6. Cluster 1 is most common and includes women with low intensity symptoms. Cluster 2 resembles classic dysmenorrhea symptoms. Clusters 3, 5, 7, and 8 include women with moderate to severe premenstrual turmoil. Cluster 4 includes women whose disrupted sleep may represent perimenstrual arousal.

This application of cluster analysis contributed to the identification of symptom profiles differentiating women's experiences with perimenstrual symptoms. Identification of several clusters of perimenstrual symptoms has provided evidence against the position that women experience a single premenstrual syndrome and supported the position that women experience several different types of symptoms during the perimenstruum. Table 27-7 provides the results of cluster analysis listing the mean values for symptom groups for each symptom cluster.

TESTING THE RELATIONSHIP BETWEEN REPEATED MEASURES

Testing the relationship between repeated measures can be accomplished through advanced statistical procedures termed *time series analysis*. Time series analysis allows the characterization of a pattern over time and the forecasting of future patterns from past patterns.

Many phenomena of interest in nursing are related to time. Change over time can be addressed in many types of analyses, but time series analysis permits investigators to analyze unique behavioral fluctuations and to forecast future observations from past patterns. Moreover, time series analysis allows both intraindividual and interindividual comparisons. Time series observations occur in temporal

TABLE 27-6. Clusters formed from identification of symptom groups

CLUSTER	N	DESCRIPTION OF SEVERITY AND TYPE
1	284	Low intensity (.4-1.3 on all symptoms)
2	8	Moderate (3-4) premenstrual bulge and mild menstrual bulge; severe menstrual discomfort (classic dysmenorrhea)
3	1	Severe (5-6) premenstrual turmoil; hermit; sleep disruption; severe menstrual out-of-sorts; moderate (3-4) premenstrual bulge; menstrual turmoil; sleep symptoms
4	7	Moderate (3-4) premenstrual and menstrual sleep disturbances
5	2	Severe (5-6) menstrual out-of-sorts; moderate (3-4) premenstrual turmoil; bulge; top-of-the-world; menstrual bulge
6	6	Moderate (3-4) premenstrual sluggishness and mild bulge, menstrual discomfort
7	2	Severe (5-6) premenstrual turmoil; moderate menstrual bulge and top-of-the-world
8	2	Menstrual (3-4) and premenstrual top-of-the-world; menstrual out-of-sorts and sleep disturbance
9	1	Severe (5-8) premenstrual hermit; menstrual discomfort; moderate (3-4) premenstrual bulge; menstrual out-of-sorts

From Woods, N., Lentz, M., Mitchell, E., Lee, K., & Taylor, D. (1987). *Prevalence of perimenstrual symptoms*. Final report submitted to National Center for Nursing Research. Washington, DC: National Institutes of Health.

TABLE 27-7. Cluster analysis results—mean values for symptom groups for each symptom cluster

CLUSTERS	PREMENSES FACTORS*						MENSES FACTORS*						N
	I	II	III	IV	V	VI	I	II	III	IV	V	VI	
1	.55	.42	.77	.36	1.29	.69	.47	.73	.50	1.27	.55	1.04	284
2	1.19	.93	3.45	.55	1.44	1.38	1.83	2.29	2.08	4.80	2.81	1.75	8
3	5.64	4.43	3.00	1.60	2.00	5.20	3.46	5.86	2.88	2.00	3.75	1.20	1
4	1.27	.59	.91	1.37	1.25	3.54	.92	.82	.95	2.37	3.43	1.71	7
5	3.05	1.93	3.60	2.50	3.50	4.00	2.77	4.50	3.13	6.20	1.63	2.30	2
6	1.14	1.64	2.90	3.87	.79	1.40	1.56	1.95	1.17	2.23	1.75	1.23	6
7	4.91	1.79	1.70	2.50	2.13	2.60	2.77	3.43	1.00	1.90	1.95	3.20	2
8	.71	.63	.56	.88	3.30	.60	1.91	2.43	1.00	1.64	3.65	1.96	5
9	2.18	7.00	3.80	1.00	.75	.50	1.18	3.29	2.13	6.00	1.00	.80	1

From Woods, N., Lentz, M., Mitchell, E., Lee, K., & Taylor, D. (1987). *Prevalence of perimenstrual symptoms*. Final report submitted to National Center for Nursing Research. Washington, DC: National Institutes of Health.
*Premenses factors: I, feelings of turmoil; II, feeling like a hermit; III, bulging; IV, sluggishness; V, on top of the world; VI, sleep disruption/pain. Menses factors: I, feelings of turmoil; II, feeling out of sorts; III, bulging/bingeing; IV, discomfort; V, sleep disruption; VI, on top of the world.

order and are assumed to be highly correlated successive values, that is, the value for time 1 is assumed to be correlated with the value for time 2 and time 3, and so on. Time series analysis requires multiple repeated observations, with a minimum 50 data points. Change over time is modeled where X_t (t = 1, 2, . . . T) and X_t to X_{t+1} are assumed to be fixed and constant intervals.

The structure of a time series contains four components: trend, or long-term movement of the time series such as the changes in weight measured annually from birth to young adulthood; fluctuation about the trend, such as daily fluctuations in weight superimposed on the long-term trend of increased weight throughout the age span; seasonal or cyclical deterministic changes such as premenstrual fluid retention and weight gain; and random residual effects such as weight gains and losses due to factors not accounted for (e.g., dieting). Once these components of the time series are identified, it is possible to apply predictive modeling techniques to the nonran-

dom components of the time series with the use of autocorrelation methods. Autocorrelation correlates X_t and X_{t+k}

where

k represents different time lags such as 0, 1, 2, . . . n

N = number of observations in the series

k < N

A high r_k (autocorrelation) indicates high association for t and (t + k). For example, when hourly observations are made that yield high r_{24} and r_{48}, a daily cycle is indicated. Based on daily observations, high values of r_7 and r_{14} indicate a weekly cycle. Temporal data can be used for both univariate and multivariate predictions, and the values for two series can be correlated.

Lee, Lentz, and Woods (1985) studied daily observations of sleep problems and fatigue recorded by women for a 90-day period. They used time series analysis to discern evidence of a menstrual cycle pattern in sleep problems and fatigue. They found that

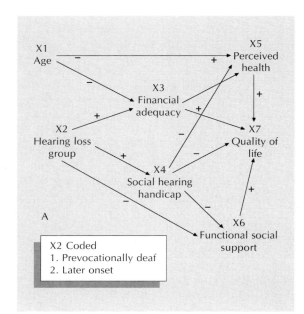
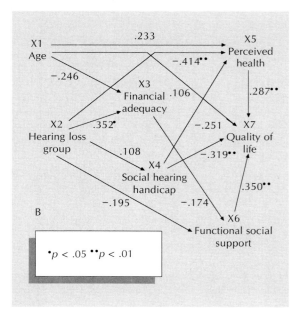

Fig. 27-4. Path analysis. **A,** Hypothesized model. **B,** Results of multiple regression analyses. Coefficients are standardized betas. (From Magilvy, K. [1985]. Reprinted with permission from *Nursing Research, 34,* 140-144. ©, 1985, American Journal of Nursing Company.)

values for r_{28} and r_{56} were high for fatigue in some women, suggesting for these symptoms a monthly cycle similar to the menstrual cycle.

TESTING COMPLEX CAUSAL MODELS

Testing complex causal models is a final application of advanced statistical methods. Two approaches that have been applied in nursing research include path analysis and linear structural relations analysis (LISREL).

Path analysis

Path analysis is a mode of interpretation of multiple regression analysis that is used to test a hypothesized model of causal relationships. The application of path analysis in nursing research is helpful in discerning a complex web of relationships that often characterize human health and human responses to health-related and illness-related situations. An application of path analysis is given in Fig. 27-4. Magilvy (1985) proposed a set of relationships explaining the quality of life of hearing-impaired women. As seen in the Fig. 27-4, *A*, she hypothesized that age and hearing loss would influence financial adequacy and social-hearing handicap, and that these, in turn, would influence perceived health and functional social support. Finally perceived health and functional social support, as well as financial adequacy and social-hearing handicap, would affect quality of life.

Magilvy (1985) initially regressed financial adequacy on age and hearing loss; next, social-hearing handicap on age and hearing loss; then perceived health on age, financial adequacy, and social-hearing handicap; then functional social support on social-hearing handicap and hearing loss group; and finally, quality of life on functional social support, perceived health, social-hearing handicap, and financial adequacy.

The coefficients given in the model in Fig. 27-4 are called "path coefficients" and represent standardized multiple regression coefficients. They indicate the strength of the relationships between the variables involved in the path. Each path coefficient was tested to determine whether it was statistically significant. Significant coefficients are indicated by asterisks (*) following the path coefficients (Fig. 27-4, *B*).

Magilvy (1985) found that only some of the relationships were statistically significant. Women with later onset of hearing loss (versus those who were prevocationally deaf) experienced better financial adequacy but poorer perceived health. Women who had a social-hearing handicap experienced poorer quality of life. Those who had better perceived health and functional social support experienced better quality of life.

Analysis of linear structural relations

Another advanced statistical technique for testing complex causal models is the linear structural relations systems, a system of advanced mathematical-statistical techniques and computer program developed by Jöreskog and Sörbom (1981) to analyze covariance structures. The analysis of covariance structures as performed by the LISREL program combines factor analysis and multiple regression analysis to examine the effects of latent variables on one another. A latent variable is a construct such as distress that is unobservable but inferred from other measurable variables. For example, distress might be inferred from scores on a measure of anxiety and depression.

LISREL analysis tests two models, a measurement model and a causal model. The measurement model uses confirmatory factor analysis and indicates the extent to which the indicators measured in the study actually identify the latent constructs. The causal model, which may be similar to the model given as an example of path analysis, is tested by a system of structural equations that relate the latent constructs, as reflected by multiple indicators of most of the constructs.

LISREL is best suited to the analysis of complex causal models that are grounded in theory. The goal is to test complex theoretical models in empirical research. LISREL requires reliable and valid measures in combination with carefully proposed theoretical relationships. Although complex, analytical strategies like LISREL can contribute to better understanding of some of the complex causal structures that explain nursing phenomena.

SUMMARY

Many advanced statistical procedures currently are being used in nursing research. These procedures,

TABLE 27-8. Multivariate statistical procedures.

NAME OF PROCEDURE	INDEPENDENT VARIABLE	DEPENDENT VARIABLE	PURPOSE
Multiple regression analysis	Two or more variables	One variable, interval level	To describe the effects (direction and strength) of two or more independent variables on a single dependent variable
Analysis of covariance (ANCOVA)	Two or more variables, one of which is an interval level covariate; covariate may be an interval level pretest score or another variable	One variable, interval level	To test the significance of differences in group means, adjusting for the effects of covariates on the dependent variable
Discriminant analysis	Two or more variables	One variable, nominal level	To determine whether or not and to what extent independent variables can discriminate between two categories of the dependent variable
Canonical correlation	Multiple variables, interval level	Multiple variables, interval level	To test the relationship between multiple independent and multiple dependent variables
Multivariate analysis of variance (MANOVA)	Multiple variables, nominal level	Multiple variables, interval level	To test the influence of multiple independent variables on multiple dependent variables
Factor analysis	Multiple variables such as multiple items on a scale	Multiple variables such as multiple items on a scale	To reduce a large set of variables to a smaller set of composite variables called "factors"
Cluster analysis	Multiple variables		To identify groups of participants that resemble one another with respect to certain variables
Path analysis	Multiple variables, interval and nominal levels	Series of single variables, interval level	To determine influence of multiple independent variables on a series of dependent variables
Time series analysis	Multiple observations of same variable(s) over time	Multiple observations of same variable(s) over time	To determine patterns of fluctuation in a variable over time; to forecast future patterns from past patterns

the types of independent and dependent variables they incorporate, and their purposes are described in Table 27-8.

Multiple regression analysis, analysis of covariance, and discriminant analysis can be used to examine the effects of several independent variables on a single dependent variable. Canonical correlation and multivariate analysis of variance can be used to examine the effects of multiple independent variables on multiple dependent variables. Factor analysis can be used to group a large set of variables into smaller sets of variables, whereas cluster analysis is used to group individuals according to the values they reflect on a certain set of variables. Time series analysis can be used to determine patterns of fluctuation within multiple repeated measures of a variable and to forecast future patterns. Path analysis and LISREL can be used to test causal models that include multiple independent and multiple dependent variables.

References

Achen, C. (1982). *Interpreting and using regression*. Beverly Hills: Sage.

Aldenderfer, M., & Blashfield, R. (1984). *Cluster analysis*. Beverly Hills: Sage.

Asher, H. (1983). *Causal modeling* (2nd ed.). Beverly Hills: Sage.

Biddle, B., & Marlin, M. (1987). Causality, confirmation, credulity and structural equation modeling. *Child Development, 58*, 4-17.

Blalock, H. (1971, 1985). *Causal models in the social sciences* (1st and 2nd eds.). Chicago: Aldine.

Blalock, H. (1972). *Social statistics*. New York: McGraw-Hill.

Bray, J., & Maxwell, S. (1985). *Multivariate analysis of variance*. Beverly Hills: Sage.

Chang, B., Uman, G. Linn, L., Ware, J., & Kane, R. (1985). Adherence to health care regimens among elderly women. *Nursing Research, 34*, 27-31.

Cohen, J. (1977). *Statistical power analysis for the behavioral sciences*. New York: Academic Press.

Cohen, J., & Cohen, P. (1983). *Applied multiple regression correlation analysis for the behavioral sciences* (2nd ed.). Hillsdale, NJ: Erlbaum.

Edwards, A. (1976). *An introduction to linear regression and correlation*. San Francisco: Freeman.

Engstrom, J. & Chen, E. (1984). Prediction of birthweight by the use of extrauterine measurements during labor. *Research in Nursing & Health, 7*, 314-323.

Everitt, B. (1980). *Cluster analysis*. New York: Halsted Press.

Ferketich, S. & Verran, J. (1984). Residual analysis for causal model assumptions. *Western Journal of Nursing Research, 6*, 41-60.

Gottman, J. (1981). *Time series analysis: A comprehensive introduction for social scientists*. New York: Cambridge University Press.

Hanley, J. A. (1983). Appropriate uses of multivariate analysis. *Annual Review of Public Health*, 155-181.

Harris, R. (1975). *A primer of multivariate statistics*. New York: Academic Press.

Heise, D. (1975). *Causal analysis*. New York: Wiley.

Herting, J. (1985). Multiple indicator models using LISREL. In H. Blalock (Ed.), *Causal models in the social sciences*. Chicago: Aldine.

Herting, J., & Costner, H. (1985). Respecification in multiple indicator models. In H. Blalock (Ed.), *Causal models in the social sciences*. New York: Aldine.

Johnson, J., Christman, N., & Stitt, C. (1985). Personal control interventions: Short- and long-term effects on surgical patients. *Research in Nursing and Health, 8*, 131-146.

Jöreskog, K., & Sörbom, J. (1981). *LISREL-V: Analysis of linear structural relationships by maximum likelihood and least squares methods*. Uppsala, Sweden: University of Uppsala.

Kang, R. (1985). *A model of parental competence*. Unpublished doctoral dissertation, University of Washington, Seattle.

Kenny, D. (1979). *Correlation and causality*. New York: Wiley.

Kim, J., & Mueller, C. (1978). *Introduction to factor analysis: What it is and how to do it*. Beverly Hills: Sage.

Klecka, W. (1980). *Discriminant analysis*. Beverly Hills: Sage.

Kleinbaum, D. & Kupper, G. (1978). *Applied multiple regression analysis*. North Scituate, MA: Duxbury Press.

Klockars, A., & Sax, G. (1987). *Multiple comparisons*. Beverly Hills, CA: Sage.

Laborde, J., & Powers, M. (1985). Life satisfaction, health control orientation, and illness-related factors in persons with osteoarthritis. *Research in Nursing and Health, 8* 183-190.

Lee, K., Lentz, M., & Woods, N. (1985). *Subjective reports of fatigue by healthy adult women*. Paper presented at Sigma Theta Tau Research Conference, Psi Chapter, Seattle, WA.

Levine, M. (1977). *Canonical analysis and factor comparison*. Beverly Hills: Sage.

Lewis-Beck, M. (1980). *Applied regression: An introduction*. Beverly Hills: Sage.

Lorr, M. (1983). *Cluster analysis for social scientists*. San Francisco: Jossey-Bass.

Magilvy, K. (1985). Quality of life of hearing-impaired older women. *Nursing Research, 34*, 140-144.

Martin, J. (1987). Structural equation modeling: A guide for the perplexed. *Child development, 58*, 33-37.

Metzger, B. & Schultz, S. (1982). Time series analysis: An alternative for nursing. *Nursing Research, 31*, 375-378.

Ostrom, C. (1978). *Time series analysis: Regression techniques*. Beverly Hills: Sage.

Pedhazer, E. (1982). *Multiple regression in behavioral research*. New York: Holt, Rinehart & Winston.

Pridham, K., & Chang, A. (1985). Parents' beliefs about themselves as parents of a new infant: Instrument development. *Research in Nursing and Health, 8,* 19-30.

Stember, M. (1986). Model building as a strategy for theory development. In P. Chinn (Ed.), *Nursing research methodology: Issues and implementation* (pp. 103-119). Rockville, MD: Aspen.

Taylor, M., & Covaleski, M. (1985). Predicting nurses' turnover and internal transfer behavior. *Nursing Research, 34,* 237-241.

Thompson, B. *Canonical correlation analysis*. Beverly Hills: Sage.

Waltz, C., & Bausell, R. (1981). *Nursing research: Design, statistics, and computer analysis*. Philadelphia: F. A. Davis.

Wildt, A., and Ahtola, O. (1978). *Analysis of covariance*. Beverly Hills: Sage.

Winer, B. (1971). *Statistical principles in experimental design*. New York: McGraw-Hill.

Woods, N. (1983). Prevalence of perimenstrual symptoms: preliminary studies. Unpublished grant proposal.

Woods, N., Lentz, M., Mitchell, E., Lee, K., & Taylor, D. (1987). *Prevalence of perimenstrual symptoms*. Final report submitted to National Center for Nursing Research. Washington, DC: National Institutes of Health.

28

USING QUALITATIVE ANALYTICAL TECHNIQUES

MARCI CATANZARO

Qualitative data are expressed in words rather than numbers. Just as the quantitative researcher does not use raw scores and frequency tables as the final report of a research project, the qualitative researcher reports more than just the words obtained through interviews, observations, or textual documents. Analysis of qualitative data is a painstaking process that requires long hours of careful work. The investigator must organize the data into patterns and cross-validate the information for interpretation. She or he must reduce and display data and draw and verify conclusions. Analysis of qualitative data is a creative process; as with other such processes, each person implements it differently.

This chapter is not prescriptive; rather, it is one way of approaching qualitative data analysis. It provides new investigators with techniques that they can modify to suit their own creative style. The chapter begins with a discussion of types of content analysis, then considers data reduction, data display, and formation of conclusions from qualitative data. Qualitative data may be generated as part of positivist-empiricist or a naturalistic-inductive study. In the latter case, a cyclical process is used to analyze data. This cyclical process involves a constant interplay between theory, concepts, and data.

CONTENT ANALYSIS

Ways to analyze the content of qualitative data have multiplied as social scientists have worked with tex-

tual material from such sources as newspapers, transcripts of speeches and interviews, books, diaries, and other written documents. *Content analysis* is useful for studying qualitative data because (1) it can be used with unstructured material, such as textual data, and (2) it is sensitive to the context and symbolic forms of the data. The researcher can use content analysis to examine existing data and can apply it to textual sources not originally generated for research.

Manifest and latent are two types of content analyses (Babbie, 1979). In *manifest content analysis* the researcher makes replicable and valid inferences by applying empirical and statistical methods to textual material (Krippendorff, 1980; Rosengren 1981; Waltz, Strickland, & Lenz, 1984). In *latent content analysis* the researcher views each passage of the textual material within the context of the entire text (Babbie, 1979; Waltz, Strickland, & Lenz, 1984).

Manifest content analysis

The investigator using manifest content analysis reviews textual material for words, phrases, descriptors, and terms central to the phenomenon under study (Field & Morse, 1985). A text is divided into units of meaning and quantified according to certain rules. The procedures for content analysis are time-consuming, but computer programs are available to search, tag, and count words and strings of words.

Holsti (1969) identified five major characteristics of manifest content analysis:

1. Analysis is based on explicitly formulated rules and procedures.
2. Analysis is a systematic process that conforms to rules about category construction, and inclusion or exclusion of content is based on consistently applied rules.
3. Analysis should permit generalization from the analyzed text to some theoretical model.
4. The object of the analysis is the manifest content of the textual material.
5. Manifest content analysis is typically a quantitative technique that is applied to qualitative data forms.

At the beginning of manifest content analysis, the investigator must decide what unit of analysis to employ. Words, themes, and time-and-space measures are examples of units of analysis. Words are easy to work with, are amenable to computer analysis, and are indicators of more abstract concepts or characteristics. Themes are sentences or propositions about some fact. Themes have more meaning than words alone but are more difficult to analyze reliably because of their complexity. Time-and-space measures require numerical counts, such as the number of words or pages or the number of minutes of discussion (Kerlinger, 1986). Table 28-1 lists examples of words, themes, and time-and-space measures.

The investigator can analyze the entire text or a random sample of the text. She or he may randomly select a starting word, phrase, or paragraph or a randomly generated number on a tape counter and analyze every *n*th unit. When books or other documents are the items for analysis, the researcher can select a random sample of all possible documents and perform further sampling within the sampled documents.

Generation of coding categories is discussed later in this chapter. In addition to categories, the researcher must establish explicit coding and scoring instructions. These rules embody the criteria for processing the content and must be as specific and complete as possible. Coding and scoring instructions must include a list of key words and examples of how to apply these criteria. For example, the investigator studying the concerns of terminally ill patients may have a category entitled "existential." Existential concerns may be defined as those that relate to death. Specific examples might include concerns about dying during surgery or other treatment procedures, plans for the future welfare of the family, and discussions of beliefs about life after death. Categories and coding instructions are tested by at least two persons, usually called "coders." The purpose of this testing is to ensure that the coding scheme and the definitions of the categories are clear. The agreement on coding among the coders is assessed for interrater reliability.

The objective of this rigor of categories, instructions, and assessment of coder agreement is to enable the researcher to confirm the reliability of the method and to analyze the data (Waltz, Strickland, & Lenz, 1984). Reliability is discussed later in this chapter.

Latent content analysis

Latent content analysis is concerned with the meaning within each passage of the textual material. Analysis of each segment of data requires the investigator

---

TABLE 28-1. Words, themes, and time and space measures

UNIT OF ANALYSIS	CHARACTERISTIC DIMENSION	EXAMPLES
Word	Parent	Mother, father, parent
Theme	Role identity	References to the character or role that is devised for self as a parent, partner, or worker
Time-and-space measure	Minutes devoted to status and role	Number of minutes during entire interview devoted to discussion of the status of parent, partner, or worker and the roles related to these

to code an incident for a category and compare it with the previously coded material in the same category. This process of comparison starts the analyst thinking about the full range of possibilities for the category: the category's dimensions, the conditions under which the category is most or least evident, the category's major consequences, and the category's relation to other categories. Each time the interviewee mentions the topic of death, for example, the coder reviews every time that death-related concerns had been coded and determines whether the current passage of the interview was consistent with previous discussions and with the meaning of death emerging from the data. Categories must arise from the data; they are never imposed on the data. Each datum is coded to create as many categories of analysis as possible. The investigator makes no attempt to quantify the coding or to determine the number of times that the data illustrate a particular code (Glaser & Strauss, 1967).

Comparison of latent and manifest content analyses

Field and Morse (1985) pointed out that manifest content analysis has numerical objectivity and therefore has procedural reliability; however, it may lack validity because the richness of the data and the context of the research are not considered. Latent content analysis may be highly valid because the underlying meanings in the communication are considered; however, it may lack reliability because of the subjective nature of the coding system. Glaser and Strauss (1967) pointed out that *constant comparative analysis*, a form of latent content analysis, is not designed to ensure that different analysts working independently with the same data will achieve the same results and code the data the same way. Rather, the issue is whether different researchers would find evidence that data could not be coded as it was.

Whether using the rigid and highly structured system of manifest content analysis, the unstructured but systematized approach of latent content analysis, or a combination of the two, the investigator must reduce qualitative data to units of workable size and display data in a way that allows analysis and formation of valid conclusions. Qualitative data often are generated as part of a naturalistic-inductive study. The cyclical rather than linear process associated with positivist-empiricist research is used (see Chapter 2).

This process requires a recurring cycle of empirical data collection, concept formation, concept development, and concept modification and integration.

REDUCING DATA

Data reduction is a process of selecting, focusing, simplifying, abstracting, and transforming raw data to simplify problems of analysis, storage, and dissemination (Miles & Huberman, 1984). Reduction begins before the actual data collection, when the researcher conceptualizes the study and makes decisions about the research question and the collection of data. Data reduction continues throughout the data collection period and ends when the final research report is completed. While working to recognize the evolving story, the researcher continuously makes decisions about which blocks of data to code and which patterns to use to summarize several blocks of data.

Conceptual framework

The *conceptual framework* of a study sets the stage and provides the first steps toward data reduction by identifying who and what will be studied and where the study will occur. The conceptual framework directs the researcher concerning the important aspects to be studied in the social setting. Many researchers may enter a hospital unit, each with a different conceptual framework: the psychologist may be interested in stress, the sociologist may study role relationships among staff members, and the epidemiologist may investigate nosocomial infections. A conceptual framework prevents the investigator from becoming overwhelmed by the social setting because it limits the events, persons, and interactions that will become the focus of the study.

The conceptual framework also provides the investigator with the first broad groups into which data will be categorized. These broad categories may be thought of as "baskets" labeled for the variables or processes that are the focus of the study. The researcher may or may not know how the facts "fit" in the basket or how they relate to each other, but she or he has at least an operational definition of what is important for the study. Baskets may be labeled for events (e.g., hospitalization), processes (e.g., obtaining assistance), or theoretical constructs (e.g., the sick role).

The specificity of the basket labels depends on how much the researcher already knows about the phenomenon of study. The nurse researcher interested in the effect of chronic illness on adult development may begin with baskets labeled "working," "parenting," "retiring," "participating in community," and so forth. The researcher who knows something about the effect of chronic illness on working may have baskets labeled "starting work," "changing jobs," and "retiring early." These baskets are based on a conceptual framework emerging from adult development theory, but they do not reflect anything about how illness influences these tasks or transitions. The labels serve to reduce all facts acquired during interviews and observation to only those relevant to the study. Baskets allow the researcher to separate data not directly related to the study.

Research questions

The specific purpose of the study, as exemplified by the research question, identifies the most important knowledge to be gained from the study. The research question in a qualitative study can be general or particular, descriptive or explanatory. In any case, the research question sets boundaries around the data to be collected. For example, will the researcher study everyone with a chronic disease, only one specific disease (e.g., diabetes), or a certain type of disease (e.g., progressive neurological)? In what context will people with chronic disease be studied (e.g., in the community or in the hospital)?

The nature of the research question also assists the researcher in setting up baskets for data reduction. The investigator interested in status may label baskets "parent" or "nurse," whereas the researcher studying roles may label the baskets "caring for children" or "caring for patients."

No investigator can study everyone, everywhere, doing everything. As noted, research questions set the boundaries of the data collection, an important component of data reduction. Questions clarify what the investigator wants to find out, from whom, and why. The researcher studying how a person with diabetes manages dietary restrictions will be interested in what foods are prepared. A study of parenting will be concerned with the task of providing meals for the family, not the specific food prepared. The research question also indicates where data are likely to be found. Data about the social interactions between patients in pain and the nurse probably will not be found in the supermarket or at a PTA meeting. The research question prevents researchers from indiscriminately collecting every datum, accumulating far more information they can ever analyze, and using valuable time in pursuing blind alleys.

Data collection

Focused data collection results in data that are more reduced. As a qualitative study progresses, data collection often becomes more specific as the investigator works to sort incoming data, organize ideas, and ask more precise questions. The line between qualitative data collection and subsequent analysis often is fuzzy. Some qualitative researchers collect all their data and then leave the social arena of study to begin analysis. This approach prevents the researcher from collecting new data to fill in gaps or to test new hypotheses that have emerged from the data. The researcher must be careful, however, not to use the initial interpretations to bias further data collection or attempt to reduce data to the extent that alternate explanations are overlooked.

Data analysis

Any qualitative study will produce quantities of data that can overwhelm the researcher if no data reduction has occurred until all the data are collected. Ongoing analysis of the data during data collection allows the researcher to alternate between thinking about the existing data and generating strategies for collecting new and often better data. Ongoing analysis keeps the investigator alert to what is happening with the data, stimulates creativity, and often energizes the entire project.

Whether the researcher chooses to engage in ongoing analysis or wait until the end, certain methods of analysis are useful for data reduction. These include summaries, coding, and writing memos.

Summaries

Preparing frequent summaries of activities in the research setting is an important step in data reduction. A summary may be written about an interview, a specific period of observations, or a document. A complete summary includes the main themes, issues, problems, and questions that arose. The box above contains a summary sheet used in a longitudinal study of the effects of progressive neurological disease on adult development. Data for this study were

EXAMPLE OF SUMMARY SHEET

ID number: _____ Date of contact: _____ Length of contact: _____

Investigator: _____ Today's date: _____

What people, events, or situations were involved?

What were the main themes or issues in the contact?

On which research questions did the contact bear most centrally?

What new hypotheses, speculations, or guesses about the situation did the contact suggest?

Where should the most energy be placed during the next contact? What sort of information should be sought?

What was this situation like for you? For example, was it particularly tiring; did it give you a feeling of satisfaction?

generated primarily through interviews.

A summary sheet is completed as soon as possible after data collection, when events are fresh in the investigator's mind. A summary allows the investigator to capture thoughtful impressions and reflections and consolidate ideas for further investigation or analysis. Succinctly written summaries are more useful than lengthy ones. The investigator can refer to the interview transcription or field notes for details of the event.

Data from a summary sheet can be used in several ways: (1) to guide planning for the subsequent data collection, (2) to suggest new or revised codes, (3) to provide communication tools between those involved in the study, and (4) to reorient the investigator to the setting when returning to the data. Sometimes summary sheets serve as a database and are coded similar to the original data.

Since summary sheets are important tools for data reduction, they must be accurate. Having someone else periodically read the interview transcription or field notes and independently fill out a summary form helps to identify and remedy systematic bias or selectivity in recording data.

Coding

Unlike numbers, words often are long, have multiple meanings, and may be meaningless when considered out of context. "The board is on the fence" can be interpreted that a piece of wood is on the backyard fence or that the decision-making body of a hospital is unable to reach a decision about increasing nurses' salaries. Words are the keystone of qualitative research and must be reduced so that they retain meanings and allow workable units. Coding field notes, transcriptions, and documents enables the investigator to assemble and retrieve words meaningful to the study and reduce the bulk of data into units that can be analyzed more readily.

The first step in coding data is to examine the data word-by-word and line-by-line, coding each segment of the data. Manifest content analysis requires the researcher to decide about the unit of analysis (word, theme, time-and-space cluster). The unit of analysis in latent content analysis is the smallest unit that contains some understanding the investigator needs. A unit of analysis may be as small as a sentence or as large as a paragraph (Lincoln & Guba, 1985).

A *code* is a category derived from the research question, and the key variable of the study, or it may emerge from the data. Codes can be generated deductively or inductively. *Deductively generated codes* are derived from the literature and from the investigator's insight before approaching the data to be analyzed. Interest in the preoperative concerns of patients scheduled for craniotomy led Markin (1985) to generate a list of concerns from reports of studies with patients undergoing other types of surgery and from her clinical experience with neurosurgical patients. She read transcripts with the intention of applying the predetermined codes to the data. This approach to coding simplifies the process of calculating intercoder reliability. In addition, it allows the researcher to count the number of responses in each category and to use a variety of descriptive statistical techniques.

Inductively generated codes emerge from the data and remain grounded in that data (Glaser, 1978). One way to generate codes inductively is to read the interview transcript or field notes and make comments in the margin about the possible analysis of data. Ideas evolve about how to assemble data into blocks and patterns as analysis continues. A disadvantage of inductively generated codes is that codes may change as the study progresses and more data become available.

An alternative that lies between using only inductively or only deductively generated codes is choosing a generic coding system that is not content specific. An example of a nonspecific coding system for data related to the meaning of role transitions is shown in the box below. The general domains identified in the box allow phenomena to be sorted into baskets that later can be recorded.

The baskets discussed earlier are a way to categorize or code data. They are labeled for the key concepts, variables, or important themes of the study. Coding allows the investigator to group related data. A participant rarely responds to questions during an open-ended interview in exactly the order and form the investigator intended. In the study of the effects of chronic illness during midlife, Mrs. K. talked about the relationship between her onset symptoms of multiple sclerosis and her pregnancy. It is evident from the line numbers of the sample transcript (see Sample Transcript box on p. 443) that data about onset symptoms and pregnancy are widely scattered throughout the interview. Placing all the passages cited in the box in a basket labeled "parenting" allowed the investigator to spot quickly everything

EXAMPLE OF NONSPECIFIC CODING SYSTEMS

Normative significance	Socially defined rules or standards of behavior that provide guidelines for the range of attitudes and behaviors
Personal significance	Personally defined rules or standards of behavior that provide guidelines for the range of attitudes and behaviors
Pattern of behavior	Ways in which an individual responds to environmental stimuli; more general than coping, which is goal directed
Socialization experiences	The structural perspectives and interactional processes experienced by the person that determine the attitudes, skills, and personal styles used in enacting roles or adapting to a change in roles
Self-concept	Descriptive perceptions of self as an object
Self-esteem	Affective and evaluative judgments made about self as an object
Social adjustment	The ability of the person to meet the demands of the environment and to experience a sense of general well-being

SAMPLE TRANSCRIPT SHOWING TEXT SEGMENTS PERTAINING TO PARTICULAR CODE

PART: I was pregnant and I first	33
started getting numbness and	34
electrical flashes down my leg.	35
COMM: Rubbing leg with hand.	37
PART: At first they thought it	38
was pressure from the pregnancy	39
on the sciatic nerve.	40
PART: Mostly, I was just scared to	151
death because I was pregnant,	152
primarily because I was pregnant.	153
PART: I was having a lot of fatigue,	165
which I think in retrospect may	166
have involved the MS, but they	167
tell you to expect fatigue with	168
pregnancy anyway.	169
PART: I started to have some	209
tingling, numbness in my fingers.	210
It was the first time I had anything	211
other than the leg. Um. I told	212
them about that, but they still felt	213
it was, um, it was pregnancy pressure.	214
PART: The pregnancy and my own	
health was	272
more important to me.	273
Something had to give, and it was not	274
going to be the pregnancy	275
PART: It was interesting that the	725
obstetrician that we consulted at	726
the hospital wanted to be very	727
conservative about it.	728
They wanted me to have the rest of	729
my prenatal care through the high-	730
risk clinic and plan on a high-risk	731
hospital birth and the whole shootin'	732
match.	733
He was born at home with a very easy	734
delivery without any interference	735
from anybody.	736

PART, Participant; COMM, Comment.

that related to parenting. The code "parenting" is descriptive; it entails no interpretation but simply labels a segment of the text.

Labels for baskets, or codes, may be names for things, cover terms, or semantic relationships. Cover terms are codes whose elements are included in the term. For example, "catheter" may be a cover term for Foley, Hickman, indwelling, condom, and intra-aortic. *Semantic relationships* indicate logical associations between terms. Spradley (1979) proposed universal semantic relationships that are useful for beginning an analysis (Table 28-2). The first column describes the type of semantic relationship; the center column contains a generalized statement of the semantic relationship; the third column shows an example of a semantic relationship derived from data on the effects of chronic illness during midlife.

The process of coding data involves seeking recurring themes in the data representing patterns that can be sorted into baskets or categories. Categories are judged by two criteria:

1. The extent to which the data placed in the category fit together in a meaningful way
2. The extent to which differences among the categories are clear

The researcher can ask the following questions regarding these two criteria:

Are the categories consistent?

When viewed together, do they seem to comprise a complete picture?

Do the categories provide a place for each relevant portion of the data?

Can the data be categorized independently by a second observer in the same way? That is, can an outside coder make sense of the categories in view of the available data and verify that data have been assigned appropriately to each category?

Are the categories relevant to those who provided the data?

Would the people studied agree that the categories appropriately reflect their issues and concerns?

A major task in the analysis of qualitative data is the identification of patterns. The process of uncovering patterns and themes is a creative process that requires carefully considered judgments about what is really significant and meaningful in the data. Just as the quantitative researcher can make type I and

TABLE 28-2. Semantic relationships for beginning constant comparative analysis

RELATIONSHIP	GENERALIZED STATEMENT	EXAMPLE
Strict inclusion	X is a kind of Y.	Father is a type of parent.
Spatial	X is a place in Y.	Seattle is a place in Washington.
	X is a part of Y.	Disciplinarian is part of being a father.
Cause-effect	X is a result of Y.	A paycheck is the result of working.
	X is a cause of Y.	Disability is a cause of early retirement.
Rationale	X is a reason for doing Y.	Love is a reason for disciplining a child.
Location	X is a place for doing Y action.	The office is a place for doing work.
Function	X is used for Y.	An automobile is used for transportation.
Means-end	X is a way to do Y.	Telephone sales is a way to do work.
Sequence	X is a step (stage) in Y.	Applying for a job is a step in becoming employed.
Attribution	X is an attribute (characteristic) of Y.	Loving is an attribute of a father.

type II errors from statistical analysis, qualitative researchers can decide something is not significant when it is, or they may attribute significance to something that is meaningless. Pattern identification requires that the investigator become fully immersed in the data, reading and rereading transcripts, field notes, and textual documents; discussing emerging findings with others; and continually returning to the data for verification. Hypotheses are generated about how data fit together, and verification of those hypotheses are sought in the data.

No definitive method exists for the search to recognize patterns in the data. Some researchers find it helpful to draw a diagram of how they believe things fit together. Such a diagram could be a concept-indicator model, in which a key concept in the data is explored to determine the links between the concept and its indicators. The relationship between the concept and the indicators can take different forms (Glaser, 1978). The pattern of indicators may be additive, so that each indicator plus all other indicators equals the concept:

$$A + B + C + D + E + \ldots = \text{Concept}$$

Data derived from study of chronic illness during midlife used this pattern of additive indicators:

Looking down + Looking suspicious + Looking too long = Eye messages

By comparing each indicator to every other indi-

cator and to the concept, a different picture becomes evident:

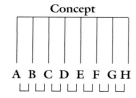

Applied to indicators of shame, this concept-indicator pattern would appear as:

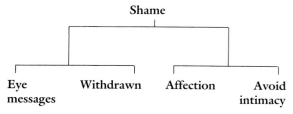

Another way to construct a concept-indicator model is to cluster the indicators into dimensions, or categories. See example below and Fig. 28-5 on p. 450.

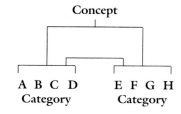

Marrying, living in, and remarrying are clustered into the category "getting coupled," and divorcing, separating, and becoming widowed are clustered in the category "getting separated."

In summary, reducing data by coding involves attaching a code to each segment of data. Codes can be derived inductively or deductively, and they may be modified as data analysis progresses. The investigator seeks recurring themes in the data and organizes the codes into patterns.

Writing memos

The use of memos or notes becomes an essential component of maintaining the investigator's sanity: they allow maximum control over experiences and become the working documents of the research. A memo is a note about facts the investigator wants to remember. Schatzman and Strauss (1973) identified three types of memos that are useful in qualitative research: methodological, observational, and theoretical.

A methodological memo might include the investigator's concerns about tactics used to collect data: reminders about timing, sequencing, stationing, staging, and maneuvering of data collection. The methodological memo might also critique the researcher's own tactics (see box below left).

An observational memo is an account of an event experienced principally through watching and listening that is deemed important enough to include in the data. An observational memo contains as little interpretation as possible and records the who, what, when, where, and how of the context or situation (see box below).

A theoretical memo is a self-conscious, controlled attempt to derive meaning from the data. It is the private declaration of the meaning the investigator believes may bear conceptual fruit. A theoretical memo provides a place for the researcher to interpret, infer, hypothesize, conjecture, or develop new concepts and links, and to relate observations to one another. The theoretical memo may serve as the medium to capture "bright" ideas that occur to the investigator at any time (showering, driving the car). It may also serve to integrate a review of the literature with the interview data (see box on p. 446).

Example of Methodological Memo

Cathy made a suggestion following her interview with 2-015 on 11/13/87: "We should add into the interview about how long the person can feel comfortable that they can leave the person alone. Can they go out of town for 2 weeks and leave it up to somebody else? Because I would have liked to have asked that question, but I didn't feel that it was my prerogative to enter new questions into the information."

Action: Communicate to Cathy that she is free to ask any questions that seem appropriate to the situation. We cannot possibly cover every contingency in the interview guide. Recheck Interview Orientation Manual. May need to revise material on the nature of unstructured interviews.

Example of Observational Memo

ID: 1-003 *Date:* 11/17/87 *Interviewer:* MC

It was difficult to find a place for the interview. The participant lives in a three-bedroom home. The living room was filled with empty and full boxes (she thinks she might move someday). One bedroom was literally packed from floor to ceiling and wall-to-wall with junk (exercise bicycle, recyclable aluminum TV trays, clothing, boxes, etc.). Nothing seemed to be organized. A second bedroom was used for storage and was piled from floor to ceiling with boxes, some open with contents hanging out. The bed was unmade, and clothes were piled on every flat surface. The kitchen counters and table were stacked with housewares and papers.

She is unable to use her walker because there isn't room to move it about.

RESPONDENT	ONSET SYMPTOMS	ACTION TAKEN	OUTCOME
100101	Numbness	Saw general practitioner	Referred to orthopedist
100201	Numbness Electric flashes	Consulted midwife	Referred to neurologist
100301	Optic neuritis	Saw general practitioner	Does not recall
100401	Waking: step, giggle, giggle, trembling hand	Made own diagnosis of Parkinson's disease	Saw doctor years later

Fig. 28-1. Matrix display of data.

EXAMPLE OF THEORETICAL MEMO

The self is partially composed of the social positions that an individual holds and enacts (Stryker, 1980). Attached to social positions are sets of normative expectations for behavior, or roles (Linton, 1936; Merton, 1957). Roles not only help define who one is, but suggest how he or she ought to behave. Role identities are reciprocal relationships that depend on recurrent interaction between the person and others.

The social positions of parent, partner, and worker seem to be the most salient in the lives of the participants. Does the set of normative expectations for behavior associated with these positions change when the parent, partner, or worker has a chronic illness? If so, how are these new expectations communicated to the person? Does the ill person describe himself or herself in terms of "usual" or "revised" role expectations?

DISPLAYING DATA

Miles and Huberman (1984) defined *data display* as "an organized assembly of information that permits conclusion drawing and action taking" (p. 21). Data display, as with data reduction, is part of qualitative data analysis. Often no clear delineation exists between data reduction and display because some

ONSET SYMPTOMS	ACTION TAKEN	OUTCOME
Sensation (N=10)	Saw MD (N=7)	Referred (N=3) Treated (N=4)
	Saw RN (N=1) Ignored (N=2)	Referred (N=1)
Movement (N=6)	Saw MD (N=1) Ignored (N=5)	Treated (N=1)
Mentation (N=1)	Saw MD (N=1)	Treated (N=1)
Integrated regulation (N=1)	Ignored	

Fig. 28-2. Summary table of data for 14 participants.

methods of data reduction require the display of data. Patient charts, digital and analog gauges of physiological measurements, and organizational charts are examples of data display familiar to nurses. They present information in a spatial format that is systematic and easily understood by the user. Unlike quantitative data, which often are displayed in the form of scatterplots, factor plots, and vector and box-and-whisker displays, qualitative data display have no standardized format. The format and shape of the entries depend on the investigator's purpose: overview the data, carry out detailed analyses, or combine parallel data (Miles & Huberman, 1984).

Data displays can take the form of matrices or fig-

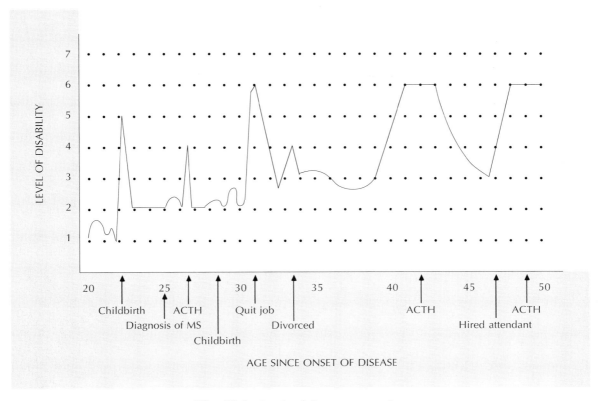

Fig. 28-3. Graph of disease progression.

ures. A *matrix* can arrange descriptive data segments around a particular event or experience. In the example shown in Fig. 28-1, short quotes and summarizing remarks are entered in the matrix with no attempt to standardize the entries by categorizing the entries or scaling them along a continuum. This matrix gives information about onset symptoms derived from 8 hours of interview data. The investigator used words from the interview transcriptions to indicate the content and display data for each study participant. The matrix allows the investigator to overview the data, see common threads, and perform more refined analysis that may lead to new displays and analyses. The matrix may also serve for case study reporting as the comments of each participant are collated in an easy to read format.

Another way to construct a matrix requires significant interpretation and transformation of data. The researcher can standardize responses and sum the components that contributed to the coding decision. For example, in the data set used in Fig. 28-1, responses about the onset symptoms could have been coded as "sensory," "movement," "consciousness," "mentation," or "integrated regulation," with verbatim quotes to substantiate the coding. Tables and charts also can be made that require the researcher to pool and interpret or evaluate responses. Summary and evaluative comments are recorded in the matrix; no quotes or other data are provided that would indicate what facts lead to the conclusions.

The research questions and the plan the investigator has for reporting the data will determine the type of matrix used to display data. When a brief, quantitative report of responses is planned, a summary table, such as shown in Fig. 28-2, is most appropriate. When case study or narrative reports are planned, more detailed information and informant quotes would need to be displayed in the matrix. The investigator may begin with a matrix that requires no interpretation and later recode the data into a matrix that requires interpretation and transformation of data.

Figures such as graphs are another way to display data. The graph in Fig. 28-3 shows the pattern of remissions and exacerbations experienced by one participant in a study of chronic illness. The graph is amplified by brief descriptions of related changes in the level of disability. One can see that each peak of disability was associated with a major life transition and that not all remissions of symptoms were responses to medication.

A flow chart is another method of displaying data. In the chronic disease study, the process of obtaining necessary health care was important. The researcher was able to design a flow chart for each participant that displayed the data to indicate the process of receiving this required health care (Fig. 28-4). In this

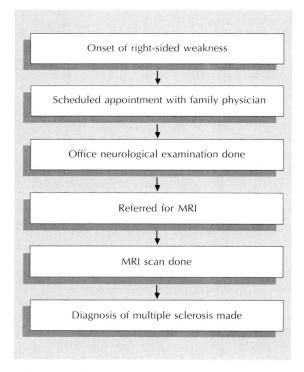

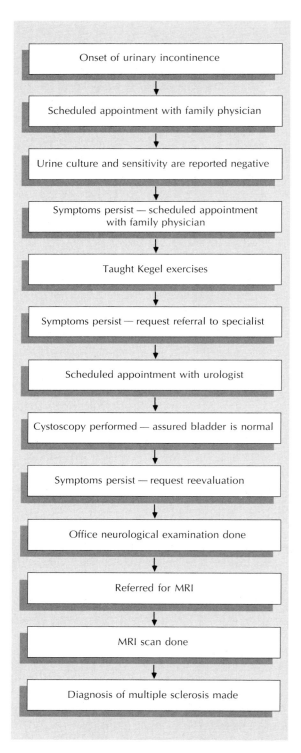

Fig. 28-4. Flow chart showing comparison of two processes of obtaining required health care.

case, diagnosis of the cause of right-sided weakness was handled with few problems, whereas the diagnosis of urinary incontinence required many telephone calls and patient appointments before neurologic disease was found as the cause.

Miles and Huberman (1984) offered advice about when to display data and many examples useful for the researcher involved in the analysis of qualitative data. The availability of a matrix or figure during data collection can save energy and time necessary to reduce transcriptions and field notes. They cautioned, however, that qualitative data evolve; later data may extend, qualify, put in perspective, or disqualify previous data. Displays almost always need to be revised, which can be a time-consuming process. Data displays also evolve; as more data are accumulated, the matrix or figure may become more complex or the headings can become more refined. Displays are rigid and can cause the investigator to force data into categories or leave data out. When the investigator takes a second and third look at data, the initial design of a matrix or figure may become irrelevant or trivial. Data must then be displayed in another way, which again takes time. Miles and Huberman suggested that the researcher construct data displays near the end of the data analysis, when they can be more contextually and empirically grounded. Also, the investigator should write down the criteria or decision rules used to select particular quotes and record how ratings or judgments were determined.

DRAWING AND VERIFYING CONCLUSIONS

The purpose of analyzing qualitative data is to draw conclusions or inferences about the meaning of the data. Miles and Huberman (1984) have identified 12 tactics for generating meaning: (1) counting, (2) noting patterns and themes, (3) seeing plausibility, (4) clustering, (5) making metaphors, (6) splitting variables, (7) searching for social processes, (8) factoring, (9) noting relations between variables, (10) finding intervening variables, (11) building a logical chain of evidence, and (12) establishing conceptual or theoretical coherence.

Counting

Qualitative research is concerned with the quality of phenomena, but quantifying facts is one way of learning about the distribution of quality. The investigator identifies themes and patterns by isolating some aspect occurring a specific number of times or in relation to another aspect. When making generalizations, the researcher has used counting to conclude that some factor happens more often or less often or that several factors are related. Miles and Huberman (1984) identified three reasons to count qualitative data: (1) to see what is present in a large piece of data, (2) to verify hunches or hypotheses, and (3) to protect against bias.

For example, the investigator may suspect that most women who had chronically ill husbands took low-status jobs. A quick calculation of the occupational status scores may show that the average level of employment for this subgroup is lower than for any other subgroup. The investigator may believe that those women who had low-status jobs lived in rural areas where job opportunities were limited. Again, counting and comparing can be used to verify or refute this hunch.

Much of qualitative analysis depends on insight and intuition. Researchers weigh information in light of their ideas, often overweighing facts in which they believe (Nisbett & Ross, 1980). Counting can force investigators to examine all the data, not just those supporting their bias.

Noting patterns and themes

Noting patterns is an intuitive process similar to clinical decision making. The process occurs constantly, but it is difficult to describe and even more difficult to teach. Recognizing patterns and themes in qualitative data occurs spontaneously as the analyst reads, rereads, and codes data or looks at the configuration of numbers generated during counting. Miles and Huberman (1984) cautioned that the researcher must not accept patterns too readily but must look for more evidence of the same pattern and evidence that would disconfirm a pattern.

In one study, husbands of chronically ill women often expressed a concern about their own use of alcohol or drugs. Was this a coping pattern of men? The researcher needed to subject this apparent pattern to skepticism, asking questions about whether the pattern made sense and whether it could predictably be found elsewhere in the data.

Seeing plausibility

Something is plausible when it is seemingly true,

honest, or trustworthy. Investigators may draw a conclusion about data because it seems true. They often experience the feeling that some idea just "feels" right; it seems to fit. Plausibility is often an initial impression that must be verified by subjecting these preliminary conclusions to other tactics of drawing and verifying conclusions. Facts that do not seem to make sense also should be verified before being discarded.

It seemed plausible that women were having more difficulty than men in obtaining a diagnosis for their neurological symptoms. The medical sociology literature had addressed the issue of gender differences in the health care received. The investigator had to search for evidence that a gender difference did exist in this sample and that factors other than gender could not account for the difference.

Clustering

Much of the data people deal with in their daily lives is grouped (clustered) in some way. Marrying, living with a partner, and remarrying can be clustered in a category called "getting coupled," and divorcing, separating, and becoming widowed are part of "getting separated." *Clustering* can be applied to events,

processes, settings, and so forth in an attempt to gain better understanding of a phenomenon (Miles & Huberman, 1984). At a low level of abstraction, the researcher is asking what factors are like or unlike each other. As analysis proceeds, clustering may be used to subsume particulars into a general class. Fig. 28-5 illustrates a cluster of codes related to living with a partner. The most general category appears on the left and the most specific on the right.

Making metaphors

A *metaphor* is a literary device that allows a person to take several particulars and make them into a single generalization. A metaphor is a figure of speech in which one thing is compared to another. As such, metaphors serve many purposes in qualitative research. They can be used to reduce data, to make patterns, to decenter the focus, and to connect findings to theory (Miles & Huberman, 1984). The metaphor "rescuer," in the transactional analysis sense, can consolidate into one package separate items of information, for example, about social relationships between the helper and the helped, about communication rituals, about the need to be needed, or about notions of helplessness.

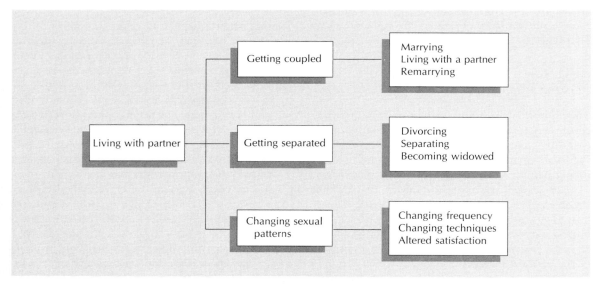

Fig. 28-5. Examples of codes related to living with a partner.

Miles and Huberman (1984) gave the following advice for researchers using metaphor:

1. Searching for metaphors too early in the study is constraining.
2. Being cognitively playful is the best way to generate metaphors; ask what is really going on in the social situation.
3. Think creatively with others; do not try to generate metaphors in isolation.
4. Know when to stop using a metaphor.

Splitting variables

The effort to integrate data and to move to a higher level of abstraction may result in identifying a variable composed of multiple variables that should not be put together. For example, retiring from work is an important variable associated with working. Sometimes people with a chronic disease retire from work because of their disability; at other times, retirement is age dependent. The issues raised by these reasons for retiring are qualitatively and quantitatively different; therefore, in the chronic disease study, retiring was separated into two variables: mature retiring (because of age) and premature retiring (because of disability).

Searching for social processes

Glaser (1978) referred to subsuming particulars into the general as looking for basic social processes. A basic social process has two or more clear stages and is described by a gerund, for example, becoming, centering, or growing. Movement from one stage to another usually depends on one or more events happening. For example, "normalizing" is a basic social process used by people with chronic illness to appear as much like peers as possible. Those involved in normalizing share a set of standards about appropriate and inappropriate behavior. Movement between "not normal" and "normal" involves stages of interaction with others in the social situation that may include degrees of openness; that is, how aware are others of the chronic disease? Efforts to keep the disease from infringing on other areas of life also may be part of normalizing. Mrs. K. attempted to normalize her birthing experience despite an obstetrician's advice (see box on p. 443, lines 725-736).

Subsuming particulars into more general classes is a conceptual and theoretical activity that requires the researcher to move back and forth between the specific categories initially labeled and the more inclusive or umbrella categories emerging as data analysis progresses (Glaser, 1978). Data are generated until a category is "saturated," that is, no new data are found that add meaning to the general category. *Saturation* is achieved when the investigator is learning nothing new about the category. The point of category saturation cannot be defined at the beginning of the research. Saturation occurs when the investigator obtains data that are repetitious of previous data. The point of saturation may be described as that sense of "I have heard all this before."

Factoring

Factoring allows the researcher to represent many variables within a smaller number of hypothetical variables. Most of the conclusion-drawing strategies already discussed are ways of pattern focusing. The investigator is essentially asking what bits of information fit together; in other words, she or he is deciding what factors go together to make this pattern. Many men in the chronic disease study identified alcohol and drug use as a problem. The researcher must ask, do men and women define substance abuse in the same way? Does this contrast between men and women make any meaningful difference? The answers to these questions allow the investigator to factor out those variables that influence patterns of substance abuse.

Noting relations

Nurse researchers are familiar with conceptual models that are depicted by boxes and arrows. Boxes contain the variables, and the arrows indicate the relationships among the boxes. The process of establishing relationships requires that investigators ask questions about how factors increase and decrease in relation to other factors. For example, does admitted overuse of alcohol increase as the spouse's disability increases? Do variables change in the same or in opposite directions? Is there a feedback loop such that a change in A results in a change in B, which results in a further change in A? Matrix displays are one way of presenting the relationship between variables. One must remember that seeing relationships does not mean that the relationship is causal. A relationship may exist between alcohol abuse and the spouse's disability, but one cannot say that the disability caused the increased use of alcohol.

Finding intervening variables

Sometimes two variables appear to go together, but the investigator's intuitive sense indicates that the connection does not make sense. Something may belong between the two variables (an intervening variable) that links them together. Does it really make sense that increasing disability in one person causes increased substance use in another? Or does another variable link the two? Perhaps environmental pressure or problem-solving orientation is the link between alcoholism and disability. Sometimes the researcher might expect two variables to be linked strongly when the data do not support such a conclusion. Is some intervening variable depressing or confounding the relationship?

Building a logical chain

The process of analyzing and drawing inferences from qualitative data is centered largely on identifying patterns within the data. These patterns are made at high analytical levels and result in the whole being greater than the sum of its parts. Building a logical chain is similar to constructing other matrices, but it demands that certain minimum conditions be met (Miles & Huberman, 1984):

1. Informants with different roles must emphasize the factors.
2. Informants must indicate the causal links either directly or indirectly.
3. The investigator must verify the claim through other sources.
4. The researcher must account for countervailing evidence.
5. The relationship must make sense.
6. The chain of events must be complete.

A logical chain is constructed by establishing the main variables in the chain and plotting their tentative relationships. The relationships then are tested against new data and subsequently are modified and refined and tested against the data again. A logical chain is a diagram of the sequence of events leading from one to the other and illustrating the steps or conditions that must be present for each subsequent step to occur in the process.

Miles and Huberman (1984) discussed two interlocking cycles: enumerative induction and eliminative induction. *Enumerative induction* involves collecting a number and variety of instances that go in the same direction. This process is also called pro-

gressive focusing. Searching for various instances of the chain of events that occur during interactions in which one person believes that others are communicating shame to him or her because of urinary incontinence is an example of enumerative induction.

Eliminative induction requires that the analyst test the hypothesis against alternatives and carefully look for qualifications that bound the generality of the case being made. *Constant comparative analysis* and structural corroborations are examples of eliminative induction. The intent of eliminative induction is to determine other factors that may appear to be, but are not, part of the chain.

Making coherence

Making conceptual or theoretical coherence requires moving from metaphors and interrelationships to theories. In other words, the researcher is linking together the findings of a study to overarching propositions that can account for the how and why of the phenomena under study (Miles & Huberman, 1984). Glaser and Strauss (1967) discussed *grounded theory* as making coherence inductively so that the resulting theory remains grounded in the real world, works in predictions and explanations, is relevant to the people concerned, and is readily modifiable. The investigator must decide the relevance of the core variable, how to integrate the theory, where to obtain the next theoretical sample, and how dense (cohesive or firm) the theory should be. Discussion of each of these steps is beyond the scope of this chapter. The theorist interested in generating grounded theory is referred to Glaser (1978) and Glaser and Strauss (1967).

CONFIRMING FINDINGS

Qualitative research often is criticized for its lack of scientific rigor in drawing valid inferences. Different analysts may look at the same data and draw different conclusions. Informants may contest some or all of the findings. An example from contemporary literature is the questioning by Freeman (1983) of Margaret Mead's classic work on Samoan adolescents. Whose judgments are right or wrong? Unfortunately, no ways are agreed on to establish the credibility of findings. Much of this chapter has been devoted to confirming inferences throughout the analysis process, but no method is available to ensure that independent analysts consistently and universally will draw the same conclusions from data. However, ways do exist to increase what Lincoln and Guba (1985) referred to as "trustworthiness." Trustworthiness can be operationalized as dealing with credibility, transferability, dependability, and confirmability.

Credibility

The credibility of findings can be increased by ensuring that the investigator spent enough time in the research setting to understand the context in which observations were made. No magic amount of time ensures credibility of findings. Lincoln and Guba (1985) suggested that the investigator needs sufficient time to understand enough about the research setting to place analysis and interpretations of data in context and to detect and take account of distortions that may creep into data. One test of time spent in the setting is to examine field notes and interpretations. If those writings are continuously predictable, either the investigator has not spent enough time in the research setting or has persisted in beliefs adopted at the beginning of the study.

Persistent observation adds the dimension of depth. The investigator must make enough observations to differentiate the relevant from the irrelevant and to describe in detail how decisions about relevance were made. Persistent observation decreases the probability that informants are putting on a front or intentionally deceiving the investigator.

Triangulation is another method of increasing credibility and research precision by measuring the same quality with multiple techniques. Denzin (1978) suggested three modes of triangulation that are useful in naturalistic-inductive studies: multiple and different sources, methods, and investigators. Multiple sources include different sources for the same information, such as more than one informant providing the same information or verification of responses from one source (informants) with another (minutes of a meeting). Multiple methods of data collection also enhance credibility. The investigator may associate observations with interview data or use written materials to gather information about what an informant has reported verbally. The investigator also can triangulate designs by combining strategies that emerge from positivist-empiricist and naturalistic-inductive paradigms. The researcher can

use multiple investigators by working with a team of investigators who have ample opportunity to interact and discuss the evolving analysis of data.

Negative case analysis is another method of establishing credibility of findings. Kidder (1981) compared negative case analysis to the activities of experimental scientists when they design subsequent studies. Negative case analysis is a series of consecutive studies within the same research project that requires the investigator to change the questions to account for unanticipated answers and observations. The hypotheses continually are refined until they account for all known cases.

A final way to establish credibility is by *informant checking*. Each level of analysis is returned to the informants for critique. The first opportunity for informant checking occurs during the interview when the investigator rephrases or reflects on the informant's comments so that the informant can verify the accuracy of interpretation. Also, another respondent or group can be asked to comment on the information obtained from other sources. Feedback can be requested from participants on coded data, analytical schemes, patterns, interpretations, and conclusions identified by the analyst. Informant checking not only provides a credibility check on the analysis process, but also offers an opportunity for the informants to share additional information. A panel of individuals can be convened to check the constructions of the analysis. Investigators are not bound to honor all criticism raised during checks; however, they must weigh each objection (Lincoln & Guba, 1985).

Transferability

External validity of studies based on a positivist-empiricist paradigm establishes the *transferability* or generalizability of study findings. External validity cannot be demonstrated in naturalistic-inductive studies; the investigator can only state the working hypotheses and describe the time and context in which they were found to hold. The description must be sufficiently inclusive to enable someone to contemplate transfer of findings to another social situation (Lincoln & Guba, 1985).

Dependability

One can argue that an investigator who has established the credibility of the qualitative analysis can disregard dependability. Lincoln and Guba (1985) argue that *dependability* must be dealt with directly. They suggested that an *inquiry audit* be used to establish the dependability of analysis. In an inquiry audit, an auditor is called in to authenticate the process of the inquiry and determine the acceptability of that process. As with a financial auditor, the inquiry auditor examines the data, findings, interpretations, and recommendations and attests that data support them. This latter process establishes confirmability, the final strategy for demonstrating trustworthiness.

Confirmability

The inquiry audit, triangulation, and the process of keeping a reflexive journal are ways of establishing that findings can be confirmed. Just as a financial audit uses a trail of records from business transactions, the *confirmability audit* uses a trail of raw data, data reduction and analysis, data reconstruction and synthesis, process notes, intentions and dispositions, and instrument development to confirm the analysis process (Lincoln & Guba, 1985). Based on work by Halpern (1983), Lincoln and Guba (1985) discussed the stages of the confirmability audit: (1) pre-entry, (2) determination of auditability, (3) formal agreement, (4) determination of trustworthiness, and (5) closure. The process of conducting a confirmability audit is complex and time consuming. Each investigator must base a decision to conduct an audit on the scope of the study and the benefits of establishing trustworthiness.

The reflexive journal is similar to the notebook used by laboratory scientists. This journal is a type of diary in which the investigator records information about himself or herself and the method of study. Information about self may include reflections about what is happening to one's values and interests because these will influence how an investigator looks at data and draws meaning from them. Methodological decisions and their rationale are recorded. For example, a researcher who was focusing on the way mothers interact with a disabled child may become interested in whether each mother interacts with the disabled child in the same way that she interacts with her other children. A decision to observe all mother-child interactions would be recorded in the journal along with the rationale for the change.

ESTABLISHING RELIABILITY

Reliability assesses the extent to which the data represent the real phenomena rather than an extraneous circumstance, a hidden idiosyncrasy of the analyst, or a surreptitious bias of a procedure (Krippendorff, 1980). The three types of reliability are stability, reproducibility, and accuracy.

Stability is the degree to which a process is constant or unchanging. Stability is assessed by code-recode designs, in which the analyst codes the same set of data twice. Intracoder disagreements from time 1 to time 2 may indicate that cognitive changes took place within the coder or that the coder had difficulty interpreting the recording instructions.

Reproducibility, also called *intercoder reliability,* intersubjective agreement, and *consensus,* is the degree to which a process can be recreated under varying circumstances. Reproducibility is assessed by having two or more individuals apply the same recording instructions independently.

Accuracy is the degree to which a process yields what it is designed to yield. Accuracy is assessed by comparing one coder's performance to what is known to be the correct performance (Krippendorff, 1980). Stability and reproducibility are much easier to implement with deductively generated codes than with inductively generated codes. Krippendorff (1980) noted that accuracy can rarely be established with qualitative data because a standard is rarely available against which to establish accuracy.

Krippendorff (1980) offers statistical procedures for arriving at a mathematical estimate of reliability. These procedures range from a simple percentage of agreement among coders to an agreement coefficient for canonical data and matrices.

MANAGING DATA

Qualitative data can easily overload the researcher. The wide range of phenomena that are observed and the extent of recorded notes (interviews, field notes) result in large quantities of data that must be managed to make analysis a reasonable undertaking. This chapter has presented ways of reducing and analyzing data that are useful in making qualitative data manageable. Additional strategies for data management include:

1. Type all verbatim interview transcriptions and

field notes on 8½ × 11–inch paper with one 3 × 4–inch side margin. This margin is used to code data and to add additional comments.

2. Make sure that each page of data contains a heading that indicates the source of data.

3. Keep data organized in files that will allow you to order and retrieve information. For example, file methodological memos separately from interview data, and keep data belonging in one analytical category separate from data in other analytical categories.

4. Write selected passages of interview data or observational notes on index cards for later sorting. Use a separate card for each data entry.

5. Use different-colored pens for various levels of coding. For example, the first coding of data may be done in blue and the next round in black.

6. Write memos on different-colored paper than raw data. Memos then can easily be spotted among piles of paper.

7. Make a duplicate copy of all data. Use one copy for coding. Keep the other in a safe place, separate from the working copies.

Computer software is available that can assist the investigator manage qualitative data. A selection of these programs for microcomputers are outlined in Appendix A. Available microcomputer programs can search for and count words or strings of words. These programs are useful for manifest content analysis. Programs, such as the Ethnograph, allow the investigator to use a microcomputer to review, mark, code, recode, display, and sort data that vary in length (Seidel, 1985).

SUMMARY

Qualitative data are obtained through interviews, observations, or textual documents. The manifest or latent content of these data can be analyzed and inferences then drawn. Codes for content analysis can be generated inductively or deductively. Whatever form of content analysis used, the investigator must select, focus, simplify, abstract, and transform raw data so that he or she can make sense of it.

The conceptual framework, the research question, the data collection process, and data analysis serve to reduce data to a workable scope. Data reduction is the process of selecting and focusing to decrease the amount of data that the investigator manipulates. Data reduction begins during the conceptual phase of the study and continues through the empirical and interpretive phases. Summary sheets, coding, and memos are techniques that can assist the qualitative investigator to reduce data. Data must be displayed in an organized manner, such as with figures, matrices, tables, or flow charts.

Finally, inferences must be drawn from data. Techniques for drawing conclusions from qualitative data are designed to identify patterns in the data and to raise the conceptual level of the codes and categories. Initially, codes are very concrete and often use the informants' words. As data are read and reread and coded and displayed, the researcher attempts to identify what is going on in the social situation and to establish patterns. Tactics for drawing inferences include counting, noting patterns and themes, seeing plausibility, clustering, making metaphors, splitting variables, searching for social processes, factoring, noting relations between variables, finding intervening variables, building a logical chain of evidence, and making conceptual or theoretical coherence. The researcher also must address issues of credibility, transferability, confirmability, stability, reproducibility, and accuracy.

REFERENCES

Babbie, E. (1979). *The practice of social research* (3rd ed.). Belmont, CA: Wadsworth Publishing.

Denzin, N. K. (1978). *Sociological methods*. New York: McGraw-Hill.

Field, P. A., & Morse, J. M. (1985). *Nursing research: The application of qualitative approaches*. Rockville, MD: Aspen.

Freeman, D. (1983). *Margaret Mead and Samoa: The making and unmaking of an anthropological myth*. Cambridge, MA: Harvard University Press.

Glaser, B. (1978). *Theoretical sensitivity*. Mill Valley, CA: Sociology Press.

Glaser, B., & Strauss, A. (1967). *The discovery of grounded theory*. Chicago: Aldine.

Halpern, E. S. (1983). Auditing naturalistic inquiries: The development and application of a model. (Unpublished doctoral dissertation, Indiana University.)

Holsti, O. R. (1969). *Content analysis for the social sciences and humanities*. Reading, MA: Addison-Wesley.

Kerlinger, F. N. (1986). *Foundations of behavioral research*. New York: Holt, Rinehart & Winston.

Kidder, L. H. (1981). *Selltiz, Wrightman and Cook's research methods in social relations* (4th ed.). New York: Holt, Rinehart & Winston.

Krippendorff, K. (1980). *Content analysis: An introduction to its methodology.* Beverly Hills, CA: Sage.

Lincoln, Y. S., & Guba, E. G. (1985). *Naturalistic inquiry.* Beverly Hills, CA: Sage.

Markin, D. (1985). Pre-surgical concerns of the patient anticipating craniotomy. (Unpublished Master's thesis, University of Washington, Seattle.)

Miles, M. B., & Huberman, A. M. (1984). *Qualitative data analysis: A sourcebook of new methods.* Beverly Hills, CA: Sage.

Nisbett, R. E., & Ross, L. (1980). *Human inference: Strategies and shortcomings of social judgment.* Englewood Cliffs, NJ: Prentice-Hall.

Rosengren, K. E. (Ed.). (1981). *Advances in content analysis.* Beverly Hills, CA: Sage.

Schatzman, L., & Strauss, A. L. (1973). *Field research: Strategies for a natural sociology.* Englewood Cliffs, NJ: Prentice-Hall.

Seidel, J. (1985). *User's manual for the Ethnograph.* Littleton, CO: Qualis Research Associates.

Spradley, J. P. (1979). *The ethnographic interview.* New York: Holt, Rinehart & Winston.

Waltz, C. F., Strickland, O. L., & Lenz, E. R. (1984). *Measurement in nursing research.* Philadelphia: Davis.

29

INTERPRETING THE FINDINGS

NANCY FUGATE WOODS

Interpretation is the final phase of conducting a research study. As in the earliest phase, the conceptual phase—in which the investigator specifies the problem, conceptual framework, purposes, and design for the study—the work goes on in the researcher's head. During the interpretative phase the investigator searches for the meaning and implications of the findings. The process begins as the researcher examines the relationships within the research study and its data, considering the design, measures, sample, and types of analysis employed in the study. The investigator examines findings for their meaning in relation to the problem, the conceptual framework, the purpose, and all research decisions and procedures made in developing and implementing the study's empirical phase. When interpreting the findings, the investigator makes inferences pertinent to the research findings and draws conclusions about these findings. During this phase the investigator also addresses the relationship between the results of the study and the conceptual framework that guided the study and seeks the broader meaning of the research data. To derive meaning from and implications of the findings, the investigator compares the results and inferences drawn from them to theory and earlier research results. Interpreting the findings from a study based on a positivist-empiricist paradigm generally occurs after all data have been collected and analyzed. This step in the research process occurs throughout a study grounded in a naturalistic-inductive paradigm. In this phase reconceptualization occurs. This, in turn, leads the investigator to the next step in the research program (Batey, 1971). Finally, the outcome of this phase guides the use of the findings in nursing practice.

The interpretation of findings is an extremely important aspect of conducting a study. Interpreting the results of a study requires confrontation with three types of validity: explanatory validity, ecological validity, and methodological validity. Explanatory validity refers to the degree to which the concepts chosen to account for the study findings do so. Explanatory validity requires examination of alternative, equally plausible explanations for the findings. Ecological validity refers to the extent to which the sample of observations in the study represents the substantive domain, the adequacy of the relationship between study design and substance being studied. Methodological validity refers to the degree to which the findings are a function of the set or methods used to test the theory (Brinberg & McGrath, 1982). In the pages that follow, we will examine several aspects of interpretation and related issues as they relate to explanatory, ecological, and methodological validity. We will begin with a discussion of the interpretation of the study findings and explanatory validity, considering the issues of proof and probability in relation to interpretation. We will examine three types of results that are difficult to interpret: negative, mixed, and serendipitous results. We will review guidelines for inferring causal relations. Next, we will examine issues of ecological and methodological validity and how the adequacy of the research design and methods may affect the findings. Finally, we will consider the relationship between the conceptual framework and the findings and the difference between statistically significant and clinically important results.

INTERPRETING RESULTS OF HYPOTHESIS TESTING

Interpreting the results of hypothesis testing requires consideration of the explanatory validity of a study. Positive, negative, mixed, and serendipitous results all require consideration of threats to validity of conclusions.

Positive findings

Interpretation of study findings is easiest when the findings confirm what the investigator anticipated. In this case the findings are consistent with the hypotheses or logic of the study's theoretical framework. This condition is described as obtaining *positive results*, meaning that the null hypothesis has been rejected. Even under these seemingly ideal conditions, the researcher needs to be conservative in celebrating the confirmation of his or her predictions. As we discussed in Chapter 26, hypothesis testing is probabilistic. This means that despite strong evidence that the null hypothesis is false, the possibility always exists that the null hypothesis is true (a type I error). The investigator must recall that proof is a deductive matter, a matter of reasoning, and that research methods are not methods of proof but methods of generating empirical data. Interpretation of positive results (as well as results that do not support the investigator's hypothesis) should include consideration of alternative hypotheses. For example, Woods (1985) hypothesized that women who performed many life roles (spouse, mother, and employee) and had little support from a partner in carrying out household activities would have the greatest number of symptoms of poor mental health. Although the null hypothesis was rejected, there could have been other explanations for the results. It might have been that these same women who had little support and performed many roles also had such poor financial support for their families that they were employed in jobs from which they received little satisfaction but held for the primary purpose of increasing their family's income. Moreover, they may have received little support from their spouses with housework because their blue-collar spouses believed that women's work was in the home.

The investigator reviews the alternative explanations for findings, attempting to determine whether any of these would be plausible in light of the research findings. Of course, one objective of this review is to rule out alternative or competing explanations when this is feasible.

Negative findings

Interpretation of *nonsignificant results*, sometimes called *negative results*, is problematic because statistical testing is oriented toward disconfirmation of the null hypothesis. Even though the research evidence suggests that the null hypothesis is true, many alternative explanations for negative results exist. Woods found that the number of roles (spouse, mother, and employee) women performed did not have an effect on mental health. Perhaps the measure of mental health was not particularly sensitive to symptoms. Perhaps certain roles, such as parenting, had effects that were apparent only at certain levels. For example, women who had several children were more symptomatic than those with one child or two children. Those with preschool children were most symptomatic. Perhaps the only thing that mattered was the woman's perception of burden associated with her roles, not simply the roles she was performing.

Because of some problem related to the empirical aspects of the study, such as measurement error or sampling bias, the null hypothesis could be false even though the research evidence fails to demonstrate a significant difference or significant relationships. This condition, referred to as type II error, generally occurs because of small sample size. When the difference between two groups or the relationship between two variables is small, the sample size for the study needs to be relatively large in order to detect them. With a small sample, small differences will not be statistically significant. This issue is related to the power of the statistical test, discussed in Chapter 26. The investigator needs to reconsider the adequacy of the sample size in light of the negative results. Perhaps with a larger sample the results would have been statistically significant if all other aspects of the study, such as conceptualization and procedures for implementation, do not suggest support for negative findings.

Another consideration in interpreting negative

results is whether a weak link existed in the research process. For example, were the hypotheses incorrectly specified? Did a problem exist in the logic guiding the study? Was the design adequate to achieve the research purposes? Did the design choice allow extraneous variables to be adequately controlled? Was correspondence poor between the concepts and their measurement? Did the study fail to reveal the proposed relationships because the concepts were poorly measured? Was the choice of analytical strategy the best for the type of data? Did the investigator choose the strongest test given the research question, design, and level of measurement? Did the investigator consider extraneous variables in the analysis to eliminate their effects on the study variables?

Perhaps the effects of women's roles on their mental health can be seen clearly only in a longitudinal study. Because women must be healthy to get into the labor force, only those women who are healthiest become and remain employed. Other women may appear less healthy, not because working at home is unhealthy, but because the groups who cannot be employed as a result of poor health are included with women who are not employed for other reasons. Often the problems related to weak links in the research process can be identified only at this stage of the research process and can be remedied only in a subsequent study.

Serendipitous findings

Serendipitous findings refer to those that the investigator did not anticipate, including those that are in opposition to the hypotheses guiding the study. For example, a nurse in a newborn nursery discovered serendipitously that infants whose beds were near the windows in the nursery experienced a lower incidence of neonatal jaundice. Her observation led to the use of light to lower bilirubin levels in newborns. Serendipitous findings can cause the investigator emotions ranging from embarrassment to elation. One can regard them as anomalous irritations or sources of discovery. As when interpreting negative results, the investigator needs to consider whether errors occurred in either the reasoning guiding the study or the methods of the study that might account for the serendipitous findings. Considering alternative theories is usually fruitful when interpreting serendipitous findings. Although they can be regarded with the spirit of discovery, serendipitous findings

need to be confirmed in other studies specifically designed to test hypotheses related to them.

Mixed findings

Mixed results constitute another type of research results. Mixed results contain some results supporting the hypotheses being tested and others that do not support them. For example, Woods (1985) had hypothesized that the number of children in a woman's family would be positively related to symptoms of poor mental health and to the number of illness episodes she experienced (1982). She found that although the number of children in a woman's family was positively related to symptoms of poor mental health, the number of children was negatively related to the number of illness episodes the women experienced. These mixed findings led her to hypothesize that although women's symptoms were mediated by stress, their actual episodes of illness were a function of the compatibility of their roles with taking on the sick role.

As with negative results or serendipitous results, the investigator considers the theoretical or methodological bases for them, carefully reviewing alternative theories and each element of the study methodology for greater understanding. Mixed results may lead the investigator to the revision of a theory or to improving the methods for studying the concepts.

DIFFERENTIATING CAUSAL AND NONCAUSAL RELATIONSHIPS

Inferring causal relationships is a major consideration in interpreting research results. Statistically significant associations, relationships, and differences do not indicate causation. In any study alternative explanations usually exist for significant associations or differences. In this section, we will examine three of these: confounding, indirect associations, and misspecification.

Confounded relationships

Spurious relationships, often referred to as *confounded relationships*, are noncausal relationships that stem not from a causal link between two variables, X and Y, but from the relationship of the two variables to a third variable (or a set of variables) that does not serve as a link in a causal chain between X and Y. For example, an investigator could find that the number of television antennas in a community is inversely related to neonatal death rate, that is, the more antennas, the lower neonatal mortality rate. Although perhaps large, the correlation does not prove that television antennas prevent neonatal deaths. In fact, the relationship probably exists because the prevalence of antennas is an indicator of affluence, which does affect neonatal death rates.

Indirect association

An *indirect association* exists when two variables are related in a causal chain but only because a third variable causes their relationship. That is, X and Y are related, but they are related because X causes Z, which causes Y. Sometimes one can trace the process by which a seemingly unrelated variable is actually part of a causal chain. For example, race and birth weight are related in that infants born to mothers of ethnic minority groups usually weigh less than those born to white mothers. On the surface we may conclude that members of certain races will always give birth to babies who weigh less than white babies. When this relationship is considered more carefully, we find that race is associated with income, which is in turn related to birth weight of the infant. Minority women tend to have lower incomes, and low income women tend to give birth to smaller infants. Thus, even though race and birth weight are significantly correlated, the relationship is an indirect one. Income is more directly related to birth weight than is race.

Misspecified relationships

Finally, a relationship may be *misspecified*. Misspecification means that the hypothesized relationship was incorrect because with the introduction of a third variable, the relationship between X and Y either disappears or changes. Returning to our example of the relationship of income and birth weight, we might find that the relationship between income and birth weight is different within different racial groups. The magnitude of the relationship between income and birth weight may be different for blacks, whites, and Asians. Specifying the relationship correctly would involve rethinking the conceptualization of the study, taking into account the different relationships for the three ethnic groups. For example, the correct specification may be that birth weight is a function of

income among all groups, but the equation

Birth weight = constant + coefficient (kg)

would require a different constant for each ethnic group to take into account the ethnic differences in body size.

GUIDELINES FOR INFERRING CAUSAL RELATIONSHIPS

Several criteria can be used in assessing whether a relationship is a causal one. Although these criteria do not provide a fail-safe mechanism for deciding that a relationship is indeed a causal one, they assist the investigator in interpreting the likelihood of X causing Y. To assess the likelihood of a causal relationship, the investigator can review a series of questions: How strong is the relationship? Is it consistent with the findings of other studies? Is it plausible that the causal variable preceded the effect variable? How specific is the relationship? Is the relationship coherent with existing knowledge? In the following pages we will explore each of these questions in greater detail.

Strength of relationship

The stronger a statistical relationship, the greater the probability that it represents a causal association. As X increases, one expects to see Y increase. The relationship between smoking and lung cancer provides a good illustration of this criterion. The more cigarettes smoked per day, the greater the incidence of lung cancer.

Consistency of relationship

When many studies using different designs and populations demonstrate a particular association, the investigator has a stronger basis for inferring a causal relationship than when the results do not conform to those from other studies. On the basis of most of the studies of preparation for surgery, we can conclude that preoperative preparation produces better health outcomes than no preparation. On the other hand, findings across studies could be consistent because the same problems of research design, measurement, or procedure could occur in multiple studies, making the evidence appear more compelling than it actually was.

Sequential relationship

The criterion of time sequence implies that the cause must have preceded the effect. The variable that is the presumed cause must plausibly have occurred before the variable that is the presumed effect. Usually this criterion is fairly easy to satisfy in experimental studies; however, in studies in which the independent variable is not manipulated, the question of sequence can be debatable. For example, disentangling whether employment produces better health in women or whether women who are healthier seek employment is difficult. Moreover, the mere occurrence of a variable antecedent in time to another variable is not a sufficient basis for inferring causality.

Specificity of relationship

The criterion of specificity refers to the degree to which one variable can predict another (e.g., the exposure to the tubercle bacillus produces tuberculosis and no other disease). However, in nursing or other fields studying human behavior, few relationships are truly predictive. One must be satisfied with considering the probability that if X occurs, so will Y.

Coherence with existing information

The relationship should be coherent with existing knowledge, making it plausible. Although the relationship's plausibility is an important consideration, its usefulness depends on the state of knowledge about a topic at any point in time. For example, Nightingale reduced the incidence of sepsis in the Crimea despite the fact that transmission of microorganisms was not understood at the time. Thus plausibility should not be used alone to dismiss assertions of causality because the state of knowledge may be inadequate to demonstrate consistency of the association with existing knowledge. In other words, a research finding like Nightingale's may be ahead of its time.

Consideration of all these criteria in combination is important when inferring that a relationship is a causal one. Making a causal inference is not a statistical operation; it is a logical operation.

ADEQUACY OF RESEARCH METHODS

Regardless of the nature of the findings—positive, negative, mixed, or serendipitous—the investigator needs to consider the adequacy of the research methods in interpreting the findings, that is, consideration of methodological validity. As we mentioned earlier, the source of the results may be due to inadequacy of the theory being tested. The hypothesized relationship or difference may be misspecified. In addition, the findings may be attributable to some aspect of the research methods that the investigator should consider modifying in future work.

Choice of indicators

The choice of indicators of the constructs (or even the theory guiding the study) may be inappropriate. Although the investigator may have selected the construct of "adjustment" of chronically ill clients and operationalized it as adherence to the regimen of diet and medication, perhaps adjustment in a chronically ill population requires nonadherence and actually manipulating the regimen to suit individual symptoms and activities of daily living. Thus perhaps "adjustment" would require indications of self-directiveness and self-governance. In this instance, the definition and indicators of adjustment did not reflect the construct of adjustment as positive adaptation to the illness, and it was not the construct of adjustment the investigator intended to study. People who had adjusted according to the operational definition might be less healthy than those who failed to demonstrate the criteria for adjustment specified in the operational definition as "adherence."

Sampling

Another explanation for spurious results is sampling. Selection of a sample that is biased with respect to some factor affecting the outcome variable may mask or exaggerate treatment effects. For example, when only the healthiest individuals participate in a study, the variability in health status is likely to be attenuated. Because of lack of variability in health status, few factors may be significantly related to health in the data even though these factors are related to health in the total population. Likewise, assignment of participants to treatment and control conditions in experimental studies can produce, before introduction of treatment, spurious results when the two groups differ systematically on some characteristic. If the treatment group is healthier than the control group before the study begins, then almost any experimental treatment will result in data that show the experimental group has much better outcomes than the control group.

A final problem related to sampling is dropout from the study. When the dropouts are differentially distributed across treatment groups—for example, when those individuals who drop out of the treatment group are sicker than those who drop out of the control group—the results may be biased. In this example the treatment should appear more effective than the control condition simply because those left in the treatment group were more healthy than those left in the control group. Ecological validity is therefore intertwined with methodological validity.

Measurement error

Measurement error, including those attributable to implementing the protocol inappropriately, also may produce spurious results. In some instances, measurement error is so great that it makes detection of small differences or associations impossible. When a very small proportion of the variance in scores is true variance, it is difficult to detect true relationships or differences. Simple errors in data collection, such as missed observations, erroneous recordings, and mechanical difficulties, may also produce spurious results. When these errors contribute to unreliability of measurement, they tend to mask differences or associations.

Inadequate statistical analysis

Inadequate statistical treatment of the data is a final source of spurious results. Using a statistical test that fails to utilize all the information in the data may interfere with discerning important differences or relationships. For example, using a measure of association that requires transforming continuous variables to categorical variables reduces the variance in the scores, thus decreasing the chance of finding a relationship between the variables.

Generalizing the results of the study

In addition to considering the elements of the research study just described, the interpretative phase of research also calls for the investigator to consider the generalizability of the study findings. Usually nursing studies are conducted with a circumscribed sample drawn from a specific population; some examples are patients admitted to a hospital for a special type of surgery, individuals who are not institutionalized but who have a special type of health problem, and in some instances individuals representing a portion of a community such as a designated neighborhood. Often human participants in nursing studies are volunteers recruited from advertisements, making it difficult to link them to an underlying population. The fact that the populations studied may be circumscribed in some way does not negate the importance of the results. What is essential is that the investigator acknowledge the population to whom the results can be safely generalized. Careful description and consideration of the characteristics of the participants and whom they represent prevent the investigator from making inappropriate generalizations to populations about which the study is not relevant. For example, in most studies of households in a community, participants will differ from those individuals who chose not to participate. Often the participants are somewhat more advantaged than the general population with respect to education and income. To prevent consumers of the research from making inappropriate inferences, acknowledging that the study results were not generated from a low income sample would be important in reporting the results. By assessing the nature of the sample studied and comparing it with the underlying population the investigator intended to study, the investigator can determine the extent to which the results can be safely generalized to the target population.

MAKING MEANING

In addition to considering the findings in relation to elements of the particular study that generated the findings, the investigator also is concerned with the broader meaning of the research data, linking the results and inferences drawn from them to related theory and to other research results.

Relating the results to theory development

In addition to considering the alternative explanations for the research results, the investigator also searches for the broader meaning of the research data. To make meaning of the findings, the investigator compares the results to other research results, as well as to explanations consistent with the theory that frames the study.

Describing the phenomenon. The conceptual framework for the study is a significant reference point for interpreting the results. When the conceptual framework is oriented toward describing a phenomenon, the interpretive work is directed toward isolating important concepts from the data. The significant contribution to nursing theory is naming and defining the relevant concepts. Gara and Tilden (1984) identified the concept of "adjusted control" to explain why women perceived their pregnancies in a positive manner. The investigators found that a common element among women who perceived their pregnancies as positive was the dimension of "adjusted," "rationalized," or "reasoned" control. They reported that "adjusted control means that those women who viewed their pregnancies as positive had achieved a feeling of control by accepting and coming to terms with their pregnancies. They had experienced a process of adjustment in order to define their pregnancies as reasonable to them" (Gara & Tilden, 1984, p. 431). The investigators cited examples that support the theoretical construct of adjusted control. Many women, when discussing the financial aspects of having a baby, said, "We'll adjust, you learn to adjust" (Gara & Tilden, 1984, p. 431).

Exploring relationships. When the conceptual framework is oriented toward exploring relationships between two or more concepts, the interpretive work is directed toward describing the relationships that were discovered. Mercer (1985) studied the process of maternal role attainment in three age-groups (15 to 19 years, 20 to 29 years, and 30 to 42 years) over the first year of motherhood. She found that the role attainment behaviors of feelings of love for the baby, gratification in the maternal role, observed maternal behavior, and self-reported ways of handling irritating child behaviors did not show a positive linear increase over the year but peaked at 4 months after birth and declined at 8 months. She also found that although age-groups functioned at different levels, their patterns of behaviors over the year did not vary, except for gratification in the role, which dropped toward the end of the first year for the youngest groups. In discussing her findings, Mercer pointed out that

the increased role skill and infant demands seemed to affect the teenagers more acutely than the older women.

The teenagers who are striving for their own independence and second individuation (Blos, 1962) may find their individuating infant's demands especially difficult. This may in part help explain their decreasing gratification in the mothering role at 8 and 12 months. Sander (1982) described the period from 5 to 9 months as one of early infant-directed activity when the infant elicits and demands responses from the mother. From 9 to 15 months the child increases these demands, and attempts to possess and manipulate the mother. Sander argued that this latter period "separates the women from the girls," since only those with a firm identity as a mother are secure in dealing with the child. (Mercer, 1985, p. 203)

As the citation illustrates, Mercer referred to theory and other research about maternal adaptation to help interpret the patterns found in her data.

Testing hypothesized relationships. When the conceptual framework is oriented toward testing hypothesized relationships or differences, the interpretation is directed toward the predicted relationships and the ways in which the data are or are not consistent with the predictions from the theory. Cronenwett (1985) tested a set of relationships between properties of the individual, properties of the social network, perceived social support, and psychological responses to parenthood. In particular, she was concerned about the elements of the support network that influenced postpartum outcomes. She found that emotional support was the best predictor of satisfaction with the parenting role and infant care for both men and women. For women, emotional support was the only significant variable. In discussing her findings, Cronenwett noted that appraisal support (provided by someone in the same situation or with similar experiences) was not a significant factor in any of the parenting outcomes. She asserted:

This result does not coincide with parent's past assessments of the importance of conversations with other new parents (Cronenwett, 1980; Kagey, Vivace, & Lutz, 1981). Appraisal support in this study may not have been significant, however, because there were few other new parents in these subjects' networks. Perhaps appraisal support is important, but is received from sources that are added after the third trimester or that are part of the larger acquaintance-level network. (Cronenwett, 1985, p. 98)

In this instance, the investigator did not find evidence to support an anticipated finding. Cronenwett discussed how her findings differ from the expected model; instead of modifying the theory to conform to her findings, she suggested some reasons for the anticipated finding not emerging in the population she studied.

Testing prescriptive theory. When the conceptual framework is oriented toward testing prescriptive theory, the interpretive work is oriented toward understanding the elements of the prescriptive theory that the study results did or did not support. Barnard and associates (1983) tested three models of providing nursing services to the families of newborns when the families had prior evidence of social and physical health problems. The Nursing Parent and Child Environment Model (NPACE) emphasized assessment of the infant, parent, and environment for planning individualized nursing care. The Nursing Support for Infant Bio-Behavior (NSIBB) was a structured curriculum that emphasized facilitating adaptation between mother and infant. The Nursing Standard Approach to Care (NSTAC) represented traditional public health nursing practice that was problem oriented and dealt primarily with physical health. The models were tested during a 3-month intervention period beginning with birth. The investigators did not demonstrate that the differences in the models' content or intensity had any influence on parent-infant adaptation or child health outcomes for the sample as a whole. They recommended that

the NSIBB model be considered for use by community health nurses. This (the NSIBB) model provides the nurse with a structure for teaching parents. The parents and infants in this program showed maintenance or improvement over time in parent-child interaction and the least decline in the infant's mental development. Ideally the program could be carried out beyond 3 months with an expansion of the theme to help parents understand their infant and support them in providing an optimum environment. We found many families who had profound stress and little support, i.e., the multiproblem and chronic problem families. For these families the intervention should be over a longer time and involve several disciplines, notably social work, psychology, and early education approaches. (Barnard et al., 1983, p. 165)

Note that the investigators considered not only the elements of the nursing models that they believed to have been particularly important but also the characteristics of the client population that are likely to interact with the nursing models tested.

Clinical and statistical significance

A final concern for nursing researchers is the clinical importance of research findings. Because nursing is a practice discipline as well as an academic discipline, nurse investigators must consider their work in relationship to its capacity to inform the delivery of human services. The fact that a finding is statistically significant does not guarantee its clinical importance. Despite the finding of a statistically significant difference in the mean blood pressure of patients who are positioned on either side, the difference may not be of any material importance. The difference must be interpreted within the framework of the study. The investigator studying a hemodynamic pattern will instantly recognize that a mean difference in blood pressure of 4 mm Hg is not likely to be of any clinical significance. Moreover, the difference is within the limits of measurement error. When large numbers of participants are studied, a smaller difference will be statistically significant than is the case when small numbers of people are studied. For this reason, considering carefully the magnitude of the difference, as well as the results of the statistical test, is important. The statistically significant difference between two groups does not ensure that it is real. Even when a p value of $<.01$ is used, the difference may still be due to chance.

Sometimes negative results are clinically significant. Consider research that shows two therapeutic approaches yield exactly the same response. Both produce improved client outcomes. Although the results of the statistical tests were not significant, the results may be very important to clinicians who learn that either approach produces the desired effects in practice.

Conceptualization and reconceptualization

The product of the interpretive phase of research is a contribution to nursing theory development. The contribution may be the description of a new construct, the discovery of a new relationship between constructs, or the specification of predictive or prescriptive theory. In many instances the contribution is the respecification of theory: the refinement of theory proposed earlier. We have seen illustrations of these contributions in the examples cited earlier. In contemporary nursing literature we are also beginning to see the evolution of research programs in which some investigators have begun by specifying important concepts and have continued their work to the point of testing prescriptive theory. Knowledge for a discipline, particularly a practice discipline, is never static. Nursing is no exception. Through the conceptualization and reconceptualization that is part of every study, the empirical work in nursing contributes to refinement of the knowledge required to provide caring services to people.

SUMMARY

Interpreting the findings of a study involves a search for their meaning in relation to the problem, conceptual framework, purpose, and all the research decisions made in developing and implementing the empirical phase of the study. Results of hypothesis testing studies may be positive, negative, mixed, or serendipitous. When the hypothesized results occur, they are termed positive results; when they do not, they are termed negative results. Mixed results occur when evidence both supports and does not support the hypothesis guiding the study. Relationships may be causal or confounded. Relationships that are causal are likely to be strong, specific, and coherent with other knowledge. In addition, it should be possible to observe a before-after time sequence between cause and effect.

The results of studies should be considered in relation to the adequacy of the study methods, including choice of indicators, sampling, measurement error, statistical analysis, and their influence on the validity of the results. Finding meaning in the results directs the investigator's attention to theory development and the reconceptualization of knowledge. Because nursing is a practice discipline, results should be examined for clinical significance.

REFERENCES

Barnard, K., Booth, C., Mitchell, S., & Telzrow, R. (1983). *Newborn Nursing Models.* (Final report of project supported by Grant No. R01-NU00719). Division of Nursing, Bureau of Health Manpower, Health Resources Administration, Department of Health and Human Services.

Batey, M. (1971). Conceptualizing the research process. *Nursing Research, 20,* 296-301.

Batey, M. (1977). Conceptualization: Knowledge and logic guiding empirical research. *Nursing Research, 26,* 324-329.

Blalock, H. (1961). *Causal inferences in nonexperimental research.* Chapel Hill: University of North Carolina Press, pp. 3-26.

Brinberg, D., & McGrath, J. (1982). A network of validity concepts within the research process. In D. Brinberg and R. Kidder (Eds.), *Forms of validity in research* (pp. 5-21). San Francisco: Jossey-Bass.

Cronenwett, L. (1985). Network structure, social support, and psychological outcomes of pregnancy. *Nursing Research, 34,* 93-99.

Diers, D. (1979). *Research in nursing practice.* Philadelphia: Lippincott.

Gara, E., & Tilden, V. (1984). Adjusted control: An explanation for women's positive perceptions of their pregnancies. *Health Care for Women International, 5,* 427-436.

Hinshaw, A. (1979). Planning for logical consistency among three research structures. *Western Journal of Nursing Research, 1,* 250-253.

Huck, S., & Sandler, H. (1979). *Rival hypotheses: Alternative explanations of data based conclusions.* New York: Harper & Row.

Kerlinger, F. (1973). *Foundations of behavioral research.* New York: Holt, Rinehart, & Winston.

Mercer, R. (1985). The process of maternal role attainment over the first year. *Nursing Research, 34,* 198-204.

Polit, D., & Hungler, B. (1983). *Nursing research: Principles and methods.* Philadelphia: Lippincott.

Selltiz, C., Wrightsman, L., & Cook, S. (1986). *Research methods in social relations.* New York: Holt, Rinehart & Winston.

Susser, M. (1973). *Causal thinking in the health sciences.* New York: Oxford University Press.

Woods, N. (1985). Employment, family roles & mental ill health in young married women. *Nursing Research, 34,* 5-10.

30

Evaluating Research Reports

Marci Catanzaro and Ellen F. Olshansky

Chapter 1 pointed out that nursing science is the body of knowledge gained through systematic study for the purpose of guiding nursing practice. As researchers proceed with the development of nursing science, they will review the literature often and for different purposes (see Chapter 4). Critical appraisal of completed research is an important part of the development of nursing theory because critique allows the investigator to move beyond a general descriptive account of the research study to a careful, systematic judgment of the study's worth. Leininger (1968) stated that: "A research critique reflects a penetrating analysis of a study in which judicious and constructive comments have been made about a piece of work" (p. 445).

The world view that we hold and the assumptions about a domain of knowledge that constitute our paradigm provide criteria for evaluating the quality of the research effort. This chapter begins by exploring the art and function of the research critique and then presents criteria for the critical analysis of nursing research that emanate from different paradigms: positivist-empiricist and naturalistic-inductive.

FUNCTION OF A CRITIQUE

The research critique provides an appraisal of completed research that helps the investigator evaluate the favorable and less favorable aspects of the study. The critic's view of the study may be different from the investigator's and may open new vistas for considering alternative hypotheses and exploring assumptions underlying the study. Leininger (1968) noted that the research critique can facilitate the scientific potential of the researcher and help the investigator move toward excellence in research. The research critique also is important to the person using the research in deciding how the study findings best can be applied to nursing practice.

EXPECTATIONS OF THE CRITIC

The critic of completed research has a very special role in that he or she is looking beyond the surface description of the study to an appraisal of the study's worth. The critic is expected to (1) maintain an objective attitude, (2) emphasize an advisory role, (3) provide constructive criticism, (4) assess the general features, strengths, and weaknesses of the study, and (5) make summary appraisals and recommendations (Leininger, 1968).

An objective attitude requires that the critic focus on the current research report and avoid basing the commentary on the personality of the investigator. The critic avoids reading between the lines of a research report. For example, the report may fail to describe how the investigator controlled for threats to internal validity. The objective critic would point out this shortcoming rather than assume that controls existed for internal validity because the investigator has a doctorate in nursing and has had many years of research experience. The critic's criteria for evaluation must be objective and comprehensive and must be applied fairly. Criteria for evaluating research reports are discussed in later sections of this chapter.

The research critic is an advisor. This advisory role requires a collegial relationship between the researcher and the critic. The purpose of the critique is to assist the investigators in enhancing their research skills and advancing toward generation of knowledge for nursing practice. The researcher and the critic must have a mutual respect for each other and a willingness to engage in a mutually beneficial exchange of ideas.

The critic must employ constructive criticism. Criticism should stimulate the researcher to use the review rather than to lose interest in investigating the topic or pursuing further research. The critic can offer criticism that is viewed as constructive by carefully selecting the words and statements used in the critique and by soliciting a second opinion from a colleague about how the investigator may interpret the choice of words.

Critique shares the same root as the word "critical," which is often interpreted to mean derogatory, disparaging, picky, or fault finding. The critic is addressing only part of the task of providing a critical analysis of research when the study's imperfections become the target of the critique. The critic is expected to assess the strengths and the weaknesses of the research. Leininger (1968) suggested that "the use of penetrating questions is an effective way to help the researcher clarify his thinking and future research strategies" (p. 447). Such questions may be directed at the research design or at the assumptions and paradigms underlying the research.

Finally, the critic is expected to provide a summary of the analysis and recommendations that will help the investigator continue to pursue excellence in research. The summaries and recommendations must be (1) congruent with analysis, (2) supported by the critic's assessment of the research, and (3) practical. An explanation to justify the criticisms is essential.

COMPONENTS OF A RESEARCH CRITIQUE

The critic, as with the investigator, has a philosophical mind-set that influences how he or she views nursing research and the domain of knowledge studied. How this mind-set influences the critique is covered in later parts of this chapter. Critics must share their paradigm so that readers of the critique will understand the perspective from which the analysis was written.

Analysis of a research report generally involves a critical examination of the total report as well as its parts. The scientific merit of research may be established through a review of the whole study and determination of the logical consistency between the theoretical, design, and analysis components of the investigation (Hinshaw, 1979a). The theoretical structure refers to the level of knowledge in the substantive area investigated. If little was known about the phenomenon of study, concept clarification is needed and a conceptual orientation for the study is appropriate. If the concepts and characteristic relationships have been defined, a theoretical framework is appropriate (see Chapter 4, Table 4-4). The problem and the purposes of the study are examined for consistency and for their relationship to the level of knowledge about the studied phenomenon. The framework for the study is viewed from two perspectives: (1) its relationship to the identified problem and purpose of the study and (2) its relationship to the research design. The framework should provide a rationale or theoretical argument underpinning the study.

The design, including the sample, data-producing instruments, and procedures, must be consistent with the descriptive, exploratory, or hypothesis-testing aspects of the study. The design also must be consistent with the theoretical model for the study and must control for the reliability and validity of the findings. The critic uses personal knowledge of the research process to make informed decisions about the quality of each part of the research design. The analysis structure flows from the theoretical structure underlying the research. Lastly, the critic considers whether the conclusions drawn by the investigator are warranted on the basis of the research design and the findings.

The critic's task is to evaluate the consistency among the three structures in the research study. Evaluating the internal consistency of a study is difficult. Hinshaw (1979b) suggested a process she called "theoretical substruction" for tracking consistency among the theoretical, design, and analysis models in a study. Theoretical substruction is a systematic assessment process that builds a picture from the verbal explanation of the theory underlying the research. The critic begins by distinguishing between the major variables under study and the control or demographic variables and identifying the level of abstraction of the concepts. This process allows the critic to understand those concepts that will be measured in the research and those more abstract phenomena that will not be measured. After identifying the concepts, the critic diagrams the relationships between the concepts.

The critic then reviews the theoretical report to determine whether the relationships are stated by the investigator and are assumed to be causal or positively or negatively correlated. The critic also determines if the investigator has indicated the expected magnitude of the relationships. The next step in theoretical substruction is to order hierarchically, according to their level of abstraction, the propositions formed by the concepts and the stated relationships. Hinshaw (1979b) noted that constructs plus stated relationships are usually the most abstract whereas stated operationalized variables and stated relationships occupy a lower level of abstraction.

Diagramming the study allows the critic to understand exactly what the researcher is investigating and to identify gaps and overlapping ideas in the study's theoretical model. The diagrams also enable the critic to follow how each of the variables was measured and whether the analysis was consistent with theoretical and design models.

Examination of each part of the research is another component of the research critique. In this approach to evaluating completed research, the critic asks specific questions about each part of the study. Although it is usually not possible or desirable to examine parts of a study in isolation, some specific questions can be asked.

The critic examines the problem statement to determine whether the problem for study is explicitly identified and stated precisely and clearly. The critic also asks whether the problem has theoretical and practical significance and if the stated problem is important to nursing science and practice.

The first question the critic asks about the conceptual framework is whether the major concepts guiding the study are identified, defined, and linked to each other. The critic also examines whether the conceptual framework accurately reflects the state of nursing science. For example, has previous empirical

and theoretical work been used to understand the problem?

The purpose of the study should specify its focus. The critic must identify and operationalize concepts or variables for the study. The purpose should be a clear outgrowth of the knowledge level in the field of study and should be consistent with the next logical step in the development of this knowledge.

The critic examines the report to determine how clearly the methods are described, then evaluates the methods to determine whether they are appropriate to the purpose. For example, is the design too complex or inadequate to accomplish the purpose? Is the population and sampling described, and is the sample representative of the groups to whom the study findings should be applied? Is the number of participants appropriate to the design? Are the procedures in keeping with the purpose of the study, and do they ensure valid and reliable data? Replication of studies in nursing is often necessary to obtain sufficiently large samples to allow generalization of findings. The critic should check that the methods are described with sufficient clarity to permit precise repetition and that the statistical treatment of the data is appropriate to the type of data collected, the population, and the sample. Evidence must show the degree of probability that statistical results could reflect a chance variation or error of measurement.

The critic reviews the conclusions to determine if they are justified by the procedures used and the data obtained. The critic must clearly differentiate conclusions supported by the data from those suggested by the data, as well as identify limitations imposed by underlying assumptions and personal opinions and impressions of the investigator.

Perhaps the most critical question in evaluating research design is whether the study has sufficient reliability and validity to warrant acceptance of the findings and their generalization to the population. In this case, *validity* refers to whether the study actually measures what the investigator intended (internal validity) and whether the results accurately represent reality (external validity). *Reliability* refers to how well the measuring instruments yield consistent results. The criteria used to assess reliability and validity are applied differently by the positivist-empiricist and the naturalistic-inductive investigator. Reliability and validity are discussed further in the following sections.

EVALUATING RESEARCH FROM A POSITIVIST-EMPIRICIST PERSPECTIVE

An important assumption of the *positivist-empiricist paradigm* is that a body of facts or principles exists that can be identified and manipulated. These facts or principles are independent of any historical or social context. Research in the positivist-empiricist tradition is oriented toward the reliable and replicable measurement of phenomena. Knowledge is generated by testing measurable hypotheses and reproducing findings. Experimental design typically is employed to infer unambiguous existence and direction of causal relations (Tinkle & Beaton, 1983).

The critic evaluating a research report from a positivist-empiricist perspective will focus on whether contextual variables have been minimized so that the results of the study may be generalized to all individuals without regard to age, gender, or situation (Baumrind, 1980). The ideal study, from a strict positivist-empiricist perspective, uses an experimental design based on control and manipulation of situational variables. Nonexperimental studies are evaluated in terms of how closely they approximate experimental studies.

The critic evaluates how well the research design controls variance. Differences between the control and experimental conditions (the independent variable) should be as great as possible. Is it obvious that the experimental intervention is different from the control intervention or from normal, unmodified experience? This is the principle of maximizing experimental variance, discussed in Chapter 11.

The critic also is concerned about how well the investigator controlled extraneous variables. Kerlinger (1986) noted that extraneous variables can be controlled by minimizing, nullifying, or isolating them. Were the research participants as homogeneous as possible in regard to extraneous variables? Evaluating the control on extraneous variables allows the critic to think creatively about all the factors that could possibly account for the findings and assess whether each of those factors or variables was controlled. Has the investigator selected the research participants at random? Have the participants been assigned to groups at random? Have the experimental treatments to groups been assigned at random?

To minimize error or random variance, the investigator must have taken steps to ensure minimum measurement error. Has the researcher controlled the conditions under which measurements were taken? How reliable were the instruments used to measure the variables?

The critic using a positivist-empiricist framework also is interested in the generalizability of the study's findings. The first question involves the *internal validity* of the study. Did the experimental manipulation account for the differences in outcome between the groups? The previous questions about control of variance determine this internal validity.

External validity involves the representativeness of the variables studied. The critic can assess the study's external validity by examining the procedures and the participants and deciding whether the research findings can reasonably be generalized beyond one particular group. This initial subjective judgment about generalizability must be verified by other studies. Is the study a conceptual replication of previous work? Are the findings congruent with previous findings? Findings that are consistent over different times and places and with different people and procedures lend themselves to generalization. How similar to the real world were the experimental conditions? The more the experimental conditions differ from the real world, the lower the external validity.

Reliable research findings are repeatable. When the exact replication of procedures produces exact results, we say that the research has external reliability. External reliability differs from external validity in that the latter involves conceptual replication of ideas with different procedures. For example, when the researcher repeats a study using exactly the same purpose, conceptual framework, and design, the researcher is establishing external reliability. When the researcher has the same conceptual framework as a previous study but uses a different research design, conceptual replication occurs, which can be used to establish external validity.

EVALUATING RESEARCH FROM A NATURALISTIC-INDUCTIVE PERSPECTIVE

Traditionally, validity and reliability are demonstrated by specific criteria based on quantitative research methods that emanate from a positivist-empiricist paradigm. However, concepts of validity and reliability apply to naturalistic-inductive research studies as well, although these concepts are demonstrated differently and must be evaluated against different criteria. The purpose of this section is to describe the specific criteria used to guide evaluation of qualitative research that evolves from a *naturalistic-inductive paradigm,* to offer criteria and guidelines for evaluating research from a naturalistic-inductive perspective, and to point out potential problem areas in evaluating qualitative research studies based on a naturalistic-inductive paradigm.

Naturalistic-inductive research differs significantly from positivist-empiricist research in the formulation of problems, the nature of goals, and the application of results, making it difficult to judge both by the same criteria (LeCompte & Goetz, 1982). In discussing the nature of goals, LeCompte and Goetz emphasized that positivist-empiricist researchers attempt to verify existing theory by finding data to match that theory, whereas naturalistic-inductive researchers attempt to generate theory that will reflect and explain the data collected. The different research processes used to accomplish these different purposes necessitate different ways of evaluating validity and reliability. Naturalistic-inductive researchers do not aim for generalization in the sense that the positivist-empiricist researcher does. However, they do aim for comparability and translatability. "Comparability," according to LeCompte and Goetz, is achieved if the researcher clearly describes the characteristics of the group studied as well as the concepts generated, enabling comparisons to be made with other groups as well as across studies. They defined "translatability" as the ability to make comparisons confidently by clearly explaining the research methods, analytic categories, and characteristics of the group studied. Thus comparability is necessary for translatability.

Criteria for evaluation

Several authors have suggested criteria for evaluating qualitative research that incorporate concepts of validity and reliability but are specific to naturalistic-inductive studies (Glaser, 1978; Glaser & Strauss, 1966; Glaser & Strauss, 1967; LeCompte & Goetz, 1982; Lincoln & Guba, 1985; May, 1986; Sandelowski, 1986; Schatzman & Strauss, 1973; Wilson 1985). Glaser and Strauss (1966, 1967) used the words "credibility," "usefulness," and "trustworthiness" when referring to criteria for evaluating the scientific merit of qualitative studies. They defined credibility as the process of ensuring that readers

understand the theoretical framework generated. Credibility should also describe the data collected in such a way that readers "can almost literally see and hear its people—but always in relation to the theory" (Glaser & Strauss, 1967, p. 228). The authors discussed usefulness of qualitative research not only as a way to generate hypotheses to be tested in later quantitative studies, but also as a worthwhile end product to help shed light on a phenomenon. Trustworthiness refers to the extent to which one can believe in the research findings.

Sandelowski (1986), drawing from and using the terminology of Lincoln and Guba (1985), identified four criteria that must be present to evaluate a qualitative study as rigorous: (1) truth value, (2) applicability, (3) consistency, and (4) neutrality.

Truth value, according to Lincoln and Guba (1985), refers to adequate representation of multiple constructions of reality. They explained that the *re*constructions by the researcher must be credible to the informants, who are the original constructors. Sandelowski used the term "credibility." This concept is similar to internal validity in a positivist-empiricist sense; one can infer that a causal relationship exists between two variables. Lincoln and Guba (1985) suggested the following techniques for demonstrating credibility:

1. Prolonged engagement with informants in the field to ensure sufficient time to build a trusting relationship with them
2. Persistent observation to provide salience and depth to the findings by studying them over time
3. Triangulation, whereby multiple sources, methods, or investigators are employed in the research process
4. Peer debriefing, whereby a colleague serves as "devil's advocate," challenging the researcher's analyses
5. Negative case analysis, in which provisional hypotheses generated are constantly modified as cases occur that negate the hypotheses as originally constructed
6. Referential adequacy, whereby some data are saved and stored for later testing against findings generated
7. Member checks, in which informants are given the opportunity to react to the researcher's analysis

Applicability refers to "fittingness," according to Sandelowski (1986), or "transferability," according to Lincoln and Guba (1985). Conceptually these terms describe the degree to which findings in one context will be similar in another. In positivist-empiricist terms, this is the concept of external validity, or generalizability. Lincoln and Guba indicated that researchers can never be sure of the degree of transferability, since they have only studied the social context from which they are attempting to transfer or generalize. The context being generalized *to* has not been studied. The authors suggest the use of "thick description" as a criterion for judging transferability, which means researchers describe the data in detail, generating working hypotheses to enable someone to consider the possibility of attempting verification in another context.

Consistency is referred to by Sandelowski (1986) as "auditability," and by Lincoln and Guba (1985) as "dependability." Both define these terms as the process by which other researchers can follow the method used in the study being evaluated and are able to find similar concepts, not contradictory ones, if they were to have access to the researcher's data, be in the same situation, and take a similar philosophical perspective. In positivist-empiricist terms, consistency is similar to reliability.

Neutrality is referred to by both Sandelowski (1986) and Lincoln and Guba (1985) as "confirmability." Confirmability depends on the existence of auditability, truth value, and applicability. This concept does not negate the intersubjectivity between researcher and informant, since that is part of the process of naturalistic-inductive research. It emphasizes the systematic nature of the research, however, such that an audit, similar to a financial audit, can be done. Lincoln and Guba, drawing from Halpern (1983), suggested that such an audit could be used to document accuracy and fairness, emphasizing the confirmability of findings. Confirmability is an attempt to parallel the positivist-empiricist concept of objectivity, although naturalistic-inductive researchers acknowledge that subjectivity is part of the research method.

Goodwin and Goodwin (1984) use the traditional terms "validity" and "reliability" in discussing criteria for evaluating qualitative research in an attempt to deemphasize the dichotomy between the two methods while recognizing differences. LeCompte and Goetz (1982) also use validity and reliability, while clearly emphasizing the differences in their meanings as they are applied to qualitative or quantitative studies.

The strategy of this section is to delineate the criteria for evaluating naturalistic-inductive research by using descriptive sentences, while incorporating concepts of validity and reliability that underlie these criteria. How each criterion is related to validity and/or reliability is explained.

Before presenting these specific criteria, it is essential to note that a good scientific study, whether naturalistic-inductive or positivist-empiricist, is conducted in a systematic manner, and evidence of this must be apparent to the critic. The researcher does this by indicating all the procedures used throughout the study, beginning with why a particular area was chosen for study, what background data and pertinent information were known about the area, why a particular research method was chosen, how subjects were obtained, and how data were collected and analyzed. Clearly, a naturalistic-inductive study is not "controlled" in the sense that a positivist-empiricist study manipulates and controls the context; however, lack of control in a quantitative sense is not equated with lack of systematization. In other words, a naturalistic-inductive study design does not control variables as a positivist-empiricist study does, but a well-done naturalistic-inductive study is conducted systematically. Thus evidence of a systematic research process is a criterion in evaluating all research.

The next sections describe specific criteria for evaluating naturalistic-inductive research. Although data collection and analysis are concurrent ongoing processes of naturalistic-inductive methodology, the criteria presented are organized into two major sections: the process (methodology) and the outcome (findings). This organization is used simply for clarity in discussing this information. Because most naturalistic-inductive studies use qualitative research methods, these terms will be used interchangeably.

Process (methodology)

One very important aspect in qualitative study is that the researcher indicates knowledge and expertise in the area chosen. This means the researcher should be familiar with the literature and know where the gaps in knowledge exist and why such a study would contribute to filling these gaps. May (1986) stated that the literature review is not meant to dictate the focus of study or the variables to be examined, since this focus is dictated by the data as they are analyzed. However, an initial literature review that shows familiarity with information on the topic is important. Further literature reviews may be done as the researcher continues with data collection and analysis. Often people have the misconception that a researcher who conducts naturalistic-inductive studies approaches "the field" as a "tabula rasa," or blank slate, without any preconceived ideas. All researchers have some notions or thoughts about a phenomenon being studied and should communicate this knowledge to their readers or consumers of their research. In addition to providing evidence of knowledge in the study area, the researcher must provide adequate rationale for approaching the study in an inductive manner using a qualitative methodology.

Researchers should also indicate how their experiences have contributed to the choice of this particular research topic as well as to the analysis of data. Glaser and Strauss (1967) referred to this as "experiential data." It is important to differentiate between experiential data used to bias the analysis and experiential data incorporated in a manner that recognizes the influence of such data on how a human being (the researcher) views the phenomenon being studied. For example, a nurse conducting research may have clinical expertise in that area, and that expertise may have contributed to her interest in conducting such research. This type of experience adds an important dimension to the research process.

The researcher should include several comparative groups in the study. This enhances the opportunity to understand the phenomenon as it may apply to other populations. The comparative groups should be systematically included in the study, which means the researcher should indicate why and at what point in the research certain groups were included. The systematic nature of this process cannot be overemphasized. Although Glaser and Strauss (1967) are known for their work with constant comparative analysis as a technique used in grounded-theory research, this concept applies to other qualitative methods as well. Lincoln and Guba (1985), referring to qualitative methods generally, as opposed to a specific kind of qualitative method, dis-

cussed interviewing several informants in order to better understand the phenomenon in question.

Along with demonstrating inclusion of several comparative groups, the researcher should provide evidence of systematic "theoretical sampling." Theoretical sampling is a process by which specific comparison groups are chosen to provide confirmation and verification of "provisional hypotheses" formulated from the analysis up to that point. Theoretical sampling is highly interrelated with and actually guides the choice of comparison groups. The researcher should make this process explicit, explaining why certain provisional hypotheses were generated, using the data to support such hypotheses, and giving a rationale for choosing a particular individual or group for theoretical sampling. Theoretical sampling is a term specific to grounded-theory methodology. Other qualitative methods, however, follow the concept of theoretical sampling, although they refer to it differently. Ethnographers, for example, discuss making a domain analysis and asking structured questions (Spradley, 1979, 1980).

Since concurrent and ongoing data collection and analysis are inherent in the process of qualitative research, the researcher should provide evidence of systematically formulating "provisional hypotheses," as well as discarding hypotheses not supported by the data. Thus there should be evidence of "open coding" and a constant "checking in" with the subjects themselves to verify or discard concepts generated through the open-coding process. This constant checking in allows for evidence of validity in a quantitative sense. By demonstrating this process, the researcher is able to give evidence of narrowing of the coding as certain codes or categories are systematically discarded when they are unsupported by further data collection. Eventually it should become clear to the reader that the investigator has become more focused in data collection and analysis, guided by initial analyses that have continued to be verified through further data collection.

As this more focused data collection process continues, eventually the researcher should be able to show evidence of having reached "theoretical saturation," whereby there is support for the construction of a "core category" or several "core categories," which repeatedly occur while less and less new information emerges. Theoretical saturation necessitates maximum variation in and verification of the data.

This means the researcher uses many comparison groups for variety, as well as for verifying concepts generated from the data. Whereas the terms "theoretical sampling" and "theoretical saturation" are specific to grounded-theory methodology, these concepts apply to qualitative research methods generally. As data are collected and analyzed, further data collection becomes more focused and systematic based on ongoing analysis. Data collection continues until the researcher is confident that enough "evidence" has been collected to present credible results. Variety addresses the issue of external validity, whereas verification addresses internal validity.

Besides systematically narrowing the focus and searching for consistent support for a core category or categories, the researcher also must attempt to discover contradictory or "negative" cases or occurrences. This means that the researcher should understand situations in the phenomenon studied that do not support the core category and that indicate a particular explanation does not hold. This process allows the researcher to understand better the conditions under which the explanation "holds up" and those under which it does not, incorporating commonalities as well as variations into a complex, dense theoretical formulation that better represents "reality."

Because the goal of qualitative research is to generate a theoretical explanation that reflects an understanding of a phenomenon, the use of various data sources is important. This enhances the probability that the theory generated does reflect the real world, since various "slices of data" (Glaser & Strauss, 1967) are incorporated into this theory. These data sources include interviews, observations, and documents such as letters or diaries kept by the research subjects. The empirical data must be integrated into the researcher's report because the reader or critic must have "evidence" for the concepts generated. In other words, the researcher is obligated to persuade the audience that the explanation constructed for a particular phenomenon of study is plausible and does reflect reality. Empirical validation is an important aspect in demonstrating internal validity.

Outcomes (findings)

The researcher should present the findings of a qualitative study in a way understandable to the critic. Statements that explain the findings must be clear and must reflect the linkages among the resulting concepts or categories, and these linkages must make sense to the critic. The findings should reflect a conceptual framework generated from and grounded in the data. An ideal conceptual framework is dense, well integrated, and modifiable because new data may necessitate changes. Because qualitative research is process oriented, the researcher should be open to modifications in the theory generated. Representative examples of data must be used to indicate the relevance of the concepts generated and the credibility of the conceptual framework constructed.

In reporting the results of a naturalistic-inductive study to a particular audience, the researcher looks for "phenomenon recognition" (Schatzman & Strauss, 1973, p. 135). This is a response to the researcher's findings in which the audience "recognizes" the theoretical explanation presented because they believe this explanation makes sense based on their experiences. A researcher may include evidence of having "gone back to the field" and elicited this phenomenon recognition from research subjects or informants. This is another way of indicating validity.

Guidelines for nurses

Based on the previous discussion of criteria for evaluating naturalistic-inductive research, several guidelines that consist of pertinent questions can help nurses evaluate and critique such research. May (1986) and Wilson (1985) discussed several questions that apply to the evaluation of a grounded-theory study. Although they specifically referred to grounded-theory methodology, these criteria are broad enough to be applicable to evaluating other naturalistic-inductive studies.

One important question concerns the research question itself. Is the question broad enough initially? Does evidence show that the initial research question has become more focused as data are collected and analyzed? Answers to these questions reflect whether or not the researcher demonstrates a systematic approach to the phenomenon under study, carefully narrowing and defining the focus based on ongoing analysis of data. These questions address the issue of internal validity.

Another important question concerns whether or not data sources are comprehensive, allowing the researcher to analyze the range and variation of phenomena under study. This question addresses the issue of external validity, or how well the findings represent the "real world."

The critic should ask whether a relationship exists between the study and the literature. May (1986) stated that one specifically must ask if the researcher has illustrated knowledge of the study area and how the analysis derived in the naturalistic-inductive study concurs with, adds to, differs from, or challenges the literature. This question also addresses the issue of external validity in that the findings are questioned in relation to other studies, which may or may not accurately represent the "real world."

The critic must also question the analysis that the researcher is presenting. Is the analysis understandable? Is it plausible? Are the concepts within the analysis well integrated with linkages evident? In naturalistic-inductive terminology, one is asking whether or not the findings actually measure what was intended; thus the critic addresses the issue of internal validity.

These questions are meant to be guidelines for critics of naturalistic-inductive studies. They provide a framework from which to analyze and evaluate such studies.

Potential problem areas

In evaluating naturalistic-inductive research, the critic must realize potential problems that exist in conducting these studies. Wilson (1985) addressed two major problems. First, the researcher may end theoretical sampling before theoretical saturation has occurred. Glaser and Strauss (1967) refer to this as "premature closure" on the data. The keen evaluator of such research must be able to detect such a problem. Strauss (1985) explained that in trying to reach saturation, the researcher maximizes differences in comparison groups (data sources) in order to maximize varieties of data and develop as many diverse properties in the categories as possible. He stated that "saturation means that no additional data are being found whereby the researcher can develop properties of the category further. As he or she sees similar instances over and over again (events, actions, conditions, consequences) the researcher becomes confident that a category is saturated. The researcher goes out of his or her way to look for groups that stretch diversity of data as far as possible, just to make certain that saturation is based on a wide range of data on the category" (Strauss, 1985).

The second major problem is lack of identification of a core category, which indicates that the researcher lacked specific direction in collecting and analyzing the data. Wilson (1985) stated that a study with this problem can be presented as descriptive research without offering a conceptual scheme or framework. The critic of such research must be able to discern this type of study from a grounded-theory study, which does result in a conceptual framework consisting of linkages among concepts generated from the data.

Application to specific study

Wilson's study (1977) of an experimental psychiatric treatment community (Soteria) is an excellent naturalistic-inductive study based on grounded-theory methodology. This section discusses her study using the criteria outlined in this chapter.

In studying a particular psychiatric treatment modality, Wilson chose an area in which she had current knowledge and expertise. Her experience as a nurse and her knowledge of the literature fulfilled the criteria of having both knowledge and expertise.

More specifically, in examining the methodology she used, she clearly conducted her research systematically. She used several comparative groups, collecting data at all periods of the day and night every day of the month. She acquired data during meals, special occasions, field trips, meetings, and visitors' arrivals. She also collected data from different persons, including long-term and new residents and staff members. The various data sources included interviews, documents related to the community, and a film about the setting. Wilson stated, "This multifaceted accumulation of data was sought in order to provide different views or vantage points from which to understand a category and to develop its properties in the analytical process" (1977, p. 107). By incorporating many data sources, Wilson also was able to examine negative cases and thus account for maximum variation in establishing conceptual categories.

The systematic nature of the methodology used is apparent. Wilson explicitly stated that she searched for variation in situations to provide new properties of the processes discovered based on substantive and theoretical concepts and their relationships. She systematically formulated provisional hypotheses to be tested as she continued her data collection and analysis. The core category of "limiting intrusion" provided a central integrative scheme, leading to selective coding and eventual theoretical saturation. Ultimately, Wilson arrived at an integrated, dense, theoretical framework centered around "limiting intrusion," a process that reflects the phenomenon whereby this psychiatric community protects itself from external mandates, regulations, rules, expectations, and values and preserves its autonomy.

SUMMARY

This chapter has discussed two perspectives from which to evaluate research: positivist-empiricist and naturalistic-inductive.

The critic viewing a research report from a positivist-empiricist perspective primarily is concerned about the reliable and replicable measurement of phenomena. Questions determine how well the investigator maximized experimental variance, controlled extraneous variance, and minimized error variance. The critic assesses the generalizability of findings in terms of the conceptual and the procedural replication that has occurred.

Specific criteria for evaluation of naturalistic-inductive research studies include truth value, applicability, consistency, and neutrality. The concepts of reliability and validity also relate to these studies. Specific criteria for evaluating qualitative research are applied to the process (methodology) and the outcome (findings) of the study and include the researcher's familiarity with the field of study and the systematic inclusion of comparative groups. The use of various data sources is essential. Research findings must be presented in a way understandable to the critic. Guidelines for evaluating naturalistic-inductive studies include the scope of the question, the comprehensive nature of data, the relationship to existing literature, and the understandability and plausibility of the presentation. Potential problem areas that the critic must be aware of are ending data collection prematurely and failing to identify the core category for collecting and analyzing data.

REFERENCES

Baumrind, D. (1980). New directions in socialization research. *American Psychologist, 35,* 639-652.

Glaser, B. G. (1978). *Theoretical sensitivity.* Mill Valley, CA: Mill Valley Press.

Glaser, B. G., and Strauss, A. L. (1966). The purpose and credibility of qualitative research. *Nursing Research, 15* (1), 56-61.

Glaser, B. G., and Strauss, A. L. (1967). *Discovery of grounded theory: Strategies for qualitative research.* Chicago: Aldine Publishing.

Goodwin, L. D., and Goodwin, W. L. (1984). Are validity and reliability relevant in qualitative evaluation research? *Evaluation and the Health Professions, 7* (4), 413-426.

Halpern, E. S. (1983). *Auditing naturalistic inquiries: The development and application of a model.* Unpublished doctoral dissertation. Indiana University.

Hinshaw, A. S. (1979a). Planning for logical consistency among three research structures. *Western Journal of Nursing Research, 1*(3), 250-253.

Hinshaw, A. S. (1979b). Theoretical substruction: An assessment process. *Western Journal of Nursing Research, 1*(4), 319-324.

Kerlinger, F. N. (1986). *Foundations of behavioral research.* New York: Holt, Rinehart & Winston.

LeCompte, M. D., and Goetz, J. P. (1982). Problems of reliability and validity in ethnographic research. *Review of Educational Research, 52* (1), 31-60.

Leininger, M. M. (1968). The research critique: Nature, function, and art. *Communicating nursing research:* Vol. 1: *The research critique* (pp. 20-31).

Lincoln, Y. S., and Guba, E. G. (1985). *Naturalistic inquiry.* Beverly Hills, CA: Sage.

May, K. A. (1986). Writing and evaluating the grounded research report. In C. Chenitz and J. Swanson (Eds.), *From Practice to Grounded Theory,* Menlo Park, CA: Addison-Wesley.

Sandelowski, M. (1986). The problem of rigor in qualitative research. *Advances in Nursing Science, 8* (3), 27-37.

Schatzman, L., and Strauss, A. L. (1973). *Field research: Strategies for a natural sociology.* Englewood Cliffs, NJ: Prentice-Hall.

Spradley, J. P. (1979). *The ethnographic interview.* New York: Holt, Rinehart & Winston.

Spradley, J. P. (1980). *Participant observation.* New York: Holt, Rinehart & Winston.

Strauss, A. L. (1985). *Qualitative analysis.* West Germany: Fink Press.

Wilson, H. S. (1977). Limiting intrusion—social control of outsiders in a healing community: An illustration of qualitative comparative analysis. *Nursing Research, 26* (2), 103-111.

Wilson, H. S. (1985). *Research in nursing.* Menlo Park, CA: Addison-Wesley.

31

DISSEMINATING AND USING
RESEARCH FINDINGS

MARCIA GRUIS KILLIEN

Research is a public enterprise. Whenever an individual undertakes a research project, the commitment includes the responsibility to communicate the completed project to others. Each investigator must decide which components to disseminate, to whom, and by what method. This chapter discusses these issues and offers specific guidelines for disseminating research by both oral and written mechanisms. Research, once disseminated, is available for use by consumers; issues related to this use of research are also discussed.

ISSUES IN DISSEMINATING RESEARCH

Dissemination as a responsibility

The importance of research to the profession of nursing is discussed in Chapter 1. The accumulation of new scientific knowledge is essential to guide nursing practice, nursing education, and nursing administration. Knowledge development is a cumulative process shared by the entire body of nursing professionals; it is not a private endeavor of the individual investigator. Dissemination of research serves scientific, professional, and public functions (Batey, 1978). Through communication of research processes and outcomes among scientists, ideas are generated, developed, tested, and refined. Thus all investigators have the responsibility to contribute to this process by disseminating their research to others for dialogue, debate, and evaluation.

The professional functions of research dissemina-

tion are concerned with influencing professional practice. The public functions involve influencing public knowledge, opinion, and public policy. Presenting or publishing one's research to serve any of these functions can be perceived as challenging, difficult, overwhelming, and rewarding. Dissemination of research is, above all, essential. As expressed by Styles (1978), ". . . the future of the profession depends on it."

Reasons for dissemination

The reasons for "going public" with one's research fall into three categories: disseminating for knowledge, disseminating for change, and disseminating for reward (McCloskey & Swanson, 1985).

By presenting and publishing their research, investigators submit their work to scrutiny by their peers and add to the scientific knowledge base of nursing (Batey, 1978). In addition, they may contribute to knowledge development in other fields. Contributions to knowledge come not only from sharing research findings but also from presenting research instruments, methodological strategies, and conceptualizations of nursing phenomena.

Disseminating for change involves the goal of benefiting others through one's research. The ultimate goal of sharing new knowledge and insights with nurse educators, nurse administrators, and nurse clinicians is to effect changes in practice. Disseminations of nursing research findings to the public may result in changes in consumers' health behaviors or knowledge or changes in public policy. These are the professional and public functions of research communication as described by Batey (1978).

Disseminating for reward acknowledges the personal benefits gained from presenting or publishing one's work. These benefits can include recognition from colleagues, a sense of personal accomplishment, opportunities for job promotion or security, and improved chances of obtaining research funding. Occasionally, publications can generate income. Also, one can benefit from the resulting development in scholarly thinking that occurs during the process of preparing a talk or manuscript and from the debate and dialogue with colleagues.

Dissemination options: product, audience, method

When considering dissemination, researchers might first consider sharing the results of a completed project. To meet the goals just discussed, they might also consider the conceptual model, instruments, design or analytical strategies, or project implementation experiences as other products of research worth disseminating to others. Sharing any of these products could contribute directly or indirectly to knowledge development. The box below lists questions the researchers can ask when making decisions about dissemination.

Although research findings are the substantive building blocks of our scientific knowledge base, development of knowledge in nursing also depends on innovations in research methodology and theory development. Sharing theories or conceptual models provides the opportunity for additional testing by other researchers. Dissemination of information about research instruments, their development, and usefulness strengthens the measures available to all researchers. Similarly, discussions of methodological innovations, issues, problems, and solutions contribute to the ongoing development of scientific rigor in nursing research. These products of nursing research, the findings, the instruments, and the processes each may be used by colleagues in nursing practice, administration, and education, as well as by nurse researchers (Stetler, 1985).

Another option is to present research while it is in progress, often as a poster presentation at a research conference. This method of dissemination informs others of current work that might influence them and also provides investigators with critical comment on their work from colleagues during the developmental stages of a research project.

QUESTIONS TO GUIDE RESEARCH DISSEMINATION DECISIONS

What do I want to achieve?
1. Contribute to knowledge development
2. Facilitate change in practice or policy
3. Obtain personal rewards and benefits

What aspects of the project do I want others to know about?
1. Theories, framework used
2. Design and methodological strategies
3. Instruments used or developed
4. Research results and conclusions
5. Practice or public policy implications
6. Pragmatic issues encountered or solved

What audience do I want to reach?
1. Nurses
   a. Scientists
   b. Administrators
   c. Educators
   d. Clinicians
2. Nonnursing professionals
   a. Scientists
   b. Practitioners
3. Public
   a. Health-care consumers
   b. Policymakers

What mode of dissemination is best?
1. Is the project in progress or completed?
2. How rapidly do I want information disseminated?
3. How wide an audience do I want to reach?
4. What resources do I want to expend (time, money, energy)?

Besides a choice of several research products to share, researchers can also select various audiences to target for dissemination efforts. Choosing an audience depends on the goal and the intended product for dissemination. Other nurse researchers are often the targeted audience. McCloskey and Swanson (1985) suggested that nurse researchers are more often motivated by the goals of dissemination for knowledge and reward than for change. Since knowledge development in nursing is primarily the responsibility of nurse researchers, they are a logical audience. Other nurse researchers can also convey significant rewards related to personal recognition, career advancement, research funding, and scholarly development. However, "if change is to occur within nursing practice, more research articles need to be published in journals read by practitioners. . . . Researchers . . . should also publish in practice journals so practitioners can be exposed to new and current knowledge in order to evaluate their clinical practice and subsequently facilitate change" (McCloskey & Swanson, 1985, p. 1).

When practitioners are targeted for dissemination of research, the communication usually pertains to research findings. However, they also might be considered as a potential audience with whom to share research instruments (e.g., questionnaires, observation guides) that could be used for client assessment in practice settings.

Nurse educators and nurse administrators are viable audiences for nursing research as well. Their responsibilities for the education of future generations of nurses and for nursing care delivery systems make them powerful agents for change.

Nurse researchers should also consider potential audiences outside the nursing profession, including scientists and health-care professionals in other disciplines. Nursing research can contribute to knowledge development in fields other than nursing, but only if that research is disseminated more broadly. Publishing in nonnursing journals and presenting at interdisciplinary meetings not only serves to disseminate new knowledge widely but also informs members of other disciplines about the type and quality of work done by nurse scientists.

Finally, the public consumer of nursing care is an important audience for research dissemination. Such efforts might be directed toward influencing change in individuals' health behavior or knowledge or toward influencing public policy.

Research can be disseminated to these various audiences through two major methods: verbal and written. The product to be shared, the target audience, and the goal are key factors influencing choice of a particular dissemination method.

The most rapid means to disseminate one's research is to discuss it during formal or informal professional meetings, public lectures, or interviews with the media. Researchers typically elect to present scientific papers at research or clinical conferences. Because these presentations are usually limited to 10 to 30 minutes, in-depth discussion of an entire project rarely is possible. However, conference participants often can ask the investigator more about the project. The content of such presentations can be targeted to the audience in attendance and might focus on conceptual or methodological issues, selected research findings, or implications for practice. The opportunity for dialogue with the audience can stimulate the researcher's thinking and help refine ideas before publication.

Many professional meetings now include the "poster session" format for presentation of research. This format combines verbal and written communication; the researcher prepares a visual display highlighting elements of the research but usually also is present to talk informally to interested observers. The poster format is ideal for sharing information about research in progress and for stimulating idea exchange among peers. The novice researcher can also use it as a nonintimidating format for dissemination.

Limitations of the preceding methods of research dissemination are that only the audience at the presentation directly benefits from the knowledge, and time constraints usually limit depth or scope of content.

Written reports of research offer the advantages of permanence and potential for reaching a wider audience. The major disadvantage of written reports is the time involved in their preparation and publication. Almost all research projects include preparation of a final written report as a requirement of either the academic program (e.g., thesis, dissertation) or the funding agency; written progress reports throughout the project might also be made. These reports usually document in great detail the entire research process, although specific requirements may vary according to the institution or funding source. The clinical agencies or institutions where the project was conducted or the research participants may also request summaries, which usually emphasize research results. The primary purpose of these types of reports is usually to document to the institution or funding agency the investigator's expertise and accountability for project completion, not to disseminate research findings widely for the goals previously discussed.

Preparation of a written report of scholarly work for publication in a journal or book is the most common method for dissemination of nursing research. This method allows specific audiences to be targeted according to the journal's usual readership (e.g., nurse scientists, practitioners in a special field, the public) and allows dissemination to national and international audiences. The review and publication schedules of most professional journals, however, involve long intervals between article submission and eventual publication. This means that research findings may be several years old by the time a reader receives the information. For example, the usual time for manuscript review and editorial decision once a manuscript is received by a journal is 1 to 3 months; the time between manuscript acceptance and publication ranges from a month to 2 or more years, with an average of 8 months (McCloskey & Swanson, 1982; Swanson & McCloskey, 1982). Publishing a book based on a research project takes even longer, involving more preparation time because of greater length and a longer production phase.

Books or monographs allow in-depth reports of an entire research project. Journal articles are briefer but can describe either an entire project, including conceptualization, methods, and results, or focus on selected aspects. Also, brief reports, technical notes, or abstracts of research are published by a variety of journals. Short abstracts (e.g., one to two pages) of research presented at professional meetings often are compiled and distributed as conference proceedings to attendees and sometimes to others on request. These written reports reach a smaller audience but often allow more rapid dissemination because of shortened production time. The abstracts, however, usually do not meet peer review criteria for "publication" and thus may not fulfill the researcher's reward or recognition goals.

Most researchers select multiple methods to disseminate their work. They may present their work in progress in a poster session, give several talks on the various aspects of the project at professional meetings, and then use the verbal presentations as the bases for papers published in journals that reach several different audiences. Although publishing identical manuscripts in several journals is considered unethical, the researcher can often appropriately develop several unique articles, each addressing different aspects of a research project or directed toward different audiences. The number of presentations and publications generated from a single project depends on the project's scope, the investigator's goals, and the time and energy devoted to dissemination efforts.

ESSENTIAL INGREDIENTS

Several principles guide the communication of research ideas, regardless of the intended audience or the mode of communication.

Focused message

The components of a research project that might be the focus of a talk or paper have been mentioned. For example, the conceptual model, the methodology, the data production instruments, the research findings, or the practice implications could each be selected as a primary focus.

Knowing the intended message helps the researcher select both the audience and the place for dissemination. For example, if the intent is to share information about the development of a new research instrument to measure a nursing phenomenon, a journal or conference targeted toward nurse scientists with an interest in that phenomenon would be an appropriate selection; a practice journal aimed at a general nursing readership would not. This latter audience would most likely be interested in the practice implications of a study rather than issues of research instrumentation and methodology.

The researcher must also know the primary message in order to maintain the emphasis on that message throughout the presentation or article. This focus helps the presenter allocate time and space among a project's components according to their contribution toward understanding the primary message. For example, if the researcher intends to emphasize research results in a 20-minute oral presentation, 15 minutes cannot be spent discussing a literature review on the research problem. With a clear focus, the presenter can decide what information is essential to understanding and interpreting the primary message (e.g., research results) and which information can be deleted or saved for another time and place.

Clarity of communication

"When you say something, make sure you have said it. The chances of your having said it are only fair," wrote William Strunk, Jr., and E. B. White in *The Elements of Style* (1979). The transmittal of ideas from one person to another requires that the sender actively consider the audience or reader to be addressed. This consideration means using commonly understood language, eliminating unnecessary words and jargon, using words with precision and consistency of meaning, and presenting ideas in a logical progression. Knowledge about the audience helps one to avoid a condescending tone and oversimplified message and not to assume inherent understanding.

Scientific writing and speaking differ from creative writing in that original use of words, streams of consciousness, personal opinion, and emotion are discouraged. This does not mean that scientific writing needs to be redundant, dull, or technically difficult to read. Using language that comes naturally and maintaining a focus on the message and the audience can make a research report both clear and interesting.

Scientific communication should be free of language that reinforces sexist or ethnic bias. Ambiguous or stereotypical word choices are inappropriate. Such errors, for example, the use of "man" as a generic noun, are often unintentional but may be perceived as demeaning or lead to inaccurate interpretation of a research report. Suggestions for alternative word choices can be found in several sources, such as the *APA Publication Manual* (American Psychological Association, 1984, p. 43).

Logical organization

Reports of research usually follow a common format, as illustrated in the box above. In journal articles this format enables readers to locate particular aspects readily and to evaluate the report for completeness. A similar format for verbal presentation can be a useful way to organize ideas. Deviations from this format may be indicated by the particular focus of the

COMPONENTS OF A RESEARCH REPORT

   I. Title page
      Title
      Author's name and affiliation
  II. Abstract
 III. Introduction
      Overview of problem under study and research strategy
      Conceptual or theoretical framework
      Background literature review
      Study purpose and rationale
 IV. Method
      Subjects
      Setting
      Variables and their measurement
      Procedures
  V. Results
      Report of data (tables, figures)
      Statistical presentation
 VI. Discussion
      Evaluation of results
      Study limitations
      Implications
VIII. References

journal or conference or by special interests or style of the presenter or audience.

A well-organized talk or paper carries the audience smoothly and logically from one idea to the next. Paragraphs are the framework for accomplishing this organization. Each paragraph presents a single topic or idea through the sentences it contains. As a rule, each paragraph begins with a sentence that introduces its focus or helps with transition to the topic. Subsequent sentences further develop the topic. In written papers, visual presentation also dictates paragraph structure. Using long paragraphs or a succession of short ones is distracting for readers; the writer may choose to break or combine paragraphs for visual as well as conceptual reasons (Strunk & White, 1979).

Communication aids

Disseminating ideas, especially technical or complex ones, is made easier by considering the audience's visual, as well as cognitive, skills. Verbal presentations can be made more clear and interesting through use of pictures, schematic diagrams, and graphs displayed on slides, handouts, or transparencies. Similarly, written papers can employ illustrations and tables to supplement the manuscript text. Use of these visual aids can serve to communicate much information economically. Although visual aids can expand on written or spoken words, each must stand alone in conveying complete thoughts. Audience readability, clarity, and simplicity are key elements for visual materials used in presentations and manuscripts.

Adherence to guidelines

Specific guidelines for content and format accompany nearly all journals, calls for abstracts, and conference presentations. Careful reading of these guidelines helps researchers to target their work to the particular focus of the journal, conference, or organization. Guidelines usually contain suggestions for how to organize and emphasize content and how to prepare it. Format instructions, such as for margins, paper length, and references, should be strictly observed.

METHODS OF DISSEMINATION

Several different methods for disseminating research have been introduced. This section discusses in greater detail the methods used most frequently: the research abstract, the journal article, the scientific paper presentation, and the research poster presentation.

The research abstract

An abstract is a brief written summary of a research project. It can vary in length from a paragraph of several sentences to two or three pages. The purpose of the abstract is to synopsize an entire project. The abstract usually is an adjunct to a more thorough presentation of the project. For example, it may be submitted in response to a "call for abstracts" issued to solicit papers for presentation at a research conference. Used in this way, the abstract serves to "market" one's research to a review or selection committee; if judged appropriate, this is followed by a more extensive presentation at the conference. Abstracts might also be compiled and distributed to participants through conference proceedings. Such a compilation assists conference participants to select which presentations to attend and also disseminates information about the research to individuals who cannot attend the complete presentation. These compilations of abstracts often reach a wider audience because they are shared with colleagues not attending the conference.

Abstracts may also serve as an introduction to a journal article or final research report. The abstract thus may be the most important paragraph of the article. It is read first and may be the *only* part of the article that is read, since readers often decide on the basis of the abstract whether to read the entire article. Abstracts also are an important mechanism for accessing and retrieving articles (APA, 1984, p. 23).

Abstracts can also stand alone and be used independent from an additional report. For example, an investigator might use an abstract to provide a summary of the project to study participants or to other interested researchers. Abstracts might appear in journals in the same way as more detailed research reports are published.

Regardless of the intended purpose, the abstract ideally should include a description of the study purpose, the sample and setting, methods, major findings, and conclusions. The depth and amount of detail reported on each component depend on the length of the abstract and its intended audience and purpose. A good abstract accurately reflects the purpose and content of the manuscript or presentation. It should be self-contained and not include terminology that requires supplemental material for understanding. Because of an abstract's brevity, each sentence must be maximally informative (APA, 1984).

Abstracts may not include actual data or statistics, but they should provide as much specific information as possible. Thus an abstract should not resemble an advertisement for a movie enticing you to attend by hinting at, but not disclosing, the plot (e.g., "significant differences were found"). Rather, specific findings are described (e.g., "the experimental group reported significantly lower levels of depression than did controls").

The key to writing a meaningful abstract is to

decide, within the space limitations, what critical elements of information are needed to communicate the essence of a study. Condensing a major work into a brief format challenges any investigator. The result is a succinct, cogent description that communicates information but invites the reader to learn more.

The journal article

The journal article is a major method of opening research to the scrutiny of the scientific and professional community. Most nursing research is disseminated in this form. Because of its potential for communication to a wide audience and its permanence, publication of research in journals is an expected part of the scientific endeavor. Two basic types of journals exist, the research journal and the practice journal.

Research journals, including *Nursing Research, Advances in Nursing Science, Research in Nursing and Health,* and *Western Journal of Nursing Research,* principally publish reports of completed research, methodological papers, or articles on theory development. Their focus is on the processes of scientific inquiry and knowledge development in nursing. Readership is comprised predominantly of nurse researchers and nurse scholars.

Practice journals focus on the informational needs of nurse clinicians, educators, and administrators related to their practice of direct patient care, teaching, or delivery of nursing services. Examples are the *American Journal of Nursing, JOGNN, Heart and Lung, Journal of Nursing Education,* and *Journal of Nursing Administration.* Although these journals do publish research articles, they represent a small proportion of the total research manuscripts published. McCloskey and Swanson (1985) surveyed all issues published in 1984 by the five practice journals just cited. The percentage of the entire manuscripts in each journal that were research reports ranged from 0% in the *Journal of Nursing Administration* to 34% in the *Journal of Nursing Education.* Overall, research articles represented 10.6% of the total articles published in these journals in 1984.

Table 31-1 lists examples of journals that publish research. Either the research or the practice journal can be an important avenue for research dissemination. The journal selected for a particular manuscript will depend on the goal for publishing (i.e., knowledge development, reward, change in practice) and the intended audience. Plans for dissemination of findings are part of the overall planning of a research project. Usually several manuscripts result from a single project; some may be targeted for dissemination to nurse scientists through research journals and others to consumers of nursing research through practice journals. As mentioned, it is not considered ethical to publish the same article in more than one journal; however, a single set of data can provide the basis for two or more different manuscripts with unique emphases (e.g., research methods, practice implications).

The process of preparing an article for publication in a journal includes the following steps: identifying the focus of the article, selecting a publication source, preparing for writing, writing the manuscript, and submitting the manuscript for review. Deciding what to write and for what audience have already been discussed as the first steps. Most journals stipulate a maximum manuscript length and have a very specific readership. Clearly focusing the article on an aspect of the research project that can be discussed in sufficient depth within limited pages is essential.

Selecting a publication source

Selecting the journal for which the manuscript is targeted *before* actually writing the article helps the author focus the manuscript's style, content, and format. First, the general type of journal (practice, research) is selected based on the intended audience. Within these two major types, numerous alternatives exist as potential outlets for a manuscript. One element to consider thoughtfully when choosing a journal is the developmental status of the research. That is, are results speculative and in need of further verification, or are they ready for application to practice? If the former is true, publication in a practice journal may be premature.

Other factors in choosing an outlet might include the journal's circulation, prestige or reputation, acceptance rates, and speed of the review and publication process.

Swanson and McCloskey (1986) summarized this information from major nursing journals; these details are also usually found in any issue of the journal. Colleagues who have published in that or similar journals can be useful sources of information and advice as well.

One helpful exercise when seeking a publication

TABLE 31-1. Nursing journals publishing research*

JOURNAL FOCUS	PERCENTAGE RESEARCH
NURSING RESEARCH	
Advances in Nursing Science	25
Nursing Research	85
Research in Nursing and Health	99
Western Journal of Nursing Research	95
NURSING ADMINISTRATION	
Journal of Nursing Administration	15
Nursing Administration Quarterly	25
Nursing Economics	30
Nursing Management	15
NURSING EDUCATION	
Journal of Nursing Education	25
Journal of Nursing Staff Development	25
Nurse Educator	15
Nursing and Health Care	10
NURSING PRACTICE	
Nursing Clinics of North America	20
AAOHN Journal	10
Public Health Nursing	50
Cardiovascular Nursing	40
Dimensions of Critical Care Nursing	20
Heart and Lung	60
Journal of Emergency Nursing	25
Journal of Gerontological Nursing	40
Nursing Homes	10
Birth	25
Children's Health Care	40

From Swanson, E., and McCloskey, J. C., Publishing opportunities for nurses. ©, 1986, American Journal of Nursing Company. Reprinted with permission from *Nursing Outlook,* Sept.-Oct., *34*(5), 227-235.
*Includes those journals in which research reports constitute 10% or more of total published manuscripts.

source is to examine several recently published issues of the journals under consideration. Have articles on similar topics been recently published? If so, this may indicate a positive interest in publishing other research on the topic and may suggest how to develop the article to build on the existing literature. Does the journal publish studies using similar designs and methods? Some journals are more likely to accept nonexperimental or small-*n* studies than others. What are the experience and credentials of authors who have published in the journal? Some journals in disciplines outside of nursing rarely accept manuscripts from nurse authors unless coauthored by a member of that discipline.

The purpose of this examination process is to select a journal in which a manuscript will have the best possible chance of being published. Finding a good "fit" between the manuscript and the journal is the goal. Several journals may meet many of the author's criteria for a source. The author selects a first choice and holds the others in reserve in the event the first-choice journal does not accept the manuscript. It is not ethical to submit the same manuscript simultaneously to several different journals.

Preparing for writing

Once the publication source is selected, preparation activities occur. A letter of inquiry or telephone call to the journal's editor might be made to ascertain the level of interest in reviewing the proposed manuscript. Whether or not this step is taken depends on the journal's policy and the author's preferences. To

TABLE 31-1. Nursing journals publishing research—cont'd

JOURNAL FOCUS	PERCENTAGE RESEARCH
NURSING PRACTICE—cont'd	
Journal of Obstetric, Gynecologic and Neonatal Nursing	35
Journal of Pediatric Nursing	50
Journal of Nurse-Midwifery	30
MCN: The American Journal of Maternal/Child Nursing	33
Pediatric Nursing	35
Issues in Mental Health Nursing	60
Journal of Psychosocial Nursing and Mental Health Services	25
American Nephrology Nurses' Association Journal	25
Cancer Nursing	50
Oncology Nursing Forum	33
AANA Journal	22
Perioperative Nursing Quarterly	10
Today's OR Nurse	20
Journal of Ophthalmic Nursing and Technology	10
Ophthalmic Nursing Forum	100
American Journal of Infection Control	40
Journal of Enterostomal Therapy	15
NITA	40
Orthopaedic Nursing	15
Plastic Surgical Nursing	10
Rehabilitation Nursing	15
PROFESSIONAL DEVELOPMENTS	
Computers in Nursing	40
Image	50
Journal of Professional Nursing	33
Nursing Outlook	20

be useful to both editor and author, a letter of inquiry should contain several elements, as outlined by Wilson (1985, pp. 518-519):

1. A lead paragraph that catches the editor's interest
2. A paragraph that tells what the article is about, what direction it will take, and what it will offer the reader
3. Facts and evidence that support the basic premise of the article and offer the author's credentials for writing the article
4. Concluding paragraph to convince the editor to publish the article and to ask if the editor is interested in its review

A letter of inquiry does not ensure publication of the manuscript; however, it can eliminate costly delays incurred in sending a manuscript to a journal that is not interested in the focus of the manuscript, regardless of quality. Also, although sending a manuscript to several journals is inappropriate, multiple letters of inquiry can be sent simultaneously. If several editors indicate interest in reviewing the manuscript, one selects from among them and writes the others, thanking them for their interest.

Another preparation activity is to obtain and review the journal's instructions for manuscript preparation. Some journals publish complete instructions in every issue; others provide them in response to written requests from prospective authors. These guidelines usually address issues of manuscript length, general format, reference format, and accompanying materials such as abstracts and biographical data on authors. Since a manuscript might be rejected on the basis of incorrect format before it is sent to reviewers, adherence to these guidelines is important. The physical appearance and the author's attention to detail might influence the subsequent review of the manuscript's scientific merit. In the absence of guidelines from the journal, the *Publication Manual of the American Psychological Association* (1984) offers specific instructions for manuscript preparation. A review of Swanson and McCloskey's recent summary (1986) of manuscript preparation and review processes of many nursing journals may also be helpful.

The question of authorship should also be addressed before writing begins. When more than one person works on a project, the colleagues must decide which names should appear for credit and what responsibilities each will assume for the manuscript. Authorship is a means to visibility, credit, acknowledgment, and reward for one's work and can have long-term consequences, such as in academic promotion and tenure decisions. No universally agreed on rules exist for allocating authorship on publications (Werley et al., 1981). The American Psychological Association suggests that authorship encompasses not only those who actually write an article but also those who make substantial scientific contributions to a study. Major contributions, including formulating the problem or hypothesis, structuring the study design, conducting data analyses, interpreting results, or writing a major portion of the paper, are acknowledged by joint authorship, with names listed in order of decreasing contribution. Other supportive contributions, such as statistical consultation or extensive clerical assistance, are usually acknowledged in footnotes but may justify authorship (APA, 1984, p. 20). Other conventions also may be followed. McCloskey and Swanson (1982) suggest the common-sense approach that the person who assumes the most work should receive the most credit.

Writing the manuscript

The process that yields good writing is unique for each person. With experience, individuals discover the components that produce success for them. For some, choosing a specific environment or materials is of critical importance. Allocation of time for thinking and writing is essential, but the necessary amount and organization of that time varies among individuals. Most writers begin with either a written or

mental outline of the paper. The components of a research report (see previous box) offer guidance for the structure of a research article.

The manuscript may be developed through one or multiple drafts. Rereading a draft after several days usually helps to uncover flaws. Obtaining initial comments from colleagues on final versions is also beneficial. Such comment can fine-tune a manuscript by identifying unclear areas. Selecting several individuals who have published but do not know the author's work can simulate a journal's review process. Review by those who represent the journal's readers (e.g., nurse clinicians) can also help appropriately focus the manuscript's content, style, and emphasis. Rewriting, based on these comments, may be time consuming but generally results in a manuscript that is more accurate, thorough, and clear and has a greater probability of being published.

Before submitting the manuscript to the journal for review, an evaluation based on the following questions may be helpful:

1. Is the topic and study design appropriate for the journal to which the manuscript is submitted?
2. Does the introduction provide the reader with an overview of what was studied and why?
3. Is the review of literature current and pertinent to the problem studied?
4. Is the conceptual or theoretical framework explicit?
5. Are the research questions or hypotheses clearly identified?
6. Are the setting and subjects for the study completely described?
7. Are the methods described in sufficient detail to permit replication?
8. Are the techniques of data analysis appropriate and clearly described?
9. Do tables and figures stand alone and supplement but not duplicate material in the text?
10. Do the conclusions and discussion derive from the findings of the study, the study limitations, and previous work in the area?
11. Are implications for practice feasible and based on clinical significance of findings?
12. Is the paper concise and interesting?
13. Are citations appropriate and complete?
14. Has the manuscript been thoroughly proofread for accuracy?

15. Are the manuscript and accompanying materials prepared according to the journal's requirements?*

Submitting for review

Journals vary in their review processes. Some rely on review by the journal's editorial staff, whereas others submit papers to peer review. In a study of 49 nursing journals, Swanson and McCloskey (1982) reported that approximately 75% classified themselves as "refereed." This process usually involves an evaluation of the merit of the manuscript by three or more individuals, selected because of their professional expertise (Clayton & Boyle, 1981). Reviewers were "blind" to the author's identity in 52% of the journals. Although a journal that does not use a peer review system may publish high-quality material, "refereed" journals are generally considered more prestigious (Swanson & McCloskey, 1982). Peer reviewers may be members of the journal's editorial review board, outside reviewers, or a combination of both. Members of established review boards are usually identified in each journal issue, whereas outside reviewers may be listed only annually. If the journal uses a review board, perusal of the names might help the author to identify the research or practice expertise areas of potential reviewers of the article. For example, review boards of practice journals may have fewer members with expertise in research but many with expertise in the practice area the author's research addresses. These latter reviewers might scrutinize the practice relevance of the manuscript more thoroughly than its research methods. Usually journals try to assign at least one reviewer with research expertise to each research manuscript received.

The review process can be lengthy, averaging about 3 months from receipt of the manuscript to notification of the author about the editorial decision (Swanson & McCloskey, 1986). The peer review usually takes longer than a process not using outside reviewers. The editorial decision is usually one of three types. In the first, the manuscript may be accepted for publication exactly as written or may be subject to minor revisions suggested by the reviewers. A second response is that the reviewers do not accept the manuscript outright but do make suggestions for rewriting the article and encourage resubmission for a second review. If these suggestions seem reasonable to the author, the revised manuscript generally has a good chance of being accepted in a second review, especially if reviewed by the same individuals who made the original suggestions for revision. Finally, the manuscript might be deemed unacceptable for publication for various reasons, ranging from relevance of the topic to the journal's readership to quality of the written manuscript. Reasons for article rejection include (McCloskey & Swanson, 1982; Wilson, 1985, p. 517):

1. The subject was recently covered or is already scheduled for a future issue.
2. The article is too technical for the journal.
3. The content is inaccurate or undocumented.
4. The work is based on a poor research design or faulty methodology.
5. Nursing concerns are not highlighted.
6. The content is unimportant.
7. The article resembles a speech or term paper in too many ways and would be difficult to change.
8. The conclusion is unwarranted by the data as presented.
9. The idea was previously published elsewhere.
10. The idea is poorly presented.

Competition for journal publication space is keen; acceptance rates reported by nursing journals range from 14% to 56% of manuscripts received. New and specialty practice journals have somewhat higher acceptance rates (Swanson & McCloskey, 1986).

Having a manuscript rejected is an experience shared by *all* authors. Most editors provide reasons for rejection and reviewers' comments to the author. If a paper has been rejected by one journal, the author should consider submission to another. Revising the manuscript after considering the first reviewers' comments and the second journal's requirements usually results in a higher-quality article.

Rapidity of research dissemination is a concern to all. New knowledge from research is sometimes several years old by the time it appears in journal articles. As already noted, the time between manuscript acceptance and publication may range from a month to 2 or more years; intervals of 6 to 12 months are common (Swanson & McCloskey, 1986). Before publication, the author usually receives page proofs showing how the manuscript will appear in print.

---

*American Psychological Association. *Publication Manual of the American Psychological Association* (3rd ed., p. 29). Washington, DC: Author. © 1984 by American Psychological Association. Adapted by permission of the publisher.

The author should review these proofs carefully for accuracy and immediately alert the publisher about any changes.

Although the journal article remains a primary method for the dissemination of nursing knowledge, it is not without limitations, particularly in regard to the time gap between discovery and dissemination. Also, the specificity of readership for each journal means that research dissemination may be restricted to either a research or a practice group unless special efforts are made to write different articles for diverse audiences. Other methods of research dissemination provide alternatives for overcoming these limitations.

The research presentation

The verbal research presentation allows the researcher to share information about a project more rapidly than does the written research article. In fact, many research articles are based on talks given at professional or scientific meetings. Research presentations vary in both length and formality. For example, the researchers may present an informal report to the staff of a clinical agency where data were collected. The investigator might present the same project at a national clinical or research conference, using a more formal, scientific paper format. Research presentations may be invited talks or may result from responding to a competitive "call for abstracts" issued by a conference planning committee.

As with the research article, the research presentation needs to be developed with a clear content focus and attention to the intended audience. The major elements to be included in an oral research presentation are the same as those for a written research article (see the box on p. 483). The elements that receive the most emphasis and time will depend on the purpose of the conference and its expected audience. For example, a research presentation at a clinical conference usually will devote more time to discussion of a study's clinical relevance and practice implications, whereas a similar presentation at a research conference may give more emphasis to research design and methods.

A research presentation differs from a written paper in that the audience cannot read and study the material presented to understand it thoroughly. Thus clarity of communication is critical. Explanations of conceptual models, research methods, or analysis strategies that are perfectly comprehensible in writing may be too technical or complex for an audience to understand when presented verbally. Simple language supplemented by visual aids (slides, handouts) that illustrate complex ideas can increase clarity.

Visual aids are useful only if they are clear and readable to the audience. Slides and overhead transparencies must contain limited information and use print large enough to be read from the back of the presentation room. Consultation from a media expert can be valuable in designing effective visual materials. Handouts, produced in sufficient quantities, can be a useful alternative because they can contain more information and can be reviewed again later by the participants.

Most presenters speak from written material, which ranges from a topical outline to a verbatim paper. Because of the technical nature of research reports, most presenters need fairly detailed notes to ensure accuracy and to maintain a time schedule for the talk. However, literally reading a paper to an audience is boring for everyone. Visual contact with the audience helps the presenter identify cues that an illustration or clarification is needed, that the talk is being heard, or that the talk is being positively received. Visual contact also helps to hold the audience's attention.

One strategy to aid in developing a presentation is to write a draft of the talk and then practice it aloud before a volunteer audience of friends or family; if necessary, a mirror can substitute. Hearing the spoken words readily points out ideas that are poorly communicated. Such a trial also assists the presenter with accurate timing. Nothing is more frustrating to an audience or presenter than running out of time before reaching the major findings of a study. Because timing can be misjudged or changed because of unexpected questions, delays, equipment problems, or altered delivery pace, it is helpful to plan in advance which points in a talk could be deleted or expanded as time permits. This strategy makes such on-the-spot transitions smooth and unnoticed by the audience. Practicing with slides or other visual aids to be used is an added benefit; juggling a slide projector, written notes, and eye contact with an audience becomes smoother with practice.

Most research presentations allow the presenter to respond to questions and comments from the audience. Preparation for a talk should include preparation for the potential questions or criticisms that may arise. It is always appropriate to acknowledge one's inability to answer a question at the moment and offer to respond to the questioner later.

The research poster presentation

The research poster presentation is an alternative format for communication at professional meetings of completed research or research in progress. Through visual displays, researchers disseminate information about their projects in a less formal setting. Usually a poster session is held in a large room or display area; each project is assigned a table, easel, or space for displaying visual materials. Attendees are free to walk among the various displays, reading the materials and discussing the research with the presenters.

Preparation for a poster session differs from a research talk in its emphasis on the visual rather than the spoken message. The organization sponsoring the poster session should provide the presenter with information about the length of the session, space and equipment available for the display (e.g., table, easel, wall space, electrical outlets), and expectations about the researcher's presence during the poster session. Often the researcher is expected to be available with the display to discuss the project with viewers. The most effective poster is informative, attractive, easily and rapidly read, and conveys essential information without needing an accompanying discussion by the researcher. Within these guidelines, the researcher then plans the display, considering the purpose and content, materials to be used, and the composition (Sexton, 1984).

The content of the display is based on the goals for dissemination, the expected audience, and the status of the research. For example, a poster based on a study in progress may emphasize the conceptual model, the design, instruments, or methods. A poster based on completed research usually emphasizes research findings and conclusions in addition to the above information. Depending on the focus of the conference and the audience, clinical application or research methodology might be emphasized. Because of space limitations for most poster sessions, the content must be limited or presented succinctly; the researcher can elaborate for those interested in more detail.

Materials used for the display are most often one or a series of posters using poster board or similar materials. Some researchers also include videotapes, slides, or other audiovisual materials in their displays; arrangements for these additional components should be made in advance with the conference planners. Considerations when choosing materials include cost, permanence (i.e., will the poster have single or multiple uses), space limitations, and transportation. Sexton (1984) offers additional helpful information related to these issues. Media departments in universities or art stores often can provide consultation on choice of materials and layout. Written materials on posters must be in large print so they can be read from a distance. Graphs, photographs, and illustrations should be considered for use whenever possible; a picture *is* worth a thousand words. An effective poster need not be elaborate or expensive, but thoughtful planning and allowing sufficient time to develop and build the poster is essential to success.

Other methods of dissemination

The research abstract, the journal article, the research presentation, and the poster presentation are major methods for disseminating nursing research. Another alternative that relies on similar principles is the publication of a research report in book format.

An innovative method for research dissemination is satellite communication. Barnard and colleagues from the University of Washington tested this method as a means to achieve rapid dissemination of nursing knowledge about infant development to nurse scientists and practitioners throughout the United States (Barnard & Hoehn, 1978). They televised presentations by nurse researchers and broadcasted them via satellite to different sites. An opportunity also existed for verbal exchange among the researchers and the audience. This method capitalized on the technology now available for communication.

Nurse researchers are also using the media (television, newspapers, consumer magazines) to disseminate nursing research to the public. The brevity of time and space for these reports limits them almost entirely to the presentation of one or two major research findings. Research methods are rarely included. The appeal is that these methods communicate to the public about the nature of nursing science and what the discipline can offer society.

UTILIZATION OF NURSING RESEARCH

Once research has been disseminated, it is available for use by other researchers, educators, administrators, and practitioners. The activity of research utilization is essential for research to accomplish the goals of furthering knowledge development and bringing about change in nursing practice, education, and delivery of care. Johnson (1977) documented that 50 years can elapse before research in a field is properly used. With the rapid rate of change in society and in nursing practice, concerned professionals cannot tolerate such an extensive lag; research findings would be obsolete before even reaching the nurse consumer.

Barriers

The nursing profession is increasingly aware that scientific nursing knowledge becomes the basis for nursing education and nursing care delivery. Several barriers to the utilization of scientific knowledge exist. These relate to the state of the knowledge base, characteristics of disseminators and consumers of nursing knowledge, and characteristics of the professional environment.

Despite the rapid increase in the amount of nursing research conducted, present knowledge still has major gaps. Basic descriptions of nursing phenomena and studies of clinical therapeutics that form the basis of nursing actions are lacking. Replication of studies has been minimal; the lack of established validity and reliability of research findings often make direct application of findings premature. Likewise, programmatic research that builds on previous work in a defined area of nursing science to develop knowledge fully has been limited; instead, single, isolated studies exist. The nature of study settings and populations also restrict practice application of much nursing research. Nursing is often a science of well-educated, ethnically homogeneous, middle-class individuals who live in university teaching settings. Although this problem is not unique to nursing science, the lack of demographic diversity of study subjects limits how much research findings can be applied to actual clinical populations.

Until very recently, few nurse investigators had the academic preparation to conduct nursing research. As the number of nurse scientists with doctoral and postdoctoral preparation increases, the work force to address the limitations of the nursing knowledge base will expand. They must focus on research central to the phenomena that concern the nursing discipline.

For utilization to occur, nurses must also be able to fulfill the role of research consumers. This role implies knowledge of and access to research in one's field, the ability to evaluate the knowledge critically for its practice relevance, and skill in knowledge utilization and change. Deficits exist in each of these areas among nurse consumers. As long as research continues to be largely disseminated in journals and at meetings with primarily nurse-researcher audiences, nurses in practice have limited access to current nursing knowledge. As McCloskey and Swanson (1985) advocated, researchers must also make an effort to disseminate their work to practice audiences if change is to occur.

Nurses in practice as clinicians, administrators, and educators often lack the necessary knowledge to evaluate research either for its scientific merit or its practice relevance. Educational programs in nursing may focus on learning current knowledge to the exclusion of learning how to evaluate and assimilate knowledge not yet uncovered. Results of a recent survey of members of a specialty nursing organization indicated that nurses functioning as clinicians had less positive attitudes toward research and were less competent in both conducting and using research than their counterparts in administrative, educational, or research positions (Killien, 1985).

The professional environment promotes the gap between knowledge generation and knowledge utilization. The clinician and nurse scientist often operate in isolation from one another, preventing the sharing of language, values, and goals (Horsley, Crane, Crabtree, & Wood 1983). Nurse researchers who are faculty members in universities are not rewarded by promotion and tenure committees for publishing in practice journals (McCloskey & Swanson, 1985). Nurses often find research reports dull and difficult to understand; research journals discourage reporting the practice observations that make a problem "real" to the clinician reader but encourage forming a theory that can be attached to that observation (Killien, 1985; Lindeman, 1984). Practice journals may omit from research-based articles salient information about design and methodology that are essential to evaluate the study for scientific merit and practice relevance (Swanson & McCloskey, 1986).

The practice setting may also present a barrier to research utilization activities. Tradition operates as a powerful "way of knowing" and may be more valued as a rationale for specific nursing practices than in research-based knowledge. Nurses may not be rewarded for engaging in activities related to research utilization, such as reading current research, attending research conferences, or documenting the research basis for written policies, procedures, or plans of care. Further, resistance to change in some practice settings, concern for allocation of scarce resources to research activities, and lack of role models or expert consultants to aid decisions and processes concerning research utilization may discourage nurses from actively pursuing such endeavors.

Factors influencing research utilization

Given these barriers, what variables in nursing practice environments are most likely to be associated with the utilization of research? Horsley (1985) identified variables related to the research knowledge, to channels for communicating knowledge, and to individual and organizational characteristics.

The nature of the knowledge is a strong influence on research utilization. Research that offers a better way of doing something or a solution to an important problem is more readily adopted than knowledge that offers insight about a phenomenon but no clear recommendation for change from the status quo. Use of knowledge or an innovation usually will not occur when the knowledge or innovation departs markedly from existing practices or knowledge in the professional environment. For knowledge to be readily used, it must be able to be tried on a limited basis and have observable outcomes so the individual nurse or the nursing care organization can determine the benefit of using the knowledge on a broader scale.

Research findings often must be transformed into a new format to be useful to the nurse consumer. The nursing care protocols developed by one research utilization project conducted at the University of Michigan are examples of the transformation of research knowledge into a practice-relevant format (Horsley, Crane, Crabtree, & Wood, 1983). Some nurses, such as master's-prepared clinical nurse specialists, may be in an excellent position to take research disseminated in journals and in research pre-

sentations and translate it into language and format meaningful to other nurse clinicians or administrators. Innovative publications such as the *Research Review* newsletter (Cronenwett, 1986) that provide research reviews abstracted for staff nurse readers also assist in overcoming communication barriers.

In every organization certain individuals are leaders in adopting new ideas and promoting change. These individuals are pivotal in research utilization. They must have the knowledge to be able to evaluate the nursing research critically for both its scientific merit and its relevance for practice in a specific setting. Individual characteristics that might influence research use include knowledge about the research evaluation process, the perception of need for new knowledge, readiness to adopt new ideas, and attitudes of openness to new ideas.

For research-based knowledge to be used at the organizational level, the organization must also have several important characteristics. These include the presence of innovative leaders who can influence the organization, the perception of need at the organizational level for the knowledge, readiness to adopt research innovations, and the necessary resources to implement a planned change process.

Models for research utilization

Several models for research utilization have been proposed. Phillips (1986) has presented a summary of these models. Two models are discussed here, the Stetler-Marram model and the Conduct and Utilization of Research in Nursing (CURN) model.

Stetler and Marram (1976) proposed a model for research utilization that described the process used for evaluating research findings for applicability in practice (Fig. 31-1). This model can be applied to research use at the level of the individual nurse as well as the organizational level. Three phases in the research utilization were proposed: validation, comparative evaluation, and decision making.

Phase 1 involves the validation of the scientific merit of an individual study. This evaluation is based on the elements of a research critique described in Chapter 30 and is summarized in the box on pp. 494 and 495.

If the study is determined to have sufficient scientific merit, phase 2, comparative evaluation, occurs. In this phase, the study of interest is assessed for its relevance to practice applicability to a specific prac-

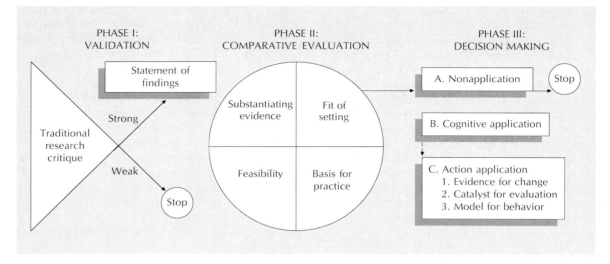

Fig. 31-1. Stetler-Marram model of steps in research evaluation for practice application. (From Stetler, C., and Marram, G., Evaluating research findings for acceptability in practice. ©, 1976, American Journal of Nursing Company. Reprinted with permission from *Nursing Outlook,* Sept., *24*[9], 559-563.)

Evaluating Research for Practice Use

A. Problem studied and literature review
  1. Scientific evaluation
     a. Is problem clearly identified?
     b. Is significance of problem discussed?
     c. Was research justified by literature?
     d. Is relationship to previous research clear?
     e. Was conceptual framework evident? Appropriate?
     f. Is specific purpose of study clear? Are variables defined? Are hypotheses stated and well founded?
  2. Practice evaluation
     a. Is this problem significant to nursing practice?
     b. Does the framework "fit" with what the nurse knows about nursing practice and the phenomenon?

B. Setting and subjects
  1. Scientific evaluation
     a. Is population described? Sample described?
     b. How were subjects recruited? Sampled?
     c. What were the sources of sampling error?
     d. Is sample size adequate?
     e. Were subjects' rights adequately protected?
     f. What was the setting for the study? Laboratory? Community? Hospital?
  2. Practice evaluation
     a. Are the patients typical? Are they similar to the patients in the nurse's setting? Could differences possibly influence results?

EVALUATING RESEARCH FOR PRACTICE USE—cont'd

    b. Is the setting typical? In what ways is it similar and different from the nurse's setting?

    c. Would patients be likely to participate if this was not a study?

C. Design

  1. Scientific evaluation

    a. What type of design was used (e.g., descriptive, correlational, longitudinal, experimental, cross-sectional)?

    b. Is design appropriate to answer question asked?

    c. Are appropriate controls included?

    d. Can confounding variables be identified?

  2. Practice evaluation

    a. Would it be possible to measure the same outcomes if findings were applied in the nurse's setting?

    b. Are methods adequately described to permit replication?

D. Instruments and measures

  1. Scientific evaluation

    a. To what extent are measures valid and reliable?

    b. Were reliability and validity tested and reported in this study?

    c. Were measures adequately described to determine their relevance to study purpose and findings?

    d. Could the measures have influenced findings?

  2. Practice evaluation

    a. Is there any assurance that these measures would be meaningful and accurate in the clinical setting?

    b. Are these data collection methods feasible in the nurse's setting?

E. Data analysis

  1. Scientific evaluation

    a. How were the data distributed (e.g., frequency distribution)?

    b. Do methods answer the questions posed?

    c. Are statistical tests appropriate and applicable to questions or hypothesis?

    d. Are data presented clearly in tables?

  2. Practice evaluation

    a. Do the data fit the clinical picture?

    b. What are the probabilities that findings are due to chance? Or to some other variable?

    c. Are findings clinically as well as statistically significant?

F. Discussion and conclusions

  1. Scientific evaluation

    a. Are conclusions stated clearly?

    b. Are conclusions based on the data presented?

    c. Are limitations and alternative explanations presented?

    d. Are findings related to the original framework and purpose of the study?

    e. Are results generalized to population studied?

    f. Are conclusions appropriate, given a. to e. above?

  2. Practice evaluation

    a. Does the nurse agree with the author's conclusion?

    b. What decision does the conclusion promote?

    c. Should the literature be further examined for more information?

    d. Do the findings replicate previous findings? Suggest innovation or change?

    e. Do the findings increase the nurse's sensitivity to the problem, but not lead to direct action?

    f. Does the nurse need more information from the researcher?

tice setting or client population, and feasibility for implementation in practice. Relevant questions to be asked about a study in this phase are outlined as well. Comparative evaluation also involves an evaluation of the substantiating evidence for a piece of knowledge. That is, do other studies exist that offer replication of study findings? Horsley, Crane, Crabtree, and Wood (1983) suggested that a minimum of two studies replicating findings are required for practice application.

Phase 3 is decision making. Based on an evaluation of both the scientific and clinical merit of research findings, the consumer may elect not to apply findings to practice, to apply the findings cognitively, or to apply the findings directly to practice (i.e., action application). Stetler and Marram (1976) described cognitive application as the use of research findings to enhance understanding of nursing practice phenomena. Such indirect, or cognitive, application is appropriate for nursing research that is at the descriptive level or lacks sufficient reliability or validity to be directly applied. For research findings that have been established and replicated, an individual or organization may elect to change existing practices to incorporate the new knowledge. Such change might include discontinuing use of existing practices, confirming or modifying existing practices, or adopting new practices based on new knowledge.

The Conduct and Utilization of Research in Nursing (CURN) project was designed to develop and test a model for using scientific nursing knowledge in practice settings (Horsley, Crane, Crabtree, & Wood, 1983). This model described research utilization as an organizational process and was based on the linkage model of problem solving by Havelock (1969). It emphasized the interaction and interdependence between the resource system developing the knowledge (the researcher) and the user system (the practice organization). Essential to research utilization in this model was the organization's commitment to the research utilization process. Six phases of the research utilization process were identified in the CURN project:

1. Identification of nursing practice problems needing solution and assessment of research bases for problem solution

2. Evaluation of the relevance of the research-based knowledge related to the identified practice problem, the organization's values and current practices, and potential costs and benefits of adopting the knowledge
3. Design of a research-based practice innovation that meets the needs of the practice problem and is consistent with the scientific limitations of the research base
4. Evaluation of the innovation in the practice setting using a clinical trial
5. Decision making to reject, modify, or adopt the innovation
6. Development of strategies to extend the innovation to appropriate nursing practice settings

This model recognizes that planned change is a complex process in an organization. When research is targeted for utilization at the organizational level, a thorough understanding of the organizational structure and climate, resources, and change dynamics is essential.

SUMMARY

The conduct of research, research dissemination, and research utilization are interdependent processes involving the total nursing community. Each process calls for individuals with unique knowledge and skills. Issues related to the dissemination of research include reasons for dissemination, potential audiences, and methods for dissemination. Essential ingredients for effective dissemination, regardless of the audience targeted or methods used are a focused message, clarity of communication, logical organization, communication aids, and adherence to guidelines. The use of research in nursing practice involves both barriers and factors that facilitate research utilization. Selected models have outlined the process of research utilization at the individual and organizational level. The Stetler-Marram model proposed three phases of research utilization: validation, comparative evaluation, and decision making. The CURN project identified six phases in a model for using scientific nursing knowledge in practice settings.

References

American Psychological Association. (1984). *Publication manual of the American Psychological Association* (3rd ed.). Washington, DC: Author.

Barnard, K. E., & Hoehn, R. E. (1978). Nursing child assessment satellite training. In R. A. Duncan (Ed.), *Biomedical communication experiments*. Washington, DC: Lister Hill National Center for Biomedical Communications, Department of Health, Education and Welfare, Public Health Service.

Batey, M. (1978) Research communication: Its functions, audiences and media. *Communicating Nursing Research, 2,* 101-109.

Clayton, B. C., & Boyle, K. (1981). The referred journal: Prestige in professional publication. *Nursing Outlook, 29,* 531-534.

Cronenwett, L. (Ed.). (1986). *Nursing research review.* Hanover, NH: Dartmouth-Hitchkok Hospital.

Havelock, R. (1969). *Planning for innovation through dissemination and utilization of knowledge.* Ann Arbor: Center for Research on Utilization of Scientific Knowledge, Institute for Social Research, The University of Michigan.

Horsley, J. A. (1985). Factors that influence research utilization. Paper presented to Council of Nurse Researchers, San Diego, CA.

Horsley, J. A., Crane, J., Crabtree, M. K., & Wood, D. J. (1983). *Using research to improve nursing practice: A guide.* New York: Grune & Stratton, Inc.

Johnson, J. E. (1977). Nursing research impact vital for profession. *American Nurse, 9,* 15.

Killien, M. (1985). Research attitudes, activities, and competence of OGN nurses. In B. Raff, & N. Paul (Eds.), *NAACOG Invitational Research Conference. Birth Defects: Original Article Series, 21*(8), 89-101.

Lindeman, C. A. (1984). Dissemination of nursing research. *Image, 16*(2), 57-58.

McCloskey, J. C., & Swanson, E. (1982). Publishing opportunities for nurses: A comparison of 100 journals. *Image, 14,* 50-56.

McCloskey, J. C., & Swanson, E. (1985). Publishing in practice journals: A responsibility of the researcher. *CNR Newsletter, 12*(3), 1-4.

Phillips, L. (1986). *A clinician's guide to the critique and utilization of nursing research.* New York: Appleton-Century-Crofts.

Sexton, D. (1984). Presentation of research findings: The poster session. *Nursing Research, 23*(6), 374-375.

Stetler, C. (1985). Research utilization: Defining the concept. *Image, 17,* 40-44.

Stetler, C. B., & Marram, C. (1976). Evaluating research findings for applicability in practice. *Nursing Outlook, 24*(9), 559-563.

Strunk, W., Jr., & White, E. B. (1979). *The elements of style* (3rd ed.). New York: Macmillan.

Styles, M. M. (1978). Why publish? *Image, 10,* 29.

Swanson, E., & McCloskey, J. C. (1982). The manuscript review process. *Image, 14,* 72-76.

Swanson, E., & McCloskey, J. C. (1986). Publishing opportunities for nurses. *Nursing Outlook, 34*(5), 227-235.

Werley, H., Murphy, P., Gosch, S., Gottesmann, H., & Newcomb, B. (1981). Research publication credit assignment: Nurses' views. *Research in Nursing and Health, 4,* 261-279.

Wilson, H. S. (1985). Disseminating research: The scholar's commitment. *Research in nursing* (pp. 501-532). Menlo Park, CA.: Addison-Wesley.

32

GENERATING A RESEARCH PROPOSAL

NANCY FUGATE WOODS

A research proposal communicates to scientists, clinicians, educators, and funding agency personnel an investigator's intended plan for conducting a study or series of studies. Research proposals convey the background for the study, the methods for conducting it, and the anticipated significance of the results. The proposal also indicates the investigator's capability to conduct the proposed research. Development of a research proposal helps clarify the investigator's thinking, requiring the researcher to make critical decisions about how to achieve the goals of the study and to anticipate the consequences of alternative decisions about the research project. A proposal not only communicates information about the proposed study, but also serves as a vehicle to generate support for the research.

This chapter explores the processes involved in developing a nursing research proposal and generating support for nursing research. The research proposal is not merely a technical document; it is also an instrument of persuasive communication, designed to convince others of the study's merit and the investigator's ability to perform the research.

PREPARING A RESEARCH PROPOSAL

Specific guidelines for preparing a research proposal are designed to guide an investigator's efforts and are usually available from the person or agency requiring the proposal. For example, an educational program, clinical service agency, and research funding agency

might have different goals in reviewing the same proposal and may require different types of information from the investigator. Nevertheless, most agencies require similar proposal components. This section considers these components and the guidelines that federal funding agencies use and the modifications in proposals that various agencies may require.

Components of a research proposal

The purpose of a research proposal is to explain in detail each aspect of the proposed study. The investigator has an opportunity to demonstrate comprehension of the topic as well as to describe plans for further inquiry. The guidelines that follow have been adapted from those currently used for federal grant proposals submitted to the National Center for Nursing Research and other agencies within the National Institutes of Health of the U.S. Public Health Service. The boxes provide examples from an actual research proposal to illustrate better each of these components.

Specific aims

This section of a proposal conveys the researcher's intentions. The purpose specifically delimits the focus of the study by clearly, precisely, and concisely specifying the variables to be studied. The researcher derives the purpose from a review of earlier work and the conceptual framework for the study. The connections between the previous work and this framework should be logical. If the state of knowledge about the topic supports the generation of hypotheses, then the aims are stated as hypotheses. If the state of knowledge is less well developed, then the aims can reflect the need for description before hypothesis testing. Specific aims reflect the special contribution that the work will make to nursing knowledge. An example of the specific aims component is given in the box on the right.

Significance

The section of a proposal describing the significance of the research contains a statement of the problem, the background information on which the proposed work rests, a critical evaluation of existing knowledge, and identification of the gaps in knowledge that the proposal is intended to fill. In this section the investigator usually states the problem being investigated and addresses the following questions:

What is the issue or concern that triggered the study?

What is the issue that demands further knowledge?

What is the scope of the problem area (e.g., how many people are affected by it and how pervasive is it)?

How would nursing science or practice be influenced by the results of the study?

Why is it an important problem?

In addition to a statement of the problem, the significance section usually contains a critical review of scientific and theoretical literature relevant to the specific question or problems being studied. It addresses such questions as:

What is already known about the problem? What is not known?

What are some of the problems or shortcomings of previous work?

How will the proposed study expand this body of knowledge?

What approaches to inquiry about the problem should have but have not yet been tried?

The review of the literature is a critical analysis of inquiry directly relevant to the question being studied. Although not necessarily exhaustive, the review should identify the current state of knowledge about the problem.

The conceptual framework presents the rationale or theoretical argument underpinning the proposed study. Providing the perspective from which the investigator views the problem, this framework is characterized by conceptual or theoretical concerns

EXAMPLE OF "SPECIFIC AIMS" COMPONENT

Symptoms occurring immediately before and during menstruation (perimenstrual symptoms, PS) affect 30% to 50% of women (1),* and account for approximately 1.5 million physician visits annually (2). To date, however, there are few published studies of the prevalence of symptoms among U.S. adult women. Existing estimates are based on highly selected groups such as students or employed women. The large national databases related to health, including the Health Interview Survey, the Health and Nutrition Examination Survey, and the National Survey of Family Growth, do not contain PS data. Moreover, our understanding of the etiology and therapeutics for PS is limited by inadequate specification of the multidimensional nature of PS. Although several lines of investigation are in progress, there is no biological hypothesis to account for the range of PS women experience. Little attention has been given to the influence of psychosocial factors on these symptoms and the disability associated with them. Variation of PS prevalence among women of differing ethnic groups has been demonstrated, yet the reasons for these differences have not been explored.

The goal of this research program is to improve understanding of the multidimensional nature of PS and the relationship between psychosocial factors and symptoms as an essential basis for developing nursing therapeutics. The specific aims of this study include:

1. Determining the prevalence of PS and associated disability in a population of women residing in King County, Washington
2. Describing the clustering of symptoms in the premenstruum and menstruum
3. Generating a typology of PS
4. Determining the relative contribution of the woman's socialization, current social context, ethnic group, gynecological history, health practices, and general health status to models explaining the variance in PS, related disability, and illness behavior

*Numbers in parentheses are references to the literature in this and subsequent boxes.

and is not merely a restatement of others' previous work. The investigator considers such questions as:

What is the state of knowledge in this problem area?

Do the phenomena still need description?

Do studies of the connections between concepts need to be done?

Does the level of sophistication warrant exploration of how multiple concepts are related?

What concepts are important in guiding the study? How are they linked?

What theoretical perspective or imagery will be used to guide the study of the problem?

This part of the proposal may blend existing theoretical traditions or may compare and contrast competing frameworks. The researcher may address the literature review and the conceptual framework separately or may integrate the discussion of these topics. (An example of the significance component of a proposal is given in the box on pp. 500 to 502.)

Preliminary studies

Preliminary studies, such as pilot studies or related studies conducted by the investigator, are described to illustrate the investigator's competence to pursue the proposed project and relevant experience in studying the topic. Publications of the investigator's earlier work are cited and often are appended to the proposal for the reviewer's reference. This component of a proposal offers the investigator the opportunity to outline her or his own contribution to knowledge in the area, as well as to illustrate how the idea for the current study grew from earlier work. An example of the preliminary studies component of a proposal is given in the box on pp. 503 and 504.

Methods of procedure

The "methods of procedure" section describes the plan for accomplishing the proposed work. This section usually consists of several components, including (1) design, (2) description of the data-producing instruments, (3) sample, (4) methods of data production, (5) protection of human subjects or (6) animals, (7) methods of analysis, and (8) time frame to conduct the study.

Design. The investigator clearly describes the type of design or designs to be used and the rationale for its (their) selection. Making the design congruent with the study's conceptualization and its specific aims or purposes is a major consideration in preparing this part of the proposal. The investigator speci-

---

Example of "Significance" Component

Perimenstrual symptoms (PS) constitute an important problem for women. Immediately before and during menstruation, many women experience symptoms such as cramps, backache, headache, weight gain, painful or tender breasts, swelling, irritability, mood swings, depression, tension, anxiety, and fatigue. Although 30% to 50% of women describe their symptoms as mild or moderate, 10% to 20% describe their symptoms as severe or disabling (1). Some suggest that PS are the primary reason for women missing work or school (3), and these symptoms frequently cause women to seek medical care (2). One of the most striking features of perimenstrual symptomatology is its variability, which is reflected both in the variety of symptoms women experience and in the large variation in the prevalence of these symptoms from one population to another (4-12). It is not clear whether variation in prevalence is due to inherent variability in age, parity, and other demographic characteristics of the groups; to variation across studies in definitions; to instruments and methods; or to systematic variation in other processes influencing the health status of the groups.

Despite the fact that dysmenorrhea and premenstrual syndrome have been studied among clinical populations for several decades, little consensus exists about what symptoms constitute these syndromes or what leads to their development. Dalton (13,14) proposed two discrete forms of PS, spasmodic and congestive dysmenorrhea, each mediated by different hormonal influences. Spasmodic dysmenorrhea occurred at the time of menstruation, with pain following the uterine and ovarian nerve distribution. Dalton attributed these symptoms to an excess of progesterone to

—— Example of "Significance" Component—cont'd

estrogen and recommended treatment with birth control pills or estrogens. Congestive dysmenorrhea occurred primarily before the onset of menstruation, and the pain involved the lower abdomen, back, and breasts and was accompanied by joint pains and headaches. Dalton believed that congestive dysmenorrhea was caused by an excess of estrogen to progesterone and recommended treatment with progesterone. Recent endocrine studies show little relationship between estrogen and progesterone levels and symptoms (15,16) and mood states (17).

Subsequent work has demonstrated that spasmodic and congestive dysmenorrhea symptoms are not mutually exclusive (18,19). Many investigators (7, 20-22) recognized the multidimensional nature of PS and encouraged the refinement of a typology of PS. Inadequate specification of the dimensions of PS as well as the complex mechanisms responsible for symptoms are no doubt responsible for the inconsistency in results of etiological studies and clinical trials and make careful description of the phenomenon an important priority.

Biological factors

Several lines of biological research are being pursued to explain PS. Evidence linking prostaglandins, particularly $PGF2\alpha$ to menstrual cramps, as well as to other systemic symptoms such as backache, nausea, vomiting, diarrhea, headache, tiredness, nervousness and dizziness is compelling. However, women with apparently normal $PGF2\alpha$ levels also complain of dysmenorrhea (23) and drugs that interfere with $PGF2\alpha$ synthesis are not universally effective (24). Prolactin and vasopressin are currently being studied for their role in producing some premenstrual and menstrual symptoms (25-29).

Another biological line of investigation has been directed at elucidating autonomic nervous system (ANS) events that may account for PS. Some investigations have shown no menstrual cycle phase differences in catecholamine excretion (adrenaline and noradrenaline), skin conductance, heart rate, and respiratory rate (30,31), whereas others suggest higher or lower levels of ANS arousal in the premenstrual phase (32,33).

Although diet and exercise are often prescribed as remedies for PS, their relationship to PS has not yet been explored systematically. Diet has been linked to estrogen levels, with vegetarian women demonstrating lower levels than non-vegetarians (34), and magnesium deficiency has been implicated as a possible cause of premenstrual tension (35). Postovulation food intake is higher in calories than that in the 10 days preceding ovulation (36). Strenuous exercise has been associated with delayed menarche and amenorrhea, though effects on symptoms have not been assessed (37,38).

Psychosocial factors

Investigations of the psychosocial factors involved in PS range from psychoanalytical formulations suggesting that PS are the result of inability to accept one's femininity (39,40) to contemporary theories about the influence of individual expectations about menstruation (41), feminine socialization (42), social attributions (43), attitudes toward menstruation, and exposure to a stressful environment (44-46) on PS. Although the prevalence of symptoms (42,47,48) varies across ethnic groups, little effort has been devoted to exploring the responsible mechanisms (social, genetic, or lifestyle).

Intervention trials

Intervention trials using hormonal agents, pyridoxine, bromocriptine, and diuretics for PS characteristically yield moderate placebo effects, suggesting that social processes can ameliorate symptom experience (49,50). In addition, therapy with systematic desensitization, biofeedback, and systematic relaxation is successful with subsets of women with dysmenorrhea or premenstrual symptoms (51-53).

A theoretical perspective that unites what is understood about the biological fluctuations underlying the menstrual cycle with psychosocial processes influencing women's experiences of symptoms and their responses to symptoms is absent from the menstrual cycle literature. In this study,

Continued.

EXAMPLE OF "SIGNIFICANCE" COMPONENT—cont'd

PS will be viewed as "symptoms" as opposed to a discrete disease entity. Current models of symptoms and illness behavior will provide the framework for the study. Mechanic (54) suggests that individuals' definitions of illness are shaped by three factors: bodily sensations, which one labels as symptoms or feelings that differ from the ordinary; cognitive definitions, which suggest some hypothesis about what the individual is feeling; and the environment, particularly social stress. Mechanic's work demonstrates that a complex set of factors influences whether women label bodily sensations as symptoms, how they label them, and the way in which they respond to them. Factors influencing the reporting of PS include the cognitive definitions women apply to their situations. These definitions are influenced by the culture which conveys to women, through socialization processes, what to expect about menstruation and symptoms, attitudes and beliefs about menstruation and its effects on one's life, and what aspects of behavior to attribute to the perimenstruum (56). Thus the woman's exposure to cultural norms about health in general, and menstruation in particular, creates a set of cognitions that influence how she labels the bodily sensations she experiences with menstruation (57).

In addition to the influence of cognitive definitions, women are continuously exposed to a social environment, which for some is adverse. The relationship between a stressful milieu and symptoms in general is well established. In addition, there is evidence that exposure to a stressful social environment is associated with a greater than expected incidence of PS (44-46). In particular, health-related stressors seem to have important effects on PS (46).

Once bodily sensations are labeled as symptoms, the individual engages in a series of deliberations about how to respond to them. Typically the person judges the nature of the symptoms in terms of presumed causality, their treatability, and likely prognosis, against standards of the culture. Severity of the symptoms is judged on the basis of factors such as associated physical manifestations, ability to conceal the symptom, and familiarity of the condition (58).

Following this process of evaluation, the person may engage in a series of responses such as altering activity by going to bed or resting, engaging in self care such as use of over the counter drugs, seeking help or advice from a lay person, or seeking help from a health professional (59). The response to symptoms is influenced by socialization as well as by the current social environment, including expectations of others and adverse conditions (54).

This general process, including perception of symptoms, evaluation of the symptoms, and response to symptoms is termed illness behavior. Each aspect of illness behavior is influenced by the culture through the process of socialization, and by the individual's current social environment.

In sum, the literature on PS reveals several important gaps. In brief, there is inadequate specification of the multidimensional nature of PS. A typology of PS is needed for further investigations of the relationship between PS and factors that amplify or alleviate symptoms. Relatively little effort has been devoted to understanding the relationship between psychosocial processes and PS. The proposed work should yield:

1. A more complete understanding of the multidimensional nature of PS
2. A typology of PS
3. An improved understanding of the psychosocial processes influencing several dimensions of PS, which may have implications for nursing therapeutics for PS
4. Insights about factors affecting PS disability and illness behavior

Example of "Preliminary Studies" Component

The aims of the preliminary studies were to:
1. Estimate the prevalence of perimenstrual symptoms (PS) in a nonclinical, noninstitutionalized population of women residing in the community
2. Determine the extent to which selected symptoms varied across menstrual cycle phases
3. Explore clustering of PS
4. Assess the effects of two approaches to measuring PS on prevalence estimated
5. Determine the consistency of PS experienced over two menstrual cycles
6. Explore the effects of parity, contraceptive use, characteristics of the menstrual cycle, and demographic characteristics on PS
7. Describe the relationship between women's socialization experiences and their PS
8. Explore the relationship between women's current social contexts and their PS

Methods

We studied a population of women residing in five southeastern city neighborhoods who varied in race and socioeconomic status. We identified each woman living in these neighborhoods who was 18 to 35 years of age, was not pregnant at the time of interview, and had not had a hysterectomy. Of 650 households, there were 241 potential participants, and 179 (74%) agreed to participate in the study.

Measures

We used the Moos Menstrual Distress Questionnaire (MDQ) (60) which had been commonly used to document the presence and severity of symptoms associated with menstruation. The MDQ contains 47 symptoms grouped into eight factors, six of which measure negative perceptions: pain, impaired concentration, behavior change, autonomic reactions, water retention, and negative affect. A seventh factor, arousal, contains positive experiences such as excitement. The eighth factor contains control symptoms that are infrequently endorsed and which reflect a general tendency to complain of a variety of symptoms. Women are asked to report their perceptions of each of the symptoms for (1) their most recent flow; (2) the week before their most recent flow; and (3) the remainder of the cycle. They are asked to use a rating scale in which responses range from 1 for "no experience of the symptom" to 6 for "acute or partially disabling." Examples of the items include: weight gain and muscle stiffness. These scales showed cycle phase differences in the sample of 839 wives of graduate students on whom the scale was normed in the mid '60s. The scales were internally consistent (correlations = .53 to .89), and had split half reliabilities of .74 to .98 (7). *Cycle phase* was defined as the MDQ dictated, such that the premenstruum included the week prior to the last menstruation, the menstruum included time during the most recent menstrual flow, and the remainder of the cycle included all residual days after accounting for the premenstruum and menstruum.

Participants

Most participants were in their late twenties and early thirties; were married, white, and employed; and had an annual family income greater than $15,000. In general, they were well educated, with most having more than a high-school education. Although most were Protestant, the women represented a variety of religious denominations. Less than half had one or more children.

Continued.

Example of "Preliminary Studies" Component—cont'd

Results

Results related to only aims 2 and 6 of the preliminary studies are presented here.

2. Variation of selected symptoms across menstrual cycle phases. There were significant differences in several of the MDQ symptom scores for the premenstruum versus the menstruum. The actual magnitude of the mean difference is small (<0.3), with the exception of cramps, with a mean cycle phase difference of 0.83. Cycle phase differences in symptoms are blunted for women taking oral contraceptives. Cramps, backache, fatigue, and tension are more prevalent during the menstruum; and weight gain, skin disorders, painful and tender breasts, swelling, irritability, mood swings, and depression are more common in the premenstruum. Correlations between severity of the symptoms for premenstrual and menstrual ratings suggest that women who experience more severe symptoms premenstrually also experience these during the menstruum (7).

6. Effects of parity, contraceptive use, characteristics of the menstrual cycle, and demographic characteristics on PS. The prevalence of PS was influenced by several characteristics of the woman's reproductive health history. Women who had been pregnant were significantly less likely to experience menstrual cramps, as were women using oral contraceptives. Women using oral contraceptives also experienced a lower rate of skin disorders. Women who used an IUD reported more premenstrual cramping than others (1).

Women who had long menstrual cycles reported more premenstrual swelling, mood swings, depression and crying than their counterparts with shorter cycles. Women with a long menstrual flow were less likely to report premenstrual cramps, menstrual irritability, premenstrual and menstrual mood swings, and premenstrual depression than those with shorter flow. Women with heavy flow reported more premenstrual and menstrual cramping, menstrual swelling, and premenstrual work/school impairment than their counterparts (1).

Several demographic characteristics were related to the prevalence of PS. Older women generally had fewer PS than their younger counterparts, including a lower prevalence of menstrual cramps, headache, depression, premenstrual irritability and napping, and crying. Married women were less likely to nap or stay in bed than single women (1).

Black women were significantly less likely than whites to experience menstrual cramps, premenstrual anxiety and premenstrual and menstrual crying. Black women reported more menstrual weight gain, headache, fatigue and swelling than their counterparts. Employed women experienced less premenstrual performance impairment but more premenstrual anxiety than their non-employed counterparts. Women with more formal education had a lower prevalence of several symptoms, including menstrual headache, premenstrual cramping, premenstrual and menstrual irritability, premenstrual and menstrual depression, and premenstrual and menstrual tension. Women with high family incomes were less likely to experience several PS, including: premenstrual weight gain, menstrual headache, premenstrual cramping, menstrual irritability, menstrual mood swings, and premenstrual tension. These findings underscore the important influence of parity, contraceptive use, menstrual cycle characteristics, and demographic characteristics on PS (1).

Our preliminary work has raised important questions about the variability in the nature of PS and clustering of symptoms into discrete dimensions. A useful approach for future descriptive work will be studying PS as a multidimensional phenomenon. In addition, we have found great variability in prevalence across measurement instruments, suggesting the limitations of both retrospective, closed-ended and prospective, open-ended measures. We have shown that measurements of PS over a single cycle are inadequate for prevalence estimates or as outcome measures in clinical trials. We have demonstrated the importance of parity, contraceptive use, menstrual cycle characteristics, and demographic factors on the prevalence of PS. Finally, we have some initial evidence for the important influence of women's socialization experience and current social milieu on reports of certain types of PS, providing impetus for the proposed work.

fies whether the design is experimental or naturalistic and describes in detail the design elements. An example of the design component of a proposal is given in the box below.

Example of "Design" Component

A cross-sectional design will be employed to estimate the prevalence of perimenstrual symptoms (PS) and related disability and to assess the relative contributions of women's gynecological history, health practices, general health status, socialization, and current social context to an explanatory model of PS, related disability, and illness behavior. The cross-sectional design is appropriate given the recurrent nature of PS and its relatively common occurrence. The primary measures of the independent variables, including gynecological history, health practices, general health status, socialization, and current social context, will be made at entry into the study. Daily measurement of the occurrence and severity of PS, related disability, and illness behavior will be made over the following 3-month period. The prospective approach to measuring PS is essential in order to overcome the influence of strong stereotypes about menstrual symptoms on prevalence estimates, to ensure accurate estimates given the lack of consistency of symptom experience from one cycle to the next, and to overcome the tendency of respondents to telescope events that are studied retrospectively (68-70). This approach will yield reports about PS in relation to the precise day of their occurrence within the cycle. Participants will be told that they are part of a study of women's health, but they will not be told about the menstrual cycle emphasis until completion of the study.

At completion of the study, retrospective measures will be used to explore each woman's perceptions related to her last two menstrual cycles, including which symptoms she believes are related to her menstrual cycle, her evaluation of her symptoms in terms of their severity and treatability, and methods she typically uses to cope with PS.

Data-producing instruments. The investigator carefully describes the indicators that will be used to reflect each concept. Operational definitions accompany each concept expressed in the purposes or hypotheses. The discussion includes estimates of the instruments' reliability and validity taken from past applications. The researcher also describes instruments constructed for the proposed study in detail and usually presents pilot study data to document the feasibility and appropriateness of the instrument for the proposed application. Means to establish the reliability and validity of new instruments are outlined. The investigator also discusses biomedical instrumentation plans in detail, offers means to maintain their calibration, and provides evidence for the reliability and validity of assays. When new methods are considered, their advantages over existing methodologies are described, as are the potential difficulties and limitations associated with particular methods. An example of a data-producing instruments component of a proposal is given in the box on pp. 506 and 507.

Sample The investigator carefully describes the target population for the study and presents the procedures for participant selection. Quantitative studies typically include estimates of sample size and power. The researcher outlines in detail the rationale for sample size, characteristics of the sample, and criteria for inclusion or exclusion. The setting and sampling approaches are described and justified. An example of the sample component of a proposal is given in the box on pp. 507 and 508.

Methods of data production. The investigator describes how data production will proceed. Topics include methods for gaining entry to a setting, what participants will be told and asked to do, and how attrition or nonparticipation will be handled. Data collection methods are clearly described. An example of a methods of data production component of a proposal is given in the box on p. 509.

Protection of human subjects. The researcher clearly and completely describes the potential risks to the participants, including physical, social, legal, or other risks, their likelihood of occurrence, and their seriousness. The relationships between the risks and benefits of participating are weighed and should be reasonable in relation to the importance of the knowledge sought in the study. The investigator describes procedures for protecting against or minimizing any potential risks, including risks to confi-

Text continued on p. 511.

EXAMPLE OF "DATA-PRODUCING INSTRUMENTS" COMPONENT

The major concepts of interest in this study include perimenstrual symptoms (PS), related disability, and illness behavior; indicators of these will constitute the dependent variables for purposes of testing an explanatory model of PS, disability, and illness behavior. In addition, current social context, feminine socialization, health practices, general health status, and gynecological history will be examined as factors that explain the variance in women's PS experience, disability, and illness behavior. Description of instruments measuring the dependent variables will precede description of instruments for measuring the independent variables. (See Table 7 for a summary of concepts, indicators, and instruments.)

Table 7
Concepts, Indicators, and Instruments

A description of the indicators and instruments for only the concepts symptom perception *and* general health status *is presented here.*

Concept/Indicators	Instruments
1. *Symptom perception*	
Perimenstrual symptoms (PS)	Item pool from Moos Menstrual Distress Questionnaire, form T, PAF, and PMTS to be incorporated as a checklist in daily diary
Inquiry into symptoms other than PS	Daily diary; open-ended item, list of general symptoms
Woman's perception of symptoms usually associated with her cycle	PS rating scale, telephone interview
4. *General health status*	
Health perceptions	Health Perceptions Questionnaire, including prior health, current health, health outlook, resistance-susceptibility, health worry-concern, and sickness orientation
General well-being	General Well-Being Scale

A description of only the instruments used to measure general health status is presented here.

4. *General Health Status.* Assessment of the participants' general health status is challenging because most measures of health status are relatively insensitive for young adults, a primarily healthy population. Health will be assessed using indicators of health perceptions and general well-being.
   a. *The Health Perceptions Questionnaire* (HPQ) is a 26-item instrument dealing with perceptions of prior health, current health, health outlook, resistance-susceptibility, health worry-concern, and sickness orientation. It was initially developed by the National Center for Health Statistics and was recently field-tested in the Rand Health Insurance Study (92). This instrument asks respondents for a general assessment of their health. Sample items include "I feel better now than I ever have before" and "When there is something going around I usually catch it." Respondents indicate on a 5-point scale whether these items are definitely true (score=1) or definitely false (score=5). Scores on each dimension usually yield sym-

EXAMPLE OF "DATA-PRODUCING INSTRUMENTS" COMPONENT—cont'd

metrical distributions. Six-week test-retest correlations indicate that the use of the HPQ is preferable to a single-item rating of health perceptions. Item-total correlations averaged greater than 0.5. Associations between age and general health ratings tend to be negative, whereas income, educational level, and being male are positively associated with general health perceptions.

b. *The General Well-Being Schedule* (GWB) was developed by Dupuy to assess psychological well-being through self-reports of well-being or distress. The GWB consists of 22 items representing six content areas: intrinsic life satisfaction; health worry, concerns, or conditions; depressed mood; behavioral, mental, or emotional control; energy level or vitality; and tension, anxiety, and stress. Respondents indicate their experience on a 1 to 6 scale. A total score is obtained by summing each item. Scores range from 0-110; 73-100 represents positive well-being, 61-72 moderate distress, and 0-60 severe distress (93). The internal consistency among the GWB items is 0.93, and 3-month test-retest coefficients are about 0.80.

EXAMPLE OF "SAMPLE" COMPONENT

Composition and sampling method. The sample will be drawn from King County, Washington, a community in which multiple ethnic groups reside. Data from the 1980 census (71) indicate the following distribution of women between the ages of 15 to 59 years:

	n
White	362, 473
Black	16,282
American Indian, Eskimo, and Aleut	3,147
Asian and Pacific Islanders[a]	21,169

[a]Including Japanese, Chinese, Filipino, Korean, Asian and Pacific Islander, Vietnamese, Hawaiian, Guamanian, and Samoan.

In addition, about 1.5% of the white population in Seattle is of Hispanic origin, with approximately 8,000 women who would meet the age criteria for our study. It is evident that the population of King County affords a unique opportunity for a multi-ethnic comparison.

Previous research on menstrual symptoms has demonstrated differences in prevalence estimates across racial-ethnic groups, yet the mechanisms are poorly understood. For example, it is not clear whether ethnic differences in PS within the same study are attributable to ethnic origin per se, to socialization processes within these groups, or to differences in health practices or life style patterns. We will therefore sample from each of the three major racial-ethnic groups in Seattle to assess whether there are differences in prevalence and, if so, whether they can be explained by other study factors.

In order to achieve representation of women from the three major racial-ethnic groups, the sample will be drawn from block groups of census tracts in King County that will maximize the likelihood of identifying women from these groups who are of premenopausal age. In addition, we will only include block groups populated by lower middle income and upper middle income respondents to avoid confounding income and racial-ethnic group membership.

Block groups in King County in which at least 40% of the women meet our age criterion (18-45

Continued.

EXAMPLE OF "SAMPLE" COMPONENT—cont'd

years) will be stratified by dominant racial-ethnic group. From the three ethnic group strata, block groups will be randomly selected to yield the desired number of households for each stratum.

Within each block group selected, all households will be enumerated using Cole's Directory for households in Seattle–King County. Each block group will consist of approximately 800-900 households. Households will be selected at random from the directory. From our previous experience in studying PS, we anticipate that 50% of the households will yield at least one woman meeting our eligibility criteria. Thus we will initially select twice as many households as the number of women desired for each stratum. An interviewer will call the phone number listed in Cole's Directory, or in the case of an unlisted phone number, will approach the household in person to determine if an eligible woman resides in the household. Ninety-six percent of the housing units in King County have telephones (72), thus most initial contacts will be made by telephone. If more than one eligible woman resides in the household, one will be selected using a table of random numbers. "No answer" numbers will be called again at other times. All eligible women will be asked to participate in the study until the desired number of participants in each ethnic group is enrolled.

Criteria for eligibility include:

Over 18 but under 45 years of age

Not pregnant at time of study

Currently menstruating (have not had a hysterectomy or oophorectomy, do not have amenorrhea)

Not currently under treatment for depression

Able to read and write English

Women who have been diagnosed with endometriosis, pelvic inflammatory disease, peptic ulcer, liver disease, cervical stenosis, hypoplastic uterus, fibroids, adenomyosis, ectopic pregnancy, pelvic mass, tubal infection, abnormal pap smears, genital herpes, or urinary tract infections, all conditions which are capable of causing pelvic or lower abdominal discomfort, will be included in the study providing they are not currently under medical care for these problems and are not currently experiencing symptoms they attribute to these problems. Infertile women will be included unless they are currently being treated for anovulation. Their histories will be recorded and taken into account in the analysis of data. Women who have had tubal ligations will be included, and their PS data will be contrasted with those of women who have not been sterilized in this fashion.

In order to assess the extent of selection bias in the sample, women who decline to participate will be asked if they would consent to complete a short form describing their demographic characteristics and a checklist of PS. Their responses will be compared to those of the participants to determine if the two groups differ significantly.

*Sample Size Estimates.** Equal allocation of subjects across each ethnic group stratum (rather than proportional allocation) will be employed to insure adequate numbers of women within each stratum to support bivariate analyses capable of detecting a moderate effect size (73,74). Also of importance in this study is a sufficient sample size to test the multivariate model of PS. A sample of 500 will provide a sufficient n to test a hypothesis including as many as 20 variables with an alpha of 0.05 and a beta of 0.20 (73).

Our previous studies of menstrual cycle symptoms yielded a 74% participation rate for household interviews without subject reimbursement. When a subset of these women was offered a $20 reimbursement for keeping a menstrual symptom diary for 2 months, 96% complied (61). Using these response rates to estimate the probable proportion of completed interviews and symptom diaries over 3 months, it is anticipated that for each 100 women asked to participate in the study approximately 70 will complete the entire study. Thus, we will recruit 900 women to insure a final sample size of 600.

*Estimates are from preliminary studies (1).

EXAMPLE OF "METHODS OF DATA PRODUCTION" COMPONENT

Trained interviewers will identify all women within selected block groups of census tracts who meet the eligibility criteria for the study. One eligible woman from each household will be asked to participate. A complete explanation of the study will be given. If the woman agrees to participate, the interviewer will arrange to conduct the first interview at the respondent's home or a place of her choice. From our previous experience with administering these instruments in an interview, we estimate the interview will not exceed 1 hour. Before the interview begins, the woman will be read the consent form outlining all parts of the study. The interviewer will then conduct the initial interview (see Table 8 for content of interview #1). At the end of the interview, the interviewer will instruct the woman in keeping the health diary for 3 months. She will then contact the woman every 2 weeks by phone regarding any questions or problems she is encountering with the diary. At the end of the 3 months, the woman will be interviewed by telephone. She will be asked to return her diary by mail and thanked for her assistance. She will be debriefed at the end of the study and told that a specific focus of the investigation is menstrual symptoms. On completion of the study, we will send the respondent a check for $30. Validity checks will be performed on 10% of all the interviews by the supervisor.

EXAMPLE OF "PROTECTION OF HUMAN SUBJECTS" COMPONENT

Participants in this study will be identified through random selection of households within selected block groups of census tracts. Nine hundred women between 18 and 45 years of age, from several ethnic backgrounds (white, Asian, and black) will be included in the study. Women who are not pregnant, who have not had a hysterectomy or oophorectomy, are not currently under treatment for depression or anovulation, and are able to read and write English will be included in the study. We anticipate these women will be in good health.

Women will be initially contacted by telephone or visited at their home by a trained interviewer. The interviewer will ascertain their eligibility for the study and explain the study. If the woman is interested in participating, the interviewer will schedule an appointment for the interview at a place chosen by the participant. At the time of the interview, the woman will be read a consent form, and her signed consent will be obtained prior to the interview. The women will be told that the study is concerned with women's health. The focus on the menstrual cycle will not be made explicit to avoid a stereotypical response set in the participants. The women will be debriefed regarding the specific focus on the menstrual cycle during the telephone interview at the end of the study. Women will be asked to: participate in a 1-hour interview; keep a health diary for 3 months; and participate in a 30-minute telephone interview at the end of the study. Women who complete all three portions of the study will be paid $30. The risks associated with the study include mild anxiety evoked by some questionnaire items, but participants will be told they may choose not to answer some questions or terminate the interview at any time.

All data will be kept in a locked file cabinet, and only numbers will be used on the questionnaires. Participants' names will not be attached to their data. Data will be accessible only to the study personnel. There are no direct benefits of participation in this study, but the results may benefit women who experience PS by increasing our understanding of the phenomena and suggesting therapies. The benefits to society include knowledge about a problem that affects a large percentage of women. In light of this, the risks appear small, and the potential outcomes may benefit many women.

EXAMPLE OF "METHODS OF DATA PRODUCTION" COMPONENT

Trained interviewers will identify all women within selected block groups of census tracts who meet the eligibility criteria for the study. One eligible woman from each household will be asked to participate. A complete explanation of the study will be given. If the woman agrees to participate, the interviewer will arrange to conduct the first interview at the respondent's home or a place of her choice. From our previous experience with administering these instruments in an interview, we estimate the interview will not exceed 1 hour. Before the interview begins, the woman will be read the consent form outlining all parts of the study. The interviewer will then conduct the initial interview (see Table 8 for content of interview #1). At the end of the interview, the interviewer will instruct the woman in keeping the health diary for 3 months. She will then contact the woman every 2 weeks by phone regarding any questions or problems she is encountering with the diary. At the end of the 3 months, the woman will be interviewed by telephone. She will be asked to return her diary by mail and thanked for her assistance. She will be debriefed at the end of the study and told that a specific focus of the investigation is menstrual symptoms. On completion of the study, we will send the respondent a check for $30. Validity checks will be performed on 10% of all the interviews by the supervisor.

From Cowan, M., & Felzer, L. (1984). Nursing implications of circadian rhythm in hypokalemia. Grant proposal submitted to the Division of Nursing, U.S. Public Health Service.

EXAMPLE OF "METHODS OF ANALYSIS" COMPONENT

In general, analysis will proceed in five phases:
1. Assessment of the internal consistency of standardized scales and those generated for this study
2. Estimation of the prevalence of several dimensions of perimenstrual symptoms (PS)
3. Generation of a typology of PS profiles
4. Assessment of the risk of experiencing each dimension of PS
5. Testing of the models for explaining the relative contribution of women's gynecological histories, health practices, general health status, socialization, and current social context to PS, related disability, and illness behavior

In the following pages, analyses designed to meet each of our specific aims will be discussed. Data reduction methods will be discussed in that context.

A description of proposed analysis for only phase 3 is presented here.

3. *Generating a typology of PS.*

Profiles of women based on their scores on the PS dimensions and individual symptoms will be developed. From our previous work we anticipate that some women will score high on each dimension, whereas others will experience intense PS on only a single dimension such as negative affect or fluid retention. Cluster analysis using the nearest or farthest neighbor technique (97) will be used to assess the empirical clustering of women by symptoms. The Clustan program (98) offers a number of clustering options and is available at the University of Washington Academic Computer Center.

It is anticipated that these analyses will yield patterns of symptoms that cluster together, as well as subsets of women who experience different dimensions of PS. These results will be compared with the earlier work of Moos (60), Dalton (12), and Abraham (20), Haskett (76), and Halbreich (22). Taken together, the patterns seen in our results and suggested by earlier work should be useful in generating etiological hypotheses for an anticipated typology of PS.

dentiality, and evaluates their effectiveness. Provisions for ensuring necessary professional intervention in the event of adverse effects to the participants are discussed where appropriate, including monitoring the data to ensure the participants' safety. When deception about the purpose of the study is used, its justification is presented and the debriefing procedure provided to participants is described.

The researcher describes in detail plans for the recruitment of participants and the consent procedures to be followed. This includes explaining the use of an intermediary to contact participants whose names otherwise would not be accessible to the investigator. The form used to obtain informed consent to participate in the study is usually appended, as is an assent form used for minors. In addition, this section outlines sources of data such as records or information obtained directly from identifiable individuals.

When the investigator includes special classes of participants such as pregnant women, children, institutionalized mentally ill, prisoners, or others who are likely to be particularly vulnerable, she or he gives the rationale for their involvement. In addition, use of an advocate for vulnerable participants is described. An example of the component of a proposal addressing the protection of human subjects is given in the box at lower left on p. 509.

Protection of animals. When using vertebrate animals in the study, the investigator must justify their use. The species, strains, ages, and numbers; the procedures for their maintenance and care; and the procedures to avoid unnecessary discomfort, pain, or injury, such as using anesthesia, analgesia, and comfortable restraining devices, are described. The box at upper left on p. 510 includes a description of animal protection procedures for a study of hypokalemia in rats.

Methods of analysis. The investigator describes how he or she will analyze the data in relation to each of the study's specific aims. The statistical procedures to be used and the reasons for their choice in relation to the type of data anticipated are specified. An example of the methods of analysis component of a proposal is given in the box at left.

Time frame. The investigator includes a time plan for data production, analysis, and interpretation, including preparation of the final report. She or he estimates the time required to accomplish each major study component (see box above).

EXAMPLE OF "TIME FRAME" COMPONENT

The following timetable is proposed for this study:

Months 01-03
  Recruit and train interviewer, supervisor, and interviewers
  Finalize instruments and complete final field testing
  Enumerate households selected from block groups

Months 04-28
  Conduct interviews
  Code and edit interview data
  Enter data into database management system

Months 24-30
  Perform preliminary data analysis

Months 30-36
  Perform final data analysis
  Report writing

Literature cited

The researchers include complete literature citations at the end of the proposal. The documentation of relevant citations provides evidence of the investigator's awareness of important work in the topic area.

Appendices

The investigator may append carefully selected materials that clarify the proposal for the reviewer's information. Usually this includes publications by the investigator or members of the research team that relate to the topic. In addition, one often includes instruments proposed for use, diagrams of organism-instrumentation systems to be employed, and other information not essential to the body of the proposal but providing important clarification of some aspects, such as technical charts or calculations. One must remember that the investigator's capability to conduct the research appears not only in the technical components of the proposal but also in the material accompanying the body of the proposal.

PRINCIPAL INVESTIGATOR/PROGRAM DIRECTOR: _____

BIOGRAPHICAL SKETCH

Give the following information for key professional personnel, beginning with the
Principal Investigator/Program Director. Photocopy this page for each person.

NAME	TITLE	BIRTHDATE *(Mo., Day, Yr.)*

EDUCATION *(Begin with baccalaureate or other initial professional education and include postdoctoral training)*

INSTITUTION AND LOCATION	DEGREE *(circle highest degree)*	YEAR CONFERRED	FIELD OF STUDY

RESEARCH AND/OR PROFESSIONAL EXPERIENCE: Concluding with present position, list in chronological order previous employment, experience, and honors. Include present membership on any Federal Government Public Advisory Committee. List, in chronological order, the titles and complete references to all publications during the past three years and to representative earlier publications pertinent to this application. **DO NOT EXCEED TWO PAGES.**

PRINCIPAL INVESTIGATOR/PROGRAM DIRECTOR: _____Woods, Nancy F._____

RESOURCES AND ENVIRONMENT

FACILITIES: Mark the facilities to be used and briefly indicate their capacities, pertinent capabilities, relative proximity and extent of availability to the project. Use "other" to describe facilities at other performance sites and at sites for field studies. Using continuation pages if necessary, include a description of the nature of any collaboration with other organizations and provide further information in the RESEARCH PLAN.

☐ Laboratory: N/A

☐ Clinical: N/A

☐ Animal: N/A

☒ Computer: The University of Washington Academic Computer Center has a CDC-6400 computer available for project use.

☒ Office: Office space for the project staff will be provided in the School of Nursing.

☐ Other (_____):

MAJOR EQUIPMENT: List the most important equipment items already available for this project, noting the location, and pertinent capabilities of each.

ADDITIONAL INFORMATION: Provide any other information describing the environment for the project. Identify support services such as consultants, secretarial, machine shop, and electronics shop, and the extent to which they will be available to the project.

PRINCIPAL INVESTIGATOR/PROGRAM DIRECTOR:

DETAILED BUDGET FOR FIRST 12 MONTH BUDGET PERIOD
DIRECT COSTS ONLY

FROM _____ THROUGH _____

PERSONNEL (Applicant organization only)

NAME	POSITION TITLE	TIME/EFFORT		DOLLAR AMOUNT REQUESTED (Omit cents)		
		%	Hours per Week	SALARY	FRINGE BENEFITS	TOTALS
	Principal Investigator					
	SUBTOTALS ⟶					

CONSULTANT COSTS

EQUIPMENT (Itemize)

SUPPLIES *(Itemize by category)*

TRAVEL

| DOMESTIC |
| FOREIGN |

PATIENT CARE NEEDS

| INPATIENT |
| OUTPATIENT |

ALTERATIONS AND RENOVATIONS *(Itemize by category)*

CONSORTIUM/CONTRACTUAL COSTS

OTHER EXPENSES *(Itemize by category)*

TOTAL DIRECT COSTS

$

PRINCIPAL INVESTIGATOR/PROGRAM DIRECTOR: _____

BUDGET FOR ENTIRE PROPOSED PROJECT PERIOD
DIRECT COSTS ONLY

BUDGET CATEGORY TOTALS		1st BUDGET PERIOD	ADDITIONAL YEARS SUPPORT REQUESTED			
			2nd	3rd	4th	5th
PERSONNEL (*Salary and fringe benefits.*) (*Applicant organization only*)						
CONSULTANT COSTS						
EQUIPMENT						
SUPPLIES						
TRAVEL	DOMESTIC					
	FOREIGN					
PATIENT CARE COSTS	INPATIENT					
	OUTPATIENT					
ALTERATIONS AND RENOVATIONS						
CONSORTIUM/ CONTRACTUAL COSTS						
OTHER EXPENSES						
TOTAL DIRECT COSTS						

TOTAL FOR ENTIRE PROPOSED PROJECT PERIOD ⟶ $

JUSTIFICATION (Use continuation pages if necessary): Describe the specific functions of the personnel and consultants. If a recurring annual increase in personnel costs is anticipated, give the percentage. For *all* years, justify any costs for which the need may not be obvious, such as equipment, foreign travel, alterations and renovations, and consortium/contractual costs. For any additional years of support requested, justify any significant increases in any category over the first 12 month budget period. In addition, for COMPETING CONTINUATION applications, justify any significant increases over the current level of support.

Investigator and team

The investigator includes information about the research team and consultants for the proposed project. Usually a biographical form is completed for each of the investigators and the consultants. These forms should include each team member's most relevant publications as well as documentation of his or her pertinent research experience. In addition, the inclusion of the team members and consultants is justified in light of their particular expertise. The box on p. 512 shows the Public Health Service form used in completing this component of the research proposal.

Resources and environment

The investigator describes the setting in which the research will be conducted, including a description of any special aspects of the facilities and equipment necessary to the project. This includes the availability of needed laboratory, clinical, animal, or computer resources (see box on p. 513).

Budget

When investigators prepare a research proposal for purposes of generating funding, inclusion of a budget statement is essential. When they are preparing a proposal for other purposes, such as an academic experience, budget preparation is extremely useful if only to provide projections to help judge the feasibility of conducting the study. Budget projections include several categories but typically contain personnel salaries and fringe benefits and estimates of the personnel time and effort. The budget also includes consultant fees and travel expenses for consultants and cost estimates associated with equipment purchase, leasing and maintenance expenses, and supplies. The researchers estimate travel costs related to data production as well as travel expenses for presentations at professional meetings. In addition, expenses necessary for alterations, renovations, and use of space to house the project are also included. The box on pp. 514 to 516 shows the Public Health Service form for completing this component of the research proposal.

Directing the proposal

When preparing a proposal, the investigator considers the intended audience and their concerns. He or she must not only provide the information the agency requires, but must also consider the particular program areas of interest to the agency. The investigator's challenge is to write the proposal so the reviewer can see the proposed work's relevance to the program emphasis of the funding agency, academic unit, or clinical setting. Sometimes the reviewers' identities are known to the investigator, but typically they are unknown. By subsequently identifying the review body, as is possible when their names are published, the investigator can assess the intended audience. The researcher should recognize that the reviewer is an intelligent scientist who may be extremely well informed or only modestly well informed about the particular topic for the study. Thus orienting the proposal to the relatively uninformed reviewer as well as to the expert in the field is important. Both usually will contribute to the judgment of the project's scientific merit.

Guidelines used for reviewing research proposals

The investigator preparing a research proposal should consider the guidelines that reviewers will be using in judging the project's scientific merit. Individual agencies publish guidelines for reviewers' comments on research grant applications to the U.S. Public Health Service (PHS). At the minimum, these guidelines include a summary of the reviewer's proposed work as well as a critique of the application, comments on the investigator, resources and environment, budget, and considerations such as involvement of human subjects, animal welfare, hazardous material, and procedures.

The guide for reviewers of PHS grant applications asks reviewers to consider the following: (1) significance and originality of the proposed study in its scientific field, (2) the validity of the hypothesis, (3) the logic of the aims, and (4) the feasibility and adequacy of the procedures. The reviewer is asked to assess whether the research is likely to produce new data and concepts and whether alternate routes to the solution of the problem have been considered. The competence of the principal investigators and key staff to conduct the proposed research, including their academic qualifications, research experience, productivity, and any other special attributes, also are judged, as are the adequacy of the resources and environment to implement the proposed work. The budget is reviewed to determine if it is realistic and justified in terms of the aims and methods. Budget modifications are recommended when appropriate.

In addition, the reviewers are asked to consider the adequacy of protection of human subjects and animal welfare. Where appropriate, potentially hazardous materials and procedures to limit risk are critically evaluated for their adequacy. The reviewers are asked to provide an overall evaluation of the strengths and limitations of the application and a recommendation of approval, disapproval, or deferral.

Before submitting a proposal for review, the investigator is well advised to seek critical evaluation of the proposal from colleagues knowledgeable in the topic area and nursing research. In addition, some agencies' staff will provide preliminary reviews of proposals prior to formal submission so that investigators can make modifications before final submission.

GENERATING SUPPORT

Necessary support for conducting research includes human resources, material resources such as equipment, and financial resources. Few studies require only the investigator's time and energy. Indeed, most undergraduate and master theses require a budget of several hundred dollars and many hours of the student's time. Some human and material resources may be available to the investigator through the employing organization, but these resources are rarely unlimited. As funding for patient care becomes increasingly scarce, the access to human and material resources for research in patient care organizations has decreased. Likewise, the economic challenges facing most universities make supplementary funding essential. For these reasons, investigators in educational, clinical, and research organizations must be able to communicate their research plans and need for support to public and private organizations that fund research.

Komnenich (1981) outlined five key elements for gaining access to research resources, whether from public or private agencies:

1. Knowledge of the funding agency or foundation providing support
2. Mechanism by which an award is made
3. Programs supported by the agency
4. Individuals who can provide information about the organization's program priorities or who can help the applicant
5. Review process for evaluating research proposals

The funding agency

Knowledge of the funding agency providing support for research and its organizational context is essential for the investigator applying for funding. Two primary sources of support for nursing research are public and private agencies.

Public funding agencies

Public agencies include the Center for Nursing Research of the National Institutes of Health (NIH); other institutes of the National Institutes of Health; the Alcohol, Drug Abuse and Mental Health Administration; and the Division of Maternal Child Health, which are all part of the PHS and are tax-supported federal agencies that fund health-related research (Fig. 32-1).

Federal agencies. Federal funding agencies are parts of complex organizations with specific missions. It is important for the investigator to comprehend the location of the agency within the larger federal organization to understand the orientation and priorities of programs within that agency.

The National Center for Nursing Research was created in 1986 by congressional mandate (PL 99-158) and is part of the NIH. The Center was developed because of the necessity for a highly placed federal agency to foster nursing research. Before 1986 the research grant funding section of the Division of Nursing was part of the Health Services and Resources Administration. The mission of the National Center for Nursing Research is to support nursing research and research training related to patient care, promotion of health, prevention of disease, and mitigation of effects of acute and chronic illnesses and disabilities. The Center has four branches, each related to a special program area: Health Promotion and Disease Prevention, Acute and Chronic Illness, Nursing Systems and Special Programs, and Research Development and Review. Studies involving ethical issues related to patient care and patient care research are included in Special Programs. Nursing research efforts funded by the National Center for Nursing Research will complement other biomedical research programs of the NIH that are primarily concerned with the cause and treatment of disease.

The NIH is a complex federal organization and part of the PHS established by Congress in 1930. It includes 11 research institutes as well as research and support divisions, the Fogarty Center for Advanced Study in Health Sciences, and the National Center

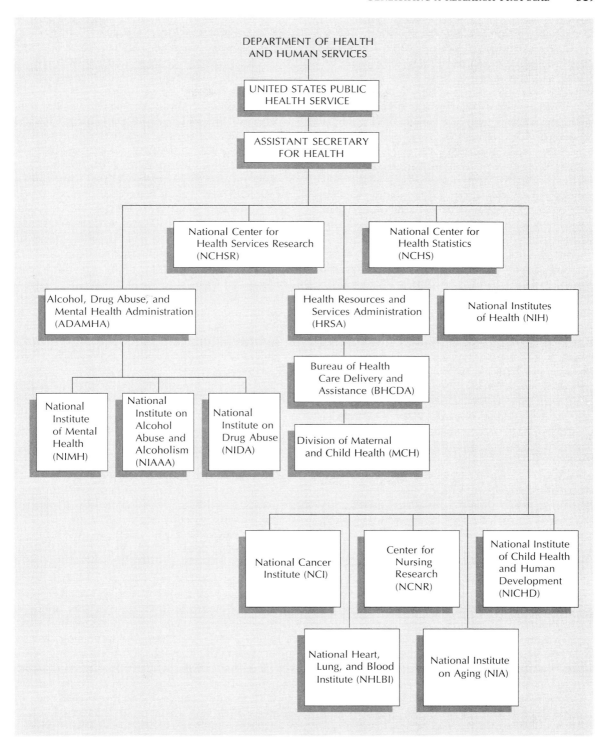

Fig. 32-1. Federal agencies funding nursing and health-related research.

for Nursing Research. The research institutes are oriented toward particular diseases such as cancer, broad research program areas such as environmental health, and anatomical areas such as the eye, heart, and lung. The mission of the NIH is to improve the health of the people of the United States by increasing understanding of processes underlying human health and by acquiring new knowledge to help prevent, detect, diagnose, and treat disease. The NIH accomplishes this mission in part by supporting research in U.S. institutions and those in other nations and by conducting research in its own laboratories and clinics. Despite its general mission statement, most of the research supported by the NIH is biomedical.

The Alcohol, Drug Abuse and Mental Health Administration (ADAMHA) is another complex organization. It consists of three institutes: the National Institute of Mental Health, National Institute on Alcohol Abuse and Alcoholism, and the National Institute of Drug Abuse. The mission of ADAMHA is to provide a national focus for the federal effort to increase knowledge and promote effective strategies to deal with health problems and issues associated with the use and abuse of alcohol and drugs and with mental illness and mental health. Among ADAMHA's research-related programs are those designed to expand knowledge of etiology, diagnosis, treatment, and prevention; train researchers and other personnel; and gather data on the extent of and national response to alcohol, drug abuse, and mental health problems.

The National Center for Health Services Research also is part of the PHS. Its mission includes research directed toward the following areas:

1. Health promotion and disease prevention, including health status measurement, organization and provider studies, analysis of public and private program interventions, and methods to increase consumer knowledge and change health attitudes and behavior
2. Technology assessment, including studies of the safety, efficacy, effectiveness, and cost effectiveness of specific technologies; development of new methods for evaluating medical technologies; and diffusion of medical technology
3. Role of market forces in health care delivery
4. Primary care, including development and testing of better designs, measures, and analytical techniques to improve primary care research and evaluation and surveillance techniques to assess quality of care and effectiveness of health promotion and disease prevention efforts
5. State and local health problems, including data and methods to project the demands for service and to forecast health care expenditures and studies to develop and evaluate decision models for allocating health care resources

The Division of Maternal Child Health, part of the PHS, is located in the Health Resources and Services Administration, Bureau of Health Care Delivery and Assistance. Its mission includes supporting (1) special maternal and child health projects of regional and national significance that contribute to improvement of services for mothers, children, and handicapped children; (2) maternal child health research and training projects; (3) genetic disease testing, counseling, and information projects; and (4) hemophilia diagnostic and treatment centers. General research priorities include:

1. Validation of currently accepted health care practices
2. Studies of innovations before they are widely adopted
3. Research on the familial, economic, cultural, and environmental factors in disease etiology
4. Analyses of the effect of federal and state health care policies
5. Continuation and expansion of routine data collection programs to monitor maternal and child health
6. Improvements of research methods

Private funding agencies

Private funding agencies include (1) family and corporate foundations created to manage the distribution of family fortunes or corporate profits according to the goals specified by the founder and interpreted by a board of trustees and (2) voluntary organizations dedicated to alleviation of a specific health problem. Private agencies funding nursing research include the American Nurses' Foundation, Sigma Theta Tau, the Robert Wood Johnson Foundation, American Cancer Society, American Heart Association, the Ford Foundation, the Rockefeller Foundation, the Kellogg Foundation, the Milbank Foundation, and a wide range of corporations, including drug, hospital supply, and insurance companies (Table 32-1).

TABLE 32-1. Private funding resources for nursing research

FUNDING AGENCY	PURPOSE	DEADLINES	FUNDING RANGE
Sigma Theta Tau (National) National Honor Society of Nursing 1200 Waterway Blvd. Indianapolis, IN 46202 (317) 634-8171	To encourage qualified nurses to contribute to the advancement of nursing through research.	March 1	$3000 (maximum)
American Nurses' Foundation 2420 Pershing Rd. Kansas City, MO 64108 (816) 474-5720	The competitive extramural grants program is designed for beginning nurse researchers. Experienced researchers will be considered for funding only if the proposal is in an area not previously investigated by the researcher.	July 1	$2500 (maximum)
Robert Wood Johnson Foundation P.O. Box 2316 Princeton, NJ 08540 (609) 452-8701 Write: Edward H. Robbins, Proposal Manager	This is the largest foundation devoted exclusively to improvement of health services, with emphasis on projects to improve access to personal health care for the most underserved population groups; to make health care arrangements more effective and affordable; and to help people maintain attainable function in their everyday lives.	Board meets in January, March, May, July, October, and December	$1000 to $1 million
Kellogg Foundation 400 North Ave. Battle Creek, MI 49016 (616) 968-1611 Write: Robert D. Sparks President	Aid is largely limited to programs concerned with application of knowledge rather than its creation through basic research. Current funding priorities include projects designed to improve human well-being through adult continuing education; health promotion and disease prevention; coordinated, cost-effective health services; and so on.	Board meets monthly	$425 to $2 million

Private-sector funding agencies vary greatly in their size and mission. The private agencies range from small, family-operated foundations awarding sums of a few hundred dollars to complex organizations awarding millions of dollars each year. The mission of the private foundations varies greatly with the specific foundation. The American Nurses Foundation, founded by the American Nurses Association in 1955, is a private, nonprofit foundation making awards for research related to clinical nursing and nursing administration. Sigma Theta Tau, a national nursing honorary founded in 1922 at Indiana University, is a private nonprofit organization that encourages qualified nurses to contribute to the advancement of nursing through research. Sigma Theta Tau has had a research fund since 1936. The Robert Wood Johnson Foundation is a private philanthropy interested in improving health in the United States. Its goals are to fund programs that improve access to personal health care for the most underserved population groups; to make health care arrangements more effective and affordable; and to help people maintain or regain maximum attainable function in their everyday lives. The Kellogg Foundation supports projects in agriculture, education, and health. In addition to these funding agencies, corporate groups such as biomedical instrumentation companies and groups such as the Licensed Beverage Industries support studies pertinent to their mission.

Mechanism of award

Both public and private agencies use a variety of award mechanisms. Grants are investigator-initiated awards that an agency makes to individuals or a team of investigators to support proposed research. The investigator develops the ideas and methods and subsequently proposes them to the agency. In contrast, *contracts* are awards made to individuals or to teams of investigators and initiated by the funding agency through a request for proposals. Agencies usually use publications to outline the program areas in which the organization desires work, such as requests for proposals to stimulate contract applications and requests for applications and program announcements to stimulate grant applications. The federal government uses both of these mechanisms. Awards are available through the federal government to support individual research projects (project grants) or a program of research with multiple individual studies (program grants). Research project grants support a discrete, specified project in an area representing the interests and competency of a principal investigator. Program project grants support a broadly based, multidisciplinary, and often long-term research program that has a well-defined, overall major goal or basic theme. Many institutes of the federal government offer small grants, usually less than $25,000, to support an investigator's early efforts. The National Institutes of Health recently initiated the First Independent Research Support & Transition Award (FIRST), which will provide an opportunity for first-time investigators to apply for support for longer periods (up to 5 years) and for funding up to $350,000. The purpose of the FIRST award is to give new investigators an adequate period to develop their capabilities and demonstrate the merit of their research ideas. These awards encourage new investigators in basic or clinical science disciplines, including those who have interrupted promising research careers, to develop their interests and capabilities in biomedical, behavioral, and nursing research. Table 32-2 lists institutes and centers with FIRST awards and small grants.

In addition to research grants, the National Center for Nursing Research provides research training support for nurse scientists. Research training grants include those made to institutions (Institutional Training Grant) and individuals (National Research Service Award). Individual predoctoral, postdoctoral, and senior fellowships (National Research Service Awards) and two care development awards—the Academic Investigator Award and Clinical Investigator Award—provide funding to promote a cadre of well-prepared nurse scientists to meet future nursing research needs.

Programs and individuals in the organization

Usually a funding agency identifies its program areas through publications describing its objectives and priorities. For example, the NIH Guide for Grants and Contracts* publishes programmatic emphases of the National Center for Nursing Research, Division

---

*Available through Grants and Contracts Guide Distribution Center, National Institutes of Health, Bldg. 31, Room B3BN10, Bethesda, MD 20205.

TABLE 32-2. Federal and private agencies with FIRST awards or small-grant programs

AGENCY	FIRST	SMALL GRANT
NATIONAL INSTITUTES OF HEALTH		
National Institute on Aging	X	
National Institute of Allergy and Infectious Diseases	X	
National Institute of Arthritis, Diabetes, and Digestive and Kidney Diseases	X	
National Cancer Institute	X	
National Institute of Child Health and Human Development	X	
National Institutes of Dental Research	X	
National Institute of Environmental Health Sciences	X	
National Eye Institute	X	
National Institute of General Medical Sciences	X	
National Heart, Lung, and Blood Institute	X	
National Library of Medicine	X	
National Institute of Neurological and Communicative Disorders and Stroke	X	
Division of Research Resources	X	
National Center for Nursing Research	X	
ALCOHOL, DRUG ABUSE, AND MENTAL HEALTH ADMINISTRATION		
National Institute on Alcohol Abuse and Alcoholism		X
National Institute on Drug Abuse		X
National Institute of Mental Health		X
PRIVATE FOUNDATIONS		
Sigma Theta Tau		X
American Nurses' Foundation		X

of Maternal Child Health, ADAMHA and the NIH. Program emphases of private foundations such as Robert Wood Johnson, Sigma Theta Tau, and American Nurses' Foundation, appear frequently in agencies' literature.

The literature describing the program areas usually identifies the individuals with program responsibility for a particular area of research. Often these individuals are available to discuss the application with the investigator until the time the individual formally submits the proposal. Although staff members are not part of the formal review process, they can give advice to the investigator while the proposal is under development. A publication entitled NIH Extramural Programs outlines program areas and individuals the investigator can contact for further information.*

---

*Available through Grants and Contracts Guide Distribution Center, National Institutes of Health, Bldg. 31, Room B3BN10, Bethesda, MD 20205.

Review process

The Center for Nursing Research, the other components of the NIH, and ADAMHA use a two-tiered review mechanism consisting of an initial review for scientific merit and a second review for programmatic emphasis (Fig. 32-2). The investigator sends self-initiated research proposals intended for any of the institutes of the NIH or for ADAMHA to the Division of Research Grants, which is part of the NIH. The Division of Research Grants personnel refer the proposal to an appropriate review body. The staff of the Division of Research Grants reviews the information in the title of the proposal and in the abstract in order to assign the proposal to the most appropriate initial review group. A group of scientists called a "study section" performs the initial review of the proposal for scientific merit. The review criteria address:

1. Scientific and technical significance and originality
2. Adequacy of the methodology to carry out the research

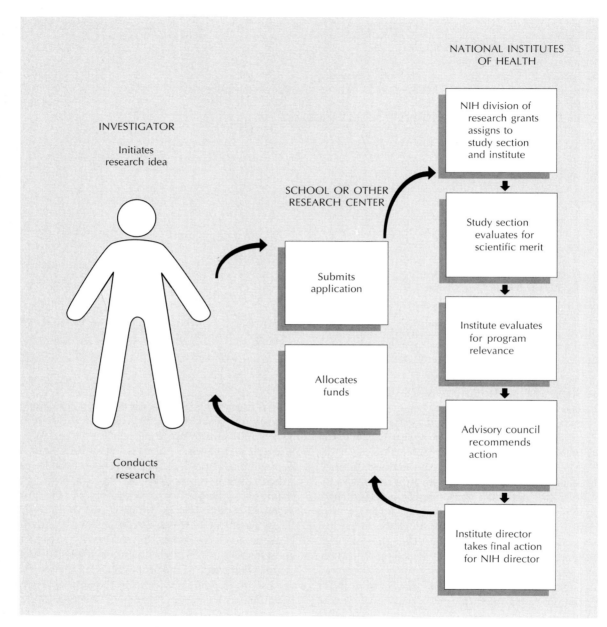

Fig. 32-2. How a research grant is made. (From National Institutes of Health. *NIH peer review of research grant applications.* Washington, DC: Department of Health and Human Services.)

3. Qualifications and experience of the principal investigator and staff
4. Reasonable availability of resources
5. Reasonableness of the proposed budget and duration
6. Other factors, such as human subjects protection, animal welfare, and biohazards

The study section may take the following actions: approval, disapproval, or deferral. Approval indicates that the application is of sufficient merit to be worthy of support. The vote for approval is equivalent to a recommendation that an award be made provided sufficient funds are available. If a proposal is approved, the study section gives it a numerical priority score: 1 is excellent and 5 is marginally acceptable.

Disapproval indicates the application is not of sufficient merit to be worthy of support. Disapproval also may be recommended when hazardous or unethical procedures are involved or when no funds can be recommended, such as a request for supplemental funding deemed unnecessary by the review group. The most common reasons proposals are disapproved include:

1. Lack of new or original ideas
2. Diffuse, superficial, or unfocused research plan
3. Lack of knowledge of published relevant work
4. Lack of experience in the essential methodology
5. Uncertainty concerning the future directions
6. Questionable reasoning in experimental approach
7. Absence of an acceptable scientific rationale
8. Unrealistically large amount of work
9. Lack of sufficient experimental detail and/or uncritical approach

Deferral indicates the study section cannot make a recommendation without additional information.

After the study section review, a national advisory council or board consisting of scholars and laypersons makes recommendations based on the study section review and relevance to the organizations' program priorities. The council may concur with the study section, modify the study section's action, defer the proposal for future consideration, or reverse a study section decision. The latter is most likely to occur when study section members were split in their decision and there is a minority report. The award is based on both scientific merit and the institute's program priorities. Final action rests with the director of the institute or center.

The NIH has chartered study sections, and the names of members in the initial review groups and the public advisory groups are published in a document entitled NIH Public Advisory Groups. The Center for Nursing Research has a chartered review group responsible for the initial scientific review of all research grants and a public advisory group for nursing.

After a grant proposal is reviewed the institute's staff prepares a summary statement, including an evaluation and recommendation of the priority score. This summary statement is available at the investigator's request after the study section meets. The summary statement, called the "pink sheet" because it is written on pink paper, is sent to both the investigator and the national advisory council for their information after the council meets. (See box on pp. 526 and 527.)

The review process employed by private funding agencies varies greatly with the specific funding agencies. Although some now use the two-tiered system already described, many agencies use internal staff review or send the proposal to outside consultants for their review. The availability of feedback to the investigator, such as the pink sheet, varies with the funding agency. Although available to investigators who apply for federal funding, this information is not usually available to applicants to private funding agencies.

After the review

Comments from reviewers often contain helpful suggestions that the investigator can use to improve the study design or methods. Reacting to criticism constructively may be difficult, particularly when the investigator does not agree with the review. Often criticisms of the research plan or the investigator's ability to carry out the project are helpful in stimulating the investigator to reconsider elements of the proposal or to seek a collaborator with more experience before the next submission. Sometimes the criticism is attributable to the reviewer's lack of understanding of the proposal. Revising the proposal to

SUMMARY STATEMENT
(Privileged Communication)

Application Number: 1 301 HD18479-01   RS
Dual Review: NU

Review Group: EPIDEMIOLOGY AND DISEASE CONTROL REVIEW

Meeting Date: JUNE 1983   1

Investigator: WOODS, NANCY F   Degree: PHD
Position:

Organization: UNIVERSITY OF WASHINGTON
City, State: SEATTLE, WASH   Requested Start Date: 01/01/84

Project Title: PREVALENCE OF PERIMENSTRUAL SYMPTOMS

Recommendation: APPROVAL

Special Note: HS INV.-CERTIFIED, NO IRG CONCERNS OR COMMENTS.

PROJECT YEAR	DIRECT COSTS REQUESTED	DIRECT COSTS RECOMMENDED	PREVIOUSLY RECOMMENDED	GRANT PERIOD
01	129,792	129,792		
02	134,988	134,988		
03	80,385	80,385		

RESUME: The aims of this study are to estimate the prevalence of perimenstrual symptoms (PS) and associated disability in a population of women residing in King County, Washington; explore the clustering of symptoms in the perimenstruum; generate a typology of PS; and assess the relative contribution of women's socialization, current social context, ethnic group, gynecological history, health practices and general health status to a model explaining the variance in PS.

This is an epidemiologically sound proposal which could be strengthened by the inclusion of biologic variables along with the psychosocial issues. A few minor design problems are noted but these can be corrected easily. However, as presented, the project will add only modestly to the previous work performed by this investigative team.

DESCRIPTIVE: Nine hundred menstruating women between 18 and 45 years of age from three ethnic groups (black, white and Asian) will be enrolled in the study through random sampling of households within selected census tracts. Women will be interviewed regarding their feminine socialization, current social context, gynecological history, health practices and general health status. They will be instructed in keeping a 90-day health diary in which they will record symptoms, disability and illness behaviors. During a telephone interview at the end of the study, they will be asked about the PS they typically experience, will rate their PS severity and treatability, and will describe coping methods they employ for PS. Pooled and stratum specific estimates of PS prevalence will be calculated. Dimensions of PS will be identified using factor analysis. Cluster analysis of cases will be used to generate a PS typology. Relative risk of experiencing PS types, given study factors, will be calculated. Multiple regression analysis will be used to test multivariate models of PS, PS disability, and illness behavior.

CRITIQUE: This is clearly a much needed study to collect basic epidemiological data on PS in the general population. The design is well-formulated and informed by some considerable pilot work, thus increasing the chances of a successful study. Some easily corrected concerns should be noted.

It is not clear why the age limit was raised from 35 to 45, thus increasing the rate of exclusion for women not currently menstruating (more than 20 percent of 45 year olds will have had a hysterectomy and/or oophorectomy).

The selection of "block groups" of census tracts is not clear. The income bounds need to be stated, as does the number of "block groups."

The final strata and sampling strategy are not clear. Is some form of quota sampling to be used? And if so, how will this be implemented to ensure random samples without selection bias? The impact of the design effect on the variances is not discussed. Another issue is that household dispositions require validity checks, not just completed interviews.

Diaries are being kept for three months to collect two complete cycles of data. Why not modify this to collect three complete cycles for equivalent cost?

Although the principal investigator has completed some research on the use of daily diaries, no reference is made to the seminal work of Lois Verbrugge who has in recent years been undertaking key research regarding the use of this instrument and is widely regarded as a national expert on the subject.

The sample size calculations appear to be inappropriate. They should be based on the precision of desired estimates, not on the basis of detecting differences between groups. What are the "comparison" and "index series" referred to in the proposal?

Finally, and most importantly, the role of biologic variables seem to be minimally discussed and hastily dismissed—especially hormonal levels. It might be of interest to examine the interrelationship of hormones to the psycho-social aspects in an interactive way to see how they might influence the nature and severity of perimenstrual symptoms.

INVESTIGATORS: Nancy Fugate Woods, the principal investigator, is a nurse who obtained her Ph.D. in epidemiology from the University of North Carolina in 1978. Her current position is Professor and Director of the Office of Nursing Research Facilitation, School of Nursing at the University of Washington, Seattle. Her past research activities have been mostly in the areas of human sexuality and problems associated with menstruation. She will devote 30 percent of her time to the project. She is the only professional for whom salary support is requested.

Consultative services are included for Janet Daling, Ph.D., who is another epidemiologist at the School of Public Health and Community Medicine of the University of Washington. Two days per year of her services are requested to assist in the sampling and analysis aspects of the study. No budget request is made for these services.

Additional consultative services are requested for Bonnie Worthington-Roberts, Ph.D., for the nutritional aspects of the project and for Karen Paige, Ph.D., a psychologist at the University of California at Davis. Three and two days per annum, respectively, will be spent by these consultants.

The research team seems well qualified and experienced in the methods and issues proposed in this project.

RESOURCES AND ENVIRONMENT: These appear adequate for the conduct of the project, largely based on the evidence provided by the prior studies described.

BUDGET: The budget seems generally appropriate although the time allocations for the consultants appears to be an underestimate of their needs.

provide a better explanation of the study and its background can remedy this problem. Sometimes the criticism is unjustified, and the investigator must ignore it. Sometimes the criticisms are made out of ignorance, and the investigator can have a good laugh about them. Most often, the investigator can learn from the reviewer's criticisms and then produce a better research product.

SUMMARY

The investigator proposing a research idea must develop that idea with care. Likewise, in this present economic climate, the investigator must devote the same amount of care to seeking support to conduct the research. Nothing substitutes for a good idea. It is extremely important for the proposal to be well developed and for the investigator to have a clear idea of the research priorities and the resources necessary to support them. Once the investigator has identified the need for support, she or he can scan the available resources. Often support exists for research within academic settings, nursing service agencies, and other organizations where the investigator may be employed. Usually this support is in the form of small grants to fund pilot research, but assistance from a senior investigator, access to laboratory space and equipment, or donation of supplies for the project may also be available.

Next, the investigator weighs the available support with the essential support for conducting the research. When a mismatch occurs between what is readily available and what is necessary, the investigator begins the search for funding resources. Often consultation with individuals in one's organization can facilitate this search. Staff in research development offices or offices dealing with grants and contracts can be extremely supportive in helping investigators identify potential sources of funding. Several references also are designed to help investigators identify sources of funding. The *Federal Register*, published daily, informs the public of the grant priorities of federal programs. The NIH Guide to Grants and Contracts, published monthly, contains information about all new federal programs and priorities.

Information about funding from the private sector is usually more difficult to obtain. Several resources are designed to acquaint investigators with private foundation resources, including the *Foundation Directory*, which provides information for more than 3000 foundations with assets of more than $1 million. The *National Data Book* includes a listing of all current U.S. foundations that award grants. Obtaining a computer search of guides to foundation grants is also possible. *Comsearch: Subjects* includes 68 separate subject listings that can be ordered as a complete set or by the particular subject of interest (e.g., nursing). The *Taft Corporate Directory* provides information on 300 company-sponsored foundations. *Corporate 500: The Directory of Corporate Philanthropy* contains information on the contribution programs of the 500 largest American corporations. In addition, the *Annual Register of Grant Agencies* lists funding agencies, including corporate groups.

Once the investigator has identified potential sources of funding, the next step is to contact the staff of the organizations. Staff can be helpful to the investigator in developing the proposal and may offer important advice about directing the proposal and defining the budget limits. The staff can also explain the review process and the specific guidelines for submitting proposals. The researcher must recognize that individual organizations have different requirements for proposals and must follow the directions for submitting proposals, including the necessary information for an adequate review. Organization staffs can also help in assessing the match between the investigator's idea and the emphasis of the funding agency. Sometimes emphasizing certain aspects of a proposal and deemphasizing others is advantageous. Sometimes the investigator would be unwise to submit a specific proposal to a certain funding agency because of a mismatch in their priorities. In this case, the alert investigator should have assessed the mismatch before investing months of work in developing a proposal for which funding is unlikely. On the other hand, staff can often offer suggestions about how to orient a proposal that is unusual for the particular funding agency.

Once the investigator has identified the agency to which to submit a proposal, she or he must obtain and follow the guidelines that specify the expectations of the organization. When reviewed without complete information, some proposals may receive poor priority scores and in some instances may be deferred for a later review once the investigator completes the application. Many funding agencies have special deadlines for submitting grants. The researcher must ascertain the review schedule to avoid missing the opportunity for an expeditious review.

References

Allen, E. (1960). Why are research grant applications disapproved? *Science, 132*, 1532-1534.

Berthold, J. (1973). Nursing research grant proposals: What influenced their approval or disapproval in two national granting agencies. *Nursing Research, 22*, 292-299.

Bloch, D., Gortner, S., & Sturdivant, L. (1978). The Nursing Research Grants Program of the Division of Nursing, United States Public Health Service. *Journal of Nursing Administration, 8,*(3), 40-45.

Campos, R. (1974). *Private monies for nursing research.* Boulder, CO: Western Interstate Commission for Higher Education.

Campos, R. (1975a). *Federal monies for health science research.* Boulder, CO: Western Interstate Commission for Higher Education.

Campos, R. (1975b). *Funding sources for research in the health sciences.* Boulder, CO: Western Interstate Commission for Higher Education.

Campos, R. (1976). Securing information on funding sources for nursing research. *Journal of Nursing Administration, 6*, 16-18.

Cole, S., Cole, J., & Simon, G. (1981). Chance and consensus in peer review. *Science, 32,*(1), 9-14.

Dixon, J. (1982). Developing the evaluation component of a grant application. *Nursing Outlook, 30*, 122-127.

Eaves, G. (1972). Who reads your project-grant application to the National Institutes of Health? *Federation Proceedings, 31,*(1), 2-9.

Eaves, G. (1973). The project-grant application of the National Institutes of Health. *Federation Proceedings, 32,*(5), 1541-1550.

Elliott, R., & Michak, J. (1972). Raising funds from foundations. *Nursing Outlook, 20,*(2), 108-110.

Fuller, E. (1982). The pink sheet syndrome. *Nursing Research, 31*, 185-186.

Geitgey, D., & Metz, E. (1969). A brief guide to designing research proposals. *Nursing Research, 18*, 339-344.

Gortner, S. (1971). Research grant applications: What they are not and should be. *Nursing Research, 20*, 292-295.

Hall, M. (1971). *Developing skills in proposal writing.* Portland, OR: DLE Media Publications.

Henley, C. (1977). Peer review of research grant applications at the National Institutes of Health. *Federation Proceedings, 36*(8), 2066-2068; *36*(9), 2186-2190; and *36*(10), 2335-2338.

Heywood, A. (1982). *The Resource Directory for Funding and Managing Nonprofit Organizations.* New York: Exxon Education Foundation.

Horgen, G. (1981). *Playing the funding game: Where it is, how to get it, keep it, increase it, and manage it.* Sacramento, CA: Human Services Development Center.

Kaiser, L. (1973). Grantsmanship in continuing education. *Journal of Nursing Education, 12*(1), 12-20.

Komnenich, P. (1981). Creating an environment for successful grant applications. In *Creating research environments in the 1980's.* Madison, WI: Midwest Nursing Research Conference Proceedings.

Krathwohl, D. (1977). *How to prepare a research proposal* (2nd ed.). Syracuse, NY: Syracuse University Book Store.

Lewis, M. (1975). *The Foundation Directory* (5th ed.). New York: Foundation Center.

Notter, L. (1973). Improving our skills in developing research protocols. *Nursing Research, 22*, 291.

Phillips, T. (1975). What is the difference between a research grant and a research contract? *Nursing Research, 24*, 388-389.

Rockefeller, J. (1973). Philanthropy and research today. In *Issues in research: Social, professional, and methodological* (pp. 50-55). Kansas City, MO: American Nurses' Association Council of Nurse Researchers.

Sexton, D. (1982). Developing skills in grant writing. *Nursing Outlook, 30*, 31-38.

Sleeper, J. (1985). The foundations. *Change, 1*, 12-26, 52-53.

Stevenson, J. (1979). Support for an emerging social institution. In F. Downs and J. Fleming (Eds.), *Issues in nursing research* (pp. 39-66). New York: Appleton-Century-Crofts.

White, V. (1975). *Grants: How to find out about them and what to do next.* New York: Plenum Press.

NEW DIRECTIONS FOR NURSING RESEARCH

MARY DUFFY AND BARBARA A. HEDIN

The issues of feminism and science, and feminism and research are not new. They arose in the social and biological sciences. Women scientists, products of educational and scientific communities steeped in the traditions of the scientific method, began to question the validity in the use of the traditional scientific methods for the study of women's concerns and science in general. In the 1930s, McClintock, a female genetic researcher, found the methods of traditional science insufficient in her attempts to explain the genetic transformation she observed. The current discussion of a feminist perspective in nursing is a product of the contemporary women's movement. At the center of the controversy is the traditional scientific method and its use of the causal model and maintenance of the status quo as opposed to the use of an approach that questions the structures and institutions of society and the roles it prescribes.

That feminist and nursing issues should come together would seem to be natural; yet an uneasy alliance has existed between the two. It was only in 1983 with the appearance of Kathleen MacPherson's article applying the feminist paradigm to nursing research that the advent of a new age in nursing research was foreshadowed. Nursing, because of its predominantly female makeup and its impact on clients' lives, has tremendous potential to effect a transformation in women's consciousness and the quality of women's lives. This supposition holds true for women as both givers and recipients of health care.

This chapter explores the interface between issues of feminism and science within nursing and offers guidelines for designing a research study from a feminist perspective.

Feminism is a perspective that describes a balanced vision of the world. This vision of a balanced world transcends behavior stereotyped as "masculine" and acceptable male behavior and "feminine" and expected and acceptable female behavior. The result is a world beyond dualism, where people are valued as individuals and encouraged to be fully human and develop characteristics that are both "feminine" and "masculine."

Feminists believe that positivist-empiricist paradigms have failed to question the structures and institutions of society that oppress women. Instead, these methodologies focus on the characteristics that facilitate the individual's adaptation to the norms of society and study existing structures and their maintenance. A feminist paradigm is founded on the belief that shortcomings exist in research methods that presume to be value free and that establish relationships between researchers and research participants based on objectivity and a hierarchical structure.

CHARACTERISTICS OF FEMINIST RESEARCH

The feminist perspective begins with a feminist consciousness. This feminist consciousness sensitizes the researcher to the vital concerns of women. Women are to be included in research as people; their concerns are more than reproductive or maternal-role issues. According to Roberts (1981), feminist research is concerned with all phases of the research process, including the language used, the sexual division of labor on the research team, and the use of the findings.

A feminist consciousness guides the researcher to investigate institutional discrimination against women. Misogyny in the health-care delivery system is one such example (Lovell, 1981; Thompson & Thompson, 1980). Normative behavior that encourages women to become economically dependent on men is another form of institutionalized sexism. A third example is the research tradition of studying gender differences rather than gender similarities.

An attitude of equality is at the root of feminist consciousness; all human beings are regarded of equal worth and treated in a manner consistent with "horizontal" rather than hierarchical relations. A feminist consciousness sensitizes the investigator to the importance of the contribution of each member of the research team and each participant in the study. The concern is to treat all participants as people and not data sources.

Feminist consciousness is more than the appearance of equality; its intent is to be fair and nondiscriminating in the treatment of all research participants. Such an intent is difficult to evaluate because it is a subjective perception of the researcher.

Feminist research has developed on two levels. The aim of the first level is to include women in research. However, not all research on women is feminist. For example, research questions that reinforce stereotypical roles for women are not feminist, although they are studies of women. An example is the study of the effects of maternal employment on child development. This research question suggests maternal employment is an option for women. The answer to this question will inform women of either the beneficial or the harmful effects of maternal employment on child development. The parallel question—What are the effects of paternal employment on child development?—is not asked, however, because of the bias that assumes fathers do not have the employment/unemployment option.

The second aim of feminist research is political and controversial: to attain the political goals of the women's movement by limiting feminist research to the study of phenomena that are of practical concern to women—day-care, family roles, occupational segregation in the workplace, and so forth. This research then applies a feminist analysis and perspective to the role and status of women in society (DuBois, Kelly, Kennedy, Korsmeyer, and Robinson, 1985; Ehrlich, 1976).

One must realize that a particular methodology is not *inherently* feminist or not feminist; rather, the means by which it is employed determines its nature. A participant-observation methodology could be mechanistically applied in a women's study in a manner antithetical to feminist principles. Thus it is not merely the application of a particular methodology that connotes feminist research, but rather the use of methodology in accordance with certain theoretical and philosophical underpinnings. Because of the interactive, inclusive, and contextual nature of feminism, limiting research to one or several specific methodologies would be wrong. Instead, in keeping with feminist principles, research demands a high degree of self-awareness and reflexivity in the course of the process as one meshes various methodologies, selected because of their congruency with research aims, with a feminist mode of researching.

Another important characteristic of feminist research is its "conscious partiality." This means that the biases already present in the researcher are acknowledged, brought into the open, and dealt with. Acknowledging these biases allows the researcher to question them and explore their validity and effect on the current study. A feminist paradigm opens people to new perspectives and to previously ignored experiences and introduces gender as a category of analysis.

We now apply these characteristics of feminist research to the design of a research study, basing the guidelines on our synthesis of feminism and the research process.

CONCEPTUALIZATION OF THE FEMINIST RESEARCH PROCESS: RESEARCHING

To begin with, one needs to consider the conceptualization of the research process itself and the end toward which it strives. Some presuppositions related to both these points influence the entire process and design of the study. The researcher asks: What is the intent of the research? Is it to discover knowledge, with the "end" being most important? Or is the belief, described in this chapter thus far, that the means—the process of the research—and the end are equally important? If the latter is the case, a more dynamic conceptualization of the research process than that traditionally described is needed.

This research process can be called "researching" and is consistent with the terms and process outlined by Rowan (1981). Rowan discusses a dialectical paradigm for research, broadly conceptualized in six steps: being, thinking, designing, encountering, making sense, and communicating. Each step is seen as a dialectical encounter with the world, that is, as engagement in reality with an awareness of and an active search for the contradictory and opposing forces operating in situations.

"Being" occurs as one recognizes that one's existing practice, such as nursing practice, seems inadequate. Dissatisfaction results, and one turns away from previously accepted ideas.

"Thinking" ensues, a creative process of invention and testing. The researcher gathers information from various sources and through varied means, processing, breaking down, and recombining material in unfamiliar relationships. Although more thinking and more information are always needed, one also must move to action.

"Designing" involves an outward movement: forming an intention and developing a thought that contradicts a current idea, then forming a concrete plan of action, a study. During this stage the tension exists between the development of adequate plans and the need for more.

"Encountering" involves both inward and outward movements. It demands confronting the previous thought; it involves action and engagement; and one's thinking is confirmed or disproved. The tension exists between the need to continue to persevere versus possible overstimulation from too much activity.

This uncertainty is followed by the "making sense" phase, in which one analyzes and contemplates the data. Although the researcher attempts to reduce and simplify the data, he or she wants additional connections to make the data more understandable until they say everything.

The analysis is not enough, however; a need arises for "communicating," an outward movement to share what has transpired. This process is wrought with the tension of finding it impossible to communicate *fully* what has gone on to anyone who has not participated in the process.

Researching, as conceptualized in this manner, is both process and outcome. Both the process and the end contribute to knowledge development. The dynamic of the research itself, not just written facts drawn at the conclusion of the study, results in knowledge. The research incorporates the knowledge gained through the process. This is praxis, or action guided by theory. Knowledge is viewed not merely as inert material to be pondered intellectually, but as a living dynamic to be experienced. The artificial division between the research process and the research findings is broken, and the knowledge gained through the research process becomes part of the research results.

This conceptualization of the research process is not meant to mystify research through the use of new terminology. The wording may lead some to think that we are saying no correlation or commensurability exists between this and the positivist-empiricist method. This is not true: being and thinking can be related to the traditional description of "defining the problem area"; designing to "explaining the methodology"; encountering to "implementing"; and making sense and communicating to "analyzing and presenting the results." The change is not so drastic that it severs all previous ties with tradition. The purpose of the change in terminology is to expand one's thinking about researching. The purpose is to break molds and encourage fresh ideas about the process and its outcome, thus creating and infusing a new consciousness. In Rowan's schema the terminology suggests an ongoing, circular process, from "being" through "communicating." This open-endedness is consistent with feminism. The research process is continuously dynamic and affects the outcomes of the study.

APPLICATION TO SPECIFIC STUDIES

This section discusses the various phases of researching just listed and relates feminist principles to them. We offer questions the researcher can reflect upon during each phase of designing a study from a feminist perspective. We also give examples of how we attempted to incorporate feminist principles in our own research. Where appropriate, we critique our research activities. We begin by presenting a brief synopsis of a study we each conducted. As we discuss the various stages of researching and refer to these studies, the reader will gain a basic understanding of their nature and content.

Hedin's research (1985, 1986) culminated in an analysis of the social, political, and economic factors that affect the nursing education system in the Federal Republic of Germany. The analysis examined a specific situation: the implementation of a university-based, experimental program for nursing instructors at the Free University of Berlin from October 1976 through June 1982.

The investigator interviewed faculty members of the experimental program, read reports of the project, and reviewed the literature to gain insight into the factors leading to the conceptualization of the program and its noncontinuance. She employed a naturalistic-inductive method of inquiry and analysis, seeking what the events meant to the participants and revealing contradictions in the situation. This method purposefully searches for contradictions in understanding and explanation to force an analysis of the structural factors that impinge on a situation and influence its meaning for an individual.

The data analysis revealed that on one level political and economic reasons existed for the program not being established as a permanent course of study at the Free University. On a deeper level, however, preventing its entrance into the realm of university education was an oppressive act toward the nursing discipline.

Habermas' critical social theory (1971) and Freire's model of oppressed group behavior and a pedagogy of the oppressed (1970, 1973) were used to provide the theoretical underpinnings for dealing with this situation of oppression to determine ways to transcend it.

Duffy's research (1984, 1986) was a grounded-theory study of the practice of primary prevention behaviors (health enhancement, disease prevention) in one-parent families headed by women. These behaviors include immunizations, stress reduction, nutrition practices, exercise, and so forth. She collected data at both the personal and the system level, since a review of the literature (Duffy, 1982) demonstrated the system barriers against women as household heads. The women were interviewed and then completed a health diary and card sort of health behaviors. The purpose of this phase was to understand how the women perceived their situations as

heads of one-parent families and to determine their practices of primary prevention behaviors. The second phase of data collection showed how society perceived women heads of one-parent families. Duffy conducted interviews with professionals who provided social services to one-parent families and informally analyzed the media for its portrayal of one-parent families headed by women.

Following content analysis, the "theory of transcending options" emerged. This theory describes the women's perceptions of the world and integrates the specific societal barriers they face, the interrelationships between the experiences of women as heads of households, and their practices of primary prevention behaviors.

Being

In the being phase of researching, one recognizes that existing practice is inadequate, which leads to dissatisfaction and a rejection of previous ideas. One experiences dissonance, which results from being in and experiencing the real world as it is and realizing that things could be different. Feminist research has its roots in the real world of its participants; it emerges from the lived experience of women. Lived experience gives the direction for selecting a research focus. These experiences can be personal, an outcome of nursing (professional) practice, or a result of interaction with other women and women's groups. The discrepancy between what is and what could be is realized by being in touch with oneself and feeling the seeds of discontent and the vibrations of disharmony that exist. "Gut-level" feelings and gestalt-type reactions allow one to perceive reality and simultaneously realize that things can be better or different. "Being" involves not only the left-brain, rational analysis of situations for discrepancies, but also the right-brain, personal and aesthetic ways of knowing.

Hedin's research stemmed from her feeling of uneasiness or disquietude when reading accounts of American nursing history in which nursing advances have been lauded as the result of nurses' hard work to achieve goals. The histories, however, seemed to give only a fragmented view; that is, they only discussed nursing history as related to nursing with little connection to the health-care system, much less to society or economic and political trends as a whole. In other words, nursing's achievements were described in a vacuum. Hedin believed that if she could view a broader picture, she could achieve a different perspective on reality that could be important to a deeper understanding of the context and allow for more effective functioning within that reality. This view led her to develop a study that dealt with the effects of the social, political, and economic context on nursing education. The intent of the study was consistent with feminism in its attempt to uncover systematic injustices against women and to conceive of ways to transform or transcend these injustices.

Duffy's research resulted from her practicing as a community health nurse, teaching community health nursing, and experiencing life as a woman. She often observed frustration in the nurse-client relationship when the client was a woman head of a one-parent family, especially if the woman received a low income. This tension occurred because of the discrepancies between what the nurse—a representative of white, middle-class society—expected from the client and what the client actually did. Duffy thought that the barriers women heads of one-parent families face may affect their ability or willingness to accept conventional health teaching regardless of their desire to do so. The intent of this study was feminist because the concerns of a group of women were its focus. These concerns—economic, political, cultural, and so forth—are central to the agenda of the women's movement. This group of women, heads of one-parent families, experiences societal discrimination against women. The purpose of this study was to identify the societal barriers that discriminate against women as heads of one-parent families and ultimately to influence the practice of primary prevention behaviors in those families.

When working in the being phase, the researcher can ask several questions that help to identify the discrepancies between what is and what can be. These include*:

1. Based on an analysis of the situation using all types of knowledge—empirical, personal, aesthetic, and so forth—what do I think is the problem needing analysis, and what do I believe is happening?
2. What contextual factors are affecting the problem?

---

*The authors acknowledge the contributions of Karabenies, Miller, Nagel-Bamesberger, Rossiter, & Thompson (1986) and Rowan (1981) in the development of these and subsequent questions in this section.

3. What societal/system factors are affecting this group of women?
4. How do I think the problem could be reconceptualized so that individual women would not be blamed or victimized for not conforming to society?
5. To whom are the problem's solution relevant?
6. What is my interest in investigating this issue?
7. Does the issue direct attention to issues of sex and gender?

Thinking

Thinking is the creative process of invention and testing and involves gathering information from many and varied sources. It is an attempt to discover if an identified problem is also a difficulty for others. It involves contact: a connection to the past (i.e., what has already been done in this area) and a connection with the present. Through reading, talking, interviews, and any other available means, the researcher collects information and assembles it in different ways. Thinking involves a dialogical encounter with people. Instead of the researcher stating, "I have an idea" (the "truth"), the researcher says, "Here is an idea, what is your reaction to it? Where can we go with it?" This latter question invites people from other situations to discuss the proposed research need or problem. The researcher seeks input from many different sources and combines and recombines the input into new ideas. The dialectic that exists in this phase is the pull between needing to take in more and more information and the need to move on, declaring that enough has been gathered. The researcher conceptualizes issues from more than one perspective and may study them from dual perspectives.

The feminist researcher requires that women, especially women who represent the population to be studied, be involved in the thinking, dialoguing, and reacting that occurs. Their involvement is the only reasonable assurance that the problem or need addressed is a concern to women. Thinking is far more than a literature review or a professional analysis of the problem.

In Hedin's study in West Germany (1985), the need to collect as much information about the context as possible seemed an almost impossible task. She felt she could never know enough about a culture *in which she did not grow up*. She had much to learn and combine through reading, interviewing, and experiencing. She attempted to determine the focus of the study in a dialogical manner. Although Hedin had anticipated studying the effect of the context on the nursing education system, she left open how this would be done. She decided on the "window" to use, that is, an incident in West German nursing history that would provide the substance for analysis after collaboration with West German nurses, so that she was not an outside researcher entirely dependent on her own interests deciding on the topic for a study in another culture. Rather, she attempted to select an area West German nurses perceived as relevant.

Questions that facilitate the thinking phase of researching affect not only the current state of knowledge but the perceptions of the population to be studied. The researcher can ask herself or himself the following questions during this phase:

1. What are the chief concerns of the population that I am interested in working with?
2. How do they (the research participants) prioritize their research needs?
3. Does the literature reflect the experiences of the population?
4. How do women conceptualize the problem or need?
5. What are the various ways of stating the problem for this issue?
6. What is the history of the development of the conceptual framework?
7. Is the conceptual framework applicable to women, or does it reflect the male experience?
8. Is the historical significance of the problem under study fully developed, including its current status?

Designing

Designing is the phase of researching in which an intention to study a problem is concretized into a study plan. Tension exists between having adequate plans versus the need for more planning. The actual design of a study in feminist research takes into account women in the sampling, nonhierarchical relations, and the experience of day-to-day real life as its starting point. Planning is carried out within the research team through dialogue as much as possible, and when appropriate, with participants or other

women or women's groups as consultants. Shared decision making is the modus operandi.

Although the feminist researcher takes responsibility for the design of the study, it is not finalized until consultation with the participants has occurred and their recommendations have been integrated into the design. For example, the participants are asked to describe the best way to study the phenomena: what method, questions, and techniques should be used to understand the problem area from the perspective of the women? One technique is to ask the participants what they would ask if they were trying to understand the phenomena.

The pilot study is one mechanism for soliciting participation from the subjects regarding the study design. Duffy's research began with a pilot study in which 17 women were first interviewed and then asked to comment on the design. She used their input to redesign the study; for example, they suggested adding the health diary. Several women were uncomfortable because they could not remember all their health practices during the interview. The diary gave them a chance to write down other behaviors they had not mentioned during the interview. Two women participating in a self-help group for single parents also suggested Duffy observe those meetings. They thought she would get a better understanding of their problems if she listened to the group discuss the stressors they faced daily.

Client-action groups (Damrosch & Lenz, 1984) would have enhanced Duffy's study, since a group of women would have provided input throughout the study from its inception to the data analysis. The group interaction would produce more fruitful input than the individual discussions between the researcher and each woman. These women would be consultants to the researcher throughout the study. The need for input from the research-team members is equally critical. A single investigator conducted this study, but a current study by Duffy involves research assistants and a secretary. The team meets regularly, and each member is encouraged to critique the study design and explore alternative ways of effectively alleviating the problems in either current or future studies. The comments from the participants regarding questionnaires, the interview, and so forth are often the substance of the critique.

The purposes of the design questions are to include all persons involved in the research team and representatives of the study population in the development of a method that best studies the problem or need. Questions the researcher can ask during the designing phase include:

1. Are the opinions of each member of the research team solicited?
2. Is discussion of research issues encouraged, or do I defend the "expert" position?
3. How can I encourage representatives of the study population to participate in all phases of the research?
4. Does the design of the study treat the participants as equals, or are they treated as objects used to collect data?
5. Does the design of the study investigate the societal- and system-level factors that affect the women?
6. Are the instruments used appropriate for the study of women?
7. Does the design allow for serendipitous findings, that is, the pursuit of intuitive clues?
8. Are my biases built into the study in any way?
9. Is the effect of context taken into account and allowed to express itself?
10. Are limitations imposed on who could be seen or on the types of questions asked? Do pressures to pursue a particular line of research exist?

Encountering

Encountering is the phase in which action and engagement occur. Tension exists between persevering and engaging in too much activity. It is an outward movement followed by and balanced by the need to pull back.

Encountering involves entering into the process of research and at the same time reflecting on it. For example, the researcher, aware of the influence of biases throughout the research process, asks: How are my biases influencing what is occurring? This reflection is essential because biases are affecting the research process, and the researcher must become aware of those biases and make them known. Reflection occurs throughout this stage, ideally through process work with others involved in the research but perhaps through dialogue with someone outside the research. An outside person who is willing to listen can review data and the research process to raise the level of the researcher's awareness.

In feminist research, dialogue with other women is used as a means to ensure that the researcher maintains a feminist consciousness. This includes not reverting to previously learned, traditional, hierarchical modes of thinking and relating to people. It also means being aware of one's values and how they are influencing the research process. For example, if interviews are being used, is a bias coming through? Sometimes someone external to the research can better identify this than the researcher.

Grounded theory guided Duffy (1982, 1986) to reflect on the data throughout the research process. For example, questions were added to the interview when a woman raised an issue not discussed previously. A second interview was added to the study design when several paths of inquiry emerged during the data analysis and each woman needed to be recontacted. However, one bias influenced this entire study. Duffy determined from the onset that differences exist in the experiences of women and men as heads of one-parent families. Purposefully she chose to study women only and sought to elicit the societal discrimination against these women. Aware of this bias, Duffy needed consultation throughout the study to differentiate between the societal discrimination that contributed to the common problems experienced by many of the women and the problems attributable to individual differences. For example, both inadequate income and job preparation were common problems. Within the group of women with low incomes and poor job skills, however, some of the women pursued changes in their lifestyles, whereas others were immobilized. These differences were individual.

The encountering phase demands reflection. Throughout this phase the researcher asks questions to reflect on the implementation of the study and the effects of her or his biases on that process. In experiencing or conducting this phase of the study, the researcher can ask:

1. Does the way I am carrying out the study make sense?
2. Am I open to my own feelings and reactions during the research process?
3. Am I communicating in a dialogical, nonhierarchical manner?
4. Am I breaking down control patterns?
5. Am I respecting the rights and dignity of colleagues and those participating in the study?

6. Am I doing any good? Any harm?
7. Am I expressing myself in an honest, authentic manner?
8. Am I following the experience where it naturally leads, but not to the detriment of study controls?
9. How are my values influencing the process?

Making Sense

In the making sense phase the researcher analyzes and reflects on the data. She attempts to reduce and simplify the data, but she still wants to add more and more connections to make them understandable. In reflecting on the data, the researcher tries to move beyond the presuppositions and assumptions unconsciously accepted by society to deeper levels of understanding and analysis. Habermas' conceptualization (1971) of emancipatory knowledge and its ability to lead to freedom from constraints requires cutting through the opaqueness that blinds persons and makes them accept existing structures and relations as "the only way" instead of "one way." In the case of feminist research, this necessitates identifying those structures and situations that perpetuate discriminatory behavior toward women and developing ways to eliminate this systematic discrimination.

Taking early analyses and interpretations of the data back to the participants for confirmation or disconfirmation is one means of making sense out of the data. The participants help the researcher to understand the meaning of the data and to determine directions for continual data analysis. The researcher may also ask consultants to react to interpretations of the data.

Those working within a feminist perspective realize they are not alone in what they are doing; they know that they need the input of other women to make sense of the world around them. They also know that more and better ideas come from working together, not from pursuing isolated efforts. Power and knowledge emerge from shared experiences and connectedness.

Hedin (1985, 1986), after analyzing and reflecting on the data in her study for the contradictions and opposing forces at work throughout all phases of the experimental program, shared these initial interpretations with study participants for their reactions and further clarification. She also shared early write-ups of the data presentation with participants for their reactions.

The researcher asks questions that open up the avenues of explanation. Conventional interpretations of the data are challenged by questioning those interpretations and looking for other avenues of explanation. The more people exposed to the data and the findings, the more likely the researcher is to elicit multiple explanations. In conducting this making sense phase, the researcher can ask the following:

1. What are the participants' responses to the data?
2. Does my interpretation of the data make sense to the participants?
3. What alternative explanations exist for the data?
4. Are the findings politically useful for women?
5. Are the data compared to theories and standards that were developed for women and not the norms based on the experiences of men?
6. Does the analysis make biased assumptions—sexist, racist, or ageist?
7. Is the analysis liberating? Does it encourage others to raise questions?

Communicating

Communicating is an outward movement, the need to share what has occurred. Tension exists in that the researcher can never *fully* communicate what went on to those who did not participate in the research. Feminist research is characterized by the obligation to share results with those who supplied the data and who were the focus of the study. At the very least, this means that participants should receive some type of written summary. Communicating may also include other ways of sharing, such as presentations to women's groups or publication of the findings in lay magazines or newsletters. The intent of feminist research is that it is done *with* and *for* women and not *to or on* them as objects. Thus it is essential that the findings be fed back to women so that, as the intent of feminist research indicates, the knowledge gained can be translated into improved quality of life for women, not merely used to fulfill a publication requirement for the academic community. Women with knowledge can make informed choices and can take action to eliminate the oppression experienced in their lives.

Hedin's study (1985) was conducted in West Germany, and although certain aspects have been publicized in the United States and copies of the research (dissertation) shared with West German nurses and made available for their perusal, Hedin felt obligated to make the results known to nurses in that country in their own language for their critique.

Duffy regularly offers to share the results of her work with women through women's groups. In addition, she sends each participant a summary of the study's results and asks them to comment on the findings. She uses a newsletter to share the study's results with women who are single parents.

The researcher must reach the professional and general audiences. Although the same material is communicated, the language and format differ according to the audience. It is important to learn which forms of media best reach each of these audiences.

When engaged in the communicating phase of feminist research, the researcher can ask the following:

1. How can I reach the audience who represented the population of women participating in the study?
2. What language do I use to communicate the results?
3. For whom am I writing—women in general, or only the academic community?

The feminist researcher is in continuous dialogue with himself or herself and others as the synthesis of feminism and research is pursued. Researchers contribute to the evolution of feminist research as they apply the principles of feminism to the research process.

SUMMARY

This chapter has discussed feminism, the relationship between feminism and nursing, and the need for a feminist perspective in nursing research. The union of feminism and nursing science has two aims: (1) increase the volume of research on women and the visibility of feminist researchers and (2) recognize, through research, the influence of societal discrimination on the concerns of women, then remedy those injustices. No one method for research is proposed. Instead, the researcher is encouraged to apply the characteristics of feminist research to the method of the study. These characteristics guide the researcher

to develop a feminist approach to science. Reflection is essential throughout the research process if the researcher is to make the transition from the tenets of traditional research to the process-oriented, emerging approach of feminism.

Although still formative, most agree that feminist research is based on horizontal relationships and shared decision making among those involved in the research; that is, it calls for a reconceptualization of science and its methods without the language and metaphors of control and domination (Bleier, 1986; Oakley, 1981). Feminist research demands a "conscious partiality" that does not presume a value-free stance and advocates active participation in actions, movements, and struggles for women's emancipation. Feminism thus makes two major contributions to science. First, women are included in studies as people and not only as maternal or reproductive beings. Second, feminist science incorporates subjective as well as empirical knowledge. Because most nurses and many of their clients are women, the issues of the relationship between feminism and science are especially relevant to nursing. Both feminism and nursing can benefit as each draws on the strengths of the other to set new directions and create a new, more balanced, more just, future.

REFERENCES

Bleier, R. (1986). *Feminist approaches to science*. Elmsford, NY: Pergamon.

Damrosch, S. P., & Lenz, E. (1984). The use of client-advisory groups in research. *Nursing Research, 33*(1), 47-49.

Dubois, E. C., Kelly, G. P., Kennedy, E. L., Korsmeyer, C. W., & Robinson, L. S. (1985). *Feminist scholarship: Kindling in the groves of academe*. Chicago: University of Illinois Press.

Duffy, M. E. (1982). When a woman heads a household. *Nursing Outlook, 30*(8), 468-473.

Duffy, M. E. (1984). Transcending options: Creating a milieu for practicing high level wellness. *Health Care for Women International, 5*, 145-161.

Duffy, M. E. (1986). Primary prevention behaviors: The female headed, one-parent family. *Research in Nursing and Health*.

Ehrlich, C. (1976). *The conditions of feminist research*. Report No. 1. Baltimore: Research Group One.

Freire, P. (1970). *Pedagogy of the oppressed* (M. Bergman Ramos, Trans.). New York: Continuum Press.

Freire, P. (1973). *Education for critical consciousness*. New York: Continuum Press.

Habermas, J. (1971). *Knowledge and human interests.* (J. J. Shapiro, Trans.). Boston: Beacon Press. (Original work published 1968.)

Hedin, B. A. (1985). Nursing education, constraints, and critical consciousness: The birth and death of a *Modellversuch* in West Germany. Unpublished doctoral dissertation, University of Utah, Salt Lake City.

Hedin, B. A. (1986, January). *Nursing education as freeing.* Paper presented at the Fourth Annual Research in Nursing Education Conference, San Francisco. Nursing education and emancipation: Applying the critical theoretical approach to nursing research. In P. Chinn (Ed.), Nursing research methodology: Issues and implementation pp. 133-146 Rockville, MD: Aspen.

Jayaratne, T. E. (1983). The value of quantitative methodology for feminist research. In G. Bowles & R. D. Klein (Eds.), *Theories of women's studies* (pp. 140-161). Boston: Routledge & Kegan Paul.

Karabenies, A., Miller, L., Nagel-Bamesberger, H., Rossiter, A., & Thompson, M. (1986). What makes a feminist social science? *Cassandra: Radical Feminist Nurses Newsjournal, 4*(1), 9-11.

Klein, R. D. (1983). How to do what we want to do: Thoughts about feminist methodology. In G. Bowles & R. D. Klein (Eds.), *Theories of women's studies* (pp. 88-104). Boston: Routledge & Kegan Paul.

Lovell, M. C. (1981). Silent but perfect "partners": Medicine's use and abuse of women. *Advances in Nursing Science, 3,* 25-40.

MacPherson, K.I. (1983). Feminist methods: A new paradigm for nursing research. *Advances in Nursing Research, 5,* 17-25.

Oakley, A. (1981). Interviewing women: A contradiction in terms. In H. Roberts (Ed.), *Doing feminist research* (pp. 30-61). Boston: Routledge & Kegan Paul.

Roberts, H. (1981). *Doing feminist research.* Boston: Routledge & Kegan Paul.

Rowan, J. (1981). A dialectical paradigm for research. In P. Reason & J. Rowan (Eds.), *Human Inquiry.* New York: Wiley.

Thompson, J. E., & Thompson, H. O. (1980). The ethics of being a female patient and a female care provider in a male-dominated health-illness system. *Issues in Health Care of Women, 2,* 25-54.

Tinkel, M. B., & Beaton, J. L. (1983). Toward a new view of science: Implications for nursing research. *Advances in Nursing Science, 5*(2), 27-36.

SOFTWARE

There are many ways to use a microcomputer (personal computer, PC) in nursing research. Word processing is the most obvious application—the researcher uses a microcomputer to type the text of a research proposal or final report of research. A microcomputer can be used to manage reference citations as the investigator reviews the literature throughout a research project. Finally, a microcomputer can be used to manage and analyze text and numerical data. Microcomputer hardware and software technology changes rapidly. New and better applications are available daily. In the table that follows there is a sampling of microcomputer software for the IBM-PC and closely compatible microcomputers. Our selection of IBM compatible software is consistent with the industry emphasis on MS-DOS and PC-DOS microcomputers. The software listed here represents a small portion of what is currently available and provides an overview of the software that is available. Many other programs are available

that space does not permit listing. We have selected programs that are widely used by nurse researchers, that are easily learned and used, and that have adequate documentation and technical support. The researcher interested in acquiring microcomputer software for his or her personal use is urged to read reviews of the current releases of software in microcomputer periodicals, such as *InfoWorld, PC Tech Journal, PC Magazine, MacUser,* and *Byte*. Other sources of current information about software may be found in *Addison-Wesley Book of IBM Software, Consumer Guide Computer Buying Guide, PC Buyers Guide,* and *ICP Software Directory*. Talking with researchers who use a particular program can provide valuable insight into the program's idiosyncrasies. The table on pp. 542-545 does not include word processing software. It does include a sampling of programs useful for managing bibliographic citations, text and numerical data, and statistical analysis.

PROGRAM NAME AND SOURCE	SYSTEM REQUIREMENTS	COST	COMMENTS
Bibliography management			
BIBLIOGRAPHY *Digital Marketing*	64KB	$125.00	Compares citations in manuscript with entries in master bibliography and constructs a bibliography of all entries in the manuscript; flexible and powerful program; no limit on length of reference titles, etc., in master bibliography; can include abstract or other notes; will alphabetize a master bibliography; arranges manuscript bibliography in alphabetical order or order of citation; will replace citations with number in manuscript; also available for CP/M systems.
Data management			
ASKSAM *Seaside Software*	128KB	$150.00	Text oriented database management system; uses variable-length fields and performs arithmetic; updates records with text editor; batch operation; imports and exports ASCII files; user defined templates and overlays
dBASE III+ *Ashton-Tate*	640KB	$695.00	Creates, uses, and modifies multiple databases; uses pull-down menus; has query system, application generator, data catalog, code encryption and linking, debugging, and assembly language calls
ETHNOGRAPH *Quallis Research Associates*		$150.00	Allows coding, recoding, and sorting of text data files into analytic categories; text can be reviewed, marked, displayed, sorted, and printed in any order; data do not need to be rectangulated for analysis and can be entered in any configuration, e.g., narrative, lists; any segment of data can be assigned up to 12 distinct code words; a segment can contain any number of lines and segments can overlap or be "nested" up to seven levels; carries a "contextual comment" to each sorted segment that identifies the larger context of the sorted segment
R:BASE *Microrim*	64-256KB	$700.00	Relational databases; updates, sorts, and qualifies data from multiple files; selectively retrieves rows of data, calculates column totals; accepts data from Lotus 1-2-3, PFS:File, dBASE II and DIF, SYLK and ASCII

PROGRAM NAME AND SOURCE	SYSTEM REQUIREMENTS	COST	FUNCTIONS	COMMENTS
Statistical				
ABSTAT *Anderson-Bell Corp*	196KB Two disk drives	$395.00	Descriptive Regression Correlations ANOVA *t* tests Crosstabs Nonparametric	Reads and writes dBase, Lotus, ASCII
A-STAT *Rosen Grandon Associates, Inc.*	48KB	$175.00-$200.00	Descriptive Regression Correlation ANOVA *t* test Crosstabs Factor analysis	Includes data base management systems; includes data transformation language and report writer with break and sum fields; available for IBM-PC jr
BIOSTATISTICS 3PC *A2Devices*	128KB	$125.00	Descriptive Regression ANOVA, MANOVA *t* tests Nonparametic	Available for IBM-PC jr
BMDP/PC *BMDP Statistical Software, Inc.*	650KB Math coprocessor 10 MB hard drive	$450.00-1500.00	Descriptive Regression Correlation ANOVA, MANOVA Time series Cluster Nonparametric	Supports missing data; 40 programs available in packages; minimally interactive; error handling clumsy and limited; reads only ASCII files
CRISP *Crunch Software Corp.*	256KB	$495.00	Descriptive Regression Correlation ANOVA *t* tests Crosstabs	Reads ASCII, DIF, dBASE II, III, Rbase 5000; sorts, merges, concatenates, copies, lists; batch processor and keystroke macros; easy to use menu interface
[Multiple programs] *Dynacomp, Inc.*	16-128KB	$20.00-100.00 each	Descriptive Regression ANOVA, MANOVA *t* tests Time series Nonparametric	22 separate packaged allows purchase of only those required; nonparametric statistics keyed to Seigal

Continued.

PROGRAM NAME AND SOURCE	SYSTEM REQUIREMENTS	COST	FUNCTIONS	COMMENTS
Statistical				
NUMBER CRUNCHER STATISTICAL SYSTEMS *NCSS*	256KB Two disk drives	$79.00-199.00	Regression ANOVA/ANCOVA *t* tests Factor analysis Time series Discriminate	Spreadsheet-like data entry; imports from ASCII files
PC STATISTICIAN *Human Systems Dynamics*	256KB	$300.00	Descriptive Regression Correlation ANOVA Crosstabs Nonparametric	Accepts Lotus 1-2-3 and VisiCalc files; includes database management system
SAS *SAS Institute, Inc.*	512KB One floppy disk 10 MB hard disk	$1500 for 1 year license	Regression ANOVA Factor analysis Discriminant	Requires Base SAS Software for PC; interactive windowing; smooth micro-to-mainframe communication; complicated if not used to mainframe version
STATA *Computing Resources Center*	256KB	$195.00 $395.00	Descriptive Regression Correlation ANOVA, MANOVA Crosstabs Nonparametric	Answers what-if questions; creates, sorts, appends, and merges data sets; creates tables and plots; copies output in file for editing; interactive analysis graphics, multiple-imaging, overlaying of images, pie/bar charts
SPSS-PC+ *SPSS, Inc.*	384-448KB 10 MB hard disk	$295.00-495.00 each	Descriptive Regression Correlation ANOVA, MANOVA *t* test Crosstabs Cluster Factor analysis Discriminate	Multiple packages can be purchased separately; full-screen editor and report generator; color graphics and tables options available; allows titling, formatting, labeling; review allows edit of listing and com-

PROGRAM NAME AND SOURCE	SYSTEM REQUIREMENTS	COST	FUNCTIONS	COMMENTS
Statistical				
				mands on screen; imports word processing, Lotus 1-2-3, dBase files; interactive and batch mode
STATISTICIAN *Quant Systems*	128KB	$350.00	Descriptive Regression ANOVA Time series	Database search and sort
STATISTICS *Basic Business Software, Inc.*	8KB	$ 75.00	Descriptive Regression Correlation ANOVA, MANOVA t tests Nonparametric	Handles permutations plus combinations
STATPAC *Walonick Associates, Inc.*	192 KB	$495.00	Descriptive Regression Correlation ANOVA, MANOVA t test Crosstabs	Batch processing; fixed or free format ASCII files; printing options include graphics
STATPAK *Northwest Analytical, Inc.*	64-128KB Two disk drives	$395.00-495.00	Descriptive Regression Correlation ANOVA t tests Crosstabs Nonparametric	Graphics; interfaces with spreadsheets and databases; available for Macintosh
STAT-PAK *AD&P Analysis Design & Programming*	4KB		Descriptive Regression Correlations Crosstabs	Modeled after SPSS
STATPRO *Penton Software, Inc.*	256KB	$795.00	Descriptive Regression ANOVA, MANOVA Time series	Integrates statistical techniques with graphics and database management capabilities; multicolor graphics
SYSTAT *Systat, Inc.*	256KB	$595.00	Descriptive Regression ANOVA, MANOVA Crosstabs Time series Cluster Nonparametric	Includes graphics and data management system; available for Macintosh; interactive

RESEARCH INSTRUMENTS

One of the recurrent tasks facing researchers is the selection of instruments to measure the variables of interest. Thousands of paper-and-pencil instruments have been developed and many biomedical instruments are in use both for clinical and research measurement. The frustration associated with locating an instrument that will measure the desired variables and that is reliable and valid has led many people to compile compendia of instruments. In this table we have reviewed some of these compendia so that the researcher is aware of some places to begin the search. Those chosen for inclusion here are ones that were readily available in our libraries. There are many others and the researcher in search of an instrument is encouraged to look for these books and others.

It is evident from this table that each compilation is organized differently and includes different information. Some provide an overview of few instruments whereas others include a comprehensive review and critique of each instrument.

Tool development is an exacting and time-consuming process. It is hoped that researchers will utilize these and other resources to identify tools useful for their research rather than undertaking the task of developing something new.

AUTHOR/DATE	NUMBER OF ENTRIES	SOURCE OF INSTRU-MENTS*	VARIABLES LISTED	DESCRIPTION OF INSTRUMENT†	PSYCHO-METRIC PROPERTIES GIVEN	BIBLIOGRAPHY‡	COMMENTS
Andrulis 1977	155	Addresses	Yes	Purpose Length Type	Yes	None	Superficial coverage
Bauer 1982	NA	NA	Yes	Type Scoring Application Administration	No	Uses	Clinical laboratory procedures
Beere 1979	235	Address Reference	Yes	Development Length Type Sample Scoring Application Administration	Yes	Development Uses	
Buros 1978	1184 listed 638 reviewed	Addresses	Yes	Given for some Development Application Length Type	Yes	Development Uses	Critiques Achievement, Intelligence Supplements earlier volumes
Chun 1975	3,000	Reference	Yes	No	No	Development Uses	Cross indexed by variables and author
Comrey 1973	1,100	References Addresses	Yes	Purpose Length Type	None	No	Abstracts reprinted from literature; vary in content
Geddes 1984	NA	None	Yes	Development Uses	No	Development Uses	Easy to read Cardiovascular measurement

Continued.

*Source of instrument: entire tool reproduced, reference to tool given, or name and address of the source.
†Description of instrument: development (origins, rationale, purposes, procedures for development); length (number of items or time to administer); type (projective, questionnaire, checklist, scale, biomedical); sample items; scoring (how scored, range of scores); application (age group, special populations); administration (qualification/training required).
‡Bibliography: uses (bibliography lists studies that have used the instrument); development (bibliography lists material on which development of the instrument was based).

AUTHOR/ DATE	NUMBER OF ENTRIES	SOURCE OF INSTRUMENTS*	VARIABLES LISTED	DESCRIPTION OF INSTRUMENT†	PSYCHOMETRIC PROPERTIES GIVEN	BIBLIOGRAPHY‡	COMMENTS
Goldman 1974	339	References	No	Purpose Length Type	None	Uses	Superficial
Israel 1984	145	125 in Vol II 20 addresses or references	Yes	Purpose Length Type Scoring Application Administration	Reference	Development Uses	Attractive layout
Johnson 1971	322	References Addresses	Yes	Length Type Scoring	Yes Reference	Development Uses	Quality of descriptions varies
Johnson 1976	900	References Addresses	Yes	Development Length Type Sample items Scoring Application Administration	Yes	Development Uses	Birth to 18 years
Keyser 1984	422	Addresses	Yes	Development Length Type Scoring Application Administration Critique	Yes	Development	4 Volumes Keyed to Sweetland, 1983 Variability in reporting Child and adult measures
Lake 1973	84	Addresses	Yes	Development Length Type Scoring Application Critique	Critique	None	List and critique of other compendia

Lyerly 1973	61	Some included References Addresses	Yes	Development Length Type Sample items Scoring Application Administration	Yes	Development Uses	Children included
Miller 1977	58	Some included References	Yes	Purpose Application	Yes	Uses	
Mitchell 1983	2,672	Name only	Yes	Application	No	Development Application	Some entries include only title and one reference
Pfeiffer 1976		Addresses	Yes	Length Sample items	Some	Some	Reviews range from nothing to several pages
Reeder 1976	77	Some included References	Yes	Development Length Type Items Scoring Administration	Yes	Development	
Robinson 1973	127	Some included References	Yes	Development Length Application Critique	Yes	Development	
Shaw 1967	176	Included	Yes	Development Length Type Sample items Scoring Application Administration	Yes	Development Uses	All references at end of book and include instruments not reviewed

Continued.

*Source of instrument: entire tool reproduced, reference to tool given, or name and address of the source.

†Description of instrument: development (origins, rationale, purposes, procedures for development); length (number of items or time to administer); type (projective, questionnaire, checklist, scale, biomedical); sample items; scoring (how scored, range of scores); application (age group, special populations); administration (qualification/training required).

‡Bibliography: uses (bibliography lists studies that have used the instrument); development (bibliography lists material on which development of the instrument was based).

AUTHOR/ DATE	NUMBER OF ENTRIES	SOURCE OF INSTRU-MENTS*	VARIABLES LISTED	DESCRIPTION OF INSTRUMENT†	PSYCHO-METRIC PROPERTIES GIVEN	BIBLIOGRAPHY‡	COMMENTS
Straus 1978	8,131	References Addresses	Yes	Length Type Sample item	No	Development Uses	Type face hard to read
Sweetland 1983	3,000	Addresses	Yes	Purpose Length Type Administration	No	None	Extensive cross-references
Walker 1973	143	Addresses	Yes	Sample items Length Type Scoring Application Administration	Yes	Development	Ages 3 to 6 Brief, easy to read
Ward 1979	140	135 included Addresses References	Yes	Development Length Type Sample items Scoring Application Administration	Yes	Development Uses	Vol I: Psychosocial Includes description, critique, copy Vol II: Physiological
Weiss 1973	NA	NA	Yes	Development Type Application	No	Development Uses	General theory underlying biomedical instrumentation

*Source of instrument: entire tool reproduced, reference to tool given, or name and address of the source.

†Description of instrument: development (origins, rationale, purposes, procedures for development); length (number of items or time to administer); type (projective, questionnaire, checklist, scale, biomedical); sample items; scoring (how scored, range of scores); application (age group, special populations); administration (qualification/training required).

‡Bibliography: uses (bibliography lists studies that have used the instrument); development (bibliography lists material on which development of the instrument was based).

REFERENCES

Andrulis, R. S. (1977). *Adult assessment: A source book of tests and measures of human behavior*. Springfield, IL: Thomas.

Bauer, J. D. (1982). *Clinical laboratory methods* (9th ed.). St. Louis: Mosby.

Beere, C. A. (1979). *Women and women's issues: A handbook of tests and measurements*. San Francisco: Jossey-Bass.

Buros, O. K. (Ed.). (1978). *The eighth mental measurement yearbook*. Highland Park, N. J.: Gryphon Press.

Chun, K-T., Cobb, S., & French, Jr., J. R. P. (1975). *Measures for psychological assessment: A guide to 3,000 original sources and their applications*. Ann Arbor, MI: Institute for Social Research, University of Michigan.

Comrey, A. L., Backer, T. E., & Glaser, E. W. (1973). *A sourcebook for mental health measures*. Los Angeles: Human Interaction Research Institute.

Geddes, L. A. (1984). *Cardiovascular devices and their application*. New York: Wiley.

Goldman, B. A., & Saunders, J. L. (1974). *Directory of unpublished experimental mental measures*. New York: Behavioral Publications.

Israel, L., Kozarevic, D., & Sartoruis, N. (1984). *Source book of geriatric assessment*. Basel: S. Karger.

Johnson, O. G. (1976). *Tests and measurements in child development: Handbook II* (Vols. 1 & 2). San Francisco: Jossey-Bass.

Johnson, O. G., & Bommarito, J. W. (1971). *Tests and measurements in child development: Handbook I*. San Francisco: Jossey-Bass.

Keyser, D. J., & Sweetland, R. C. (1984). *Test critiques* (Vols. 1-4). Kansas City, MO: Test Corporation of America.

Lake, D. G., Miles, M. B., & Earle, Jr., R. B. (1973). *Measuring human behavior: Tools for the assessment of social functioning*. New York: Teachers College Press.

Lyerly, S. B. (1973). *Handbook of psychiatric rating scales* (2nd ed.). Rockville, MD: National Institutes of Mental Health.

Miller, D. C. (1983). *Handbook of research design and social measurement* (4th ed.). New York: McKay.

Mitchell, J.V. (Ed.). (1983). *Tests in print III: An index to tests, test reviews, and the literature on specific tests*. Lincoln: University of Nebraska Press.

Pfeiffer, J. W., Heslen, R., & Jones, J. E. (1976). *Instrumentation in human relations training* (2nd ed.). San Diego, CA: University Associates.

Reeder, L. G., Ramacher, L. G., & Gorelnik, S. (1976). *Handbook of scales and indices of health behavior*. Pacific Palisades, CA: Goodyear Publishing Co.

Robinson, J. P., & Shaver, P. R. (1973). *Measures of social psychosocial attitudes*. Ann Arbor, MI: Institute for Social Research, University of Michigan.

Shaw, M. E., & Wright, J. M. (1967). *Scales for the measurement of attitudes*. New York: McGraw-Hill.

Straus, M. A., & Brown, B. W. (1978). *Family measurement techniques: Abstracts of published instruments, 1935-1974* (rev. ed.). Minneapolis: University of Minnesota Press.

Sweetland, R. C., & Keyser, D. J. (Eds.). (1983). *Tests: A comprehensive reference for assessment in psychology, education, and business*. Kansas City, MO: Test Corporation of America.

Walker, D. K. (1973). *Socioemotional measures for pre-school and kindergarten children*. San Francisco: Jossey-Bass.

Ward, M. J., & Lindeman, C. (Eds.). (1979). *Instruments for measuring nursing practice and other health care variables*. Hyattsville, MD: DHEW Publication No. HRA 78-53 (Vol. 1 and HRA 78-54 [Vol. 2]).

Weiss, M. D. (1973). *Biomedical instrumentation*. Philadelphia: Chilton.

GLOSSARY

accessible population That aggregate of participants that meets the criteria for inclusion in the study and that is available to the investigator.

accuracy The reliability and validity of the estimates obtained from the sample.

acrophase The clock time at which a peak value occurs within a circadian rhythm.

aesthetics Knowledge gained through subjective experience that cannot be formulated according to logic or reasoning alone because it involves perceptions of unique characteristics of an individual rather than universals that characterize a large group of individuals.

agency The person(s) attempting to bring about a desired aim by performing a given prescription, including not only the professional involved, but all those who have the internal and external resources to perform the prescription, such as family members, visitors, and other professionals.

alpha level Probability of making a type I error; level of significance; p value.

amplitude The extent of change between the peak and trough values of the parameter studied in terms of a circadian rhythm.

analysis of covariance (ancova) Analysis that describes the relationship between a continuous dependent variable and one or more categorical variables, while controlling for the effect of one or more continuous independent variables.

association Relationship between two or more variables.

analysis of variance (anova) An inferential statistical test used to test the significance of differences between the means of two or more groups.

anchors Specifications that define scale steps. They are usually specified at the beginning of the form and in some cases for each item.

artifactual associations Spurious associations that result from problems in research design, measurement problems, peculiarities of the sample under study, and confounding variables.

assay A method for physically detecting the presence of a substance. In a bioassay, the substance is in a cell, tissue, or body fluid.

assumption A statement of principle that is accepted as true on the basis of logic or reason.

asymmetrical distribution A frequency distribution that, when displayed graphically, consists of two halves that are not mirror images of one another.

average duration Descriptive statistic calculated by dividing the total duration of a behavior by the total frequency of that behavior.

axiom A summary of empirical evidence linking two concepts.

backward elimination Procedure in which all predictors are entered first into multiple regression equations, and then variables are deleted one at a time, after an assessment of whether the decrease in the multiple correlation coefficient is statistically significant.

baseline assessment Description of the participant's initial status, usually including personal characteristics plus health characteristics and prognostic factors that would influence further measures or the response to a treatment trial.

baseline stability The ability of an instrument to maintain a constant baseline value without drift.

batch processing mode Means of communicating with a computer in which the investigator submits a program or a group of programs in one batch, and the programs are executed simultaneously rather than interactively.

beneficence An obligation to secure the benefits of research by (1) doing no harm to participants in the process, and (2) maximizing possible benefits and minimizing possible harms.

beta weights The weights that would need to be applied to the independent variables in a regression equation to predict the value of the dependent variable.

bias The difference between the true but unknown value for the population and its estimate based on data from the sample. Systematic distortion of the research findings.

bimodal distribution A distribution having two peaks.

blinding In a clinical trial, having the caregivers and/or the participants unaware that they are participating in a trial.

broad-range theory A theory that takes into account all of nursing. Because of the scope, such a theory cannot be tested by conventional empirical methods; grand theory.

canonical correlation Statistical procedure designed to analyze the relationship between two or more independent and two or more dependent, interval-level variables.

card reader Machine that transforms codes punched on computer cards into electrical impulses the computer can interpret.

case studies Intensive, systematic investigations of a single individual, group, community, or some other unit, typically conducted under naturalistic conditions, in which the investigator examines in-depth data related to background, current status, environmental characteristics and interactions among individuals, groups, and communities.

causal direction Principle in causation that states that changes in X produce changes in Y.

central processing unit (CPU) Element of a computer that controls and coordinates all computer activities.

chi square test Statistical test used to test hypotheses about the association between variables that can be divided into categories (nominal or categorical variables).

chronobiology Field of study that emphasizes the dimension of time for understanding human biology and for characterizing the time dimension of human health.

circadian pattern biological pattern occurring within a 24-hour period.

clarity Property that describes how well the boundaries of the theory are communicated and the sense of orderliness and consistency throughout the theory.

clinical trial Planned experiment involving participants, usually patients, to determine the most appropriate therapy by comparing one therapeutic approach with another therapeutic approach, usually standard care.

closed loop systems A system in which the output partially determines the input; part of the output is "fed back" and participates as input to the system.

cluster analysis Procedure used to classify people or things by using multivariate statistical procedures.

cluster sampling Technique that involves successive random sampling of units, beginning with the largest units and followed by smaller and smaller units.

clustering In qualitative analysis the grouping together of related events, processes, or settings to gain better understanding of a phenomenon.

code Category derived from the research question and the key variables of the study.

code book A directory for use while coding data that lists the kinds of data the investigator anticipates or collects.

coefficient of determination Proportion of the variance in the dependent variable accounted for by the independent variables included in the regression equation.

coherency In prescriptive theory the consistency between the theoretical specification of the prescription and its implementation.

cohort Group of persons who share a common experience within a defined time period. The collective group or groups of individuals enrolled in a longitudinal study.

cohort effect Effect of being a member of one of varying groups sampled at different times, e.g., those born during a specific era.

comparative survey Research design that contrasts the experiences of two or more groups of individuals, usually selected to resemble one another as much as possible in areas not addressed by the study, yet differing with regard to the particular variable(s) being studied. May be studied at a single or multiple time points; often termed comparative descriptive survey.

compiler Program that translates programing language into machine language.

computer hardware Electronic equipment that processes, controls, and stores data.

computer software Instructions and procedures required to operate a computer.

concept An abstract characteristic, category, or label of an object, person, or event to be studied. An abstract way of referring to the real world, which may have a different meaning depending on feelings, values, attitudes, and perceptions.

conceptual framework Network of concepts and relationships within which research questions are asked and data are integrated.

conceptually-derived techniques Techniques of data aggregation using coding categories based on the researcher's *a priori* ideas about which codes can be lumped together.

concurrent design Naturalistic research design in which the researcher measures the antecedent and consequent variables simultaneously. Also known as cross-sectional design.

concurrent validity A type of criterion validity that represents the degree of correlation of two measures of the same concept administered at the same point in time.

confidence interval Interval estimate that measures the variability associated with the point estimate.

confidence limit One of two boundary points between which the researcher has a specified level of confidence that the population parameter lies.

confirmability audit A method of assessing the confirmability of results by completing the stages of pre-entry, determination of auditability, formal agreement, determination of trustworthiness, and closure.

confounded relationship Noncausal relationships stemming from the relationship of 2 variables to a third variable; spurious relationship.

consensual validation The process by which a panel of experts judges the validity of an instrument.

consistency Criterion that implies that terms are repeatedly used to express the same thought, or that the meaning of a concept and observable reality are in accord.

constant comparative analysis A form of latent content analysis that continually compares new data with previous data.

constitutive definitions Explanation of a construct based on other constructs.

construct A concept invented for a special scientific purpose, the construct has theoretical meaning but no empirical meaning unless it is linked to an observational term. On the abstract-concrete continuum, a concept that is neither directly nor indirectly observable.

construct validity A way of describing how the scores from a measurement instrument interrelate with other variables; since the theory guiding a research study suggests which characteristics and traits should be related and which should be unrelated, a new measure that shows this pattern of relationships and nonrelationships is said to have construct validity.

content analysis A method used for studying qualitative data that is sensitive to the context and symbolic forms of the data.

content validity The adequacy of the sampling of the domain under study by a measurement instrument.

context In prescriptive theory the variables that influence progress toward the therapeutic goal, including sociopolitical and organizational realities.

contingency table A two-dimensional frequency distribution in which the frequencies of two variables are cross-tabulated. Most commonly used to describe relationships between two nominal or categorical variables.

contract Award made to individual or team of investigators and initiated by the funding agency through a request for a proposal.

control condition Condition used in contrast to an experimental treatment.

control group In an experiment, the group that does not receive the experimental treatment, but instead receives no treatment or a treatment that does not include the experimental variable.

convenience sample A sample obtained by accessing individuals who are easy to identify and contact.

convergence of evidence A strategy for assessing construct validity in which investigators look for uniformity of evidence from different sources, each of which measures the same construct.

correlation The relationship between two variables that are of ordinal, interval, or ratio level measurement.

correlational survey A research design that relates multiple variables measured at a single time point in a sample from a designated population; allows the investigator to assess the extent to which changes in one phenomenon correspond to changes in another. Usually a sample representing a wide cross-section of the population of interest is sought.

counterbalanced design Experimental design in which respondents have multiple treatments and the order of treatments is varied systematically to control for the effects of treatment order.

covariation In causation, the principle that states that when X (the cause) changes, Y (the effect) will also change.

criterion referenced measures Techniques appropriate for determining whether or not an individual has acquired a set of behaviors or mastered a specific task.

criterion validity The relationship between a new measure and an established measure of the same phenomenon. Assessment based on comparing the score of the new measure with an established standard of measurement for that variable.

critical social theory paradigm Paradigm derived from the belief that reality has as its ultimate foundation the negotiated agreement of the community. Its goal is political or social change; its proponents view the purpose of research as understanding the multiple truths that together explain the situation in which people live.

Cronbach's alpha The most commonly used method of assessing internal consistency reliability; based on the intercorrelation or covariance of all items in a scale examined simultaneously.

cross-sectional designs Research design that involves selecting a representative sample from the population of interest and observing all the phenomena (including the putative cause and effect) of interest at the same point in time.

crossover trials The same individual is included in both treatment and control conditions or in multiple treatment conditions in the same study.

cultural group The study sample in an ethnographic study, defined as those who share knowledge, customs, objects, events, and activities.

cumulative scales Scales that consist of items constructed so that the person who agrees with item 2 also agrees with item 1, but not necessarily with item 3; cumulative scale construction requires developing a number of items of increasing intensity regarding some construct, usually an attitude.

data display Part of qualitative data analysis; organized data presentation that facilitates arriving at conclusions and acting.

data matrix Method of arranging data; usually constructed so that data from each case appear in one or more rows with the variables occupying designated columns.

data modification Procedure that transforms the original data to another form but does not necessarily reduce the data to a smaller number of units.

data reduction Translation of information from several variables to a smaller number of variables to simplify problems of analysis, storage, and dissemination to other scholars.

deductive reasoning Reasoning that proceeds from a general law to a conclusion that is specific or particular to a situation.

deductively generated codes Codes derived from the literature and the investigator's insight before the data has been analyzed.

degrees of freedom In tests of statistical significance, the number of sample values that cannot be calculated from knowledge of other values and a calculated statistic (e.g., by knowing sample variance, all but one value is free to vary). Degrees of freedom (df) is often $N - 1$, but formulas are specified for each test.

Delphi technique Questionnaire strategy in which a panel of experts complete consecutive questionnaires generated on the basis of the answers to the previous questionnaires; designed to achieve a consensus among the panel of experts.

dependability See stability.

dependent variable The variable the investigator measures in response to the causal (treatment or independent) variable; outcome variable.

derivable consequences The extent to which the theory results in or produces valued nursing outcomes.

descriptive longitudinal study A research design used to observe stability or change over time and involving repeated observations over time.

descriptive statistics Statistics that provide precise, standard ways to summarize, understand, and communicate complex information; the "facts" on which an analysis is based, the summary of the key characteristics of the sample being studied.

descriptive survey A research design that involves collecting information from a sample resembling the total population of interest to the investigator.

dichotomous response questions Questions providing a grammatical structure that suggests a "yes" or "no" response.

dichotomous scale Scale that provides only two responses, such as "yes" or "no."

differential loss of participants Loss of participants from one or more treatment or control groups before an experiment has been completed, thereby causing difficulty in interpreting the relationship between the independent variable and the dependent variable; experimental mortality.

differential selection Systematic differences in the allocation of participants to treatment and control groups.

direct association Causal relationship in which the cause (X) produces the effect or outcome (Y) without the influence of any intermediate variable.

discriminance A strategy for assessing construct validity that refers to the ability to differentiate the construct under study from other similar constructs.

discriminant analysis Analysis that allows investigators to examine the effects of multiple independent variables on a categorical or nominal dependent variable; the purpose of discriminant analysis is to determine how one or more independent variables can be used to discriminate among different categories of the nominal dependent variable.

discriminant function Equation that includes the variables that best discriminate between groups and is derived by maximizing the ratio of the variance between groups to variance within groups.

disproportional sampling strategy Sampling strategy in which the investigator selects a number of elements from different strata that do not reflect the proportion of those elements found in the population. The purpose is to ensure adequate representation of individuals from different strata in a study.

double-barreled questions Questions containing two or more separate ideas, demanding two separate responses from the participant and creating confusion as to the actual intent of the question.

double-blind trial Neither the participant nor the person responsible for the care component of a clinical trial knows which treatment the participant is receiving.

drift In coding, the tendency to code differently as the coding process continues.

dynamics In prescriptive theory the motivating factors in performing and sustaining the activities that produce the goal.

effect size The magnitude of the findings, such as the degree to which the phenomenon is present in the population being studied or the degree of departure from the null hypothesis.

effectors In a closed loop system, the element(s) that act(s) in some way to vary the characteristic that is being regulated.

eigenvalue A value equal to the sum of the squared weights for each factor in a factor analysis.

element The most basic unit of a population about which information in a study can be collected.

empirical indicators The instruments or experimental conditions used in a study; observables associated with a given concept that link constitutively defined concepts to the real world.

empirical precision Property requiring that concepts contained in the theory be linked with observable reality, particularly if the theory is intended to be used for predicting and controlling some aspect of practice.

empirically-derived techniques Techniques of data aggregation used when the underlying relationships among the coding categories are not readily apparent to the researcher.

empirics Knowledge about the experienced (empirical) world, generally organized into laws and theories that help to describe, predict, and explain phenomena.

enumerative induction Collecting a number and variety of instances that go in the same direction; progressive focusing.

equivalence The degree of similarity between two or more forms of a measuring instrument.

error variance Variance in Y that is attributable not to a competing cause (extraneous variance) but to measurement error; random variance.

ethics The moral component of nursing knowledge that guides difficult decisions that must be made within an increasingly complex health services context.

ethnography A broad, detailed study of the lifeways of people of a particular cultural or subcultural group.

event-triggered observational system Approach to observational methods in which the observer begins recording behaviors when an event of interest occurs or changes.

experimental variance. The variance in the dependent variable attributable to the experimental treatment (X).

experiments Studies in which the investigator manipulates a putative cause and measures an effect.

explanatory theory A reasoned argument for why certain events happen that is made up of concepts and propositions.

exploratory data analysis An approach to data analysis that emphasizes familiarity with data as a means of understanding what they convey.

external criticism In historical research the lower form of criticism, which examines sources of data to determine their authenticity.

external equilibrium systems Systems that react to or act on the environment and that usually can be observed as physical behaviors.

external validity The extent to which the findings observed in one set of data can be generalized to other potential samples or to the entire population.

extraneous variable Variable that confuses the relationship between the independent and dependent variables. The investigator tries to control the variable through the research design or the statistical procedures.

extraneous variance The variance in the dependent variable caused by some unwanted influence other than the independent variable.

F *ratio* Statistic obtained by contrasting variation between groups with variation within groups.

face validity The extent to which the measurement appears to be measuring the item under study.

factor Underlying dimension that variables have in common.

factor analysis Multivariable statistical procedure designed to identify one or more new composite variables called factors; it is commonly used to reduce a large set of variables to a smaller number of summary measures.

A method of assessing convergence and discriminance that gives information about the extent to which a set of items measures the same underlying construct or dimension of the construct.

factor extraction Phase of factor analysis that consists of intercorrelation of variables to identify clusters of highly correlated variables within the matrix, resulting in an unrotated factor matrix.

factor loadings The weights representing the degree to which each item of an instrument loads on a particular factor.

factor rotation Second phase of factor analysis, in which factors are rotated to distinctly associate clusters of items with factors.

factor scores Scores computed by using the factor loadings as coefficients and multiplying them by the participants' scores on the individual items.

factorial experiment Design option in which the investigator simultaneously manipulates two or more independent variables, permitting analysis of two or more factors at the same time and providing information on whether the factors interact with one another.

feasibility An assessment based on human and cost-benefit comparisons.

first order change A difference that occurs in a given system that itself does not change.

fixed alternative question A form of question that provides a fixed set of responses from which the respondent must choose one of the responses provided.

fluorometry Method for assessing the concentrations of certain chemicals that, when illuminated by light of a short wavelength (ultraviolet range), emit light of a longer wavelength, a phenomenon call fluorescence.

formative evaluation The measurement and judgments made before or during implementation of an intervention to control, assure, or improve the quality of the performance or delivery of the intervention.

forward stepwise multiple regression analysis Procedure in which the independent variable that is correlated most highly with the dependent variable is entered first into the equation, followed by the one with the next highest correlation with the dependent variable until all the independent variables have been included in the regression equation.

frequency distribution A form of description in which the values of a particular variable are arranged from lowest to highest and the frequency with which each value appears in the population studied is revealed.

frequency polygon A frequency distribution technique that involves plotting the number of times a given value appears in the data (the frequency) on a vertical axis, and the value of the variable (or score) on the horizontal axis, and then connecting the points with straight lines.

frequency response The variation in sensitivity (amount of change in output for a given change in input) over the frequency range of the measurement. An instrument should be able to respond rapidly enough to reproduce all frequency components of the waveform with equal sensitivity.

Friedman test Nonparametric test used when several measures are obtained from a single sample or when the investigator has studied paired groups.

futuristic design Naturalistic research design in which the researcher measures the antecedent and consequent variables in their order of occurrence; longitudinal design; panel design; prospective design.

gamma Nonparametric measure of association.

generality Property that ensures that the empirical facts and situations to which the theory applies are not limited.

generalizations A summary of observed facts arrived at systematically (empirically) or derived from logical and abstract thinking (theoretically).

generational effect Effect of being born in a specific period of time.

grand theory See broad-range theory.

grounded theory Methodology in which constructs or theories are generated from data and remain grounded in the real world.

hierarchical multiple regression analysis Procedure for entry of variables in multiple regression equations in which the investigator enters the variables into the equations in a certain order, according to theoretical justification.

histogram A form of frequency polygon in which the frequency of a particular score is plotted with a bar.

historical approach Theory based on the idea that in order to understand any phenomenon one must begin with what went before, that is, the background, the context out of which it emerged.

historical controls Individuals who have been treated with standard measures in the past and are used as a comparison group in a clinical trial.

historical design Naturalistic research design in which the researcher measures the consequent or outcome variable first and then looks backward in time to antecedent events; retrospective design; case-referent design.

historical research The critical investigation of events, developments, and experiences of the past, the careful weighing of evidence of the validity of sources of information about the past, and the interpretation of the weighed evidence.

history With respect to internal validity, the effects of secular trends or events external to the study on the observations made in the study.

holistic analysis Assessment of a research report to determine if logical consistency exists between the components of the study.

holistic case design In case studies, using a unit of analysis that cannot or will not be divided into components.

homeostasis The constant conditions maintained by the body for its proper function; also known as steady state.

hypotheses Tentative statements of relationship that can be tested empirically.

incidence The proportion of individuals who experience a phenomenon during the course of the study.

incremental intervention Successively adding varying strengths of the independent variable.

independent variable The intervention, treatment, or condition that the investigator manipulates in an experimental study. Also known as the treatment or causal variable.

indirect association (indirect relationship) Causal relationship in which the cause (X) is encompassed by another variable. The relationship between two variables in a causal chain is caused by a third variable.

indirect observation term A property that must be inferred; a concept that cannot be observed directly but that can be inferred from empirical indicators.

inductive reasoning From a set of particular observations, the investigator makes a generalization about the phenomenon being studied.

inductively generated codes Codes emerging from the data and remaining grounded in those data.

inferential statistics Statistics with which the investigator is able to estimate a characteristic of the population from the sample examined.

informant checking Asking informants in a qualitative research study to verify the researcher's analysis.

input devices Equipment through which the researcher transforms data into a form the computer can process; equipment that allows the investigator to provide commands and information about how a computer should function.

input evaluation In evaluation research, assessing (a) relevant capabilities of individuals involved in a program; (b) strategies for achieving objectives; and (c) ways of implementing the strategies.

input media Material onto which the investigator enters information via an input device. Includes magnetic tape, disk, diskettes (floppy disks).

inquiry audit A person unfamiliar with the research authenticates the process of the inquiry and attests to the fact that data support the findings, interpretations, and recommendations.

interaction effect The effect of two or more independent variables acting in combination rather than independently of one another; the effect of one factor is not consistent over all levels of another individual factor.

interactive mode Capability of some computer programs to provide feedback to input almost immediately.

intercoder reliability See reproducibility.

interinvestigatory affirmation The process of repeating the same study with many subjects.

internal criticism In historical research the higher form of criticism that establishes the true meaning of the content.

internal regulatory systems Systems inside the body that regulate phenomena to maintain the constant conditions of the internal environment for cells.

internal validity The extent to which the investigator is able to reach unambiguous conclusions about the relationship between the independent and dependent variables.

interobserver agreement Degree to which two coders using the same system and observing the same behavior actually make the same record.

interquartile range A measure of variability representing the range of scores that encompasses the middle 50% of the scores, leaving 25% above and 25% below it.

interrater reliability Relationship between the levels of accuracy when two or more individuals are applying the same instrument.

interval estimation A statistic that allows investigators to calculate with a certain degree of confidence a range of values within which the population value lies.

interval scale Scale on which distances are equally spaced in relation to the magnitude of the phenomenon being measured, but absolute amounts are not known. The zero point for the scale is arbitrary, not absolute; equal-interval scale.

ipsative control Technique in which the participant in a study is able to serve as his or her own control; based on comparing the participant's original set of values with the participant's own subsequent values on repeated measurements over time.

isomorphism Identity or similarity of form; in measurement theory isomorphism relates to the correspondence of sets of objects to reality.

item total correlations An estimate of internal consistency reliability that is a function of the degree of interrelatedness of all items in a scale that measures only a single dimension. Consists of a group of single correlations between each item and the total score for the entire scale. Indicates the extent to which the individual items relate to the total score for the entire instrument.

judgmental sample See purposive sample.

justice Principle that requires that fair procedures be used in the identification and selection of research participants within the framework of the proposed research so that no one group is disproportionately used as subjects for study.

Kendall's tau Nonparametric correlation coefficient for ordinal or categorical data.

known groups approach A method of assessing construct validity that requires administration of an instrument to groups who would be expected to differ on the construct under study.

Kruskal Wallis test Nonparametric test performed with ordinal data and based on the assignment of ranks to the scores for the various groups.

Kuder-Richardson (KR-20) A coefficient that gives an estimate of internal consistency reliability of a dichotomous scale.

latency The time lapse between change of condition and change in behavior.

latent content analysis A method of studying qualitative data that views each passage of the textual material within the context of the entire text.

leptokurtotic distribution A distribution with a very sharp peak.

level of significance See alpha level.

linearity The degree to which variation in the output of an instrument follows input variation. Linearity should be obtained at least over the most usual range of inputs even though it may not occur for the entire range of possible inputs.

literature controls Data about subjects obtained from previously published studies.

literature review A summary of earlier work on one topic or topics of related interest. Contains a critical analysis of earlier work that identifies what is known and not known about a topic. Although not exhaustive, it includes discussion of the most important works in the area.

location (of a distribution) The point at which a distribution is anchored.

longitudinal study Study that requires obtaining repeated measures over time.

magnitude estimation A measurement technique requiring participants to match numbers, lengths of a line, or hand-grip to stimuli.

main effects In multifactor analysis of variance, the effects of a single factor.

manifest content analysis A method of making replicable and valid inferences by applying empirical and statistical methods to textual material.

manipulation check A check, usually in the form of follow-up, to determine the effectiveness of manipulating the treatment variable.

Mann Whitney U test Nonparametric statistical test that tests the hypothesis that the two independent groups come from populations having different distributions rather than merely different medians.

matching Technique in selecting participants designed to control extraneous variance. Each participant in the treatment group is matched to one or more participants in a no-treatment group on the basis of one or more variables.

matrix A device for data display in qualitative research that arranges descriptive data segments around a particular event or experience.

maturation Threat to internal validity; changes in the individuals being studied that are expected to occur with age, regardless of the study.

MAX-CON-MIN principle Abbreviation for the principle guiding the design of experiments, which stands for: MAX—maximize experimental variance; CON—control extraneous variance; MIN—minimize error variance.

mean A measure of central tendency, which is the arithmetic average of all the scores.

meaning adequacy Criterion for operationalizing a concept that refers to the congruence that must exist between the meaning denoted by a concept and the indicators selected to represent the concept.

measurand The physical quantity, characteristic, or condition that is to be measured in a system output.

measure of central tendency A measure that describes the center of the distribution or the most typical values in the distribution.

measurement The assignment of some numerical value to objects or events to represent the kind or amount of some characteristic of those objects or events. Measurement, as used in this context, includes qualitative measurement, in which objects are assigned to categories that represent the kind of characteristics they possess and that are mutually exclusive and exhaustive.

measurement norms The values (e.g., mean, standard deviation, and range of values) obtained when using a measure.

median Measure of central tendency, which is the value that marks the midpoint of the distribution; half of the cases fall above and half below the median.

median test Statistical test that assesses the research hypothesis that the two compared groups derive from populations with different medians.

memory Element of the computer that stores program instructions and data while the program is executing.

mesor The average value of the parameter whose rhythm is being studied.

meta-analysis A variety of analytic strategies that permit an investigator to summarize mathematically the results of several studies by calculating the size of the effect of the independent variable on the dependent variable.

metaphor comparison of two unlike things; taking several particulars and making a single generalization of them.

middle-range theory A theory whose scope is limited enough to allow empirical testing. It is generalizable but specific enough to be tested.

misspecified relationship An incorrectly hypothesized relationship (e.g., the relationship between two variables changes when a third variable is introduced).

mixed results Research findings that partially support the hypothesis being tested and partially do not support the hypothesis.

modality Characteristic that describes the number of peaks in the values of a distribution.

mode A measure of central tendency, which is the most frequently occurring value in a distribution.

monotonic relationship Correlation in which an increase in X is associated with an increase or a decrease in Y throughout the entire range of X.

multifactor analysis of variance Statistical determination of the influence of two or more independent variables on a dependent variable.

multimodal distribution A distribution having multiple peaks.

multiple case design In case studies, the use of two or more cases.

multiple comparison test Tests used to compare different pairs of means or variances, used in conjunction with analysis of variance.

multiple correlation coefficient The correlation between the independent variables, taken as a group, and the dependent variable.

multiple regression analysis Multivariate statistical method used to describe the extent, direction, and strength of the relationship between several independent variables and a single dependent variable.

multitrait-multimethod approach A method of assessing convergence and discriminance that requires examining the relationship between indicators that should measure the same and different constructs, and those measured by different measures.

multivariate Designs in which investigators study multiple independent and/or dependent variables.

multivariate analysis of variance (manova) Statistical analysis that allows the investigator to take into account the variation in more than one independent and dependent variable simultaneously.

multivariate statistical procedures Statistical techniques designed to help the investigator consider multiple variables simultaneously.

narrow-range theory Theory that addresses one situation at one point in time. Because of its limited scope, it has limited utility beyond that situation.

naturalistic survey design Design in which investigators test hypotheses based on observations of phenomena as they naturally occur.

naturalistic-inductive paradigm Paradigm in which it is assumed that science is necessarily historical and that facts and principles are embedded in both historical and cultural contexts. Truth is seen as dynamic and derived from human interaction with real social and historical settings.

negative case analysis In establishing credibility in qualitative research, a process that requires the researcher to analyze unanticipated answers and observations.

negative-feedback system A regulatory system whereby a change in the characteristic being regulated toward normal reduces effector output.

negative results Research findings that are inconsistent with the hypothesis or logic in the study's theoretical framework; the null hypothesis is accepted; nonsignificant results.

negatively skewed distribution A distribution that, when it is displayed graphically, has the longer tail pointing toward the left (and the lower values of the variable).

nominal measurement The assignment of numbers to represent categories or classes of things; the numbers represent the phenomenon's membership in a category that is mutually exclusive of other categories. The numbers have no quantitative value and are used only as labels.

nonspuriousness Principle of causation guaranteeing that plausible alternative explanations for the observed relationship between X and Y have been eliminated, that is, other variables that cause changes in Y are not responsible for the effect of X on Y.

nonequivalent control group design Design in which the groups are naturally occurring collectives and thus are not allocated randomly to the treatment and control groups at the same point in time; equivalence therefore cannot be assumed.

nonmonotonic relationship Correlation that changes directions so that an increase in X may be associated with an increase in Y over part of the distribution but with a decrease in Y over other parts of the distribution.

nonparametric test A class of statistical test that is not based on the estimation of a parameter for the underlying population, usually does not require that the variable is normally distributed, and can be applied when the data are nominal or ordinal.

nonprobability sampling Sampling strategies that do not ensure that each element in the population has the same chance of inclusion in the sample.

nonsignificant results See negative results.

norm-referenced measurement approaches Techniques appropriate for evaluating the performance of an individual relative to some other individuals in a group.

normal curve A type of distribution that is bell-shaped, symmetrical, unimodal, and not too peaked (with a mean of 0). Half of the observations lie above the mean and half below it; normal distribution; Gaussian curve.

normative theory Theory developed to describe, explain, or predict values as opposed to empirical phenomena.

null hypothesis Assertion that no difference or relationship exists between variables.

nursing science The body of scientific knowledge that guides nursing practice.

oblique rotation Factor rotation in which the rotated axes are allowed to depart from a 90 degree angle, producing correlated factors.

observation term On the abstract-concrete continuum, a property that is a directly observable, empirical referent.

observational study Study that asks questions about overt behaviors or events and then answers those questions by having human observers record those behaviors or events over a period of time or a series of occurrences.

observed value The actual value obtained when using a particular instrument; contains the "true" value and error.

open-ended question A form of question that does not provide a fixed set of responses but allows the respondent to answer the question in his or her own words.

open-loop system A regulatory system in which the input to the system is not affected by the system output.

operational definitions Definitions that assign meaning to a construct by specifying the activities or operations necessary to measure it. Also called epistemic definitions, rules of correspondence or rules of interpretation, they are measurement-oriented interpretations of constitutive definitions.

ordinal measurement Form of measurement that requires that objects can be rank-ordered on some operationally defined characteristic. Numbers represent rank-order on some attribute; the number is assigned to represent membership in a mutually exclusive and exhaustive category that can be ordered according to the amount of the attribute possessed.

orthogonal rotation Rotation that keeps the factors at right angles to one another, or independent, so that the factors are uncorrelated with one another.

outliers Points that are remote from other values on the graph of a distribution.

output devices Means by which information is transmitted from the computer's CPU back to the investigator. Includes CRT screen, tape, disk, diskette, punched cards, and printer.

P value See alpha level.

panel design A longitudinal research design that involves observations on many entities but at relatively few times. It allows the investigator to assess not only change over time, but also the differences and similarities in two or more cohorts over time.

paradigm A way of looking at the world that presents a set of philosophical assumptions about the world that are interrelated in a way that helps break down the complexity of the real world and that guides inquiry (see also functions 1–6 on p. 22).

parameter One characteristic of a population.

parametric test A class of statistical test usually requiring the variables to be normally distributed in the population, the measurements to be on at least an interval scale, and at least one parameter to be estimated.

path analysis Statistical procedure that allows the investigator to determine the influence of multiple independent variables on a series of dependent variables.

patiency In prescriptive theory, the recipients of the prescriptions.

pattern The configuration of a phenomenon; the repetitive and regular occurrences of a phenomenon.

perfect relationship A correlation in which it is possible to predict the value of one variable, given the value of the other variable.

persistence Dynamic equilibrium seen in living systems; an ongoing series of first-order changes.

personal knowledge A subjective, concrete, and existential pattern of knowledge concerned with promoting wholeness and integrity in personal encounters and engagement with another person.

phenomena Observable facts or events that reflect concepts.

phenomenology A method of study that attempts to understand human experience through analysis of the participant's description of an experience.

platykurtotic distribution A distribution that has a flattened peak.

plethysmography Procedure used for recording volume variations.

point estimation Statistical technique that allows the investigator to use information from a random sample to determine a single numerical value that would be a good indicator of the value of an underlying parameter.

population An aggregate of elements sharing some common set of criteria.

population mean The mean for the underlying population; it is estimated based on sample means.

positive results Research findings consistent with the hypothesis or logic in the study's theoretical framework; the null hypothesis is rejected.

positively skewed distribution A distribution that, when it is displayed graphically, has the longer tail pointing toward the right (and the higher values of the variable).

positivist-empiricist paradigm Paradigm in which it is assumed that a body of facts or principles exists to be discovered or understood, independent of any historical or social context. Universal, abstract, and general principles are sought in order to understand phenomena, and investigations are outcome-oriented.

post hoc test Additional test, such as one of the tests used after analysis of variance, completed after a procedure; literally, "after this."

postulate A statement of presumed relationship between concepts.

power of a statistical test The probability that the test will lead to the rejection of the null hypothesis; the ability of the test to detect small but important findings, such as differences or associations.

practice theory Theory that is validated in natural practice settings and guides the delivery of nursing care.

precision Criterion that specifies that the description of the operationalization be explicit and specific. In a measurement device, the number of distinguishable alternatives from which a given result is selected (e.g., the number of decimal places that can be read on a meter).

predictability See stability.

prediction Specification of the necessary and sufficient variables that will produce a desired outcome.

predictive theory A set of statements that interrelates necessary and sufficient variables to forecast what will happen even though one does not know why the outcome occurs.

predictive validity A type of criterion validity that represents the degree of correlation between the measure of the concept and some future measure of the same or a similar concept.

prescriptive theory Theory whose aims include controlling, promoting, and changing nursing phenomena. Its elements include the aim, or goal, prescriptions to produce the goal, and a survey list.

prevalence The proportion of individuals who have ever experienced a particular phenomenon.

primary analysis The initial analysis of data, whether those data were collated originally to achieve a research purpose or for another purpose.

principal components analysis Procedure used to extract factors in which weights for the first factor are defined so that their average squared weight is maximum; a maximum amount of variance is extracted by the first factor, and the second factor is formed such that the maximum amount of variance is extracted from what remains after the first factor has been extracted.

principle of discontinuity Test in which the percentage of variance explained by the factor, or the eigenvalues, is graphed. When a sharp dropoff occurs in the percentage of variance explained, the factors following the dropoff are usually omitted: also known as scree test.

probability In historical methodology, an event or phenomenon whose authenticity is established by only one primary source.

probability sampling Sampling strategy in which every element in the population has a known, non-zero probability of being included in the sample, with the goal of ensuring that the sample represents the population of interest. Procedures of selection involve some form of random selection in choosing the sampling elements.

problem statement A focused description of the area under investigation that presents the unanswered question and provides information about where specific answers are needed.

process evalution Formative evaluation that provides feedback data, relating to the program's implementation, to guide modifications.

program Set of instructions written for a specific computer; software.

programer Person who writes computer instructions (programs).

programing language Sets of commands for computers that allow programers to construct simpler programs than those required when machine language is used.

proportional stratified sample Type of stratified sample in which the investigator chooses a number of elements from the various strata in proportion to their numbers in the population.

proposition Statement that indicates a relationship between concepts.

prospective design Research design that involves sampling from a population of interest to obtain a representative group, and observing the sample on at least two occasions over a designated period of time.

psychometric properties The technical quality of the measure, particularly evidence of reliability and validity of the instrument, and procedures used in developing and testing the measure.

public funding agencies All tax-supported federal agencies that fund health-related research.

purpose The specific aim or goal of the research study, the task to be accomplished, not the problem to be solved.

purposive sample Sample in which the investigator handpicks the cases based on his or her judgment of the extent to which the potential participants meet the selection criteria; also know as judgmental sample.

Q-sort Procedure used to determine respondents' judgments about the degree to which they disagree or agree with a particular idea.

qualitative measurement A process of classification that involves assigning objects to categories that represent variations of the concept being studied.

quantitative measurement The assignment of some number from one set to another set of objects or events based on a rule.

quasiexperiments Research design that has the features of manipulation and control, but in which participants are not randomly assigned to the treatment and control groups.

quota sample A sample aimed at ensuring adequate representation of underlying groups, such as age and ethnic groups, within a population.

radiochemical binding studies Assays used to identify substances or elements by complexing them with radioactively labeled molecules.

radioincorporation studies Assays in which cellular function or structure is observed by internalization of a radioactively labeled molecule.

random digit dialing A special variation of cluster sampling in which all existing telephone numbers in an area are generated as the sampling frame.

random error Errors of measurement that are highly variable and unpredictable.

randomization list In a clinical trial, a list of consecutive random treatment assignments kept by a person who does not treat the participants or evaluate the treatment; in evaluation research, studies in which a comparison is made to some standard of acceptability.

randomization test Nonparametric test that is not influenced by serial dependency and, therefore, is useful in small sample designs having multiple applications of conditions over time (A-B-A-B design). Determines whether the data in any condition differs significantly from that in any other condition.

range Computed by subtracting the lowest score from the highest score in the distribution. In a measurement device, all the levels of input variation (intensity, amplitude, and frequency) over which the device is expected to operate.

ratio level measures Measures that have all the characteristics of nominal, ordinal, and interval scales, but also have absolute zero, meaning an absolute absence of the phenomenon. Thus magnitude from zero to some point on the scale is known.

reactivity A threat to the external validity of the study in which the participants' responses to the attention of being studied may interfere with their involvement in the study and introduce bias into the results.

real duration The actual length of time that a behavior or event occurred on an occasion.

real frequency The actual number of times a behavior or event occurred on an occasion.

reliability The proportion of true variance to total variance in a measure. Criterion that refers to reproducibility of the observations and operations.

reliability coefficient Used to convey the degree of reliability; the relationship between true variance, error variance, and total variance. Determined by the equation:

$$\text{reliability} = 1 - \frac{\text{Error variance}}{\text{Total variance}}$$

reproducibility (in a measurement device) The ability of an instrument to give the same output for equal inputs applied over some period of time. The degree to which a process can be recreated under varying circumstances.

retrospective designs Naturalistic research design that begins with the selection of representative samples from at least two groups—one group having the effect that is being studied and another group not having the effect—and proceeds to study the participants to determine the putative causes.

revelatory case One that provides an investigator with the opportunity to observe and analyze a phenomenon previously inaccessible to scientific investigation.

R_n test of ranks A nonparametric test that is useful in small sample studies with multiple baselines. Evaluates the hypothesis that no difference in ranking of behavior change exists among the various baselines.

sample A subset of the population of interest.

sample or subgroup mean A statistic used to express the "average" of a set of scores (along with the median and the mode), which is computed as the sum of all the scores divided by their number.

sampling The process of selecting a subset of the population in a way that represents the entire population.

sampling distribution A theoretical distribution that would occur if one repeatedly drew a large number of random samples from a population and replaced the units used for each sample each time.

sampling error The tendency for statistical estimates to fluctuate from one sample to the next.

sampling frame An enumeration list of each element of the population from which the sample will be selected.

sampling unit The entity used for selecting the sample.

saturation In qualitative research, the point at which the investigation finds no new data to add meaning to the general category.

scale A set of symbols or numerals constructed so that the set can be assigned by rule to characteristics of individuals to whom the scale is applied. The symbols or numerals are applied based on the individual's possession of the characteristic the scale is supposed to measure.

scaling The assignment of a numerical score to an attribute, based on the combination of several measurements to form a single composite score.

scalogram analysis Procedure used to determine if a cumulative scale is unidimensional and reproducible; if it is possible to reproduce the items that a subject could perform from knowing the total score, then the scale is said to have a high degree of reproducibility.

schedule The questions that make up a questionnaire or an interview guide.

scientific-empirical theory Theory that seeks to describe, explain, and predict the empirical world and that is evaluated through empirical testing.

second order change A change of state that changes the entire system rather than merely its components.

secondary analysis The study of problems through analysis of data originally collected for another purpose.

semantic differential scale Scale designed to measure the meaning of concepts to the individual; it requires the individual to rate a concept on a bipolar scale.

semantic relationship The logical connection between words.

sensitivity The ability of a measuring instrument to make sufficiently fine distinctions to suit the purpose of the measure.

sensitivity-specificity An approach to assessing convergence and discriminance that evaluates both the instrument's ability to detect true instances of the phenomenon (sensitivity) and its ability to detect instances in which the phenomenon is not present (specificity).

sensor In a closed loop system, the element that senses or detects the operative level of the characteristic that is regulated.

sequential comparison design In small sample research, the use of the subject's baseline as the control condition with the sequential introduction of the experimental condition.

sequential-analysis Analysis used when the investigator has a hypothesis regarding the ways in which specific behavior codes occur in relation to other behavior codes; also called lag sequential-analysis.

serendipitous findings Research results that the investigator did not anticipate.

serial dependency Within an individual, the high correlation of repeated measures over time.

setting The physical conditions under which the investigation is to take place, whether naturalistic or controlled.

sign test Nonparametric statistical test used when data are paired but do not meet the assumptions for the paired t test.

significance level The probability that the investigator will mistakenly reject the null hypothesis when it is true; in other words, will infer that a statistically significant difference or association exists when it does not.

simple random sample A sampling strategy in which the investigator, using a table of random numbers, or some other means, selects numbers, then matches the series of random numbers to the enumeration list of possible sampling elements to identify a subset of the elements for inclusion in the sample.

skewed distribution Asymmetrical distribution.

small N experimental design Design based on principles of designing valid experiments with one or a few participants.

small sample research Research involving a small number of participants.

Spearman's rho Nonparametric correlation coefficient for ordinal data; determined by ranking individual scores on each variable.

specificity The ability of the measuring device to detect only those phenomena that represent the event of interest and ignore competing or extraneous phenomena.

split-half reliability A measure of internal consistency reliability that correlates the scores on two halves of an instrument.

split-middle technique A variant of time series analysis that requires plotting a line of data points that splits the data at the median of each condition and thus provides visual evidence of continuity or discontinuity across phases.

spread of a distribution The variability or dispersion of values in the distribution, the width of the distribution, and the distance between values.

spurious associations A relationship in which two variables are associated, but the association exists because of the influence of a third variable; see confounded relationship.

stability Measuring instrument's property of producing the same results on repeated measurement occasions; dependability; predictability.

standard deviation Statistic for summarizing the average deviation about the mean of a distribution; the square root of the variance.

standard error of the mean Standard deviation of a distribution of sample means from the population means.

standard scores The determination of exactly how far away from the mean any given score lies; z scores.

statement of purpose Reflections of what the investigator intended to accomplish in the study.

statistic A characteristic of a sample.

statistical inference Process of estimating parameters from statistics, generalizing from the sample to the population.

statistical power analysis Technique for estimating how effective a test will prove in rejecting false null hypotheses.

statistical regression Phenomenon that sometimes occurs in groups selected because they represent extremes. The participants' scores on an instrument are likely to change in the direction of the mean simply because extreme scores are unstable.

statistical significance Refers to results that are unlikely to be attributable to chance.

stem and leaf display A frequency distribution technique in which the column to the left of a vertical line gives the highest digit in the distribution of scores and the rows to the right of the vertical line reflect the individual digits.

stem statement The attitude or other phenomenon to be rated on a scale.

strain gauge Resistive element that increases in length while decreasing in cross-sectional area when a force is applied, thus causing a change in the resistance.

stratified random sampling A type of sampling in which the investigator first divides the population into subgroups called "strata" and then obtains a random sample from each stratum, with the goal of ensuring that subgroups of the population are represented.

structuralism Approach to knowledge in which data is used to explain and to interpret the larger issues.

study protocol This formal document usually contains detailed specifications of a clinical trial procedure as it relates to each participant.

summated rating scale A set of scales, each expressing some attitude or value, to which the participant responds with varying degrees of intensity on a scale ranging between extremes. Scores for all scales are summed or averaged to yield each individual's score.

summative evaluation Measurements and judgments that permit conclusions about the effects of a program.

survey list In prescriptive theory, includes the theory, agency, patiency, framework, terminus, procedure, and dynamics.

symmetrical distribution A distribution that, when displayed graphically, consists of two halves that are mirror images of one another.

system of care In prescriptive theory, "a set of agents doing work with patients in a given sociopolitical context, using certain sources of motivation or energy toward measurable end points, all in the service of achieving some desired goal" (Diers, 1979).

systematic variance Variance in a measure attributable to factors such as relatively stable characteristics of the study population. Can also occur if the instrument is calibrated improperly.

systematic random sample A sampling strategy in which the investigator selects every kth case from an enumeration of all elements, rather than simply in random order.

systematic replication The attempt to determine the enduring factors in the experiment by systematically altering some conditions to discover those circumstances under which one's findings among subjects are similar.

t test Statistical test used to assess differences between groups. For a dependent sample, a t test is used to compare two measures obtained from the same individuals.

target population The population that the researcher wishes to study and about which he or she wishes to make a generalization.

terminus In prescriptive theory, the product of the activity; it reflects the outcome of the procedure on health and the effects on the cost of care, the caretakers, and the nature of other health professionals' practices.

testing effects Changes in values for a dependent variable as a consequence of repeated testing.

test-retest reliability Reliability estimated by administering the measure once and again later at a specified time to the same individuals.

theoretical simplicity Property that describes the number of concepts in a theory and their interrelationships; ideally, a theory has a minimum number of descriptive components; parsimony.

theoretical term A complex global property that is impossible to observe and whose meaning depends on its use in the theory.

theory A systematic vision of reality; a set of inter-related concepts that is useful for prediction and control.

theory-generating research Research designed to discover and describe phenomena and the relationships between phenomena as observed in the empirical world.

theory-testing research Research that provides a means for investigators to determine how accurately the theory accounts for the empirical world.

time series analysis Method of analysis in which multiple observations of a variable are made over time to determine patterns of fluctuation and to forecast future patterns on the basis of past patterns. Observations occur in temporal order and are assumed to be highly correlated successive values.

time series design A longitudinal research design that involves multiple repeated observations on a single entity or a small number of entities at relatively many points of time. The unit of analysis is the time point.

time-and-space-measures A type of measurement used in manifest content analysis in which the investigator numerically counts such things as words, pages, or the number of minutes of a discussion.

time-sharing Computer processing mode that permits parts of several different computer programs to be executed at the same time.

time triggered strategies Approach to observational methods in which the observer records behaviors at certain predetermined times.

total variance In a score, the information from the true values and the measurement errors.

transferability The generalizability of study findings.

treatment group In an experiment, the group that receives the independent variable.

trend An assessment based on the slope of the data (increasing or decreasing); useful when dealing with a phenomenon in which frequency is not constant.

triangulation A strategy to increase the precision of research measurement by measuring the same phenomenon with multiple techniques.

triple-blind trial The person interpreting the trial results, the therapist, and the evaluator are all blind to the group assignment of the participants.

true variance Information from the true values; obtained only under the ideal conditions of no measurement error.

type I error Occurs when the null hypothesis is true for the population, but the investigator rejects the null hypothesis in favor of the research hypothesis.

type II error Null hypothesis is accepted as true when it is in fact false; often occurs because of low power and measurement error.

unimodal distribution A distribution having only a single peak.

unit of analysis The primary focus of analysis for the study, often an individual, but possibly an observation, family, group, organization, community, or some larger social unit.

univariate Designs that address only one phenomenon or variable.

utility Need for the operationalization to be useful within the context of the investigation and the discipline of nursing.

validity Determination of whether the measure being used actually assesses the phenomenon that the theory and research questions imply.

validity of an estimate The extent to which the estimate of a population parameter differs from the true value of the population.

variance A commonly used summary of the variability of a distribution for interval- and ratio-level data; involves finding the mathematical difference of each score from the mean, squaring each of these differences, and dividing the sum by the number of scores in the distribution.

visual analog scale A measurement technique designed to obtain interval-level data; requires respondents to select a point on a linear scale to indicate the intensity of their feelings, opinions, or beliefs.

Wilcoxon signed rank test Similar to the sign test but involves calculating the difference between paired scores and ranking this difference.

within-subject analysis Analysis focused on variations within data obtained from the same participant.

z scores See standard scores.

AUTHOR INDEX

INDEX